W9-CBF-897

Polymicrobial Diseases

Polymicrobial
Diseases

Edited by

Kim A. Brogden
Respiratory Diseases of Livestock Research Unit
National Animal Disease Center
Agricultural Research Service
U.S. Department of Agriculture
Ames, Iowa

Janet M. Guthmiller
Department of Periodontics
and Dows Institute for Dental Research
College of Dentistry
The University of Iowa
Iowa City, Iowa

ASM
PRESS

Washington, D.C.

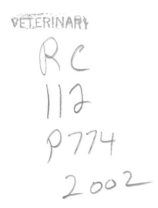
Address editorial correspondence to ASM Press, 1752 N Street NW,
Washington, DC 20036, USA

Send orders to ASM Press, P.O. Box 605, Herndon, VA 20172, USA
Phone: (800) 546-2416 or (703) 661-1593
Fax: (703) 661-1501
E-mail: books@asmusa.org
Online: www.asmpress.org

Library of Congress Cataloging-in-Publication Data

Polymicrobial diseases / edited by Kim A. Brogden, Janet M. Guthmiller.
p. cm.
Includes bibliographical references and index.
ISBN 1-55581-244-9

1. Communicable diseases. 2. Fungi-bacteria relationships. I. Brogden, Kim A. II.
Guthmiller, Janet M.

RC112.P774 2002
616'.01—dc21

2002016407

10 9 8 7 6 5 4 3 2 1

Cover photos: Scanning electron micrographs of human gingival plaque showing a mixed
biofilm of rods and cocci. An occasional erythrocyte and leukocyte can also be seen. Cour-
tesy of John E. Laffoon and Janet M. Guthmiller, College of Dentistry, University of Iowa,
Iowa City, Iowa.

CONTENTS

CONTRIBUTORS

Abelardo Araujo
Centro de Pesquisa Hospital Evandro Changas, Ministerio da Saude, Av. Brasil,
4365, Manguinhos, Cep., Rio de Janeiro 21045-900, Brazil

Lauren O. Bakaletz
Division of Molecular Medicine, College of Medicine and Public Health,
The Ohio State University, and Children's Research Institute, Columbus, OH 43205

Yves Benhamou
Service d'Hépato-Gastroentérologie, Groupe Hospitalier, Hôpital Pitié-Salpêtrière,
75651 Paris, France

Steven R. Bolin
Department of Pathobiology and Diagnostic Investigation, College of Veterinary
Medicine, Michigan State University, East Lansing, MI 48824

Susan L. Brockmeier
Respiratory Diseases of Livestock Research Unit, National Animal Disease Center,
USDA Agricultural Research Service, Ames, IA 50010

Kim A. Brogden
Respiratory Diseases of Livestock Research Unit, National Animal Disease Center,
USDA Agricultural Research Service, Ames, IA 50010

Itzhak Brook
Department of Pediatrics, Georgetown University School of Medicine,
Washington, DC 20007

Jennifer A. Conlon
Biocor Animal Health, 2720 North 84th St., Omaha, NE 68134

Vincent Di Martino
Service d'Hépato-Gastroentérologie, Groupe Hospitalier, Hôpital Pitié-Salpêtrière,
75651 Paris, France

Donatella Donati
Viral Immunology Section, Neuroimmunology Branch, National Institute
of Neurological Disorders and Stroke, National Institutes of Health, Bethesda,
MD 20892, and Dipartimento di Biologia Molecolare, Sezione di Microbiologia,
Università di Siena, via Laterina 8, 53100 Siena, Italy

L. Julia Douglas
Division of Infection and Immunity, Institute of Biomedical and Life Sciences,
University of Glasgow, Glasgow G12 8QQ, United Kingdom

David R. Drake
Dows Institute for Dental Research and Department of Endodontics,
College of Dentistry, University of Iowa, Iowa City, IA 52242

Robert S. Fujinami
Department of Neurology, University of Utah School of Medicine,
Salt Lake City, UT 84132

Eduardo Gotuzzo
Alexander von Humboldt Institute of Tropical Medicine, Universidad Peruana
Cayetano Heredia, Lima, Peru

Janet M. Guthmiller
Department of Periodontics and Dows Institute for Dental Research,
College of Dentistry, University of Iowa, Iowa City, IA 52242

Patrick G. Halbur
Veterinary Diagnostic and Production Animal Medicine, College of Veterinary Medicine,
Iowa State University, Ames, IA 50011

William W. Hall
Department of Medical Microbiology, Conway Institute of Biomolecular
and Biomedical Research, University College Dublin, Belfield, Dublin 4, Ireland

Phillip E. Hay
Department of Genitourinary Medicine, St. George's Hospital Medical School,
Cranmer Terrace, London SW17 0QT, United Kingdom

Douglas C. Hodgins
Department of Pathobiology, Ontario Veterinary College, University of Guelph,
Guelph, Ontario N1G 2W1, Canada

Raul E. Isturiz
Centro Medico de Caracas and Centro Medico Docente La Trinidad,
Caracas, Venezuela

Steven Jacobson
Viral Immunology Section, Neuroimmunology Branch, National Institute
of Neurological Disorders and Stroke, National Institutes of Health,
Bethesda, MD 20892

Howard F. Jenkinson
Department of Oral and Dental Science, University of Bristol Dental School,
Bristol BS1 2LY, United Kingdom

Alistair J. Lax
Oral Microbiology, Guy's King's and St Thomas' Dental Institute,
King's College London, London SE1 9RT, United Kingdom

Jane E. Libbey
Department of Neurology, University of Utah School of Medicine,
Salt Lake City, UT 84132

Tibor Magyar
Veterinary Medical Research Institute, Hungarian Academy of Sciences,
H-1143 Budapest, Hungary

John A. Marshall
Victorian Infectious Diseases Reference Laboratory, Locked Bag 815,
Carlton South, Victoria 3053, Australia

Joseph Moussalli
Service d'Hépato-Gastroentérologie, Groupe Hospitalier, Hôpital Pitié-Salpêtrière,
75651 Paris, France

Robert P. Myers
Service d'Hépato-Gastroentérologie, Groupe Hospitalier, Hôpital Pitié-Salpêtrière,
75651 Paris, France

Karen F. Novak
Center for Oral Health Research, Division of Periodontics, College of Dentistry,
University of Kentucky, Lexington, KY 40536

Thierry Poynard
Service d'Hépato-Gastroentérologie, Groupe Hospitalier, Hôpital Pitié-Salpêtrière,
75651 Paris, France

Vlad Ratziu
Service d'Hépato-Gastroentérologie, Groupe Hospitalier, Hôpital Pitié-Salpêtrière,
75651 Paris, France

Noreen Sheehy
Department of Medical Microbiology, Conway Institute of Biomolecular
and Biomedical Research, University College Dublin, Belfield,
Dublin 4, Ireland

Patricia E. Shewen
Department of Pathobiology, Ontario Veterinary College, University of Guelph,
Guelph, Ontario N1G 2W1, Canada

Jørgen Slots
School of Dentistry, MC 0641, University of Southern California,
Los Angeles, CA 90089-0641

Harry Smith
Medical School, University of Birmingham, Birmingham B15 2TT,
United Kingdom

David R. Soll
Department of the Biological Sciences, University of Iowa, Iowa City,
IA 52242

Clive Sweet
School of Biosciences, University of Birmingham, Birmingham B15 2TT,
United Kingdom

Marie Hélène Tainturier
Service d'Hépato-Gastroentérologie, Groupe Hospitalier, Hôpital Pitié-Salpêtrière,
75651 Paris, France

Hidehiro Takahashi
Department of Pathology, National Institute of Infectious Diseases, Tokyo, Japan

Eileen L. Thacker
Veterinary Medical Research Institute, Iowa State University, Ames, IA 50011

PREFACE

The veterinary, medical, and dental literature is filled with reports of diseases involving more than one etiologic agent. These have come to be known as polymicrobial diseases. Polymicrobial diseases in animals and humans are more common than generally realized, and many perceived "single-etiologic-agent diseases," when examined closely, contain polymicrobial etiologies. These include respiratory diseases, gastroenteritis, conjunctivitis, keratitis, hepatitis, Lyme disease, multiple sclerosis, genital infections, intra-abdominal infections, and pertussis.

Polymicrobial Diseases is a collection of chapters from investigators researching a variety of diseases with multiple etiologies. These diseases can be categorized as those originating from polyviral infections, polybacterial infections, viral and bacterial infections, and polymicrobial mycotic infections, and those that result in immunosuppression. The book begins with a section on an integrated view of polymicrobial diseases in animals and humans, including a representative list of these diseases, the etiologic agents, and the underlying mechanisms of pathogenesis (chapter 1). Also included in this section is a chapter on the in vitro methods for the study of polymicrobial diseases (chapter 2). Section II contains information on polyviral infections in animals (chapter 3), infections with multiple hepatotropic viruses (chapter 4), multiple retroviral infections (chapter 5), and viruses associated with multiple sclerosis (chapter 6). Section III discusses polybacterial infections, including bacterial vaginosis (chapter 7), periodontal disease (chapter 8), abscesses (chapter 9), and atrophic rhinitis in swine (chapter 10). Section IV comprises polymicrobial diseases involving viruses and bacteria. These are infections seen in respiratory diseases in humans (chapter 11) and animals (chapters 12 and 13), otitis media (chapter 14), and intestinal disorders (chapter 15). The emerging role of viruses in periodontal disease is also discussed (chapter 16). Section V discusses polymicrobial infections involving fungi (chapter 17) and *Candida* interactions with bacterial biofilms (chapter 18). Section VI focuses on polymicrobial diseases that result from microbe-induced immunosuppression (chapter 19), which often allows other microbes to become established (chapter 20). In conclusion, section VII summarizes the state of polymicrobial infections in animals and humans (chapter 21).

Polymicrobial infections share underlying mechanisms of pathogenesis, and these are presented in chapter 1. First, stress, physiologic abnormalities, and metabolic disease favor the colonization of multiple organisms. Second, alterations induced in the mucosa by one organism favor the colonization of others. Third, synergistic triggering of proinflammatory cytokines increases the severity of disease, reactivates latent infections, or favors the colonization of other microorganisms. Fourth, sharing of determinants among organisms allows activities that organisms do not possess individually. Finally, suppression of the immune system by one organism allows the colonization of others.

We hope that *Polymicrobial Diseases* will stimulate great interest and spur discussion among its readers and draw together investigators from various fields to assess the mechanisms underlying the pathogenesis of these complex infections. This book provides an overview of our current knowledge of mixed infections in both animals and humans, and we believe that it will serve as a useful reference in this area. The emphasis is on identifying polymicrobial diseases, understanding the complex etiology of these diseases, recognizing difficulties in establishing methods for their study, identifying mechanisms of disease pathogenesis, and assessing appropriate methods of treatment. In some instances, the mechanisms of disease are not well known; in others, the mechanisms of pathogenesis have been under intense investigation. Our intent is to present another edition of this book dealing with the specific mechanisms of polymicrobial infection, host response to infection, predisposition and/or risk factors for the diseases, and pathogenesis of polymicrobial disease.

KIM A. BROGDEN
JANET M. GUTHMILLER

INTRODUCTION

I

POLYMICROBIAL DISEASES OF ANIMALS AND HUMANS

Kim A. Brogden

Polymicrobial diseases represent the clinical and pathologic manifestations induced by the presence of multiple microorganisms. These are serious diseases whose etiologic agents are sometimes difficult to diagnose and treat. They are often called complex infections (136), complicated infections (26), dual infections (15, 76, 82, 186), mixed infections (40), secondary infections (179), coinfections (1, 51, 106, 123), synergistic infections (87), concurrent infections (186), or polymicrobial infections (65, 75). The multiple etiologies often induce a characteristic set of clinical signs and lesions referred to as "complexes" or syndromes. Examples include bovine respiratory disease complex (4, 126), porcine respiratory disease complex (24, 174, 176), and acquired immunodeficiency syndrome (70). Polymicrobial etiologies of multiple sclerosis in humans (39, 77, 125), poult enteritis mortality syndrome in turkeys (76, 139, 188), papillomatous digital dermatitis in dairy cattle (33, 59, 177), and postweaning multisystemic wasting syndrome in pigs (2, 3, 97) are strong suspects but yet to be proven.

Polymicrobial disease is a rapidly emerging and highly researched area, yet it represents a neglected concept. For example, in recent reviews of host-pathogen interactions, the basic concepts of virulence and pathogenicity were redefined (36, 37), and new definitions were based on a pathogen's ability to cause damage as a function of the host's immune response (37). Virulence was defined as a property of the pathogen, which is modulated by host susceptibility and resistance, and disease was defined as a complex outcome, which can arise because of pathogen-mediated damage, host-mediated damage, or both (37). Unfortunately, these were "single etiologic agent" concepts not seriously addressing polymicrobial infections and diseases.

In this book, we focus on the common theme of polymicrobial infections and, in part I, present an integrated view of polymicrobial diseases in animals and humans including a representative list of these diseases, the etiologic agents, and the underlying mechanisms of pathogenesis (chapter 1). Also included is a chapter describing the difficulties in establishing methods for their study (chapter 2). Part II discusses polyviral infections in animals (chapter 3), infections with multiple hepatotropic viruses (chapter 4), multiple retroviral infections (chapter 5), and viruses associated with

Kim A. Brogden, Respiratory Diseases of Livestock Research Unit, National Animal Disease Center, USDA Agricultural Research Service, Ames, IA 50010.

multiple sclerosis (chapter 6). Part III discusses polybacterial infections and includes bacterial vaginosis (chapter 7), periodontal disease (chapter 8), abscesses (chapter 9), and atrophic rhinitis in swine (chapter 10). Part IV discusses polymicrobial diseases involving viruses and bacteria. These are the infections seen in respiratory disease in humans (chapter 11) and animals (chapters 12 and 13), otitis media (chapter 14), and intestinal disorders (chapter 15). An emerging role of viruses in periodontal disease is also discussed (chapter 16). Part V includes chapters on polymicrobial mycotic infections (chapter 17) and *Candida* interactions with bacterial biofilms (chapter 18). Part VI discusses polymicrobial diseases that result from microbe-induced immunosuppression (chapter 19), often allowing other microbes to become established (chapter 20). Part VII summarizes the state of polymicrobial infections in animals and humans (chapter 21).

HISTORICAL PERSPECTIVE

Polymicrobial diseases are not new, and infections involving numerous pathogens were recognized early in the 20th century (87, 161). In animals, foot rot (160) and chronic nonprogressive pneumonia (40, 91, 92) in sheep were among the first diseases found to have multiple etiologies. Respiratory disease in cattle was also shown early to have multiple etiologies (66, 161), which are still being characterized (67, 164, 165). More recently, atrophic rhinitis in swine (128) and porcine respiratory disease complex (25, 68, 163, 168) have been included, the latter because of the emergence of porcine reproductive and respiratory syndrome virus (57, 180).

In humans, acute necrotizing ulcerative gingivitis (87) and respiratory disease were recognized very early as having polymicrobial etiology. In the 1920s, the polymicrobial etiology of respiratory disease was firmly established, and *Haemophilus influenzae* or *Streptococcus pneumoniae* were routinely found in individuals with viral respiratory disease (79). A similar relationship was seen during the influenza pandemics in 1918, 1957, and 1968–1969. Detailed accounts were reported earlier (12, 38, 79). In the 1968–1969 pandemic alone, a threefold increase in *Staphylococcus aureus* pneumonia occurred (153). Later studies confirmed the polymicrobial etiology of respiratory disease (64, 79, 81, 121, 130) and otitis media (79). In otitis media with middle ear effusion, coinfections with bacteria were detected in 65% of cases (81).

ETIOLOGIC AGENTS

Polymicrobial diseases in animals and humans are more common than generally realized, and many perceived "single etiologic agent diseases," when examined closely, contain polymicrobial etiologies (Table 1). These include respiratory diseases, gastroenteritis, conjunctivitis, keratitis, hepatitis, Lyme disease, multiple sclerosis, genital infections, intra-abdominal infections, and pertussis.

Polymicrobial diseases can be categorized as those originating from polyviral infections, polybacterial infections, viral and bacterial infections, polymicrobial mycotic infections, and those that result in immunosuppression (Table 2). In respiratory diseases (chapters 11 to 13), abscesses (chapter 9), and periodontal disease (chapters 8, 16, and 18), the list of potential etiologic agents is very extensive. For example, in bovine respiratory disease complex, up to 13 viruses and 12 bacteria have been described. These include infectious bovine rhinotracheitis virus, bovine viral diarrhea virus, bovine respiratory syncytial virus, parainfluenza virus, bovine herpesvirus 4, malignant catarrhal fever virus, bovine adenovirus, bovine rhinovirus, bovine reovirus, bovine calicivirus, bovine coronavirus, bovine parvovirus, or bovine enterovirus; and *Mannheimia haemolytica*, *Pasteurella multocida*, *Haemophilus somnus*, *Arcanobacterium pyogenes*, *Mycoplasma bovis*, *Mycoplasma dispar*, *Mycoplasma hyorhinis*, *Ureaplasma diversum*, *Chlamydia* spp., *Mycobacterium bovis*, *S. pneumoniae*, or *S. aureus* (4, 10, 34, 67, 94, 109, 126, 137, 165). Once the upper respiratory tract is colonized, large numbers of bacteria can enter the lung and induce severe fibrinonecrotic pneumonia (126, 182). Similarly,

TABLE 1 Reports of polymicrobial infection and disease

Infection and disease	Comments
Animals	
Bovine respiratory disease complex	Up to 13 viruses and 12 bacteria have been described (4, 67)
Bovine gastroenteritis	Polymicrobial disease involving *Salmonella enterica* serovar Dublin, *S. enterica* serovar Typhimurium, coronavirus, and bovine virus diarrhea virus (1, 19, 186)
Ovine conjunctivitis	*Branhamella ovis, Mycoplasma conjunctivae,* and *Chlamydia psittaci* (53)
Ovine foot rot	Multistrain infections of *Dichelobacter nodosus* (89) and mixtures of other bacteria
Ovine pneumonia	Multistrain infections of *Mycoplasma ovipneumoniae* (40) and mixtures of other viruses and bacteria (26)
Porcine atrophic rhinitis	*Pasteurella multocida* and *Bordetella bronchiseptica* (128, 144)
Porcine gastroenteritis	Infection with bovine viral diarrhea virus and transmissible gastroenteritis virus (185)
Porcine respiratory disease complex	Up to 5 viruses and 8 bacteria have been described (24, 25, 163, 168)
Poult enteritis mortality syndrome	Coronavirus and *Escherichia coli* (76)
Infectious coryza	*Haemophilus paragallinarum* and *Ornithobacterium rhinotracheale* (18)
Humans	
Asthma	*Chlamydia psittaci, Chlamydia pneumoniae,* and *Mycoplasma pneumoniae* may play a role in the pathogenesis of asthma (7)
Chicken pox	15% of children with invasive group A streptococcal disease had prior varicella-zoster virus infection (103)
Gastroenteritis	A combination of viruses and bacteria (16)
Genital infections	22.7% of 494 women had mixed chlamydial, bacterial, viral, and fungal infections (112)
Hepatitis	Infections with hepatitis B, C, and D viruses (47, 189)
Infectious keratitis	Polymicrobial infection after surgery (75)
Intra-abdominal infections	Intra-abdominal infections and abscesses contain aerobic and anaerobic gram-positive and gram-negative microorganisms (27–32)
Lyme disease	11% of patients may also have babesiosis (101)
Multiple sclerosis	Epstein-Barr virus and retrovirus (77)
Necrotizing fasciitis	Gram-positive, gram-negative, aerobic, and anaerobic bacteria common (65)
Otitis media	When virus was isolated from middle ear effusion, coinfection with bacteria was detected in 65% of cases (9, 81)
Periodontal infections	A combination of viruses, bacteria, and fungi (113, 131, 132, 159)
Pertussis	In 58% of patients, the nasopharynx has been colonized with species of pathogenic bacteria other than *Bordetella pertussis* (166, 171)

TABLE 2 Reported examples of polymicrobial diseases

Example	Reference(s) for disease
Agents of polyviral diseases	
Bovine viral diarrhea virus and transmissible gastroenteritis virus	185
Bovine viral diarrhea virus and bovine coronavirus	1
Cytopathic bovine viral diarrhea virus and noncytopathic bovine viral diarrhea virus	19
Epstein-Barr virus and retrovirus	77
Hepatitis B, C, and D viruses	47, 117, 189
HTLV-1, HTLV-2, and/or HIV-1 or HIV-2	74, 106, 152, 172
Hepatitis B or C virus and HIV-1	5, 8
Porcine circovirus type 2 and epidemic diarrhea virus	82
Porcine circovirus type 2 and porcine reproductive and respiratory syndrome virus	2
Porcine circovirus type 2 and porcine parvovirus	3, 97
Small round virus and turkey coronavirus	139, 188
Agents of polybacterial diseases	
Bacteroides spp., *Clostridium* spp., *Escherichia coli*, *Fusobacterium* spp., *Klebsiella pneumoniae*, *Peptostreptococcus* spp., *Porphyromonas* spp., *Prevotella* spp., *Propionibacterium acnes*, *Proteus* spp., *Pseudomonas* spp., *Staphylococcus aureus*, *Streptococcus* spp.	27–32, 65, 112
Branhamella ovis and *Mycoplasma conjunctivae*	53
Bordetella pertussis, *Streptococcus pneumoniae*, *S. aureus*, *Haemophilus influenzae*	171
Multiple *Mycoplasma ovipneumoniae* genotypes	40
Multiple *Dichelobacter nodosus* genotypes	89
Multiple *Haemobartonella felis* genotypes	181
Polymicrobial diseases involving viruses and bacteria	
Bovine shipping fever	4, 47, 67
Bovine viral diarrhea virus and *Salmonella enterica* serovar Dublin or *S. enterica* serovar Typhimurium	186
Herpes simplex virus, *Streptococcus epidermidis*, and *Fusarium solani*	75
HIV and *Mycobacterium tuberculosis*	46, 154
Influenza virus and *S. aureus*	38
Norwalk-like virus and *Aeromonas sobria*	16
Norwalk-like virus and *E. coli*	16
Hemorrhagic enteritis virus and *E. coli*	129, 135
Porcine reproductive and respiratory syndrome virus and *Haemophilus parasuis*	163
Porcine reproductive and respiratory syndrome virus and *Mycoplasma hyopneumoniae*	168
Turkey coronavirus and enteropathogenic *Escherichia coli*	76
Varicella-zoster virus and *Streptococcus pyogenes*	103

continues

TABLE 2   *Continued*

Example	Reference(s) for disease
Polymicrobial diseases involving fungi and parasites	
Candida albicans and oral streptococci	132
C. albicans and *S. aureus*	120
Candida dubliniensis and *Fusobacterium nucleatum*	88
Cryptosporidium parvum and *Cryptosporidium muris*	169
Dictyocaulus spp. and gastrointestinal nematodes	84
HIV and *C. albicans*	175
Lyme disease and babesiosis	101
Nocardia asteroides and *Cryptococcus neoformans*	155
Schistosoma haematobium and *Schistosoma mansoni*	61
Polymicrobial diseases as a result of microbe-induced immunosuppression	
Infectious bursal disease virus	149, 157, 158
Hemorrhagic enteritis virus	140, 141, 149
Chicken anemia virus	146
Avian leukosis virus	62
Reticuloendotheliosis virus	62
Avian reovirus	157
Avian *S. enterica* serovar Typhimurium	80
Border disease virus	151
Bovine respiratory syncytial virus	95, 96
Porcine reproductive and respiratory syndrome virus	57
Ehrlichia phagocytophila	102
Bovine viral diarrhea virus	34, 85, 138
HIV and *Histoplasma capsulatum*	78

in porcine respiratory disease complex, up to five viruses and eight bacteria have been described and include porcine reproductive and respiratory syndrome virus, swine influenza virus, pseudorabies virus, porcine respiratory coronavirus, or porcine circovirus as well as *Mycoplasma hyopneumoniae, Bordetella bronchiseptica, Actinobacillus pleuropneumoniae, P. multocida, Haemophilus parasuis, Streptococcus suis, Actinobacillus suis,* or *A. pyogenes* (24, 25, 68, 162, 163, 168). In abscesses, aerobic, anaerobic, gram-positive, and gram-negative bacteria are present (27–32). The predominant aerobic and facultative bacteria are *Escherichia coli* and *Streptococcus* spp., and the predominant anaerobes are *Bacteroides* spp., *Peptostreptococcus* spp., *Clostridium* spp., and *Fusobacterium* spp. In periodontal disease, a vast combination of bacteria, viruses, and possibly fungi are present (99, 113, 131, 132, 134, 159). Although periodontal disease is a major cause of tooth loss in adults (45, 86), pe-

riodontal infections are now thought to play a significant role in systemic health. Numerous systemic infections are thought to originate in the oral cavity (156), which may lead to an increased risk of systemic disease including coronary heart disease (13, 55, 118, 124).

MODELS

Reproducing polymicrobial disease is often difficult. In some cases, polymicrobial disease can be induced by simply administering comixtures of microorganisms. This approach was successful in inducing experimental chronic nonprogressive pneumonia (40, 91, 92). In other cases, disease can only be induced by sequential administration of causative agents. This approach was successful in inducing respiratory disease in sheep (26, 51, 52, 105) and swine (25). In swine, *P. multocida* could not be isolated from pigs challenged with *P. multocida* alone or after inoculation with porcine reproductive and respiratory syndrome virus. However, *P. multocida* could be isolated from pigs challenged sequentially with porcine reproductive and respiratory syndrome virus, *B. bronchiseptica,* and *P. multocida.* Finally, physical stress may be required. In cattle, abrupt changes in temperature (56, 90) and exercise (6) increase the numbers of *M. haemolytica* in the nasopharynx, thus increasing the susceptibility of cattle to respiratory infection.

A number of models have been described to study in vivo and in vitro polymicrobial interactions in periodontal disease. In vivo models allow the study of host response to infection. Ligature-induced models of periodontitis in nonhuman primates (58), dogs (115), and rodents have helped identify the profiles of gingival crevicular fluid mediators and their relationship to gingival inflammation. In vitro models allow for the study of the oral bacterial interactions in suspension in continuous culture chemostat systems (20), constant depth film fermenters (183), and flow cells (100). These techniques have identified the parameters involved in the formation of plaque, the interactions among members of the resident flora, factors involved in the transition of the biofilm from a commensal to a pathogenic relationship with the host, and the mode of action of antimicrobials and antiplaque agents (21). More detailed information is available in chapter 2.

COMMON UNDERLYING MECHANISMS OF PATHOGENESIS

Despite the spectrum of etiologic agents in Tables 1 and 2, five common underlying mechanisms exist that can lead to disease. First, physical, physiologic, or metabolic abnormalities including stress can predispose the host to polymicrobial disease (17, 41, 65). Second, alterations induced in the mucosa by one organism favor the colonization of others (79). Third, synergistic triggering of proinflammatory cytokines increases severity of disease, reactivates latent infections, or favors the colonization of other microorganisms. Fourth,

sharing of determinants among organisms allows activities that neither organism possesses individually (161). Finally, obliteration of the immune system by one organism allows the colonization of others.

Stress, Physiologic Abnormalities, and Metabolic Disease Favor the Colonization of Multiple Organisms

Stress is a strong predisposing factor increasing the susceptibility of animals and humans to polymicrobial diseases. In animals, common stresses include heat, crowding, limited space, exposure to inclement weather, poor ventilation with high levels of moisture and barnyard gases, handling and transport, castration and docking, weaning and change in feed, exhaustion and hunger during transportation, excessive dust in feedlots, high loads of parasites, and mixing of animals from different sources (43, 69, 98, 114). Stressed animals usually have increased body temperature; increased heart rate; increased plasma cortisol, glucose, free fatty acids, β-hydroxybutyrate, and urea; decreased body weight; and decreased hydration (93, 98, 133, 167).

In humans, stress is also a strong predisposing factor increasing the susceptibility of individuals to polymicrobial diseases. Respiratory tract infections (17, 41, 72, 73), necrotizing ulcerative gingivitis (147), and oral infections are often used as examples. Physiologic and psychological stress increases an individual's susceptibility to upper respiratory tract infections (17, 41, 72). The stress and hassles of life events, the moderating effects of psychological coping style, social support, and family environment all influence susceptibility (41). High-stress groups experience significantly more episodes and symptom days of respiratory illness than low-stress groups (72). However, sex (female) and age also seem to be important correlates of respiratory illness (72).

Physiologic abnormalities can favor polymicrobial diseases, but only a few examples exist. In pastured and feedlot cattle, acute interstitial pneumonia is precipitated by a predisposing metabolic event that often develops into a polymicrobial disease (83, 107, 108). During anaerobic ruminal fermentation of tryptophan, 3-methylindole is produced and is absorbed across the ruminal and intestinal wall and disseminated throughout the body. Metabolism of 3-methylindole produces free radicals that contribute to cellular injury in Clara and type I alveolar epithelia in the lung. A metabolite of 3-methylindole, 3-methyleneindolenine also induces damage by covalently binding to cellular macromolecules. In some cases, cellular injury is insufficient to induce acute interstitial pneumonia without the presence of other factors, but it is thought to predispose cattle to concurrent bronchopneumonia in a mechanism involving tumor necrosis factor alpha (TNF-α) and interleukin-1β (IL-1β).

Finally, polymicrobial diseases occur in individuals with coexisting metabolic diseases. Individuals with diabetes are at risk for advanced periodontal disease (122).

Alterations in the Mucosa by One Organism Favor the Colonization of Another

Bacterial infections of mucosal surfaces may, in some instances, contribute to increased adherence and replication of other microbes. C. albicans adheres more readily to epithelial cells preincubated with staphylococcal serine protease perhaps by enzymatically altering receptors on mucosal epithelium (120). These same proteases are also thought to increase the severity of viral influenza by cleaving the viral hemagglutinin (38).

Similarly, viral infections of mucosal surfaces contribute to increased incidence of secondary bacterial infections (79). First, viruses physically damage respiratory epithelium and impair ciliary clearance of bacteria. This is seen in respiratory syncytial virus (170) and influenza virus infections (178). Second, viruses alter epithelial cell surfaces thus creating receptors for bacterial adherence (38, 79, 121). For example, during replication of influenza virus, neuraminidase and hemagglutinin are inserted into the host cell membranes serving as receptors for S. pneumoniae. Pneumococcal adherence can be blocked by treating influenza A virus-infected cells with antiviral antibodies (150) or neuraminidase (54). Similarly, during replication of respiratory syncytial virus (RSV), glycoproteins F and G are inserted into the host cell membranes serving as receptors for Neisseria meningitidis (142). Increased amounts of CD14, CD15, and CD18 are also produced which enhance the adherence of nonpiliated N. meningitidis (143). H. influenzae and S. pneumoniae adhere more readily to RSV-infected cells via P5 fimbriae-binding and platelet-activating factor, respectively. In the latter, RSV infection induces the production of TNF-α and IL-1α (48, 49), which activates production of platelet-activating factor on endothelial surfaces.

During infectious bovine rhinotracheitis virus infection in vivo, neutrophil elastase cleavage of epithelial cell surface fibronectin and exposure of receptors was thought to increase colonization of M. haemolytica (23). Elastase activity in nasal mucus of sick calves increased about 15-fold within 3 days and peaked about 60-fold over baseline by 7 days after virus exposure. Increased elastase activity preceded colonization by M. haemolytica and decreasing elastase activity preceded decreasing M. haemolytica concentration in the nasal secretions (23).

Synergistic Triggering of Proinflammatory Cytokines Increases Severity of Disease, Reactivates Latent Infections, or Favors the Colonization of Another Organism

Synergistic induction and release of proinflammatory cytokines can lead to extensive clinical and pathologic polymicrobial disease in situations where neither individual organism induces high and sustained cytokine levels alone. An excellent example of this mechanism is the lipopolysaccharide (LPS)-induced release of TNF-α and IL-1 from virus-infected cells. In vitro, mouse-adapted influenza virus, which induces minimal TNF-α in leukocyte cultures, primes cells for massive TNF-α secretion after exposure to H. influenzae LPS (127). Similarly, influenza virus alone induces a massive TNF-

α accumulation in leukocytes, but efficient translation into bioactive protein occurs on further stimulation by LPS (14). In vivo, an enhanced serum TNF-α response was observed when influenza-infected mice were given an intravenous dose of LPS (116). Similarly, pigs exposed to both porcine respiratory coronavirus and LPS from *E. coli* O111:B4 developed severe respiratory disease (174) with significantly enhanced TNF-α and IL-1 levels. The effects of separate virus or LPS inoculations were subclinical and failed to induce high and sustained cytokine levels.

Polymicrobial infections are associated with transient bursts of human immunodeficiency virus (HIV) viremia in patients (123) involving LPS from systemic gram-negative bacterial infections (123), gut-associated bacterial translocation (123), or periodontal pathogens (11). Systemic up-regulation of monocyte proinflammatory cytokine secretion by LPS is thought to induce activation of HIV-1 from latently infected resting CD4$^+$ T cells (123). To demonstrate this, supernatants from macrophages exposed to LPS induced the in vitro activation of HIV-1 from latently infected, resting CD4$^+$ T cells obtained from HIV-infected individuals. Depletion of proinflammatory cytokines from the supernatant markedly reduced the ability of the supernatant to induce replication of HIV-1. Similarly, Lore et al. (110) demonstrated that infection of cultured dendritic cells, in vitro, with macrophage-tropic HIV-1 did not induce detectable cytokine or chemokine protein expression in these cells. However, LPS stimulation of HIV-1-infected dendritic cells resulted in significantly increased levels of cells producing TNF-α and IL-1β but reduced IL-1 receptor antagonist (IL-1ra). This suggests that gram-negative bacterial infection in HIV-1-infected individuals may result in endotoxin-mediated reactivation of HIV-1 in bystander CD4 CD45RO T cells caused by the increased production of proinflammatory cytokines in dendritic cells.

In patients with advanced HIV infections, systemic up-regulation of monocyte proin-

flammatory cytokine secretion might also occur by LPS from periodontal pathogens (11). Indeed, cultured monocytes from HIV-infected patients, incubated with *Porphyromonas gingivalis* or *Fusobacterium nucleatum* LPS, produced greater amounts of TNF-α, IL-1β, and IL-6 than monocytes from uninfected controls.

TNF-α and IL-1 also alter the expression of epithelial and endothelial cell receptors thus facilitating bacterial adherence (50). TNF-α and IL-1 increase the expression of E selectin and globotriosylceramide on vascular endothelial cells (148, 173). Similarly, these cytokines also increase glycoconjugate receptors on type II alveolar epithelium and vascular endothelium, facilitating the 30% and 70% increased attachment of *S. pneumoniae,* respectively (50). Enhanced *S. pneumoniae* adherence was associated with the appearance of new receptor specificity for GlcNAc within the Ga1NAcβ1-3Gal receptor family (50). Reciprocal changes in pneumococcal adhesive ligands matched the changes in the eucaryotic cell surface in those strains that achieved successful colonization.

Sharing of Determinants among Organisms Allows Activities that Neither Organism Possesses Individually

In 1982, Smith proposed a concept to explain how nonpathogenic or weakly pathogenic microorganisms can interact synergistically to cause harmful, even fatal, infections (161). Ovine foot rot, bovine shipping fever, periodontal disease, and abdominal abscesses were assigned to this group (161). The underlying mechanism for pathogenic synergy was thought to be the sharing of determinants among determinant-deficient organisms. Although little progress has been made in this area since then, many recent observations strongly support this concept. This may occur in multistrain infections of *Mycoplasma ovipneumoniae* (40, 91, 92). Sheep with severe lesions had three to four distinct *M. ovipneumoniae* genotypes, whereas sheep with lesser lesions had only two distinct genotypes (40). Other multistrain infections include *Hemobartonella felis* (181), bovine virus diarrhea virus (19), *Trichophyton rubrum* (60), and *Dichelobacter nodosus* (89). In the latter study, the proportions of protease-type *D. nodosus* S1, U1, and T strains in samples of foot rot lesion material were 58, 22, and 18%, respectively, at a ratio that remained constant during two apparent peaks in foot rot transmission. Although strain S1 was the dominant protease type in new clinical lesions, the occurrence of S1 strains did not increase relative to U1 and T strains. Strains S1, U1, and T remained in equilibrium despite changes in environment, genetic types in the population of S1 strains, and host resistance to foot rot. All these studies suggest that a single member of the multistrain population cannot alone produce the full complement of factors needed for disease production. Together, the full complement of factors can be attained. To what extent this concept occurs in other polymicrobial diseases such as periodontal disease and abscesses is still to be determined.

Tuomanen proposed a specific mechanism for the sharing (or piracy) of determinants (171), and this concept also helps explain the synergy between nonpathogenic or weakly pathogenic microorganisms to cause harmful, even fatal, infections (161). *Bordetella pertussis* produces a 220-kDa filamentous hemagglutinin capable of binding with ciliary glycoconjugates by its lectin domain, glycoconjugates in respiratory mucus by its heparin-binding domain, erythrocytes by its heparin-binding domain and N-terminal lectin domains, and leukocyte integrins by its RGD and factor X-like domains (50). *B. pertussis* also produces a 105-kDa pertussis toxin with the A-B architecture (50). *B. pertussis* infection is frequently associated with secondary infections caused by *H. influenzae, S. pneumoniae,* and *S. aureus.* Adherence of these other pathogens to cilia is usually low. In contrast, these bacteria adhere remarkably well to human cilia pretreated with *B. pertussis* or pertussis toxin (171). *B. pertussis* apparently secretes its adhesins into the environment and then recaptures them. Likewise, heterologous species of bacteria can bind to *B.*

pertussis adhesins; this piracy may contribute to superinfection in mucosal diseases such as whooping cough. Recently, *P. multocida* was found to have open reading frames that encode large proteins with homology to the virulence-associated filamentous hemagglutinin of *B. pertussis* (119). Whether *P. multocida* and *B. bronchiseptica* (44) share filamentous hemagglutinin leading to cocolonization (25) will have to be determined.

Obliteration of the Immune System by One Organism Allows the Colonization of Others

In poultry, infectious bursal disease virus (149, 157, 158) and hemorrhagic enteritis virus (140, 141, 149) induce an acute infection followed by immunosuppression, resulting in lowered resistance to a variety of infectious agents by destroying immunoglobulin-producing cells and altering antigen-presenting and helper T-cell functions. Chicken anemia virus (146), avian leukosis virus, reticuloendotheliosis virus (62, 111), *Salmonella enterica* serovar Typhimurium (80), and *Bordetella avium* (145) also induce immunosuppression resulting in secondary coinfections.

In pigs, porcine reproductive and respiratory syndrome virus infection destroys circulating lymphocytes, reduces numerous alveolar macrophages, and reduces mucociliary clearance of commensals (57). This leads to secondary infections with *M. hyopneumoniae, P. multocida, H. parasuis,* or *S. suis* (25, 57, 163, 168).

In ruminants, bovine respiratory syncytial virus depresses the proliferative responses of normal ovine peripheral blood lymphocytes to mitogens (95, 96). Persistent infections with bovine viral diarrhea virus also increase the vulnerability of cattle to secondary infections (138). The virus replicates in all the major lymphocyte subpopulations and in accessory cells, resulting in leukopenia that is often a sequel of infection (85). The envelope glycoprotein Erns, an RNase, totally inhibits mitogen-induced proliferation of porcine, bovine, and ovine lymphocytes and strongly inhibits protein synthesis of lymphocytes without cell membrane damage and apoptosis of lymphocytes (35).

In humans, human T-cell leukemia virus type 1 (HTLV-1) results in extensive immunosuppression leading to infections by polymicrobial diseases involving other viruses (74, 106, 152, 172), bacteria, fungi (22, 78, 184), protozoans, and parasites (71). Similarly, HIV infection induces extensive immunosuppression (42, 46, 63, 187) resulting in infections with other viruses (5, 8, 74, 77, 106, 152, 172); bacteria, especially *Mycobacterium avium* complex and *Mycobacterium tuberculosis* (46, 154); fungi (22, 70, 78, 175, 184); protozoans (104); and parasites (104). After primary infection, acute viremia occurs and is characterized by major expansions of certain subsets of CD8$^+$ T cells (63). The virus binds to and infects a range of CD4$^+$ leukocytes, depending on the coreceptor specificity. In addition, inappropriate immune activation and elevated secretion of certain proinflammatory cytokines occur during HIV infection; these cytokines play a role in the regulation of HIV expression in the tissues. T-cell-tropic HIV strains tend to bind to the CXCR-4 chemokine receptor (46), whereas macrophage-tropic strains tend to bind to the CCR-5 chemokine receptor (42, 187). Immunosuppression is induced in many ways. Besides depletion of virus–infected T cells, antigen-specific T-cell clones can be selectively deleted by mechanisms such as defective antigen presentation by HIV-infected macrophages (46). HIV infection of CD4$^+$ T cells also results in inducing the secretion of proinflammatory cytokines that the virus uses to its own replicative advantage (42). All this leads to falling T-cell counts, B-cell dysregulation, and macrophage dysfunction (46). Opportunistic infections exploit this immunosuppressed environment.

CONCLUSIONS

Polymicrobial diseases in animals and humans are induced by polyviral infections (chapters 3 to 6), polybacterial infections (chapters 7 to 10), polymicrobial infections involving viruses and bacteria (chapters 11 to 16), polymicrobial infections involving fungi and parasites (chapters 17 and 18), and polymicrobial infections as a result of microbe-induced immunosuppression (chapters 19 and 20). They are serious diseases whose etiologic agents are sometimes difficult to diagnose and treat. Five common mechanisms of disease pathogenesis exist. First, physical, physiologic, or metabolic abnormalities and stress predispose the host to polymicrobial disease. Second, one organism induces changes in the mucosa that may favor the colonization of others. Third, microorganisms or their products trigger proinflammatory cytokines to increase the severity of disease, reactivate latent infections, or favor the colonization of other microorganisms. Fourth, organisms may share determinants among each other, which gives them the ability to damage tissue. Finally, one organism can alter the immune system, which allows the colonization of the host by other microorganisms. Many areas of study in polymicrobial diseases are in their infancy, and we hope that this text will stimulate interest and work in this evolving field.

REFERENCES

1. **Alenius, S., R. Niskanen, N. Juntti, and B. Larsson.** 1991. Bovine coronavirus as the causative agent of winter dysentery: serological evidence. *Acta Vet. Scand.* **32:**163–170.

2. **Allan, G. M., F. McNeilly, J. Ellis, S. Krakowka, B. Meehan, I. McNair, I. Walker, and S. Kennedy.** 2000. Experimental infection of colostrum deprived piglets with porcine circovirus 2 (PCV2) and porcine reproductive and respiratory syndrome virus (PRRSV) potentiates PCV2 replication. *Arch. Virol.* **145:** 2421–2429.

3. **Allan, G. M., F. McNeilly, B. M. Meehan, J. A. Ellis, T. J. Connor, I. McNair, S. Krakowka, and S. Kennedy.** 2000. A sequential study of experimental infection of pigs with porcine circovirus and porcine parvovirus: immunostaining of cryostat sections and virus isolation. *J. Vet. Med. Ser. B* **47:**81–94.

4. **Allen, J. W., L. Viel, K. G. Bateman, E. Nagy, S. Rosendal, and P. E. Shewen.** 1992. Serological titers to bovine herpesvirus 1, bovine viral diarrhea virus, parainfluenza 3 virus, bovine respiratory syncytial virus and Pasteurella

haemolytica in feedlot calves with respiratory disease: associations with bacteriological and pulmonary cytological variables. *Can. J. Vet. Res.* **56:**281–288.

5. **Allory, Y., F. Charlotte, Y. Benhamou, P. Opolon, Y. Le Charpentier, T. Poynard, and the MULTIVIRC Group.** 2000. Impact of human immunodeficiency virus infection on the histological features of chronic hepatitis C: a case-control study. *Hum. Pathol.* **31:**69–74.

6. **Anderson, N. V., Y. D. Youanes, J. G. Vestweber, C. A. King, R. D. Klemm, and G. A. Kennedy.** 1991. The effects of stressful exercise on leukocytes in cattle with experimental pneumonic pasteurellosis. *Vet. Res. Commun.* **15:**189–204.

7. **Atmar, R. L.** 1999. Chlamydia species and Mycoplasma pneumoniae. *Curr. Infect. Dis. Rep.* **1:**73–79.

8. **Avila, M. M., E. Casanueva, C. Piccardo, D. Liberatore, G. Cammarieri, M. Cervellini, I. Gojman, and O. Libonatti.** 1996. HIV-1 and hepatitis B virus infections in adolescents lodged in security institutes of Buenos Aires. *Pediatr. AIDS HIV Infect.* **7:**346–349.

9. **Bakaletz, L. O.** 1995. Viral potentiation of bacterial superinfection of the respiratory tract. *Trends Microbiol.* **3:**110–114.

10. **Baker, J. C., J. A. Ellis, and E. G. Clark.** 1997. Bovine respiratory syncytial virus. *Vet. Clin. N. Am. Food Anim. Pract.* **13:**425–454.

11. **Baqui, A. A., M. A. Jabra-Rizk, J. I. Kelley, M. Zhang, W. A. Falkler, Jr., and T. F. Meiller.** 2000. Enhanced interleukin-1 beta, interleukin-6 and tumor necrosis factor-alpha production by LPS stimulated human monocytes isolated from HIV+ patients. *Immunopharmacol. Immunotoxicol.* **22:**401–421.

12. **Barker, W. H., and J. P. Mullooly.** 1982. Pneumonia and influenza deaths during epidemics: implications for prevention. *Arch. Intern. Med.* **142:**85–89.

13. **Beck, J., R. Garcia, G. Heiss, P. S. Vokonas, and S. Offenbacher.** 1996. Periodontal disease and cardiovascular disease. *J. Periodontol.* **67:**1123–1137.

14. **Bender, A., H. Sprenger, J. H. Gong, A. Henke, G. Bolte, H. P. Spengler, M. Nain, and D. Gemsa.** 1993. The potentiating effect of LPS on tumor necrosis factor-alpha production by influenza A virus-infected macrophages. *Immunobiology* **187:**357–371.

15. **Bergstrom, R. C., B. A. Werner, and L. R. Maki.** 1980. Dual infections in sheep: Trichostrongylus colubriformis and Corynebacterium pseudotuberculosis. *Int. Goat Sheep Res.* **1:**190–194.

16. **Bettelheim, K. A., D. S. Bowden, J. C. Doultree, M. G. Catton, D. Chibo, N. J. Ryan, P. J. Wright, I. C. Gunesekere, J. M. Griffith, D. Lightfoot, G. G. Hogg, V. Bennett-Wood, and J. A. Marshall.** 1999. Combined infection of Norwalk-like virus and verotoxin-producing bacteria associated with a gastroenteritis outbreak. *J. Diarrhoeal Dis. Res.* **17:**34–36.

17. **Biondi, M., and L. G. Zannino.** 1997. Psychological stress, neuroimmunomodulation, and susceptibility to infectious diseases in animals and man: a review. *Psychother. Psychosom.* **66:**3–26.

18. **Blackall, P. J.** 1999. Infectious coryza: overview of the disease and new diagnostic options. *Clin. Microbiol. Rev.* **12:**627–632.

19. **Bolin, S. R.** 1995. The pathogenesis of mucosal disease. *Vet. Clin. N. Am. Food Anim. Pract.* **11:**489–500.

20. **Bowden, G. H.** 1999. Controlled environment model for accumulation of biofilms of oral bacteria. *Methods Enzymol.* **310:**216–224.

21. **Bradshaw, D. J., and P. D. Marsh.** 1999. Use of continuous flow techniques in modeling dental plaque biofilms. *Methods Enzymol.* **310:**279–296.

22. **Brandt, M. E., M. A. Pfaller, R. A. Hajjeh, E. A. Graviss, J. Rees, E. D. Spitzer, R. W. Pinner, L. W. Mayer, and the Cryptococcal Disease Active Surveillance Group.** 1996. Molecular subtypes and antifungal susceptibilities of serial Cryptococcus neoformans isolates in human immunodeficiency virus-associated cryptococcosis. *J. Infect. Dis.* **174:**812–820.

23. **Briggs, R. E., and G. H. Frank.** 1992. Increased elastase activity in nasal mucus associated with nasal colonization by Pasteurella haemolytica in infectious bovine rhinotracheitis virus-infected calves. *Am. J. Vet. Res.* **53:**631–635.

24. **Brockmeier, S. L., M. V. Palmer, and S. R. Bolin.** 2000. Effects of intranasal inoculation of porcine reproductive and respiratory syndrome virus, *Bordetella bronchiseptica,* or a combination of both organisms in pigs. *Am. J. Vet. Res.* **61:**892–899.

25. **Brockmeier, S. L., M. V. Palmer, S. R. Bolin, and R. B. Rimler.** 2001. Effects of intranasal inoculation with Bordetella bronchiseptica, porcine reproductive and respiratory syndrome virus, or a combination of both organisms on subsequent infection with Pasteurella multocida in pigs. *Am. J. Vet. Res.* **62:**521–525.

26. **Brogden, K. A., H. D. Lehmkuhl, and R. C. Cutlip.** 1998. *Pasteurella haemolytica* complicated respiratory infections in sheep and goats. *Vet. Res.* **29:**233–254.

27. **Brook, I., and E. H. Fraizer.** 1993. Role of anaerobic bacteria in liver abscesses in children. *Pediatr. Infect. Dis. J.* **12:**743–747.

28. **Brook, I., and E. H. Frazier.** 1997. The aerobic and anaerobic bacteriology of perirectal abscesses. *J. Clin. Microbiol.* **35:**2974–2976.

29. **Brook, I., and E. H. Frazier.** 2000. Aerobic and anaerobic microbiology in intra-abdominal infections associated with diverticulitis. *J. Med. Microbiol.* **49:**827–830.

30. **Brook, I., and E. H. Frazier.** 1998. Aerobic and anaerobic microbiology of chronic venous ulcers. *Int. J. Dermatol.* **37:**426–428.

31. **Brook, I., and E. H. Frazier.** 1996. Aerobic and anaerobic microbiology of infected hemorrhoids. *Am. J. Gastroenterol.* **91:**333–335.

32. **Brook, I., and E. H. Frazier.** 1998. Aerobic and anaerobic microbiology of retroperitoneal abscesses. *Clin. Infect. Dis.* **26:**938–941.

33. **Brown, C. C., P. D. Kilgo, and K. L. Jacobsen.** 2000. Prevalence of papillomatous digital dermatitis among culled adult cattle in the southeastern United States. *Am. J. Vet. Res.* **61:**928–930.

34. **Brownlie, J.** 1990. The pathogenesis of bovine virus diarrhoea virus infections. *Rev. Sci. Tech. Off. Int. Epizoot.* **9:**43–59.

35. **Bruschke, C. J., M. M. Hulst, R. J. Moormann, P. A. van Rijn, and J. T. van Oirschot.** 1997. Glycoprotein Erns of pestiviruses induces apoptosis in lymphocytes of several species. *J. Virol.* **71:**6692–6696.

36. **Casadevall, A., and L. A. Pirofski.** 2000. Host-pathogen interactions: basic concepts of microbial commensalism, colonization, infection, and disease. *Infect. Immun.* **68:**6511–6518.

37. **Casadevall, A., and L. A. Pirofski.** 1999. Host-pathogen interactions: redefining the basic concepts of virulence and pathogenicity. *Infect. Immun.* **67:**3703–3713.

38. **Cate, T. R.** 1998. Impact of influenza and other community-acquired viruses. *Semin. Respir. Infect.* **13:**17–23.

39. **Cermelli, C., and S. Jacobson.** 2000. Viruses and multiple sclerosis. *Viral Immunol.* **13:**255–267.

40. **Clarke, J. K., G. Ionas, and M. R. Alley.** 1992. Mixed infection with one species of microorganism. *Vet. Rec.* **130:**20.

41. **Cobb, J. M., and A. Steptoe.** 1996. Psychosocial stress and susceptibility to upper respiratory tract illness in an adult population sample. *Psychosom. Med.* **58:**404–412.

42. **Cohen, O. J., A. Kinter, and A. S. Fauci.** 1997. Host factors in the pathogenesis of HIV disease. *Immunol. Rev.* **159:**31–48.

43. **Cole, N. A.** 1996. Metabolic changes and nutrient repletion in lambs provided with electrolyte solutions before and after feed and water deprivation. *J. Anim. Sci.* **74:**287–294.

44. **Cotter, P. A., M. H. Yuk, S. Mattoo, B. J. Akerley, J. Boschwitz, D. A. Relman, and J. F. Miller.** 1998. Filamentous hemagglutinin of *Bordetella bronchiseptica* is required for efficient establishment of tracheal colonization. *Infect. Immun.* **66:**5921–5929.

45. **Coventry, J., G. Griffiths, C. Scully, and M. Tonetti.** 2000. ABC of oral health: periodontal disease. *BMJ* **321:**36–39.

46. **Cowley, S.** 2001. The biology of HIV infection. *Lepr. Rev.* **72:**212–220.

47. **Crespo, J., J. L. Lozano, B. Carte, B. de las Heras, F. de la Cruz, and F. Pons-Romero.** 1997. Viral replication in patients with concomitant hepatitis B and C virus infections. *Eur. J. Clin. Microbiol. Infect. Dis.* **16:**445–451.

48. **Cundell, D., H. R. Masure, and E. I. Tuomanen.** 1995. The molecular basis of pneumococcal infection: a hypothesis. *Clin. Infect. Dis.* **21:**204–212.

49. **Cundell, D. R., N. P. Gerard, C. Gerard, I. Idanpaan-Heikkila, and E. I. Tuomanen.** 1995. Streptococcus pneumoniae anchor to activated human cells by the receptor for platelet-activating factor. *Nature* **377:**435–438.

50. **Cundell, D. R., and E. Tuomanen.** 1995. Attachment and interaction of bacteria at respiratory mucosal surfaces, p. 3–20. *In* J. A. Roth, C. A. Bolin, K. A. Brogden, F. C. Minion, and M. J. Wannemuehler (ed.), *Virulence Mechanisms of Bacterial Pathogens,* 2nd ed. ASM Press, Washington, D.C.

51. **Cutlip, R. C., H. D. Lehmkuhl, and K. A. Brogden.** 1993. Chronic effects of coinfection in lambs with parainfluenza-3 virus and *Pasteurella haemolytica. Small Ruminant Res.* **11:**171–178.

52. **Cutlip, R. C., H. D. Lehmkuhl, K. A. Brogden, and N. J. Hsu.** 1996. Lesions in lambs experimentally infected with ovine adenovirus serotype 6 and *Pasteurella haemolytica. J. Vet. Diagn. Investig.* **8:**296–303.

53. **Dagnall, G. J.** 1994. The role of Branhamella ovis, Mycoplasma conjunctivae and Chlamydia psittaci in conjunctivitis of sheep. *Br. Vet. J.* **150:**65–71.

54. **Davison, V. E., and B. A. Sanford.** 1981. Adherence of *Staphylococcus aureus* to influenza A virus-infected Madin-Darby canine kidney cell cultures. *Infect. Immun.* **32:**118–126.

55. **DeStefano, F., R. F. Anda, H. S. Kahn, D. F. Williamson, and C. M. Russell.** 1993. Dental disease and risk of coronary heart disease and mortality. *Br. Med. J.* **306:**688–691.

56. **Diesel, D. A., J. L. Lebel, and A. Tucker.** 1991. Pulmonary particle deposition and airway mucociliary clearance in cold-exposed calves. *Am. J. Vet. Res.* **52:**1665–1671.

57. **Done, S. H., and D. J. Paton.** 1995. Porcine reproductive and respiratory syndrome: clinical disease, pathology and immunosuppression. *Vet. Rec.* **136:**32–35.

58. **Ebersole, J. L., D. Cappelli, S. C. Holt, R. E. Singer, and T. Filloon.** 2000. Gingival crevicular fluid inflammatory mediators and bacteriology of gingivitis in nonhuman primates related to susceptibility to periodontitis. *Oral Microbiol. Immunol.* **15:**19–26.

59. **el-Ghoul, W., and B. I. Shaheed.** 2001. Ulcerative and papillomatous digital dermatitis of the pastern region in dairy cattle: clinical and histopathological studies. *Dtsch. Tierarztl. Wochenschr.* **108:**216–222.

60. **Ellis, D., D. Marriott, R. A. Hajjeh, D. Warnock, W. Meyer, and R. Barton.** 2000. Epidemiology: surveillance of fungal infections. *Med. Mycol.* **38:**173–182.

61. **Ernould, J. C., K. Ba, and B. Sellin.** 1999. Increase of intestinal schistosomiasis after praziquantel treatment in a Schistosoma haematobium and Schistosoma mansoni mixed focus. *Acta Trop.* **73:**143–152.

62. **Fadly, A. M.** 1997. Avian retroviruses. *Vet. Clin. N. Am. Food Anim. Pract.* **13:**71–85.

63. **Fauci, A. S., G. Pantaleo, S. Stanley, and D. Weissman.** 1996. Immunopathogenic mechanisms of HIV infection. *Ann. Intern. Med.* **124:**654–663.

64. **Floret, D.** 1997. Virus-bacteria co-infections. *Arch. Pediatr.* **4:**1119–1124. (In French.)

65. **Fontes, R. A., Jr., C. M. Ogilvie, and T. Miclau.** 2000. Necrotizing soft-tissue infections. *J. Am. Acad. Orthop. Surg.* **8:**151–158.

66. **Frank, G. H.** 1979. *Pasteurella haemolytica* and respiratory disease in cattle, p. 153–160. *In Proceedings of the 83rd Annual Meeting of The United States Animal Health Association.*

67. **Fulton, R. W., C. W. Purdy, A. W. Confer, J. T. Saliki, R. W. Loan, R. E. Briggs, and L. J. Burge.** 2000. Bovine viral diarrhea viral infections in feeder calves with respiratory disease: interactions with Pasteurella spp., parainfluenza-3 virus, and bovine respiratory syncytial virus. *Can. J. Vet. Res.* **64:**151–159.

68. **Galina, L., C. Pijoan, M. Sitjar, W. T. Christianson, K. Rossow, and J. E. Collins.** 1994. Interaction between Streptococcus suis serotype 2 and porcine reproductive and respiratory syndrome virus in specific pathogen-free piglets. *Vet. Rec.* **134:**60–64.

69. **Gilmour, N. J. L.** 1980. Pasteurella haemolytica infections in sheep. *Vet. Q.* **2:**191–198.

70. **Gottlieb, M. S., R. Schroff, H. M. Schanker, J. D. Weisman, P. T. Fan, R. A. Wolf, and A. Saxon.** 1981. Pneumocystis carinii pneumonia and mucosal candidiasis in previously healthy homosexual men: evidence of a new acquired cellular immunodeficiency. *N. Engl. J. Med.* **305:**1425–1431.

71. **Gotuzzo, E., C. Arango, A. de Queiroz-Campos, and R. E. Isturiz.** 2000. Human T-cell lymphotropic virus-I in Latin America. *Infect. Dis. Clin. N. Am.* **14:**211–239, x–xi.

72. **Graham, N. M., R. M. Douglas, and P. Ryan.** 1986. Stress and acute respiratory infection. *Am. J. Epidemiol.* **124:**389–401.

73. **Grandin, T.** 1997. Assessment of stress during handling and transport. *J. Anim. Sci.* **75:**249–257.

74. **Guimaraes, M. L., F. I. Bastos, P. R. Telles, B. Galvao-Castro, R. S. Diaz, V. Bongertz, and M. G. Morgado.** 2001. Retrovirus infections in a sample of injecting drug users in Rio de Janeiro City, Brazil: prevalence of HIV-1 subtypes, and co-infection with HTLV-I/II. *J. Clin. Virol.* **21:**143–151.

75. **Gupta, V., T. Dada, R. B. Vajpayee, N. Sharma, and V. K. Dada.** 2001. Polymicrobial keratitis after laser in situ keratomileusis. *J. Refract. Surg.* **17:**147–148.

76. **Guy, J. S., L. G. Smith, J. J. Breslin, J. P. Vaillancourt, and H. J. Barnes.** 2000. High mortality and growth depression experimentally produced in young turkeys by dual infection with enteropathogenic Escherichia coli and turkey coronavirus. *Avian Dis.* **44:**105–113.

77. **Haahr, S., and M. Munch.** 2000. The association between multiple sclerosis and infection with Epstein-Barr virus and retrovirus. *J. Neurovirol.* **6**(Suppl. 2)**:**S76–S79.

78. **Hajjeh, R. A.** 1995. Disseminated histoplasmosis in persons infected with human immunodeficiency virus. *Clin. Infect. Dis.* **21**(Suppl. 1)**:**S108–S110.

79. **Hament, J. M., J. L. Kimpen, A. Fleer, and T. F. Wolfs.** 1999. Respiratory viral infection predisposing for bacterial disease: a concise review. *FEMS Immunol. Med. Microbiol.* **26:**189–195.

80. **Hassan, J. O., and R. Curtiss III.** 1994. Virulent *Salmonella typhimurium*-induced lymphocyte depletion and immunosuppression in chickens. *Infect. Immun.* **62:**2027–2036.

81. **Heiskanen-Kosma, T., M. Korppi, C. Jokinen, S. Kurki, L. Heiskanen, H. Juvonen, S. Kallinen, M. Sten, A. Tarkiainen, P. R. Ronnberg, M. Kleemola, P. H. Makela, and M. Leinonen.** 1998. Etiology of childhood pneumonia: serologic results of a prospective, population-based study. *Pediatr. Infect. Dis. J.* **17:**986–991.

82. **Hirai, T., T. Nunoya, T. Ihara, K. Kusanagi, and K. Shibuya.** 2001. Dual infection with PCV-2 and porcine epidemic diarrhoea virus in neonatal piglets. *Vet. Rec.* **148:**482–484.

83. **Hjerpe, C. A.** 1983. Clinical management of respiratory disease in feedlot cattle. *Vet. Clin. N. Am. Large Anim. Pract.* **5:**119–142.

84. **Hoskin, S. O., P. R. Wilson, W. A. Charleston, and T. N. Barry.** 2000. A model for study of lungworm (Dictyocaulus sp.) and gastrointestinal nematode infection in young red deer (Cervus elaphus). *Vet. Parasitol.* **88:**199–217.

85. **Howard, C. J.** 1990. Immunological responses to bovine virus diarrhoea virus infections. *Rev. Sci. Tech. Off. Int. Epizoot.* **9:**95–103.

86. **Hujoel, P. P., B. G. Leroux, H. Selipsky, and B. A. White.** 2000. Nonsurgical periodontal therapy and tooth loss. A cohort study. *J. Periodontol.* **71:**736–742.

87. **Ingham, H. R., and P. R. Sisson.** 1984. Pathogenic synergism. *Microbiol. Sci.* **1:**206–208.

88. **Jabra-Rizk, M. A., W. A. Falkler, Jr., W. G. Merz, J. I. Kelley, A. A. Baqui, and T. F. Meiller.** 1999. Coaggregation of Candida dubliniensis with Fusobacterium nucleatum. *J. Clin. Microbiol.* **37:**1464–1468.

89. **Jelinek, P. D., L. J. Depiazzi, D. A. Galvin, I. T. Spicer, M. A. Palmer, and D. R. Pitman.** 2000. Occurrence of different strains of Dichelobacter nodosus in new clinical lesions in sheep exposed to footrot associated with multistrain infections. *Aust. Vet. J.* **78:**273–276.

90. **Jones, C. D. R.** 1987. Proliferation of *Pasteurella haemolytica* in the calf respiratory tract after abrupt change in climate. *Res. Vet. Sci.* **42:**179–186.

91. **Jones, G. E., J. S. Gilmour, and A. G. Rae.** 1982. The effect of *Mycoplasma ovipneumoniae* and *Pasteurella haemolytica* on specific pathogen-free lambs. *J. Comp. Pathol.* **92:**261–266.

92. **Jones, G. E., J. S. Gilmour, and A. G. Rae.** 1982. The effects of different strains of *Mycoplasma ovipneumoniae* on specific pathogen-free and conventionally-reared lambs. *J. Comp. Pathol.* **92:**267–272.

93. **Kannan, G., T. H. Terrill, B. Kouakou, O. S. Gazal, S. Gelaye, E. A. Amoah, and S. Samake.** 2000. Transportation of goats: effects on physiological stress responses and live weight loss. *J. Anim. Sci.* **78:**1450–1457.

94. **Kapil, S., and R. J. Basaraba.** 1997. Infectious bovine rhinotracheitis, parainfluenza-3, and respiratory coronavirus. *Vet. Clin. N. Am. Food Anim. Pract.* **13:**455–469.

95. **Keles, I., A. K. Sharma, Z. Woldehiwet, and R. D. Murray.** 1999. The effects of bovine respiratory syncytial on normal ovine lymphocyte responses to mitogens or antigens in vitro. *Comp. Immunol. Microbiol. Infect. Dis.* **22:**1–13.

96. **Keles, I., Z. Woldehiwet, and R. D. Murray.** 1998. In-vitro studies on mechanisms of immunosuppresion associated with bovine respiratory syncytial virus. *J. Comp. Pathol.* **118:**337–345.

97. **Kennedy, S., D. Moffett, F. McNeilly, B. Meehan, J. Ellis, S. Krakowka, and G. M. Allan.** 2000. Reproduction of lesions of postweaning multisystemic wasting syndrome by infection of conventional pigs with porcine circovirus type 2 alone or in combination with porcine parvovirus. *J. Comp. Pathol.* **122:**9–24.

98. **Knowles, T. G., S. N. Brown, P. D. Warriss, A. J. Phillips, S. K. Dolan, P. Hunt, J. E. Ford, J. E. Edwards, and P. E. Watkins.** 1995. Effects on sheep of transport by road for up to 24 hours. *Vet. Rec.* **136:**431–438.

99. **Kolenbrander, P. E.** 1993. Coaggregation of human oral bacteria: potential role in the accretion of dental plaque. *J. Appl. Bacteriol.* **74:**79S–86S.

100. **Kolenbrander, P. E., R. N. Andersen, K. Kazmerzak, R. Wu, and R. J. Palmer, Jr.** 1999. Spatial organization of oral bacteria in biofilms. *Methods Enzymol.* **310:**322–332.

101. **Krause, P. J., S. R. Telford III, A. Spielman, V. Sikand, R. Ryan, D. Christianson, G. Burke, P. Brassard, R. Pollack, J. Peck, and D. H. Persing.** 1996. Concurrent Lyme disease and babesiosis. Evidence for increased severity and duration of illness. *JAMA* **275:**1657–1660.

102. **Larsen, H. J., G. Overnes, H. Waldeland, and G. M. Johansen.** 1994. Immunosuppression in sheep experimentally infected with Ehrlichia phagocytophila. *Res. Vet. Sci.* **56:**216–224.

103. **Laupland, K. B., H. D. Davies, D. E. Low, B. Schwartz, K. Green, A. McGeer, and the Ontario Group A Streptococcal Study Group.** 2000. Invasive group A streptococcal disease in children and association with varicella-zoster virus infection. *Pediatrics* **105:**E60.

104. **Lebbad, M., H. Norrgren, A. Naucler, F. Dias, S. Andersson, and E. Linder.** 2001. Intestinal parasites in HIV-2 associated AIDS cases with chronic diarrhoea in Guinea-Bissau. *Acta Trop.* **80:**45–49.

105. **Lehmkuhl, H. D., J. A. Contreras, R. C. Cutlip, and K. A. Brogden.** 1989. Clinical and microbiologic findings in lambs inoculated with *Pasteurella haemolytica* after infection with ovine adenovirus type 6. *Am. J. Vet. Res.* **50:**671–675.

106. **Lewis, M. J., V. W. Gautier, X. P. Wang, M. H. Kaplan, and W. W. Hall.** 2000. Spontaneous production of C-C chemokines by indi-

viduals infected with human T lymphotropic virus type II (HTLV-II) alone and HTLV-II/HIV-1 coinfected individuals. *J. Immunol.* **165:**4127–4132.

107. **Loneragan, G. H., D. H. Gould, G. L. Mason, F. B. Garry, G. S. Yost, D. L. Lanza, D. G. Miles, B. W. Hoffman, and L. J. Mills.** 2001. Association of 3-methyleneindolenine, a toxic metabolite of 3-methylindole, with acute interstitial pneumonia in feedlot cattle. *Am. J. Vet. Res.* **62:**1525–1530.

108. **Loneragan, G. H., D. H. Gould, G. L. Mason, F. B. Garry, G. S. Yost, D. G. Miles, B. W. Hoffman, and L. J. Mills.** 2001. Involvement of microbial respiratory pathogens in acute interstitial pneumonia in feedlot cattle. *Am. J. Vet. Res.* **62:**1519–1524.

109. **Lopez, A., M. G. Maxie, L. Ruhnke, M. Savan, and R. G. Thomson.** 1986. Cellular inflammatory response in the lungs of calves exposed to bovine viral diarrhea virus, Mycoplasma bovis, and Pasteurella haemolytica. *Am. J. Vet. Res.* **47:**1283–1286.

110. **Lore, K., A. Sonnerborg, J. Olsson, B. K. Patterson, T. E. Fehniger, L. Perbeck, and J. Andersson.** 1999. HIV-1 exposed dendritic cells show increased pro-inflammatory cytokine production but reduced IL-1ra following lipopolysaccharide stimulation. *AIDS* **13:**2013–2021.

111. **Lutticken, D.** 1997. Viral diseases of the immune system and strategies to control infectious bursal disease by vaccination. *Acta Vet. Hung.* **45:**239–249.

112. **Mardh, P. A., K. Tchoudomirova, S. Elshibly, and D. Hellberg.** 1998. Symptoms and signs in single and mixed genital infections. *Int. J. Gynaecol. Obstet.* **63:**145–152.

113. **Mardirossian, A., A. Contreras, M. Navazesh, H. Nowzari, and J. Slots.** 2000. Herpesviruses 6, 7 and 8 in HIV- and non-HIV-associated periodontitis. *J. Periodontal Res.* **35:**278–284.

114. **Martin, W. B.** 1996. Respiratory infections of sheep. *Comp. Immunol. Microbiol. Infect. Dis.* **19:**171–179.

115. **Martuscelli, G., J. P. Fiorellini, C. C. Crohin, and T. H. Howell.** 2000. The effect of interleukin-11 on the progression of ligature-induced periodontal disease in the beagle dog. *J. Periodontol.* **71:**573–578.

116. **Masihi, K. N., H. Hintelmann, K. Madaj, and G. Gast.** 1995. Production of lipopolysaccharide-induced tumour necrosis factor during influenza virus infection in mice coincides with viral replication and respiratory oxidative burst. *Mediat. Inflamm.* **4:**181–185.

117. **Mathurin, P., V. Thibault, K. Kadidja, N. Ganne-Carrie, J. Moussalli, M. El Younsi, V. Di Martino, F. Lunel, F. Charlotte, M. Vidaud, P. Opolon, and T. Poynard.** 2000. Replication status and histological features of patients with triple (B, C, D) and dual (B, C) hepatic infections. *J. Viral Hepat.* **7:**15–22.

118. **Mattila, K. J., M. S. Nieminen, V. V. Valtonen, V. P. Rasi, Y. A. Kesaniemi, S. L. Syrjala, P. S. Jungell, M. Isoluoma, K. Hietaniemi, and M. J. Jokinen.** 1989. Association between dental health and acute myocardial infarction. *Br. Med. J.* **298:**779–781.

119. **May, B. J., Q. Zhang, L. L. Li, M. L. Paustian, T. S. Whittam, and V. Kapur.** 2001. Complete genomic sequence of Pasteurella multocida, Pm70. *Proc. Natl. Acad. Sci. USA* **98:**3460–3465.

120. **Miedzobrodzki, J., and A. B. Macura.** 1993. Effect of Staphylococcal proteinase on adherence of Candida albicans to mucous membrane cells in vitro. *Med. Dosw. Mikrobiol.* **45:**245–247. (In Polish.)

121. **Mills, E. L.** 1984. Viral infections predisposing to bacterial infections. *Annu. Rev. Med.* **35:**469–479.

122. **Moore, P. A., T. Orchard, J. Guggenheimer, and R. J. Weyant.** 2000. Diabetes and oral health promotion: a survey of disease prevention behaviors. *J. Am. Dent. Assoc.* **131:**1333–1341.

123. **Moriuchi, H., M. Moriuchi, S. B. Mizell, L. A. Ehler, and A. S. Fauci.** 2000. In vitro reactivation of human immunodeficiency virus 1 from latently infected, resting CD4+ T cells after bacterial stimulation. *J. Infect. Dis.* **181:**2041–2044.

124. **Morrison, H. I., L. F. Ellison, and G. W. Taylor.** 1999. Periodontal disease and risk of fatal coronary heart and cerebrovascular diseases. *J. Cardiovasc. Risk* **6:**7–11.

125. **Moses, H., Jr., and S. Sriram.** 2001. An infectious basis for multiple sclerosis: perspectives on the role of Chlamydia pneumoniae and other agents. *BioDrugs* **15:**199–206.

126. **Mosier, D. A.** 1997. Bacterial pneumonia. *Vet. Clin. N. Am. Food Anim. Pract.* **13:**483–493.

127. **Nain, M., F. Hinder, J. H. Gong, A. Schmidt, A. Bender, H. Sprenger, and D. Gemsa.** 1990. Tumor necrosis factor-alpha production of influenza A virus-infected macrophages and potentiating effect of lipopolysaccharides. *J. Immunol.* **145:**1921–1928.

128. **Nakai, T., K. Kume, H. Yoshikawa, T. Oyamada, and T. Yoshikawa.** 1988. Adherence of Pasteurella multocida or Bordetella

bronchiseptica to the swine nasal epithelial cell in vitro. *Infect. Immun.* **56:**234–240.

129. **Newberry, L. A., J. K. Skeeles, D. L. Kreider, J. N. Beasley, J. D. Story, R. W. McNew, and B. R. Berridge.** 1993. Use of virulent hemorrhagic enteritis virus for the induction of colibacillosis in turkeys. *Avian Dis.* **37:**1–5.

130. **Nichol, K. P., and J. D. Cherry.** 1967. Bacterial-viral interrelations in respiratory infections of children. *N. Engl. J. Med.* **277:**667–672.

131. **Offenbacher, S.** 1996. Periodontal diseases: pathogenesis. *Ann. Periodontol.* **1:**821–878.

132. **O'Sullivan, J. M., H. F. Jenkinson, and R. D. Cannon.** 2000. Adhesion of Candida albicans to oral streptococci is promoted by selective adsorption of salivary proteins to the streptococcal cell surface. *Microbiology* **146:**41–48.

133. **Palme, R., C. Robia, W. Baumgartner, and E. Mostl.** 2000. Transport stress in cattle as reflected by an increase in faecal cortisol metabolite concentrations. *Vet. Rec.* **146:**108–109.

134. **Paster, B. J., S. K. Boches, J. L. Galvin, R. E. Ericson, C. N. Lau, V. A. Levanos, A. Sahasrabudhe, and F. E. Dewhirst.** 2001. Bacterial diversity in human subgingival plaque. *J. Bacteriol.* **183:**3770–3783.

135. **Pierson, F. W., C. T. Larsen, and C. H. Domermuth.** 1996. The production of colibacillosis in turkeys following sequential exposure to Newcastle disease virus or Bordetella avium, avirulent hemorrhagic enteritis virus, and Escherichia coli. *Avian Dis.* **40:**837–840.

136. **Post, K. W., N. A. Cole, and R. H. Raleigh.** 1991. In vitro antimicrobial susceptibility of Pasteurella haemolytica and Pasteurella multocida recovered from cattle with bovine respiratory disease complex. *J. Vet. Diagn. Investig.* **3:**124–126.

137. **Potgieter, L. N.** 1997. Bovine respiratory tract disease caused by bovine viral diarrhea virus. *Vet. Clin. N. Am. Food Anim. Pract.* **13:**471–481.

138. **Potgieter, L. N.** 1995. Immunology of bovine viral diarrhea virus. *Vet. Clin. N. Am. Food Anim. Pract.* **11:**501–520.

139. **Qureshi, M. A., M. Yu, and Y. M. Saif.** 2000. A novel "small round virus" inducing poult enteritis and mortality syndrome and associated immune alterations. *Avian Dis.* **44:**275–283.

140. **Rautenschlein, S., and J. M. Sharma.** 2000. Immunopathogenesis of haemorrhagic enteritis virus (HEV) in turkeys. *Dev. Comp. Immunol.* **24:**237–246.

141. **Rautenschlein, S., M. Suresh, and J. M. Sharma.** 2000. Pathogenic avian adenovirus type II induces apoptosis in turkey spleen cells. *Arch. Virol.* **145:**1671–1683.

142. **Raza, M. W., C. C. Blackwell, M. M. Ogilvie, A. T. Saadi, J. Stewart, R. A. Elton, and D. M. Weir.** 1994. Evidence for the role of glycoprotein G of respiratory syncytial virus in binding of Neisseria meningitidis to HEp-2 cells. *FEMS Immunol. Med. Microbiol.* **10:**25–30.

143. **Raza, M. W., O. R. El Ahmer, M. M. Ogilvie, C. C. Blackwell, A. T. Saadi, R. A. Elton, and D. M. Weir.** 1999. Infection with respiratory syncytial virus enhances expression of native receptors for non-pilate Neisseria meningitidis on HEp-2 cells. *FEMS Immunol. Med. Microbiol.* **23:**115–124.

144. **Register, K. B., R. M. Lee, and C. Thomson.** 1998. Two-color hybridization assay for simultaneous detection of Bordetella bronchiseptica and toxigenic Pasteurella multocida from swine. *J. Clin. Microbiol.* **36:**3342–3346.

145. **Rimler, R. B., and R. A. Kunkle.** 1998. Bacterin-induced protection of turkeys against fowl cholera following infection with Bordetella avium. *Avian Dis.* **42:**752–756.

146. **Rosenberger, J. K., and S. S. Cloud.** 1998. Chicken anemia virus. *Poult. Sci.* **77:**1190–1192.

147. **Rowland, R. W.** 1999. Necrotizing ulcerative gingivitis. *Ann. Periodontol.* **4:**65–73.

148. **Rozdzinski, E., W. N. Burnette, T. Jones, V. Mar, and E. Tuomanen.** 1993. Prokaryotic peptides that block leukocyte adherence to selectins. *J. Exp. Med.* **178:**917–924.

149. **Saif, Y. M.** 1998. Infectious bursal disease and hemorrhagic enteritis. *Poult. Sci.* **77:**1186–1189.

150. **Sanford, B. A., A. Shelokov, and M. A. Ramsay.** 1978. Bacterial adherence to virus-infected cells: a cell culture model of bacterial superinfection. *J. Infect. Dis.* **137:**176–181.

151. **Sawyer, M. M.** 1992. Border disease of sheep: the disease in the newborn, adolescent and adult. *Comp. Immunol. Microbiol. Infect. Dis.* **15:**171–177.

152. **Schutten, M., M. E. van der Ende, and A. D. Osterhaus.** 2000. Antiretroviral therapy in patients with dual infection with human immunodeficiency virus types 1 and 2. *N. Engl. J. Med.* **342:**1758–1760.

153. **Schwarzmann, S. W., J. L. Adler, R. J. Sullivan, Jr., and W. M. Marine.** 1971. Bacterial pneumonia during the Hong Kong influenza epidemic of 1968–1969. *Arch. Intern. Med.* **127:**1037–1041.

154. **Servilio, J.** 1995. HIV/TB dual infection cause for concern. *Positively Aware* **6:**8.

155. **Shafiq, M., P. E. Schoch, B. A. Cunha, and M. D. Iliescu.** 2000. Nocardia asteroides and Cryptococcus neoformans lung abscess. *Am. J. Med.* **109:**70–71.

156. **Shah, H. N., S. E. Gharbia, D. M. Andrews, J. C. Williams, N. Mehta, and K. Gulabivala.** 1996. Oral pathogens as contributors to systemic infections. *Trends Microbiol.* 4:372–374.

157. **Sharma, J. M., K. Karaca, and T. Pertile.** 1994. Virus-induced immunosuppression in chickens. *Poult. Sci.* 73:1082–1086.

158. **Sharma, J. M., I. J. Kim, S. Rautenschlein, and H. Y. Yeh.** 2000. Infectious bursal disease virus of chickens: pathogenesis and immunosuppression. *Dev. Comp. Immunol.* 24:223–235.

159. **Slots, J., and A. Contreras.** 2000. Herpesviruses: a unifying causative factor in periodontitis? *Oral Microbiol. Immunol.* 15:277–280.

160. **Smith, G. R., S. A. Barton, and L. M. Wallace.** 1991. Further observations on enhancement of the infectivity of Fusobacterium necrophorum by other bacteria. *Epidemiol. Infect.* 106:305–310.

161. **Smith, H.** 1982. The role of microbial interactions in infectious disease. *Philos. Trans. R. Soc. Lond. B.* 297:551–561.

162. **Solano, G. I., E. Bautista, T. W. Molitor, J. Segales, and C. Pijoan.** 1998. Effect of porcine reproductive and respiratory syndrome virus infection on the clearance of Haemophilus parasuis by porcine alveolar macrophages. *Can. J. Vet. Res.* 62:251–256.

163. **Solano, G. I., J. Segales, J. E. Collins, T. W. Molitor, and C. Pijoan.** 1997. Porcine reproductive and respiratory syndrome virus (PRRSv) interaction with Haemophilus parasuis. *Vet. Microbiol.* 55:247–257.

164. **Storz, J., C. W. Purdy, X. Lin, M. Burrell, R. E. Truax, R. E. Briggs, G. H. Frank, and R. W. Loan.** 2000. Isolation of respiratory bovine coronavirus, other cytocidal viruses, and Pasteurella spp from cattle involved in two natural outbreaks of shipping fever. *J. Am. Vet. Med. Assoc.* 216:1599–1604.

165. **Storz, J., L. Stine, A. Liem, and G. A. Anderson.** 1996. Coronavirus isolation from nasal swab samples in cattle with signs of respiratory tract disease after shipping. *J. Am. Vet. Med. Assoc.* 208:1452–1455.

166. **Strangert, K.** 1970. Clinical course and prognosis of whooping-cough in Swedish children during the first six months of life. A study of hospitalized patients 1958–67. *Scand. J. Infect. Dis.* 2:45–48.

167. **Swanson, J. C.** 1995. Farm animal well-being and intensive productive systems. *J. Anim. Sci.* 73:2744–2751.

168. **Thacker, E. L., P. G. Halbur, R. F. Ross, R. Thanawongnuwech, and B. J. Thacker.** 1999. *Mycoplasma hyopneumoniae* potentiation of porcine reproductive and respiratory syndrome virus-induced pneumonia. *J. Clin. Microbiol.* 37:620–627.

169. **Torres, J., M. Gracenea, M. S. Gomez, A. Arrizabalaga, and O. Gonzalez-Moreno.** 2000. The occurrence of Cryptosporidium parvum and C. muris in wild rodents and insectivores in Spain. *Vet. Parasitol.* 92:253–260.

170. **Tristram, D. A., W. Hicks, Jr., and R. Hard.** 1998. Respiratory syncytial virus and human bronchial epithelium. *Arch. Otolaryngol. Head Neck Surg.* 124:777–783.

171. **Tuomanen, E.** 1986. Piracy of adhesins: attachment of superinfecting pathogens to respiratory cilia by secreted adhesins of *Bordetella pertussis*. *Infect. Immun.* 54:905–908.

172. **Vallinoto, A. C., V. N. Azevedo, D. E. Santos, S. Caniceiro, F. C. Mesquita, W. W. Hall, M. O. Ishak, and R. Ishak.** 1998. Serological evidence of HTLV-I and HTLV-II coinfections in HIV-1 positive patients in Belem, state of Para, Brazil. *Mem. Inst. Oswaldo Cruz* 93:407–409.

173. **van de Kar, N. C., L. A. Monnens, M. A. Karmali, and V. W. van Hinsbergh.** 1992. Tumor necrosis factor and interleukin-1 induce expression of the verocytotoxin receptor globotriaosylceramide on human endothelial cells: implications for the pathogenesis of the hemolytic uremic syndrome. *Blood* 80:2755–2764.

174. **Van Reeth, K., H. Nauwynck, and M. Pensaert.** 2000. A potential role for tumour necrosis factor-alpha in synergy between porcine respiratory coronavirus and bacterial lipopolysaccharide in the induction of respiratory disease in pigs. *J. Med. Microbiol.* 49:613–620.

175. **Vargas, K., S. A. Messer, M. Pfaller, S. R. Lockhart, J. T. Stapleton, J. Hellstein, and D. R. Soll.** 2000. Elevated phenotypic switching and drug resistance of *Candida albicans* from human immunodeficiency virus-positive individuals prior to first thrush episode. *J. Clin. Microbiol.* 38:3595–3607.

176. **Veenhuizen, M. F.** 1998. Three bacterial pathogens in the porcine respiratory disease complex. *Compendium* 20:S11–S21.

177. **Walker, R. L., D. H. Read, K. J. Loretz, and R. W. Nordhausen.** 1995. Spirochetes isolated from dairy cattle with papillomatous digital dermatitis and interdigital dermatitis. *Vet. Microbiol.* 47:343–355.

178. **Walsh, J., L. Dietlein, F. Low, G. Burch, and W. Mogabgab.** 1960. Bronchotracheal response in human influenza. *Arch. Intern. Med.* 108:376–388.

179. **Warr, G. A., and G. J. Jakab.** 1983. Pulmonary inflammatory responses during viral

pneumonia and secondary bacterial infection. *Inflammation* **7**:93–104.

180. **Wensvoort, G., C. Terpstra, J. M. Pol, E. A. ter Laak, M. Bloemraad, E. P. de Kluyver, C. Kragten, L. van Buiten, A. den Besten, F. Wagenaar, J. M. Broekhuijsen, P. L. J. M. Moonen. T. Zetstra, E. A. de Boer, H. J. Tibben, M. F. de Jong, P. van 't Veld, G. J. R. Groenland, J. A. van Gennep, M. T. Voets, J. H. M. Verheijden, and J. Braamskamp.** 1991. Mystery swine disease in The Netherlands: the isolation of Lelystad virus. *Vet. Q.* **13**:121–130.

181. **Westfall, D. S., W. A. Jensen, W. J. Reagan, S. V. Radecki, and M. R. Lappin.** 2001. Inoculation of two genotypes of Hemobartonella felis (California and Ohio variants) to induce infection in cats and the response to treatment with azithromycin. *Am. J. Vet. Res.* **62**:687–691.

182. **Whiteley, L. O., S. K. Maheswaran, D. J. Weiss, T. R. Ames, and M. S. Kannan.** 1992. Pasteurella haemolytica A1 and bovine respiratory disease: pathogenesis. *J. Vet. Intern. Med.* **6**:11–22.

183. **Wilson, M.** 1999. Use of constant depth film fermentor in studies of biofilms of oral bacteria. *Methods Enzymol.* **310**:264–279.

184. **Woods, C. W., C. McRill, B. D. Plikaytis, N. E. Rosenstein, D. Mosley, D. Boyd, B. England, B. A. Perkins, N. M. Ampel, and R. A. Hajjeh.** 2000. Coccidioidomycosis in human immunodeficiency virus-infected persons in Arizona, 1994–1997: incidence, risk factors, and prevention. *J. Infect. Dis.* **181**:1428–1434.

185. **Woods, R. D., R. A. Kunkle, J. F. Ridpath, and S. R. Bolin.** 1999. Bovine viral diarrhea virus isolated from fetal calf serum enhances pathogenicity of attenuated transmissible gastroenteritis virus in neonatal pigs. *J. Vet. Diagn. Investig.* **11**:400–407.

186. **Wray, C., and P. L. Roeder.** 1987. Effect of bovine virus diarrhoea-mucosal disease virus infection on salmonella infection in calves. *Res. Vet. Sci.* **42**:213–218.

187. **Wu, L., W. A. Paxton, N. Kassam, N. Ruffing, J. B. Rottman, N. Sullivan, H. Choe, J. Sodroski, W. Newman, R. A. Koup, and C. R. Mackay.** 1997. CCR5 levels and expression pattern correlate with infectability by macrophage-tropic HIV-1, in vitro. *J. Exp. Med.* **185**:1681–1691.

188. **Yu, M., M. M. Ismail, M. A. Qureshi, R. N. Dearth, H. J. Barnes, and Y. M. Saif.** 2000. Viral agents associated with poult enteritis and mortality syndrome: the role of a small round virus and a turkey coronavirus. *Avian Dis.* **44**:297–304.

189. **Zarski, J. P., B. Bohn, A. Bastie, J. M. Pawlotsky, M. Baud, F. Bost-Bezeaux, J. Tran van Nhieu, J. M. Seigneurin, C. Buffet, and D. Dhumeaux.** 1998. Characteristics of patients with dual infection by hepatitis B and C viruses. *J. Hepatol.* **28**:27–33.

CONTINUOUS-CULTURE CHEMOSTAT SYSTEMS AND FLOWCELLS AS METHODS TO INVESTIGATE MICROBIAL INTERACTIONS

David R. Drake and Kim A. Brogden

2

Polymicrobial diseases are difficult to reproduce and to study. In vivo and in vitro models are often used to study specific microbial interactions or parameters associated with infection and disease. In vivo models can determine (i) the predisposing conditions and situations leading to polymicrobial disease, (ii) the complex interactions among microorganisms in these diseases, (iii) the complex interactions between microorganisms and the host, and (iv) the mechanisms of pathogenesis leading to the clinical signs and lesions characteristic of the disease. Many of these in vivo models are discussed throughout the book and therefore are outside of the scope of this chapter. Here we focus on the in vitro techniques that have identified mechanisms of interspecies and intergeneric cooperation among microorganisms.

IN VITRO MODELS

A traditional approach taken through the years in the study of almost all aspects of microbial physiology, metabolism, expression of viru-

lence factors, and interaction with immune cells has been the batch-culture technique. Multiple ways in which bacteria can be grown in this manner exist, including test tubes, flasks, large vessels, etc. This has been traditional mainly because of the ease of preparing bacterial cultures and the ability to do so in almost any laboratory. Sophisticated equipment is not needed to prepare a batch culture of an organism. Although it is easy to obtain a bacterial suspension in this manner, however, numerous disadvantages of working with these cells exist. First and foremost, bacteria under their normal conditions in nature, whether in infections in a susceptible host or involved in the development of plaque in the oral cavity, simply do not grow at the rate they do in batch culture. Studies have shown, in fact, that bacteria freshly isolated from infections do not express the same profile of cell wall proteins as they do in batch culture. Moreover, many examples are available of bacteria that phenotypically adapt to antimicrobials in batch culture, or lose resistance upon subculturing. It is a well-known phenomenon that bacteria lose virulence and many other characteristics if they are subjected to extensive batch subculture.

Most batch cultures involve bacteria cultivated in a continuous culture (49). Here, planktonic cultures in a fermentor are fed with

David R. Drake, Dows Institute for Dental Research and Department of Endodontics, College of Dentistry, University of Iowa, Iowa City, IA 52242. *Kim A. Brogden,* Respiratory Diseases of Livestock Research Unit, National Animal Disease Center, USDA Agricultural Research Service, Ames, IA 50010.

Polymicrobial Diseases, Edited by Kim A. Brogden and Janet M. Guthmiller,
© 2002 ASM Press, Washington, D.C.

a nutrient solution to maintain a bacterial population in the exponential or log phase of growth (Fig. 1A). The continuous culture reaches "balanced growth" in which the levels of bacteria, bacterial products, media components, and waste products are constant (5). This condition is referred to as "steady-state" growth (49). The culture volume and the cell concentration are both kept constant by allowing fresh, sterile medium to enter the culture vessel at the same rate that "spent" medium, containing cells, is removed from the growing culture. Under these conditions, the rate at which new cells are produced in the culture vessel is exactly balanced by the rate at which cells are being lost through the overflow from the culture vessel (49).

One type of system that is widely used for continuous cultivation is the chemostat (49). This system depends on the fact that the concentration of an essential nutrient within the culture vessel controls the growth rate of the cells. In general, one nutrient is limited to an amount that restricts growth, and the culture is removed at the same rate as nutrients are added. Steady-state bacterial growth often forms films called biofilms on various surfaces placed in these chambers (Fig. 1B). These include acrylic, glass, or hydroxylapatite attached to titanium wire or a glass rod and immersed below the surface of the culture medium (5). Hydroxyapatite surfaces are often used because they reflect the chemical composition of enamel surfaces. Biofilms are microbial stacks or columns of microcolonies often embedded in extracellular polymeric matrix (13). The biofilm is permeable and contains pores or channels in interconnected mushroom or tulip shapes (30).

Biofilms are now thought to be the natural, environmental form of bacterial growth (2, 11, 14) as well as the form often seen in certain diseases (13) including periodontal disease (chapter 8), otitis media (chapter 14), and cystic fibrosis (53). Next we present two of the most common in vitro methods used to investigate microbial interactions: continuous-culture chemostat systems and flowcells.

Continuous–Culture Chemostat Systems

An approach that provides a spectrum of exciting possibilities for studying bacteria under conditions that more closely resemble the way they grow naturally is continuous culture (Table 1). The foundation of chemostat theory was originally described by Monod (44) in France and Novick and Szilard (45) in the United States, with the mathematical nuances refined by Herbert (21) in the United Kingdom. A description of the mathematical derivations can be found elsewhere (24). In summary, when steady-state conditions are reached in the chemostat, the dilution rate (D) is equal to the specific growth rate (μ). Therefore, one can easily calculate the mean doubling time or generation time of the microorganism in culture. The key result of such a system is that bacterial growth can be manipulated to achieve slow growth rates, which more closely resemble those found in nature. By doing so, studies have shown that bacteria grown under these conditions express cell wall proteins and respond to environmental stimuli much like cells in vivo. One can begin to see how studying bacteria grown under these conditions can be powerful indeed. Moreover, a powerful approach using this methodology has been the study of mixed cultures. Many interactions have been studied, from how communities of organisms interact and develop through time to the effect of environmental insults on the homeostasis of bacterial communities (3–9, 24, 26, 27, 33–40, 51, 52, 54, 57). Excellent examples of the use of continuous-culture techniques have been in the field of oral microbiology. Marsh et al. (35) studied the influence of growth rate and nutrient limitation on the microbial composition of a community of organisms in a chemostat. Samples of human plaque were used to inoculate the chemostats, grown under glucose-excess or glucose-limiting conditions. A complex mixture of end products was analyzed, along with the cell yields, pH, and changes in the community as the composition changed over time. The results of this study can be found elsewhere; the key point to be made here is that it

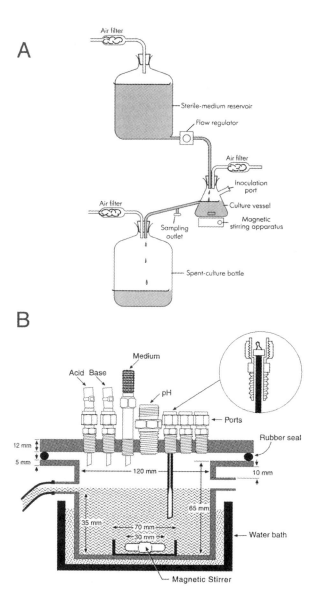

FIGURE 1   A general setup to grow microorganisms in continuous culture (A) and a basic fermentor vessel (B) containing substratum ports and support rods for biofilm accumulation. In this setup, cultures in the vessel are fed with a nutrient solution to maintain bacterial populations in the exponential or log phase of growth. The culture volume and the cell concentration are both kept constant by allowing fresh, sterile medium to enter the culture vessel at the same rate that "spent" medium, containing cells, is removed from the growing culture. Figures are reproduced from reference 49 with permission from McGraw Hill (A) and from reference 1 with permission from Academic Press (B).

TABLE 1 Variations of continuous-culture chemostat systems and flowcells for the study of mixed bacterial cultures

Method of culture	References
Continuous-flow chemostat: microbial cultures are allowed to adhere to the surfaces of materials suspended in thefermentor vessel	1, 5, 16
Robbins device: microbial cultures flow through a tubular section made of glass, metal, or clear plastic containing removable studs	16, 25
Rototorque: two concentric cylinders rotate at a set speed to generate a set shear rate, and microbial growth is matched by biomass removal	5, 16
Constant-depth film fermentors: microbial growth occurs in cutouts inserted into a flat plate. The medium flows over the plate and a wiper blade removes any growth that exceeds a maximum thickness	16, 58
Flowcells: microbial growth occurs on glass coverslips and forms extensive biofilms. The laminar flow of media through the cell can be controlled and induces a defined, constant environment. Biofilms can be viewed by time-resolved, nondestructive means.	5, 29, 47, 48, 56

was determined that the continuous-culture system could be an invaluable tool to study the ecology of dental plaque. Subsequent studies by this research group focused on many aspects of plaque-community development (9, 10, 19, 39–42).

To define how communities develop and change as a result of environmental insults, it was important to establish methods for achieving reproducible, complex communities of oral bacteria in the chemostat. Marsh et al. (35) did this through a series of studies involving defined inocula of nine commonly isolated organisms from supragingival plaque. Again, the details of these studies can be found elsewhere (35). Note, one can study oral microbial development using continuous-culture methods, and complex communities of organisms can be reproducibly obtained for long periods of study. These groundbreaking studies have opened the door for additional work focusing on not only the effects of environmental changes, but also on the effect of antimicrobials.

Having established the ability to study mixed populations of oral bacteria, investigators focused on the different groups of organisms associated with different oral diseases. In the field of cariology, it was of great interest to determine how communities changed in response to excess sugar and concomitant production of lactic acid by the mutans group streptococci. Studies by Bradshaw et al. (9) focused on the effects of carbohydrate pulses and pH on population shifts. Later studies looked at the effect of low fluoride concentrations on these communities of organisms (10). Collectively, these studies had a substantial impact on the field and once again demonstrated the power of being able to study microbial community development under continuous-culture conditions, i.e., controlling nutrient concentrations and growth rates.

Several studies have been conducted to look at the effects of antimicrobials on communities of oral bacteria (59). Studies by Bradshaw et al. (8) focused on the compounds triclosan and zinc citrate, alone and in combination. A novel approach was taken in these studies. The compounds were added to the chemostat by pulsing (a high initial concentration, which decreases over time) or dosing (concentration of inhibitor increases over time). This dual approach simulates how oral bacterial communities are exposed to antimicrobials in the oral cavity. Similar studies have been done with the effects of antibiotics on communities of organisms associated with periodontal disease (22). These studies found that, under certain, defined conditions, antimicrobials that had been previously characterized as broad spectrum in activity exerted more selectivity in their impact on complex communities of organisms. This increased selectivity was discovered only because of the power of the mixed, continuous-culture methodology that was used in the investigations.

The next evolution of the continuous-culture methodology to study communities of organisms has been the focus on biofilms. An enormous volume of literature still exists on the development of bacterial biofilms and their study during the past 5–10 years. Two recent volumes of *Methods in Enzymology* have been dedicated solely to microbial growth in biofilms and the techniques for studying them (17, 18). The importance of studying biofilms cannot be overstressed; essentially all oral diseases caused by microorganisms are a result of perturbations of the homeostasis of mixed microbial communities growing in a biofilm state (7, 32).

A classical system used to study biofilms in conjunction with continuous-culture systems is the Robbins device (25). This device is an artificial, multiport sampling catheter. It contains sampling ports whereby silicon disks are inserted in such a manner that they lie on the inner surface and are subject to the flow of media and bacteria. In many cases, this sampling system is attached to the effluent line of a chemostat so that cells growing at defined growth rates and nutrient conditions are then used as inocula for the biofilms. The biofilms can be studied through time, be exposed to antimicrobials, assayed for elaboration of various enzymes and by-products, and studied as to the response of immune cells. Thus, one has the benefit of cells grown under conditions more closely resembling those in the oral cavity and other sites in the body, and the ability to study biofilms developing under these precisely regulated conditions.

Other modified continuous-culture systems for the study of biofilms have been developed (Table 1). Bowden (1) describes a modified chemostat that has ten sampling rods that can be inserted into the lid, allowing for surfaces within the chemostat on which biofilms can form. Thus, once again, the model allows for the important environmental control of nutrient concentrations, pH, gaseous environment, and shear forces. Advantages of this model include the ability to compare equivalent biomasses of planktonic and biofilm cells grown under identical environmental conditions. One can reproducibly obtain biofilms that are equivalent from experiment to experiment.

Several other modifications of the continuous-culture system for studying biofilms have been reviewed (17, 18). Constant-depth film fermentors are similar in design to the modified chemostat described above, but with notable differences in terms of the volume of media, the sampling, and the control of the depth of biofilms (58). These systems have been used to study the effect of antimicrobials on biofilm formation, the effect of repeated pulsing of antimicrobials on biofilms, and the effect of various nutrients on the susceptibility of biofilms to antimicrobials (58).

Considerable valuable information has been gained throughout the years on the development of oral microbial communities and their response to antimicrobials. Look at the excellent, recent review by Bradshaw and Marsh (5) of the evolution of these model systems from the monoculture chemostat to the complex, mixed continuous-culture system studying gene expression in biofilms. These model systems have allowed us to determine how bacteria interact in a developing community and react to environmental stimuli. Such studies have shown how the concept of community homeostasis is critically important in the maintenance of oral health.

The chemostat has been of particular value in studies of the human oral microbiota and of other microbiota in humans (5). It provides control of environmental conditions and allows variation of one parameter at a time so that cause-and-effect relationships can be established (5), in particular, in the ecology of dental plaque in health and disease. Under highly controlled and reproducible conditions, they permit modeling of specific events that occur in vivo (5). However, they do not attempt to reproduce, or as a true model, cannot reproduce all the physical properties of the habitat (5).

Flowcells
Planktonic (free-swimming) bacteria attach, colonize, and persist on surfaces in natural, clinical, and industrial settings (2, 11, 14, 30). Once attached, they form biofilms consisting of pillarlike multicellular structures, in a hydrated polymeric matrix (13), interspersed with fluid-filled channels (14, 30). Gene expression in biofilm cells is similar to that in free-living cells, and only about 1% of genes show differential expression between these two modes of growth; about 0.5% of genes are activated and about 0.5% are repressed in biofilms (56). However, few significant differences exist (56). For example, pili and flagella are reported to be involved in attachment and microcolony formation of planktonic *Pseudomonas aeruginosa,* and these genes are repressed in biofilm cells (56). Many microbial communities are often composed of multiple species that interact with each other and their environment. The determination of biofilm architecture, particularly the spatial arrangement of microcolonies (clusters of cells) relative to one another, has profound implications for the function of these complex communities (14). Biofilms are implicated in the pathogenesis of cystic fibrosis pulmonary infections (53), corneal infections (50), burn wound infections (50), otitis media, periodontal disease (12, 28, 46), and implantable medical devices (12, 50).

Flowcells are currently used to cultivate and study biofilms. Expression of extracellular quorum-sensing signals (extracellular chemical signals that cue cell-density-dependent gene expression) to coordinate biofilm formation (43, 53, 55), receptors (15), metabolic interactions (48), metabolic interdependence (48),

horizontal gene transfer among species (20), phylogenetic groupings, mechanisms of antimicrobial resistance (31, 56), and competition among members of the biofilm (48) can all be assessed.

Flowcells are essentially perfusion chambers used for the observation of growth of stationary cells (Fig. 2). Two recent designs have been extensively described by Palmer and colleagues (23, 29, 47, 48). One cell is designed to observe microbial growth from the top (47). This cell has 4-mm^2 parallel grooves milled into a Plexiglas base stopping a few millimeters short of the cell ends. Microscopy coverslips are then used to cover the grooves forming a closed channel. Inlet and outlet openings are bored into ends of the cell through to the channel, and tubing is then cemented into the holes. Another cell is designed to view microbial growth from either the top or bottom (47). Microscopy coverslips are used to cover both the top and the bottom of a closed channel that is formed by a molded silicon rubber gasket. Elbow-shaped inlet and outlet ports are molded out of silicon. This design has two channels and has the same dimensions as a standard microscope slide, thereby making it compatible with most microscope stage hardware.

The flowcell is connected to a medium reservoir (Fig. 2A) containing broth or other biological fluid such as saliva (47, 48). A pump, placed on the outflow tube of the flowcell, is used to draw media through the cell and into a waste collection vessel. This basic setup optimizes the results and eliminates complications such as the occurrence of air bubbles in the flowcell (frequently generated on the downstream side of the pump) and flowcell contamination. The microorganism(s) to be grown can be aseptically injected directly into the flowcell through the silicon tubing.

As biofilms form on the glass of the flowcell (Fig. 2B), they are frequently examined by various forms of microscopy. Frequently, confocal microscopy is used (47) to examine biofilms in flowcells with a Plexiglas base because transmitted light is not required. However, if cell monolayers are examined with high-resolu-

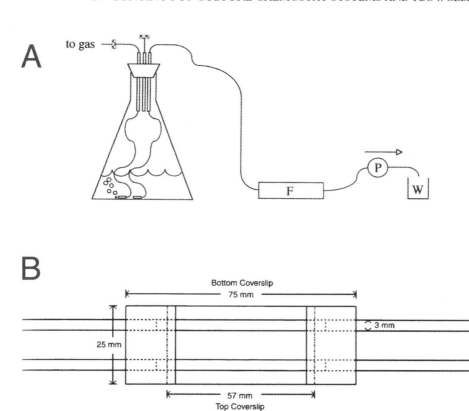

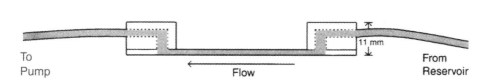

FIGURE 2 (A) A general setup to grow microorganisms in a continuous flowcell system. In this setup, the flow-cell (F) is connected by silicone rubber tubing to a reservoir and a pump (P). Fresh, sterile medium is drawn through the flowcell by the pump to a waste container (W) immediately downstream. (B) The biofilm forms on the upper glass of the flowcell and is viewed by using a confocal scanning laser microscope. Figures are reproduced from reference 47 with permission from Academic Press (A) and from reference 29 with permission from Annual Reviews (B).

tion, transmitted-light, phase-contrast optics, then the working distance of the lens and the travel of the substage condenser are important in setting the total thickness of the flowcell, and the flowcell must have glass as the base and as the top (47). Observation of colonization on the opposite coverslip is impossible with high-magnification, oil-immersion optics because the working distances of such lenses are too small. Epifluorescence microscopy techniques are also used to observe cells and eliminate the restrictions imposed by phase-contrast Koehj-ler illumination (47). Each of these techniques has advantages and disadvantages that involve the size and total thickness of the flowcell; the substage condenser; and the working distance, numerical aperture, and magnification of the microscope objective lens.

Overall, flowcells offer many advantages (47). They can be made inexpensively from a variety of materials. The laminar flow of media through the cell can be controlled and induces a defined, constant environment. Finally, the flowcell construction allows for visual assessment of biofilm formation by time-resolved, nondestructive means. Affluent and effluent media can be sampled. Unfortunately, flowcells do have some disadvantages (47). Sterilization can be difficult and dependent on the common materials used for flowcell construction. Autoclaving, gas sterilization, and disinfection procedures can be used to varying levels.

CONCLUSION

This chapter briefly describes two methods used to investigate microbial interactions in vitro, continuous-culture chemostat systems and flowcells. Biofilms form in each of the two models that can be used to identify mechanisms of interspecies and intergeneric cooperation among microorganisms applicable to polymicrobial diseases. Chemostat studies can be used to assess the responses of steady-state cultures to stresses applied by the experimenter. The steady state can be easily perturbed and allows unequivocal data on the effect of any perturbation. Flowcells offer additional advantages and the effects of treatment on biofilms can be visually assessed by time-resolved, nondestructive means or measured in sampled, effluent waste media. Both of these systems have identified synergistic and mutualistic interactions among microorganisms resulting in unique mechanisms of attachment and metabolic interdependence. These methods are rapidly gaining acceptance and are used to study biofilm diseases, particularly the interactions among members of the resident flora, factors involved in the transition of the biofilm from a commensal to a pathogenic relationship with the host, and the mode of action of antimicrobials.

REFERENCES

1. **Bowden, G. H.** 1999. Controlled environment model for accumulation of biofilms of oral bacteria. *Methods Enzymol.* **310:**216–224.

2. **Bower, C. K., M. A. Daeschel, and J. McGuire.** 1998. Protein antimicrobial barriers to bacterial adhesion. *J. Dairy Sci.* **81:**2771–2778.

3. **Bradshaw, D. J., and P. D. Marsh.** 1998. Analysis of pH-driven disruption of oral microbial communities in vitro. *Caries Res.* **32:**456–462.

4. **Bradshaw, D. J., and P. D. Marsh.** 1994. Effect of sugar alcohols on the composition and metabolism of a mixed culture of oral bacteria grown in a chemostat. *Caries Res.* **28:**251–256.

5. **Bradshaw, D. J., and P. D. Marsh.** 1999. Use of continuous flow techniques in modeling dental plaque biofilms. *Methods Enzymol.* **310:**279–296.

6. **Bradshaw, D. J., P. D. Marsh, C. Allison, and K. M. Schilling.** 1996. Effect of oxygen, inoculum composition and flow rate on development of mixed-culture oral biofilms. *Microbiology* **142:**623–629.

7. **Bradshaw, D. J., P. D. Marsh, K. M. Schilling, and D. Cummins.** 1996. A modified chemostat system to study the ecology of oral biofilms. *J. Appl. Bacteriol.* **80:**124–130.

8. **Bradshaw, D. J., P. D. Marsh, G. K. Watson, and D. Cummins.** 1993. The effects of triclosan and zinc citrate, alone and in combination, on a community of oral bacteria grown in vitro. *J. Dent. Res.* **72:**25–30.

9. **Bradshaw, D. J., A. S. McKee, and P. D. Marsh.** 1989. Effects of carbohydrate pulses and pH on population shifts within oral microbial communities in vitro. *J. Dent. Res.* **68:**1298–1302.

10. **Bradshaw, D. J., A. S. McKee, and P. D. Marsh.** 1990. Prevention of population shifts in oral microbial communities in vitro by low fluoride concentrations. *J. Dent. Res.* **69:**436–441.

11. **Brown, M. R., and J. Barker.** 1999. Unexplored reservoirs of pathogenic bacteria: protozoa and biofilms. *Trends Microbiol.* **7:**46–50.

12. **Chen, C.** 2001. Periodontitis as a biofilm infection. *J. Calif. Dent. Assoc.* **29:**362–369.

13. **Costerton, J. W., P. S. Stewart, and E. P. Greenberg.** 1999. Bacterial biofilms: a common cause of persistent infections. *Science* **284:**1318–1322.

14. **Davey, M. E., and G. A. O'Toole.** 2000. Microbial biofilms: from ecology to molecular genetics. *Microbiol. Mol. Biol. Rev.* **64:**847–867.

15. **Demuth, D. R., D. C. Irvine, J. W. Costerton, G. S. Cook, and R. J. Lamont.** 2001. Discrete protein determinant directs the species-specific adherence of Porphyromonas gingivalis to oral streptococci. *Infect. Immun.* **69:**5736–5741.

16. **Dibdin, G., and J. Wimpenny.** 1999. Steady-state biofilm: practical and theoretical models. *Methods Enzymol.* **310:**296–322.

17. **Doyle, R. J. (ed.).** 2001. *Methods in Enzymology,* vol. 310. *Biofilms.* Academic Press, San Diego, Calif.

18. **Doyle, R. J. (ed.).** 2001. *Methods in Enzymology,* vol. 337. *Microbial Growth in Biofilms. Part B: Special Environments and Physicochemical Aspects,* Academic Press, San Diego, Calif.

19. **Gerritse, J., F. Schut, and J. C. Gottschal.** 1992. Modelling of mixed chemostat cultures of an aerobic bacterium, *Comamonas testosteroni,* and an anaerobic bacterium, *Veillonella alcalescens:* comparison with experimental data. *Appl. Environ. Microbiol.* **58:**1466–1476.

20. **Ghigo, J. M.** 2001. Natural conjugative plasmids induce bacterial biofilm development. *Nature* **412:**442–445.

21. **Herbert, D.** 1961. Continuous culture of microorganisms. *SCI Monograph 12.* Butterworths, London, United Kingdom.

22. **Hoeven, J. S., and C. W. A. van den Kiebom.** 1991. Effects of propicillin on mixed continuous cultures of periodontal bacteria. *Antimicrob. Agents Chemother.* **35:**1717–1720.

23. **Jubb, K. V. F., P. C. Kennedy, and N. Palmer** 1985. The respiratory system, p. 520–528. *In* K. V. F. Jubb, P. C. Kennedy, and N. Palmer (ed.), *Pathology of Domestic Animals,* 3rd ed., vol. 2. Academic Press, San Diego, Calif.

24. **Keevil, C. W.** 2001. Continuous culture models to study pathogens in biofilms. *Methods Enzymol.* **337:**104–122.

25. **Kharazmi, A., B. Giwercman, and N. Hoiby.** 1999. Robbins device in biofilm research. *Methods Enzymol.* **310:**207–215.

26. **Kinniment, S. L., J. W. Wimpenny, D. Adams, and P. D. Marsh.** 1996. Development of a steady-state oral microbial biofilm community using the constant-depth film fermenter. *Microbiology* **142:**631–638.

27. **Kinniment, S. L., J. W. Wimpenny, D. Adams, and P. D. Marsh.** 1996. The effect of chlorhexidine on defined, mixed culture oral biofilms grown in a novel model system. *J. Appl. Bacteriol.* **81:**120–125.

28. **Kolenbrander, P. E.** 2000. Oral microbial communities: biofilms, interactions, and genetic systems. *Annu. Rev. Microbiol.* **54:**413–437.

29. **Kolenbrander, P. E., R. N. Andersen, K. Kazmerzak, R. Wu, and R. J. Palmer, Jr.** 1999. Spatial organization of oral bacteria in biofilms. *Methods Enzymol.* **310:**322–332.

30. **Kuchma, S. L., and G. A. O'Toole.** 2000. Surface-induced and biofilm-induced changes in gene expression. *Curr. Opin. Biotechnol.* **11:**429–433.

31. **Mah, T. F., and G. A. O'Toole.** 2001. Mechanisms of biofilm resistance to antimicrobial agents. *Trends Microbiol.* **9:**34–39.

32. **Marsh, P. D.** 1995. The role of microbiology in models of dental caries. *Adv. Dent. Res.* **9:**244–254.

33. **Marsh, P. D.** 1991. Sugar, fluoride, pH and microbial homeostasis in dental plaque. *Proc. Finn. Dent. Soc.* **87:**515–525.

34. **Marsh, P. D., and D. J. Bradshaw.** 1990. The effect of fluoride on the stability of oral bacterial communities in vitro. *J. Dent. Res.* **69:**668–671.

35. **Marsh, P. D., J. R. Hunter, G. H. Bowden, I. R. Hamilton, A. S. McKee, J. M. Hardie, and D. C. Ellwood.** 1983. The influence of growth rate and nutrient limitation on the microbial composition and biochemical properties of a mixed culture of oral bacteria grown in a chemostat. *J. Gen. Microbiol.* **129:**755–770.

36. **Marsh, P. D., A. S. McDermid, C. W. Keevil, and D. C. Ellwood.** 1985. Effect of environmental conditions on the fluoride sensitivity of acid production by S. sanguis NCTC 7865. *J. Dent. Res.* **64:**85–89.

37. **Marsh, P. D., A. S. McDermid, C. W. Keevil, and D. C. Ellwood.** 1985. Environmental regulation of carbohydrate metabolism by *Streptococcus sanguis* NCTC 7865 grown in a chemostat. *J. Gen. Microbiol.* **131:**2505–2514.

38. **Marsh, P. D., A. S. McDermid, A. S. McKee, and A. Baskerville.** 1994. The effect of growth rate and haemin on the virulence and proteolytic activity of *Porphyromonas gingivalis* W50. *Microbiology* **140:**861–865.

39. **McDermid, A. S., P. D. Marsh, C. W. Keevil, and D. C. Ellwood.** 1985. Additive inhibitory effects of combinations of fluoride and chlorhexidine on acid production by *Streptococcus mutans* and *Streptococcus sanguis. Caries Res.* **19:**64–71.

40. **McDermid, A. S., A. S. McKee, D. C. Ellwood, and P. D. Marsh.** 1986. The effect of lowering the pH on the composition and metabolism of a community of nine oral bacteria grown in a chemostat. *J. Gen. Microbiol.* **132:**1205–1214.

41. **McDermid, A. S., A. S. McKee, and P. D. Marsh.** 1987. A mixed-culture chemostat system to predict the effect of anti-microbial agents on the oral flora: preliminary studies using chlorhexidine. *J. Dent. Res.* **66:**1315–1320.

42. **McKee, A. S., A. S. McDermid, D. C. Ellwood, and P. D. Marsh.** 1985. The establishment of reproducible, complex communities of oral bacteria in the chemostat using defined inocula. *J. Appl. Bacteriol.* **59:**263–275.

43. **Miller, M. B., and B. L. Bassler.** 2001. Quorum sensing in bacteria. *Annu. Rev. Microbiol.* **55:**165–199.

44. **Monod, J.** 1950. La technique de culture continue. Théorie et applications. *Ann. Inst. Pasteur* (Paris) **79:**390–410.

45. **Novick, A., and L. Szilard.** 1950. Experiments with the chemostat on spontaneous mutations of bacteria. *Proc. Natl. Acad. Sci. USA* **36:**708–719.

46. O'Toole, G., H. B. Kaplan, and R. Kolter. 2000. Biofilm formation as microbial development. *Annu. Rev. Microbiol.* **54**:49–79.

47. Palmer, R. J., Jr. 1999. Microscopy flowcells: perfusion chambers for real-time study of biofilms. *Methods Enzymol.* **310**:160–166.

48. Palmer, R. J., Jr., K. Kazmerzak, M. C. Hansen, and P. E. Kolenbrander. 2001. Mutualism versus independence: strategies of mixed-species oral biofilms in vitro using saliva as the sole nutrient source. *Infect. Immun.* **69**:5794–5804.

49. Pelczar, M. J., Jr., E. C. S. Chan, and N. R. Krieg. 1986. *Microbiology,* 5th ed. McGraw-Hill Publishing Company, New York, N.Y.

50. Rumbaugh, K. P., J. A. Griswold, and A. N. Hamood. 2000. The role of quorum sensing in the in vivo virulence of *Pseudomonas aeruginosa. Microbes Infect.* **2**:1721–1731.

51. Saunders, K. A., and J. Greenman. 2000. The formation of mixed culture biofilms of oral species along a gradient of shear stress. *J. Appl. Microbiol.* **89**:564–572.

52. Saunders, K. A., J. Greenman, and C. McKenzie. 2000. Ecological effects of triclosan and triclosan monophosphate on defined mixed cultures of oral species grown in continuous culture. *J. Antimicrob. Chemother.* **45**:447–452.

53. Singh, P. K., A. L. Schaefer, M. R. Parsek, T. O. Moninger, M. J. Welsh, and E. P. Greenberg. 2000. Quorum-sensing signals indicate that cystic fibrosis lungs are infected with bacterial biofilms. *Nature* **407**:762–764.

54. Smalley, J. W., A. J. Birss, A. S. McKee, and P. D. Marsh. 1998. Hemin regulation of hemoglobin binding by *Porphyromonas gingivalis. Curr. Microbiol.* **36**:102–106.

55. Swift, S., J. A. Downie, N. A. Whitehead, A. M. Barnard, G. P. Salmond, and P. Williams. 2001. Quorum sensing as a population-density-dependent determinant of bacterial physiology. *Adv. Microb. Physiol.* **45**:199–270.

56. Whiteley, M., M. G. Bangera, R. E. Bumgarner, M. R. Parsek, G. M. Teitzel, S. Lory, and E. P. Greenberg. 2001. Gene expression in *Pseudomonas aeruginosa* biofilms. *Nature* **413**:860–864.

57. Whiteley, M., J. R. Ott, E. A. Weaver, and R. J. McLean. 2001. Effects of community composition and growth rate on aquifer biofilm bacteria and their susceptibility to betadine disinfection. *Environ. Microbiol.* **3**:43–52.

58. Wilson, M. 1999. Use of constant depth film fermentor in studies of biofilms of oral bacteria. *Methods Enzymol.* **310**:264–279.

59. Zelver, N., M. Hamilton, B. Pitts, D. Goeres, D. Walker, P. Sturman, and J. Heersink. 1999. Measuring antimicrobial effects on biofilm bacteria: from laboratory to field. *Methods Enzymol.* **310**:608–628.

POLYVIRAL DISEASES

BOVINE VIRAL DIARRHEA VIRUS IN MIXED INFECTIONS

Steven R. Bolin

3

Bovine viral diarrhea virus (BVDV) is classified in the *Pestivirus* genus within the *Flaviviridae* family, which also contains the *Flavivirus* and *Hepacivirus* genera (160). The host range for BVDV includes most even-toed ungulates, and the virus is distributed worldwide. Although many species of animals are susceptible to infection with BVDV, domestic cattle seem to be the primary host, and BVDV is considered an economically important pathogen of cattle in most regions of the world. Two biotypes of BVDV, cytopathic and noncytopathic, occur in nature. The viral biotypes are identified by cytopathic effect in susceptible cell cultures. Cytopathic BVDV induces cytoplasmic vacuolation, cell rounding, detachment from the cell sheet, and death of cells (65, 159). The cytopathic effect usually occurs within 2 to 3 days of infection of the cell culture. In contrast, noncytopathic BVDV establishes a visually inapparent persistent infection in cell culture (94). Although noncytopathic BVDV is ubiquitous in nature and frequently isolated from bovine tissues, cytopathic BVDV is rare and seldom isolated unless accompanied by noncytopathic BVDV.

Infection of cattle with BVDV induces three disease conditions that range from clinically inapparent to clinically severe. The conditions are termed congenital persistent infection, mucosal disease, and acute bovine viral diarrhea (BVD) (6, 72). Congenital persistent infection is a sequel to fetal infection with noncytopathic BVDV. Neonatal persistently infected calves may show growth retardation and ill thrift, and they may remain "poor doers" for life. Death or culling from the herd before 1 year of age is common among persistently infected cattle (76). However, some persistently infected cattle seem healthy at birth and survive for several years. Mucosal disease is a sequel of congenital persistent infection and is caused by a "mixed" infection of noncytopathic BVDV and cytopathic BVDV. Acute BVD occurs after birth and is induced by primary postnatal infection with either cytopathic or noncytopathic BVDV. Acute BVDV may result in respiratory, enteric, and/or reproductive disease. The severity of disease varies from clinically inapparent to fatal and depends on the virulence of the viral strain, physical and environmental stressors, and intercurrent infection with other pathogens.

During acute or persistent infection with BVDV, viral replication occurs in a variety of cell types located in the integument, alimentary

Steven R. Bolin, Department of Pathobiology and Diagnostic Investigation, College of Veterinary Medicine, Michigan State University, East Lansing, MI 48824.

Polymicrobial Diseases, Edited by Kim A. Brogden and Janet M. Guthmiller,
© 2002 ASM Press, Washington, D.C.

canal, nervous system, respiratory tract, and immune system (19). Although many cell types are permissive for viral replication, BVDV has a predilection for cells of the immune system (thymocytes, lymphocytes, monocytes, macrophages, and dendritic cells). Viral replication in lymphoid cells may directly, or indirectly, alter immune function and enhance severity of disease during mixed infections of BVDV or mixed infections of BVDV with other pathogens (19, 128). This chapter provides examples of mixed infections involving BVDV and discusses the role BVDV may have in enhancing disease processes during a mixed infection.

MUCOSAL DISEASE: A MIXED INFECTION OF BVDV

Clinical Disease and Lesions

Mucosal disease was first reported in 1953 as an acute and highly fatal disease of cattle (135). Manifestations of acute mucosal disease included pyrexia, anorexia, lethargy, hypersalivation, mucopurulent nasal discharge, profuse watery diarrhea containing mucus and fresh or clotted blood, dehydration, erosive lesions of the nares and oral cavity, mucosal erosions and ulcerations of the gastrointestinal tract, and death within days of onset of clinical disease. Mucosal disease also may take a chronic course that results in a less severe disease which persists for weeks to months and is manifested by inappetence, intermittent to chronic diarrhea, and weight loss. Cattle that have chronic mucosal disease appear unthrifty, may show lameness due to laminitis or interdigital necrosis, and may develop alopecia and hyperkeratinization. Acute or chronic mucosal disease usually occurs in cattle younger than 3 years of age (42, 95, 102, 106, 142, 156).

A thorough discussion of the gross and microscopic lesions associated with acute and chronic mucosal disease may be found in a recent review (19). In brief, gross lesions seen in mucosal disease may include erosions and ulcerations in the mouth and on the tongue, linear erosions and ulcerations in the esophageal mucosa, and edema and ulceration of the abomasum. Mucosal erosions and ulcerations over the Peyer's patch regions of the small intestine, at the ileocecal junction, in the proximal spiral colon, and on the rugae of the rectum are found frequently and considered highly suggestive of mucosal disease. Thymic atrophy, conjunctivitis, and eczema also may be seen. The severity of gross lesions varies considerably among cattle that die of either acute or chronic mucosal disease.

Microscopic lesions associated with mucosal disease include scattered cellular necrosis in the stratum spinosum of keratinized epithelium, cellular necrosis of intestinal crypts, and marked depletion of lymphoid cells in Peyer's patches. The thymic cortex may contain numerous apoptotic and disintegrating thymocytes. Lesions in lymph nodes are variable and include depletion of lymphocytes in the periphery of the node, as well as in the paracortical and cortical regions of lymphoid follicles. It is difficult, if not impossible, to differentiate acute and chronic mucosal disease on the basis of type or location of lesions postmortem (19, 167). Differentiation between clinical forms of mucosal disease is arbitrary and based on severity and duration of disease.

Congenital Persistent Infection with Noncytopathic BVDV

Congenital persistent infection with noncytopathic BVDV is required for mucosal disease to occur. Clinically inapparent persistent infection with noncytopathic BVDV was first discovered in healthy cattle that lacked virus-neutralizing antibody after natural or experimental exposure with BVDV (49, 102, 103). The immunotolerant cattle were rare but readily identified, because their herd mates or experimental cohorts had a high titer of virus-neutralizing antibody in serum. Persistent infection with noncytopathic BVDV was a consistent finding when virus isolation was performed on clinical specimens obtained from the immunotolerant cattle. The immunotolerance was specific for BVDV and not caused by a general immune failure, because an immune response against other viral and bacterial pathogens was evoked readily (49,

78, 113). Persistent infection and immunotolerance are established during the first 4 months of gestation, before onset of immunocompetence in the fetus (38, 103, 113). Infection of the fetus with noncytopathic BVDV after the 4th month of development causes production of virus-neutralizing antibody, and the calf is born free of virus. Experimental exposure of the fetus with cytopathic BVDV does not lead to persistent infection (18, 38, 52, 113), and naturally occurring persistent infection with cytopathic BVDV has not been identified.

Persistent infection is transmitted consistently from persistently infected cows to their offspring during gestation (113). Persistently infected bulls seldom transmit persistent infection to their offspring (88). Although vertical transmission of persistent infection from dam to offspring is important epidemiologically, it is not the most common means by which persistently infected cattle occur. Most persistently infected calves are born to healthy cows that experience primary infection with BVDV in early gestation. The number of pregnant cattle in a herd that are susceptible to primary infection with BVDV usually is small, because most cattle are exposed with BVDV, or are vaccinated against BVDV, before the first breeding. Antibody made in response to infection with BVDV persists in serum for at least 3 years, and probably for life (61). That antibody usually protects the fetus from transplacental infection. The high prevalence of antibody against BVDV in cattle combined with the short period in gestation that a fetus is susceptible to persistent infection results in persistently infected cattle being uncommon (26, 56, 77, 79, 81, 155, 168). The distribution of persistently infected cattle is clustered. Most herds are free of persistently infected cattle, a few herds contain a small number of persistently infected cattle, and very few herds contain ten or more persistently infected cattle.

Mixed Infections of BVDV

Mucosal disease is induced experimentally by exposure of persistently infected cattle with cytopathic BVDV, thereby establishing a mixed infection of noncytopathic and cytopathic BVDV (27, 39). Signs of mucosal disease usually develop 2 to 3 weeks after exposure of persistently infected cattle with cytopathic BVDV, and both noncytopathic and cytopathic BVDV strains are isolated from tissues harvested postmortem. Similarly, both noncytopathic and cytopathic BVDV are isolated from intestine or lymphoid tissues harvested from cattle involved in field outbreaks of mucosal disease (46, 80, 112). Most pairs of noncytopathic and cytopathic BVDV isolated from field outbreaks of mucosal disease are antigenically alike (46, 80), and antibody against BVDV is seldom detected in serum obtained before death of the animal (84, 101, 154). This suggests that immunotolerance to BVDV is a critical factor in the pathogenesis of mucosal disease (36). Immunotolerance would allow a mixed infection of BVDV strains that are antigenically alike to progress unabated, leading to severe clinical disease. In contrast, a mixed infection of BVDV strains that are antigenically different might break immunotolerance and stimulate an immune response that would prevent disease or reduce its severity.

Under experimental conditions, mixed infections of BVDV that are antigenically different stimulate production of virus-neutralizing antibody that likely protected some cattle from mucosal disease (12, 24, 27, 28, 40, 44, 55, 60, 99, 105, 119, 151). However, many persistently infected cattle reported to have produced antibody against BVDV after infection with cytopathic BVDV also were reported to have died of mucosal disease. Logically, antibody failed to protect some cattle, because the immune response against cytopathic BVDV in those cattle was not sufficient and/or not timely, and the disease progressed to its fatal conclusion instead of being prevented. Pairs of BVDV that are antigenically and genetically dissimilar occasionally are isolated from field outbreaks of mucosal disease (141). Thus, experimental and field data indicate that antigenic similarity between BVDV generally occurs in mucosal disease, but it is not required to induce mucosal disease.

Research into the nature of immunotolerance in persistently infected cattle has been limited. An early report suggested immunotolerance was directed primarily at viral proteins in the lipid envelope and that a cross-reactive immune response occurred after infection with cytopathic BVDV (24). The proteins in the viral envelope contain epitopes involved in viral neutralization, so failure of immune recognition of those proteins would favor persistent infection. However, some persistently infected cattle have produced neutralizing antibody against their own noncytopathic BVDV (27, 32, 45). This apparent break of immunotolerance might be attributed to the quasispecies nature of RNA viruses. The rapid rate of mutation occurring in the RNA of BVDV could lead to emergence of antigenic variants in the swarm of persistent noncytopathic BVDV that would stimulate an immune response. Diversity in predicted amino acid sequence of the immunologically important viral envelope protein E2 (Fig. 1) has been detected in BVDV isolated from a persistently infected animal (45). Emergence of antigenic variants that stimulate a cross-reactive antibody response would explain identification of persistently infected cattle that lack, or have very low concentrations of, infective BVDV in their serum (32, 45). Thus, immunotolerance in persistently infected cattle apparently is restricted to the strain of noncytopathic BVDV that infects the animal and may be further restricted to certain viral proteins or epitopes on those proteins. Also, immunotolerance can be broken by infection with cytopathic BVDV, or by the emergence of antigenic variants within the pool of persistent noncytopathic BVDV in the animal.

Origin of Cytopathic BVDV in Mucosal Disease

Isolation of antigenically alike pairs of BVDV from cattle that died of mucosal disease led to the theory that cytopathic BVDV originates from noncytopathic BVDV (46, 80). Cytopathic BVDV is genetically and antigenically similar to noncytopathic BVDV except for the expression of a nonstructural protein, now termed NS3 (54, 89, 124). The NS3 protein is derived from the carboxy-terminal portion of the nonstructural protein NS2-3, which is produced by both noncytopathic and cytopathic BVDV (Fig. 1). Several genetic alterations have been identified that allow expression of the NS3 protein by cytopathic BVDV. Those alterations include insertion of cellular RNA into the NS2-3-coding region, duplication and rearrangement of viral sequences inserted into the NS2-3-coding region, duplication of a few bases of the NS2-coding region and insertion of those bases downstream and out of the reading frame, deletion of genes encoding the structural viral proteins creating defective cytopathic particles, point mutations within the NS2-coding region, and recombi-

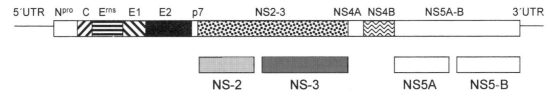

FIGURE 1 The genomic organization of BVDV. The pestivirus genomic RNA lacks a 5′ cap and 3′ poly(A) tail. The long 5′-untranslated region (UTR) has an internal ribosome entry site for initiation of translation. The viral structural proteins are named C (the capsid protein), E^{rns}, E1, and E2. (The last three proteins are in the viral envelope.) Viral-neutralizing antibody reacts primarily with E2, but some viral-neutralizing antibody reacts with E^{rns}. Antigenic similarity between BVDV usually is assessed by using monoclonal or polyclonal antibody against E2. Both noncytopathic BVDV and cytopathic BVDV produce the nonstructural protein NS2-3. However, the NS2-3 protein of cytopathic BVDV is cleaved to form the NS-2 and NS-3 proteins. Expression of the NS3 protein is considered the molecular marker for cytopathic BVDV (see references 53, 90, and 117).

TABLE 1 Origin of cytopathic BVDV in cattle persistently infected with noncytopathic BVDV, form of mucosal disease induced, production of virus-neutralizing antibody, and viral isolation post mortem

Origin of cytopathic BVDV	Full-length genomic RNA or subgenomic RNA (defective particle)	Outcome of mixed infection	Production of antibody	Isolation of cytopathic BVDV
Persistent noncytopathic BVDV	Full-length viral RNA, alteration of NS2-3-coding sequence	Acute or chronic mucosal disease	No	Yes
Persistent noncytopathic BVDV	Mutation results in subgenomic RNA, viral envelope protein-coding region deleted	Acute or chronic mucosal disease	No	No, coisolation of defective particle and noncytopathic BVDV, cytopathic effect variable and not stable in cell culture
Persistent noncytopathic BVDV, recombination with external cytopathic BVDV	Full-length viral RNA, segment of RNA from external cytopathic BVDV inserted into NS2-3 coding region of noncytopathic BVDV	Late-onset mucosal disease	Yes, against external cytopathic BVDV	Yes, second cytopathic BVDV that was derived from the persistent noncytopathic BVDV. External cytopathic BVDV not isolated postmortem.
External source, vaccine or another persistently infected animal that has mucosal disease	Full-length viral RNA from vaccine or from mucosal disease, or subgenomic RNA from mucosal disease	No disease, acute or chronic mucosal disease	Yes	Cytopathic BVDV may or may not be isolated. Antibody may neutralize cytopathic virus and prevent its isolation.

nation with NS2–3 sequences from cytopathic BVDV (9–11, 53, 69, 89–91, 115–118, 133, 134, 139, 162). With the exception of defective particles, genetic alterations that cause change in viral biotype do not alter the viral envelope proteins that contain epitopes involved in viral neutralization. Thus, most pairs of noncytopathic and cytopathic BVDV isolated from cases of mucosal disease are "antigenically similar" in viral neutralization assays or in monoclonal antibody binding assays directed at viral envelope proteins.

The cytopathic BVDV that induces mucosal disease in a persistently infected animal may originate spontaneously from the persistent noncytopathic BVDV or it may originate from an external source (Table 1). Most often, the cytopathic BVDV in a case of mucosal disease originates from the persistent noncytopathic BVDV because of spontaneous genetic alterations that allow expression of the NS3 viral protein. Under experimental conditions, inoculation of persistently infected cattle with cytopathic BVDV that is derived from the persistent noncytopathic BVDV leads to mucosal disease within 2 to 4 weeks, and antibody against BVDV is not detected. Under natural conditions, the period from creation of cytopathic BVDV to onset of mucosal disease is unknown. The anatomical site where the cytopathic BVDV first appears might affect spread of the virus in the animal and, consequently, the duration of the mixed infection and severity of disease.

Cytopathic BVDV similar to the persistent noncytopathic BVDV also may be created by recombination of the noncytopathic BVDV with a cytopathic BVDV of external origin. Cytopathic BVDV of external origin usually is antigenically distinct from the persistent noncytopathic BVDV and stimulates an immune response. In most cases, that immune response clears the cytopathic virus from the body before disease occurs. Occasionally, genetic recombination occurs between the noncytopathic BVDV and cytopathic BVDV before the cytopathic BVDV is cleared from the body. This creates a second cytopathic BVDV that is similar to the persistent noncytopathic BVDV except for a small segment of RNA contributed by the first cytopathic BVDV (11, 60, 63, 139, 151). Creation of the second cytopathic BVDV starts a new mixed infection against which the existing immune response is ineffective. Several weeks to months separate infection with the first cytopathic BVDV from mucosal disease induced by the second cytopathic BVDV (27, 37, 62, 63, 100, 119, 139, 151, 152, 165). Mucosal disease induced after a prolonged second mixed infection is termed late-onset mucosal disease. This disease is similar clinically to acute mucosal disease, but microscopic lesions suggest the pathogenetic mechanisms involved may differ between acute-onset and late-onset mucosal disease. Vascular wall necrosis and perivascular lymphocytic infiltration in the intestine are consistently found in late-onset mucosal disease and seldom reported in other forms of mucosal disease (100).

Cytopathic BVDV of external origin may induce mucosal disease in the absence of recombination with the persistent noncytopathic BVDV. Postvaccinal mucosal disease is an example of cytopathic BVDV from an external source inducing mucosal disease in cattle in the field. Persistently infected cattle often go un-detected in a herd and are vaccinated with modified live cytopathic BVDV during routine herd vaccination. The persistently infected cattle usually produce antibody and disease does not occur. Occasionally, acute mucosal disease occurs 2 to 4 weeks after vaccination (114, 123, 144). Postvaccinal mucosal disease is rare and has not been reported after use of inactivated-virus vaccines. Mucosal disease also can occur if persistently infected cattle of different origins are mixed. Cytopathic BVDV spontaneously created in one animal may be transmitted to a second animal whose persistent noncytopathic BVDV is genetically and antigenically different from that of the first animal. The first animal develops mucosal disease caused by an antigenically genetically similar pair of BVDV strains, and the second animal develops mucosal disease caused by a pair of BVDV strains that are antigenically and genetically different from each other (140, 167). The degree of antigenic difference between noncytopathic BVDV and cytopathic BVDV may determine whether acute mucosal disease, chronic mucosal disease, or late-onset mucosal disease occurs (36). This hypothesis has proven difficult to validate experimentally (105).

Pathogenic Mechanisms in Mucosal Disease

Although information on the virologic aspects and morphologic abnormalities associated with mucosal disease is plentiful, little information exists on the functional abnormalities that contribute to the disease process at the tissue or cellular level. The obvious starting point for studies on pathogenetic mechanisms associated with mucosal disease is the persistently infected animal. The association of noncytopathic BVDV with cells of the immune system and the effect persistent infection has on immune function have received some attention. In persistently infected cattle, noncytopathic BVDV infects monocytes, macrophages, B lymphocytes, BoCD4$^+$, and BoCD8$^+$ T lymphocytes, and $\gamma\delta^+$ T lymphocytes (13, 14, 17, 18, 30, 31, 107, 153). Although a relatively high proportion of cells are infected, the numbers of circulating white blood cells are within normal limits and lymphoid tissues seem normal morphologically (19). Compared with healthy cattle, the concentration of circulating immunoglobulin G2 (IgG2), lymphocyte blastogenesis response to mitogen stimulation, and neutrophil antibacterial responses are diminished and suppressor cell activity is increased in persistently infected cattle (35, 50, 93, 146). Thus, immune function is altered in persistently infected cattle, but immune cell populations are normal in number and structure.

Marked lymphocytic depletion and alteration of lymphatic tissue morphology occur in mucosal disease, particularly in the gut-associated lymphoid tissue (97, 100, 135, 136, 157, 167). Compared with apparently healthy persistently infected cattle, the number of T lymphocytes in blood is reduced in cattle that have mucosal disease (28). In tissues, numbers of IgA^+ and IgM^+ plasma cells are reduced in the lamina propria of the intestine; macrophages become the predominant lymphoid cell type, numbers of $BoCD4^+$ T lymphocytes and B lymphocytes are reduced in gut-associated lymphoid follicles, and numbers of intraepithelial $BoCD8^+$ and $\gamma\delta^+$ T lymphocytes are reduced in small and large intestine (15, 96, 97). In a manner similar to apparently healthy persistently infected cattle, viral antigen is widely distributed among various tissues and cell types in mucosal disease (13, 15, 16, 70, 98–100, 167). However, much of that viral antigen likely is produced by the persistent noncytopathic BVDV.

Clinical disease does not occur until infection with cytopathic BVDV is well established, so the sequential spread and final distribution of cytopathic BVDV in mucosal disease likely are critical factors in the disease process. The tonsils appear to be important early sites of replication of cytopathic BVDV of external origin in persistently infected cattle that are exposed with virus by the oral-nasal route (99). Cytopathic BVDV quickly spreads from the tonsil to other lymphoid tissues, likely carried to those tissues by circulating mononuclear cells. During systemic spread of cytopathic

BVDV, the gut-associated lymphoid tissue is targeted as an initial site for viral replication. Within a few days of infection, cytopathic BVDV is found in follicular dendritic cells and B lymphocytes in Peyer's patches. The cytopathic BVDV likely causes destruction of the B lymphocytes, because they are absent late in the course of disease and an accumulation of cell debris marks their normal location (99). Ultrastructural changes observed in lymphoid follicles early in the course of disease suggest loss of B lymphocytes is caused by apoptosis (157). Several investigators, who have shown that cytopathic BVDV, but not noncytopathic BVDV, induces apoptosis in infected cell cultures, support this (73, 149, 150, 161, 171). Late in the course of mucosal disease, cytopathic BVDV accumulates in the intestinal epithelium and likely causes cell death in the intestinal crypts. Loss of intestinal epithelial cells and/or disturbed myenteric ganglion cell function may be responsible for the profuse diarrhea seen in mucosal disease (99, 167). Cell death caused by replication of cytopathic BVDV is an obvious explanation for lesions seen in mucosal disease. However, altered cell function induced by the mixed infection of BVDV may result in cytokine imbalances that would contribute to lesion formation and have an important role in the disease process (19).

MIXED INFECTIONS WITH BVDV IN RESPIRATORY DISEASE

Acute BVD

Primary postnatal infection with BVDV is the cause of acute BVD. Typically, noncytopathic BVDV is isolated from cases of acute BVD. Cytopathic BVDV may induce acute BVD, but cytopathic BVDV is rare and seldom isolated from cases of acute BVD unless mucosal disease has occurred in the herd to serve as a source of virus. Most BVDV strains are not virulent, so acute BVD often is a clinically inapparent to mild disease. Manifestations of acute BVD frequently are limited to slight elevation in body temperature, transient inappetence, leukopenia, transient decrease in milk production, and increased incidence of reproductive failure (2, 6, 72). Some noncytopathic BVDV strains are virulent and cause clinically severe disease manifested by high fever, depression, inappetence, diarrhea, leukopenia, thrombocytopenia, hemorrhaging, dehydration, and death (29, 43, 47, 48, 58, 137, 163). Clinical signs and postmortem lesions associated with severe acute BVD may resemble acute mucosal disease. However, the nature of the disease outbreak allows differentiation between diseases. Few cattle are affected in an outbreak of mucosal disease and those cattle often are within 2 to 3 months of each other in age. In an outbreak of severe acute BVDV, numerous cattle may be affected, and those cattle may range in age from a few days to several years.

The Role of BVDV as a Respiratory Pathogen

Interstitial pneumonia has been seen in a limited number of field cases of respiratory disease that occurred as the result of acute BVD and in a few cattle with experimentally induced acute BVD (7, 8, 131). Conclusive experimental evidence that uncomplicated infection with BVDV causes severe respiratory disease in cattle, however, is lacking (71, 127). Difficulty in reproduction of severe respiratory disease with BVDV under experimental conditions may reflect choice of viral strain, age of experimental animal, method of viral exposure, or absence of environmental stressors present under field conditions.

Although few reports suggest that BVDV causes disease of the lower respiratory tract, several reports indicate that mild disease of the upper respiratory tract is induced by either noncytopathic or cytopathic BVDV (8, 129, 131, 166). After an initial infection of the upper respiratory tract, BVDV likely is spread to other tissues by infected mononuclear white blood cells. Lymphoid tissue is the primary target of BVDV in an acute infection and, compared with other tissues, viral replication in lymphoid tissue is maximum (34, 41). However, substantial viral titers also have been reported in lung where the virus is detected in bronchus–associated lymphoid tissue (109, 166). Replication of BVDV in lymphoid tissue may interfere with normal local and systemic immune functions, thereby weakening immune defense mechanisms and enhancing disease processes induced by respiratory pathogens. Several serologic studies show that recent infection with BVDV is associated with respiratory disease in the field (64, 67, 110, 111, 138). Rise in titer of antibody against BVDV often is associated with a concomitant rise in antibody titer against other respiratory pathogens, suggesting mixed infection is an important factor in bovine respiratory disease that involves BVDV.

Pathogenic Mechanisms of BVDV in Mixed Respiratory Infections

In acute BVD, virus is isolated from white blood cells and lymphoid tissue. Replication of BVDV in cells of the immune system impairs immune function. Occurrence of acute BVD is associated with reduction in number of T lymphocytes in blood and diminished function of T lymphocytes, as measured in vitro and in vivo (3, 25, 57, 92, 126, 147, 158). Circulating monocytes, alveolar macrophages, and polymorphonuclear leukocytes also show impaired function when harvested during an experimental infection of cattle with BVDV, or after exposure with BVDV in vitro (85, 104, 148, 164). Several investigators have noted perturbation of cytokine production and/or cytokine activity (4, 5, 83, 108, 149, 164).

In addition to causing diminished or altered immune responses, BVDV may affect other host defense mechanisms. Exposure of tracheal-ring cultures with BVDV inhibited ciliary activity of tracheal epithelial cells (145). Exposure of cultured alveolar macrophages with BVDV enhanced their procoagulant activity, which could lead to increased fibrin deposition in the lung (121). Impaired immune cell function, disruption of nonspecific host defense mechanisms, and alteration of local environment in tissues would allow other infectious agents easier access to lung, less interference with propagation, and an enriched environment for propagation. Finally, there is evidence that noncytopathic BVDV inhibits apoptosis, which might prolong a mixed viral infection by interfering with cellular self-destruct mechanisms that limit viral replication (73, 149, 150, 161, 171).

Several reports suggest that BVDV is a synergistic agent in mixed infections of the respiratory tract. Viral pathogens most frequently linked with BVDV in respiratory disease include bovine herpesvirus 1 (BHV-1), parainfluenza virus 3 (PI-3V), and bovine respiratory syncytial virus (BRSV). Those viruses have been coisolated with BVDV from lung or have been shown by serologic tests to infect cattle simultaneously with BVDV under field conditions (64, 67, 68, 138, 143). Compared with disease caused by a single pathogen, mixed infections of BVDV and BRSV, BVDV and BHV-1, or BVDV and *Mannheimia haemolytica* cause more severe disease, delayed and reduced antibody response, greater dissemination of virus, prolonged viral shedding, and more severe lesions (34, 59, 66, 125, 130, 131). Concurrent infection of calves with BRSV and BVDV results in a more pronounced alteration in leukocyte populations in lymphoid tissue than occurs in single infections with either virus (33). Coinfection of alveolar macrophages in vitro with BVDV and BRSV results in a synergistic depression of Fc receptor expression, phagosome-lysosome fusion, secretion of chemotactic factors, production of O_2^-, and production of IgM (66, 104). Taken together, field and experimental data indicate the contribution BVDV makes to respiratory disease is to alter or impair local and systemic defense mechanisms. By doing this, BVDV allows other pathogens to propagate to higher numbers and to persist for an extended period, leading to severe disease.

MIXED INFECTIONS WITH BVDV IN ENTERIC OR REPRODUCTIVE DISEASE

Enteric Disease
Few reports are available on mixed infections of BVDV and other agents in either enteric or reproductive disease. Depression and fever in neonatal calves experimentally inoculated with both BVDV and bovine rotavirus were more pronounced than in calves infected with rotavirus alone (51). The average number of days calves had diarrhea also was increased in the mixed infection of BVDV and bovine rotavirus. In both experimentally induced and naturally occurring mixed infections of BVDV and *Salmonella enterica* serovar Typhimurium, severity of enteric disease was increased and shedding of *Salmonella* was prolonged (122, 170). Experimental inoculation of cesarean section-derived, colostrum-deprived piglets with both attenuated transmissible gastroenteritis virus and either of two strains of BVDV led to more severe signs of disease and more extensive lesions than in piglets inoculated with each virus separately (169). Although most reports focus on the role of BVDV as a synergistic agent, some evidence reveals that BRSV may enhance the severity of enteric disease caused by BVDV (125). As with respiratory disease, it is thought that the effects of BVDV on immune function are responsible for enhanced enteric disease in mixed infections.

Reproductive Disease
Mixed infection of BVDV with *Leptospira borgpetersenii* serovar hardjo, *Coxiella burnetii,* or *Campylobacter fetus* reportedly leads to more severe lesions in the aborted fetus and more cattle aborting than usual for a single infection with those agents (82, 120, 132). In one survey, aborted fetuses infected with *Arcanobacterium pyogenes, Bacillus* spp., and fungi were often coinfected with BVDV (86, 87). Because those bacterial agents are considered opportunistic pathogens of the reproductive tract and fetus, intercurrent infection with BVDV may have allowed fetal infection. Some serologic evidence suggests that the protozoan parasite *Neospora caninum* also may interact with BVDV to induce abortion (1, 22). However, the number of cattle involved was small, and additional supporting evidence is needed to determine the effects this mixed infection may have on reproduction. As in

disease of other organ systems, immunosuppression induced by BVDV in the dam, or in the fetus, may contribute to increased severity of fetal lesions or to enhanced transmission of opportunistic fetal pathogens across the placental barrier.

CONCLUSION

Mixed infection of BVDV in mucosal disease is the culmination of a complex disease process that starts as a fetal infection, may involve immunotolerance, or may involve an immune response that does not protect the animal. This intriguing disease will continue to be investigated. Knowledge gained from study of immunotolerance and immunosuppression in persistently infected cattle, and from study of the sequential progression of lesions and altered cell function in mucosal disease, can be applied to mixed infections of BVDV and other pathogens. Although virulent strains of BVDV are capable of inducing severe disease in uncomplicated infections, less virulent strains of the virus are far more prevalent in nature. Low- and moderate-virulence strains of BVDV contribute to outbreaks of severe disease when they participate in mixed infections with other pathogens. Immunosuppression induced by BVDV during an acute infection long has been thought important in enhancing severity of disease in mixed infections of BVDV and other pathogens. In addition to affecting immune defense mechanisms, noncytopathic BVDV may inhibit apoptosis, which would delay or prevent cell death as a means for limiting spread of an infectious agent in vivo.

The probability of a pathogen participating in a mixed infection depends, in part, on the prevalence of the infectious agent. Numerous studies indicate that BVDV is prevalent in most cattle populations and that economic loss attributed directly, or indirectly, to the virus necessitates its control (74, 75). Persistently infected cattle that continually shed virus provide a natural reservoir for BVDV and allow the virus constant opportunity for transmission to other cattle. Prevention of disease induced by BVDV is accomplished by vaccination, removal of persistently infected cattle from the herd, and use of biosecurity measures that limit spread of the virus (20, 21, 23, 72, 74). Use of various control measures for BVDV may be restricted by size of the herd, geographic location of the production unit, management issues, and regulatory policies. However, control of BVDV is readily accomplished at the herd level when prophylactic methods are adopted.

REFERENCES

1. **Alves, D., B. McEwan, M. Hazlett, G. Maxie, and N. Anderson.** 1996. Trends in bovine abortions submitted to the Ontario Ministry of Agriculture, Food and Rural Affairs, 1993–1995. *Can. Vet. J.* **37:**287–289.

2. **Ames, T. R.** 1986. The causative agent of BVD: its epidemiology and pathogenesis. *Vet. Med.* **81:**848–869.

3. **Archambault, D., C. Beliveau, Y. Couture, and S. Carman.** 2000. Clinical response and immunomodulation following experimental challenge of calves with type 2 noncytopathogenic bovine viral diarrhea virus. *Vet. Res.* **31:**215–227.

4. **Atluru, D., S. Gudapaty, W. Xue, F. Gurria, M. M. Chengappa, D. S. McVey, H. C. Minocha, and S. Atluru.** 1992. In vitro inhibition of 5-lipoxygenase metabolite, leukotriene B4, in bovine mononuclear cells by bovine viral diarrhea virus. *Vet. Immunol. Immunopathol.* **31:**49–59.

5. **Atluru, D., W. Xue, S. Polam, S. Atluru, F. Blecha, and H. C. Minocha.** 1990. In vitro interactions of cytokines and bovine viral diarrhea virus in phytohemagglutinin-stimulated bovine mononuclear cells. *Vet. Immunol. Immunopathol.* **25:**47–59.

6. **Baker, J. C.** 1995. The clinical manifestations of bovine viral diarrhea infection. *Vet. Clin. N. Am. Food Anim. Pract.* **11:**425–445.

7. **Baszler, T. V., J. F. Evermann, P. S. Kaylor, T. C. Byington, and P. M. Dilbeck.** 1995. Diagnosis of naturally occurring bovine viral diarrhea virus infections in ruminants using monoclonal antibody-based immunohistochemistry. *Vet. Pathol.* **32:**609–618.

8. **Baule, C., G. Kulcsar, K. Belak, M. Albert, C. Mittelholzer, T. Soos, L. Kucsera, and S. Belak.** 2001. Pathogenesis of primary respiratory disease induced by isolates from a new genetic cluster of bovine viral diarrhea virus type I. *J. Clin. Microbiol.* **39:**146–153.

9. **Becher, P., M. Orlich, M. Konig, and H. J. Thiel.** 1999. Nonhomologous RNA recombination in bovine viral diarrhea virus: molecular characterization of a variety of subgenomic RNAs isolated during an outbreak of fatal mucosal disease. *J. Virol.* **73:**5646–5653.

10. **Becher, P., M. Orlich, and H. J. Thiel.** 1998. Ribosomal S27a coding sequences upstream of ubiquitin coding sequences in the genome of a pestivirus. *J. Virol.* **72:**8697–8704.

11. **Becher, P., M. Orlich, and H. J. Thiel.** 2001. RNA recombination between persisting pestivirus and a vaccine strain: generation of cytopathogenic virus and induction of lethal disease. *J. Virol.* **75:**6256–6264.

12. **Bezek, D. M., D. Stoffregen, and M. Posso.** 1995. Effect of cytopathic bovine viral diarrhea virus (BVDV) superinfection on viral antigen association with platelets, viremia, and specific antibody levels in two heifers persistently infected with noncytopathic BVDV. *J. Vet. Diagn. Investig.* **7:**395–397.

13. **Bielefeldt Ohmann, H.** 1988. BVD virus antigens in tissues of persistently viraemic, clinically normal cattle: implications for the pathogenesis of clinically fatal disease. *Acta Vet. Scand.* **29:**77– 84.

14. **Bielefeldt Ohmann, H.** 1987. Double-immunolabeling systems for phenotyping of immune cells harboring bovine viral diarrhea virus. *J. Histochem. Cytochem.* **35:**627–633.

15. **Bielefeldt Ohmann, H.** 1988. In situ characterization of mononuclear leukocytes in skin and digestive tract of persistently bovine viral diarrhea virus-infected clinically healthy calves and calves with mucosal disease. *Vet. Pathol.* **25:**304–309.

16. **Bielefeldt Ohmann, H.** 1983. Pathogenesis of bovine viral diarrhea: distribution and significance of BVDV antigen in diseased calves. *Res. Vet. Sci.* **34:**5–8.

17. **Bielefeldt Ohmann, H., B. Bloch, W. C. Davis, and J. Askaa.** 1988. BVD-virus infection in peripheral blood mononuclear cells from persistently viraemic calves studied by correlative immunoelectron microscopy. *Zentbl. Vetmed. Reine B* **35:**477–492.

18. **Bielefeldt Ohmann, H., L. Ronsholt, and B. Bloch.** 1987. Demonstration of bovine viral diarrhoea virus in peripheral blood mononuclear cells of persistently infected, clinically normal cattle. *J. Gen. Virol.* **68:**1971–1982.

19. **Bielefeldt-Ohmann, H.** 1995. The pathologies of bovine viral diarrhea virus infection. A window on the pathogenesis. *Vet. Clin. N. Am. Food Anim. Pract.* **11:**447–476.

20. **Bitsch, V., K. E. Hansen, and L. Ronsholt.** 2000. Experiences from the Danish programme for eradication of bovine virus diarrhoea (BVD) 1994–1998 with special reference to legislation and causes of infection. *Vet. Microbiol.* **77:**137–143.

21. **Bitsch, V., and L. Ronsholt.** 1995. Control of bovine viral diarrhea virus infection without vaccines. *Vet. Clin. N. Am. Food Anim. Pract.* **11:**627–640.

22. **Bjorkman, C., S. Alenius, U. Manuelsson, and A. Uggla.** 2000. Neospora caninum and bovine virus diarrhoea virus infections in Swedish dairy cows in relation to abortion. *Vet. J.* **159:**201–206.

23. **Bolin, S. R.** 1995. Control of bovine viral diarrhea infection by use of vaccination. *Vet. Clin. N. Am. Food Anim. Pract.* **11:**615–625.

24. **Bolin, S. R.** 1988. Viral and viral protein specificity of antibodies induced in cows persistently infected with noncytopathic bovine viral diarrhea virus after vaccination with cytopathic bovine viral diarrhea virus. *Am. J. Vet. Res.* **49:**1040–1044.

25. **Bolin, S. R., A. W. McClurkin, and M. F. Coria.** 1985. Effects of bovine viral diarrhea virus on the percentages and absolute numbers of circulating B and T lymphocytes in cattle. *Am. J. Vet. Res.* **46:**884–886.

26. **Bolin, S. R., A. W. McClurkin, and M. F. Coria.** 1985. Frequency of persistent bovine viral diarrhea virus infection in selected cattle herds. *Am. J. Vet. Res.* **46:**2385–2387.

27. **Bolin, S. R., A. W. McClurkin, R. C. Cutlip, and M. F. Coria.** 1985. Response of cattle persistently infected with noncytopathic bovine viral diarrhea virus to vaccination for bovine viral diarrhea and to subsequent challenge exposure with cytopathic bovine viral diarrhea virus. *Am. J. Vet. Res.* **46:**2467–2470.

28. **Bolin, S. R., A. W. McClurkin, R. C. Cutlip, and M. F. Coria.** 1985. Severe clinical disease induced in cattle persistently infected with noncytopathic bovine viral diarrhea virus by superinfection with cytopathic bovine viral diarrhea virus. *Am. J. Vet. Res.* **46:**573–576.

29. **Bolin, S. R., and J. F. Ridpath.** 1992. Differences in virulence between two noncytopathic bovine viral diarrhea viruses in calves. *Am. J. Vet. Res.* **53:**2157–2163.

30. **Bolin, S. R., and J. F. Ridpath.** 1990. Frequency of association of noncytopathic bovine viral diarrhea virus with bovine neutrophils and mononuclear leukocytes before and after treatment with trypsin. *Am. J. Vet. Res.* **51:**1847–1851.

31. **Bolin, S. R., J. M. Sacks, and S. V. Crowder.** 1987. Frequency of association of noncytopathic bovine viral diarrhea virus with mononuclear leukocytes from persistently infected cattle. *Am. J. Vet. Res.* **48:**1441–1445.

32. **Brock, K. V., D. L. Grooms, J. Ridpath, and S. R. Bolin.** 1998. Changes in levels of viremia in cattle persistently infected with bovine viral diarrhea virus. *J. Vet. Diagn. Investig.* **10:**22–26.

33. **Brodersen, B. W., and C. L. Kelling.** 1999. Alteration of leukocyte populations in calves concurrently infected with bovine respiratory syncytial virus and bovine viral diarrhea virus. *Viral Immunol.* **12:**323–334.

34. **Brodersen, B. W., and C. L. Kelling.** 1998. Effect of concurrent experimentally induced bovine respiratory syncytial virus and bovine viral diarrhea virus infection on respiratory tract and enteric diseases in calves. *Am. J. Vet. Res.* **59:**1423–1430.

35. **Brown, G. B., S. R. Bolin, D. E. Frank, and J. A. Roth.** 1991. Defective function of leukocytes from cattle persistently infected with bovine viral diarrhea virus, and the influence of recombinant cytokines. *Am. J. Vet. Res.* **52:**381–387.

36. **Brownlie, J.** 1991. The pathways for bovine virus diarrhoea virus biotypes in the pathogenesis of disease. *Arch. Virol. Suppl.* **3:**79–96.

37. **Brownlie, J., and M. C. Clarke.** 1993. Experimental and spontaneous mucosal disease of cattle: a validation of Koch's postulates in the definition of pathogenesis. *Intervirology* **35:**51–59.

38. **Brownlie, J., M. C. Clarke, and C. J. Howard.** 1989. Experimental infection of cattle in early pregnancy with a cytopathic strain of bovine virus diarrhoea virus. *Res. Vet. Sci.* **46:**307–311.

39. **Brownlie, J., M. C. Clarke, and C. J. Howard.** 1984. Experimental production of fatal mucosal disease in cattle. *Vet. Rec.* **114:**535–536.

40. **Bruschke, C. J., A. Haghparast, A. Hoek, V. P. Rutten, G. H. Wentink, P. A. van Rijn, and J. T. van Oirschot.** 1998. The immune response of cattle, persistently infected with noncytopathic BVDV, after superinfection with antigenically semi-homologous cytopathic BVDV. *Vet. Immunol. Immunopathol.* **62:**37–50.

41. **Bruschke, C. J., K. Weerdmeester, J. T. Van Oirschot, and P. A. Van Rijn.** 1998. Distribution of bovine virus diarrhoea virus in tissues and white blood cells of cattle during acute infection. *Vet. Microbiol.* **64:**23–32.

42. **Buckner, R., and H. D. Grunder.** 1995. Clinical, serological and virological findings in cattle with acute, sub-acute and chronic mucosal disease. *Bovine Pract.* **29:**119–124.

43. **Carman, S., T. van Dreumel, J. Ridpath, M. Hazlett, D. Alves, E. Dubovi, R. Tremblay, S. Bolin, A. Godkin, and N. Anderson.** 1998. Severe acute bovine viral diarrhea in Ontario, 1993–1995. *J. Vet. Diagn. Investig.* **10:**27–35.

44. **Collen, T., A. J. Douglas, D. J. Paton, G. Zhang, and W. I. Morrison.** 2000. Single amino acid differences are sufficient for CD4(+) T-cell recognition of a heterologous virus by cattle persistently infected with bovine viral diarrhea virus. *Virology* **276:**70–82.

45. **Collins, M. E., M. Desport, and J. Brownlie.** 1999. Bovine viral diarrhea virus quasispecies during persistent infection. *Virology* **259:**85–98.

46. **Corapi, W. V., R. O. Donis, and E. J. Dubovi.** 1988. Monoclonal antibody analyses of cytopathic and noncytopathic viruses from fatal bovine viral diarrhea virus infections. *J. Virol.* **62:**2823–2827.

47. **Corapi, W. V., R. D. Elliott, T. W. French, D. G. Arthur, D. M. Bezek, and E. J. Dubovi.** 1990. Thrombocytopenia and hemorrhages in veal calves infected with bovine viral diarrhea virus. *J. Am. Vet. Med. Assoc.* **196:**590–596.

48. **Corapi, W. V., T. W. French, and E. J. Dubovi.** 1989. Severe thrombocytopenia in young calves experimentally infected with noncytopathic bovine viral diarrhea virus. *J. Virol.* **63:**3934–3943.

49. **Coria, M. F., and A. W. McClurkin.** 1978. Specific immune tolerance in an apparently healthy bull persistently infected with bovine viral diarrhea virus. *J. Am. Vet. Med. Assoc.* **172:**449–451.

50. **Coulibaly, C. O. Z., B. Liess, G. Trautwein, and G. Schleuter.** 1986. Quantitative analysis of immunoglobulins G1 and G2 in blood samples of cattle persistently infected with bovine virus diarrhoea virus. *J. Vet. Med. Ser. B* **33:**685–696.

51. **de Verdier Klingenberg, K.** 2000. Enhancement of clinical signs in experimentally rotavirus infected calves by combined viral infections. *Vet. Rec.* **147:**717–719.

52. **Done, J. T., S. Terlecki, C. Richardson, J. W. Harkness, J. J. Sands, D. S. Patterson, D. Sweasey, I. G. Shaw, C. E. Winkler, and S. J. Duffell.** 1980. Bovine virus diarrhoea-mucosal disease virus: pathogenicity for the fetal calf following maternal infection. *Vet. Rec.* **106:**473–479.

53. **Donis, R. O.** 1995. Molecular biology of bovine viral diarrhea virus and its interactions with the host. *Vet. Clin. N. Am. Food Anim. Pract.* **11:**393–423.

54. **Donis, R. O., and E. J. Dubovi.** 1987. Differences in virus-induced polypeptides in cells infected by cytopathic and noncytopathic biotypes of bovine virus diarrhea-mucosal disease virus. *Virology* **158:**168–173.

55. **Donis, R. O., and E. J. Dubovi.** 1987. Molecular specificity of the antibody responses of cattle

naturally and experimentally infected with cytopathic and noncytopathic bovine viral diarrhea virus biotypes. *Am. J. Vet. Res.* **48:**1549–1554.

56. **Edwards, S., T. W. Drew, and S. E. Bushnell.** 1987. Prevalence of bovine virus diarrhoea virus viraemia. *Vet. Rec.* **120:**71.

57. **Ellis, J. A., W. C. Davis, E. L. Belden, and D. L. Pratt.** 1988. Flow cytofluorimetric analysis of lymphocyte subset alterations in cattle infected with bovine viral diarrhea virus. *Vet. Pathol.* **25:**231–236.

58. **Ellis, J. A., K. H. West, V. S. Cortese, S. L. Myers, S. Carman, K. M. Martin, and D. M. Haines.** 1998. Lesions and distribution of viral antigen following an experimental infection of young seronegative calves with virulent bovine virus diarrhea virus-type II. *Can. J. Vet. Res.* **62:**161–169.

59. **Elvander, M., C. Baule, M. Persson, L. Egyed, A. Ballagi-Pordany, S. Belak, and S. Alenius.** 1998. An experimental study of a concurrent primary infection with bovine respiratory syncytial virus (BRSV) and bovine viral diarrhoea virus (BVDV) in calves. *Acta Vet. Scand.* **39:**251–264.

60. **Fray, M. D., M. C. Clarke, L. H. Thomas, J. W. McCauley, and B. Charleston.** 1998. Prolonged nasal shedding and viraemia of cytopathogenic bovine virus diarrhoea virus in experimental late-onset mucosal disease. *Vet. Rec.* **143:**608–611.

61. **Fredriksen, B., T. Sandvik, T. Loken, and S. A. Odegaard.** 1999. Level and duration of serum antibodies in cattle infected experimentally and naturally with bovine virus diarrhoea virus. *Vet. Rec.* **144:**111–114.

62. **Fritzemeier, J., I. Greiser-Wilke, L. Hass, E. Pituco, V. Moennig, and B. Liess.** 1995. Experimentally induced "late onset" mucosal disease: characterization of the cytopathic viruses isolated. *Vet. Microbiol.* **46:**285–294.

63. **Fritzemeier, J., L. Haas, E. Liebler, V. Moennig, and I. Greiser-Wilke.** 1997. The development of early vs. late onset mucosal disease is a consequence of two different pathogenic mechanisms. *Arch. Virol.* **142:**1335–1350.

64. **Fulton, R. W., C. W. Purdy, A. W. Confer, J. T. Saliki, R. W. Loan, R. E. Briggs, and L. J. Burge.** 2000. Bovine viral diarrhea viral infections in feeder calves with respiratory disease: interactions with Pasteurella spp., parainfluenza-3 virus, and bovine respiratory syncytial virus. *Can. J. Vet. Res.* **64:**151–159.

65. **Gillespie, J. H., K. M. Lee, J. A. Baker, and K. McEntee.** 1960. A cytopathogenic strain of virus diarrhea virus. *Cornell Vet.* **50:**73–79.

66. **Graham, D. A., M. Elvander, B. M. Adair, and M. Merza.** 1998. Influence of concurrent BVDV infection on the IgM response of calves experimentally infected with bovine respiratory syncytial virus. *Vet. Rec.* **143:**198–199.

67. **Graham, D. A., J. McShane, K. A. Mawhinney, I. E. McLaren, B. M. Adair, and M. Merza.** 1998. Evaluation of a single dilution ELISA system for detection of seroconversion to bovine viral diarrhea virus, bovine respiratory syncytial virus, parainfluenza-3 virus, and infectious bovine rhinotracheitis virus: comparison with testing by virus neutralization and hemagglutination inhibition. *J. Vet. Diagn. Investig.* **10:**43–48.

68. **Greig, A., I. R. Gibson, P. F. Nettleton, and J. A. Herring.** 1981. Disease outbreak in calves caused by a mixed infection with infectious bovine rhinotracheitis virus and bovine virus diarrhoea virus. *Vet. Rec.* **108:**480.

69. **Greiser-Wilke, I., L. Haas, K. Dittmar, B. Liess, and V. Moennig.** 1993. RNA insertions and gene duplications in the nonstructural protein p125 region of pestivirus strains and isolates in vitro and in vivo. *Virology* **193:**977–980.

70. **Greiser-Wilke, I., E. Liebler, L. Haas, B. Liess, J. Pohlenz, and V. Moennig.** 1993. Distribution of cytopathogenic and noncytopathogenic bovine virus diarrhea virus in tissues from a calf with experimentally induced mucosal disease using antigenic and genetic markers. *Arch. Virol.* **7**(Suppl.)**:**295–302.

71. **Grooms, D. L.** 1998. Role of bovine viral diarrhea virus in the bovine respiratory disease complex. *Bovine Pract.* **32:**7–12.

72. **Grooms, D. L., J. C. Baker, and T. R. Ames** 2002. Diseases caused by bovine virus diarrhea virus, p. 707–714. *In* B. P. Smith (ed.), *Large Animal Internal Medicine: Diseases of Horses, Cattle, Sheep, and Goats,* 3rd ed. Mosby, St. Louis, Mo.

73. **Hoff, H. S., and R. O. Donis.** 1997. Induction of apoptosis and cleavage of poly(ADP-ribose) polymerase by cytopathic bovine viral diarrhea virus infection. *Virus Res.* **49:**101–113.

74. **Houe, H.** 1999. Epidemiological features and economical importance of bovine virus diarrhoea virus (BVDV) infections. *Vet. Microbiol.* **64:**89–107.

75. **Houe, H.** 1995. Epidemiology of bovine viral diarrhea virus. *Vet. Clin. N. Am. Food Anim. Pract.* **11:**521–547.

76. **Houe, H.** 1993. Survivorship of animals persistently infected with bovine virus diarrhoea virus (BVDV). *Prev. Vet. Med.* **15:**275–283.

77. **Houe, H., J. C. Baker, R. K. Maes, H. Wuryastuti, R. Wasito, P. L. Ruegg, and J. W. Lloyd.** 1995. Prevalence of cattle persistently

infected with bovine viral diarrhea virus in 20 dairy herds in two counties in central Michigan and comparison of prevalence of antibody-positive cattle among herds with different infection and vaccination status. *J. Vet. Diagn. Investig.* **7:**321–326.

78. **Houe, H., and I. Heron.** 1993. Immune response to other agents of calves persistently infected with bovine virus diarrhoea virus (BVDV). *Acta Vet. Scand.* **34:**305–310.

79. **Houe, H., and A. Meyling.** 1991. Prevalence of bovine viral diarrhoea (BVD) in 19 Danish dairy herds and estimation of incidence of infection in early pregnancy. *Prev. Vet. Med.* **11:** 9–16.

80. **Howard, C. J., J. Brownlie, and M. C. Clarke.** 1987. Comparison by the neutralisation assay of pairs of non-cytopathogenic and cytopathogenic strains of bovine virus diarrhoea virus isolated from cases of mucosal disease. *Vet. Microbiol.* **13:**361–369.

81. **Howard, C. J., J. Brownlie, and L. H. Thomas.** 1986. Prevalence of bovine virus diarrhoea virus viraemia in cattle in the UK. *Vet. Rec.* **119:**628–629.

82. **Jeffery, M., and R. A. Hogg.** 1988. Concurrent bovine virus diarrhoea virus and *Campylobacter* fetus infection in an aborted bovine fetus. *Vet. Rec.* **122:**89–90.

83. **Jensen, J., and R. D. Schultz.** 1991. Effect of infection by bovine viral diarrhea virus (BVDV) in vitro on interleukin-1 activity of bovine monocytes. *Vet. Immunol. Immunopathol.* **29:** 251–265.

84. **Kahrs, R. F., R. Bartholomew, J. A. House, and G. M. Ward.** 1970. Epidemiological investigation of bovine diarrhea-mucosal disease in an unvaccinated dairy herd. *Cornell Vet.* **60:**16–22.

85. **Ketelsen, A. T., D. W. Johnson, and C. C. Muscoplat.** 1979. Depression of bovine monocyte chemotactic responses by bovine viral diarrhea virus. *Infect. Immun.* **25:**565–568.

86. **Kirkbride, C. A.** 1992. Etiologic agents detected in a 10-year study of bovine abortions and stillbirths. *J. Vet. Diagn. Investig.* **4:**175–180.

87. **Kirkbride, C. A.** 1992. Viral agents and associated lesions detected in a 10-year study of bovine abortions and stillbirths. *J. Vet. Diagn. Investig.* **4:**374–379.

88. **Kirkland, P. D., S. G. Mackintosh, and A. Moyle.** 1994. The outcome of widespread use of semen from a bull persistently infected with pestivirus. *Vet. Rec.* **135:**527–529.

89. **Kummerer, B. M., and G. Meyers.** 2000. Correlation between point mutations in NS2 and the viability and cytopathogenicity of Bovine viral diarrhea virus strain Oregon analyzed with an infectious cDNA clone. *J. Virol.* **74:**390–400.

90. **Kummerer, B. M., D. Stoll, and G. Meyers.** 1998. Bovine viral diarrhea virus strain Oregon: a novel mechanism for processing of NS2-3 based on point mutations. *J. Virol.* **72:**4127–4138.

91. **Kummerer, B. M., N. Tautz, P. Becher, H. Thiel, and G. Meyers.** 2000. The genetic basis for cytopathogenicity of pestiviruses. *Vet. Microbiol.* **77:**117–128.

92. **Lamontagne, L., P. Lafortune, and M. Fournel.** 1989. Modulation of the cellular immune responses to T-cell-dependent and T cell-independent antigens in lambs with induced bovine viral diarrhea virus infection. *Am. J. Vet. Res.* **50:**1604–1608.

93. **Larsson, B.** 1988. Increased suppressor cell activity in cattle persistently infected with bovine virus diarrhoea virus. *J. Vet. Med. Ser. B* **35:**271–279.

94. **Lee, K. M., and J. H. Gillespie.** 1957. Propagation of virus diarrhea virus of cattle in tissue culture. *Am. J. Vet. Res.* **18:**952–955.

95. **Lee, S. C., I. E. Borgmann, and N. A. Gobin.** 1994. A severe outbreak of mucosal disease in central Alberta. *Can. Vet. J.* **35:**641–642.

96. **Liebler, E. M., C. Kusters, and J. F. Pohlenz.** 1996. Experimental mucosal disease in cattle: changes in the number of lymphocytes and plasma cells in the mucosa of the small and large intestine. *Vet. Immunol. Immunopathol.* **55:** 93–105.

97. **Liebler, E. M., C. Kusters, and J. F. Pohlenz.** 1995. Experimental mucosal disease in cattle: changes of lymphocyte subpopulations in Peyer's patches and in lymphoid nodules of large intestine. *Vet. Immunol. Immunopathol.* **48:** 233–248.

98. **Liebler, E. M., J. Waschbusch, J. F. Pohlenz, V. Moennig, and B. Liess.** 1991. Distribution of antigen of noncytopathogenic and cytopathogenic bovine virus diarrhea virus biotypes in the intestinal tract of calves following experimental production of mucosal disease. *Arch. Virol. Suppl.* **3:**109–124.

99. **Liebler-Tenorio, E. M., I. Greiser-Wilke, and J. F. Pohlenz.** 1997. Organ and tissue distribution of the antigen of the cytopathogenic bovine virus diarrhea virus in the early and advanced phase of experimental mucosal disease. *Arch. Virol.* **142:**1613–1634.

100. **Liebler-Tenorio, E. M., A. Lanwehr, I. Greiser-Wilke, B. I. Loehr, and J. Pohlenz.** 2000. Comparative investigation of tissue alterations and distribution of BVD-viral antigen in cattle with early onset versus late onset mucosal disease. *Vet. Microbiol.* **77:**163–174.

101. **Liess, B., H.-R. Frey, H. Kittsteiner, F. Baumann, and W. Neumann.** 1974. Obser-

vations and investigation on mucosal disease of cattle, a late stage of BVD-MD virus infection with immunobiologic explanation and criteria of a slow virus infection. *Dtsch. Tierarztl. Wochenschr.* **81:**481–487.

102. **Liess, B., H. R. Frey, S. Orban, and S. M. Hafez.** 1983. Bovine virus diarrhea (BVD)—"mucosal disease": persistent BVD field virus infection in serologically selected cattle. *Dtsch. Tierarztl. Wochenschr.* **90:**261–266.

103. **Liess, B., S. Orban, H. R. Frey, G. Trautwein, W. Wiefel, and H. Blindow.** 1984. Studies on transplacental transmissibility of a bovine virus diarrhoea (BVD) vaccine virus in cattle. II. Inoculation of pregnant cows without detectable neutralizing antibodies to BVD virus 90–229 days before parturition (51st to 190th day of gestation). *Zentbl. Vetmed. Reihe B* **31:**669–681.

104. **Liu, L., H. D. Lehmkuhl, and M. L. Kaeberle.** 1999. Synergistic effects of bovine respiratory syncytial virus and non-cytopathic bovine viral diarrhea virus infection on selected bovine alveolar macrophage functions. *Can. J. Vet. Res.* **63:**41–48.

105. **Loehr, B. I., H. R. Frey, V. Moennig, and I. Greiser-Wilke.** 1998. Experimental induction of mucosal disease: consequences of superinfection of persistently infected cattle with different strains of cytopathogenic bovine viral diarrhea virus. *Arch. Virol.* **143:**667–679.

106. **Loken, T., H. Gamlem, and O. Lysbakken.** 1989. An outbreak of mucosal disease in a dairy herd. *Acta. Vet. Scand.* **30:**321–327.

107. **Lopez, O. J., F. A. Osorio, C. L. Kelling, and R. O. Donis.** 1993. Presence of bovine viral diarrhoea virus in lymphoid cell populations of persistently infected cattle. *J. Gen. Virol.* **74:**925–929.

108. **Markham, R. J., and M. L. Ramnaraine.** 1985. Release of immunosuppressive substances from tissue culture cells infected with bovine viral diarrhea virus. *Am. J. Vet. Res.* **46:**879–883.

109. **Marshall, D. J., R. A. Moxley, and C. L. Kelling.** 1996. Distribution of virus and viral antigen in specific pathogen-free calves following inoculation with noncytopathic bovine viral diarrhea virus. *Vet. Pathol.* **33:**311–318.

110. **Martin, S. W., K. G. Bateman, P. E. Shewen, S. Rosendal, J. G. Bohac, and M. Thorburn.** 1990. A group level analysis of the associations between antibodies to seven putative pathogens and respiratory disease and weight gain in Ontario feedlot calves. *Can. J. Vet. Res.* **54:**337–342.

111. **Martin, S. W., E. Nagy, D. Armstrong, and S. Rosendal.** 1999. The associations of viral and mycoplasmal antibody titers with respiratory disease and weight gain in feedlot calves. *Can. Vet. J.* **40:**560–570.

112. **McClurkin, A. W., S. R. Bolin, and M. F. Coria.** 1985. Isolation of cytopathic and noncytopathic bovine viral diarrhea virus from the spleen of cattle acutely and chronically affected with bovine viral diarrhea. *J. Am. Vet. Med. Assoc.* **186:**568–569.

113. **McClurkin, A. W., E. T. Littledike, R. C. Cutlip, G. H. Frank, M. F. Coria, and S. R. Bolin.** 1984. Production of cattle immunotolerant to bovine viral diarrhea virus. *Can. J. Comp. Med.* **48:**156–161.

114. **McKercher, D. G., J. K. Saito, G. L. Crenshaw, and R. B. Bushnell.** 1968. Complications in cattle following vaccination with a combined bovine viral diarrhea-infectious bovine rhinotracheitis vaccine. *J. Am. Vet. Med. Assoc.* **152:**1621–1624.

115. **Meyers, G., T. Rumenapf, N. Tautz, E. J. Dubovi, and H. J. Thiel.** 1991. Insertion of cellular sequences in the genome of bovine viral diarrhea virus. *Arch. Virol. Suppl.* **3:**133–142.

116. **Meyers, G., D. Stoll, and M. Gunn.** 1998. Insertion of a sequence encoding light chain 3 of microtubule-associated proteins 1A and 1B in a pestivirus genome: connection with virus cytopathogenicity and induction of lethal disease in cattle. *J. Virol.* **72:**4139–4148.

117. **Meyers, G., N. Tautz, E. J. Dubovi, and H. J. Thiel.** 1991. Viral cytopathogenicity correlated with integration of ubiquitin-coding sequences. *Virology* **180:**602–616.

118. **Meyers, G., and H.-J. Theil.** 1996. Molecular characterization of pestiviruses. *Adv. Virus Res.* **47:**53–118.

119. **Moennig, V., H. R. Frey, E. Liebler, J. Pohlenz, and B. Liess.** 1990. Reproduction of mucosal disease with cytopathogenic bovine viral diarrhoea virus selected in vitro. *Vet. Rec.* **127:**200–203.

120. **Murray, R. D.** 1991. Lesions in aborted fetuses and placenta associated with bovine viral diarrhoea virus infection. *Arch. Virol. Suppl.* **3:**217–224.

121. **Olchowy, T. W., D. O. Slauson, and P. N. Bochsler.** 1997. Induction of procoagulant activity in virus infected bovine alveolar macrophages and the effect of lipopolysaccharide. *Vet. Immunol. Immunopathol.* **58:**27–37.

122. **Penny, C. D., J. C. Low, P. F. Nettleton, P. R. Scott, N. D. Sargison, W. D. Strachan, and P. C. Honeyman.** 1996. Concurrent bovine viral diarrhoea virus and Salmonella

typhimurium DT104 infection in a group of pregnant dairy heifers. *Vet. Rec.* **138**:485–489.

123. **Peter, C. P., D. E. Tyler, and F. K. Ramsey.** 1967. Characteristics of a condition following vaccination with bovine virus diarrhea vaccine. *J. Am. Vet. Med. Assoc.* **150**:46–52.

124. **Pocock, D. H., C. J. Howard, M. C. Clarke, and J. Brownlie.** 1987. Variation in the intracellular polypeptide profiles from different isolates of bovine virus diarrhoea virus. *Arch. Virol.* **94**:43–53.

125. **Pollreisz, J. H., C. L. Kelling, B. W. Brodersen, L. J. Perino, V. L. Cooper, and A. R. Doster.** 1997. Potentiation of bovine repiratory syncytial virus infection in calves by bovine viral diarrhea virus. *Bovine Pract.* **31**:32–38.

126. **Pospisil, Z., M. Machatkova, J. Mensik, L. Rodak, and G. Muller.** 1975. Decline in the phytohemagglutinin responsiveness of lymphocytes from calves infected experimentally with bovine viral diarrhoea-mucosal disease virus and parainfluenza 3 virus. *Acta Vet. Brno* **44**:369–375.

127. **Potgieter, L. N.** 1997. Bovine respiratory tract disease caused by bovine viral diarrhea virus. *Vet. Clin. N. Am. Food Anim. Pract.* **13**:471–481.

128. **Potgieter, L. N.** 1995. Immunology of bovine viral diarrhea virus. *Vet. Clin. N. Am. Food Anim. Pract.* **11**:501–520.

129. **Potgieter, L. N., M. D. McCracken, F. M. Hopkins, and J. S. Guy.** 1985. Comparison of the pneumopathogenicity of two strains of bovine viral diarrhea virus. *Am. J. Vet. Res.* **46**:151–153.

130. **Potgieter, L. N., M. D. McCracken, F. M. Hopkins, and R. D. Walker.** 1984. Effect of bovine viral diarrhea virus infection on the distribution of infectious bovine rhinotracheitis virus in calves. *Am. J. Vet. Res.* **45**:687–690.

131. **Potgieter, L. N., M. D. McCracken, F. M. Hopkins, R. D. Walker, and J. S. Guy.** 1984. Experimental production of bovine respiratory tract disease with bovine viral diarrhea virus. *Am. J. Vet. Res.* **45**:1582–1585.

132. **Pritchard, G. C., E. D. Borland, L. Wood, and D. G. Pritchard.** 1989. Severe disease in a dairy herd associated with acute infection with bovine virus diarrhoea virus, *Leptospira hardjo* and *Coxiella burnetii*. *Vet. Rec.* **124**:625–629.

133. **Qi, F., J. F. Ridpath, and E. S. Berry.** 1998. Insertion of a bovine SMT3B gene in NS4B and duplication of NS3 in a bovine viral diarrhea virus genome correlate with the cytopathogenicity of the virus. *Virus Res.* **57**:1–9.

134. **Qi, F., J. F. Ridpath, T. Lewis, S. R. Bolin, and E. S. Berry.** 1992. Analysis of the bovine

viral diarrhea virus genome for possible cellular insertions. *Virology* **189**:285–292.

135. **Ramsey, F. K., and W. H. Chivers.** 1953. Mucosal disease of cattle. *N. Am. Vet.* **34**:629–633.

136. **Ramsey, F. K., and W. H. Chivers.** 1957. Pathology of a mucosal disease of cattle. *J. Am. Vet. Med. Assoc.* **130**:381–383.

137. **Rebhun, W. C., T. W. French, J. A. Perdrizet, E. J. Dubovi, S. G. Dill, and L. F. Karcher.** 1989. Thrombocytopenia associated with acute bovine virus diarrhea infection in cattle. *J. Vet. Intern. Med.* **3**:42–46.

138. **Richer, L., P. Marois, and L. Lamontagne.** 1988. Association of bovine viral diarrhea virus with multiple viral infections in bovine respiratory disease outbreaks. *Can. Vet. J.* **29**:713–717.

139. **Ridpath, J. F., and S. R. Bolin.** 1995. Delayed onset postvaccinal mucosal disease as a result of genetic recombination between genotype 1 and genotype 2 BVDV. *Virology* **212**:259–262.

140. **Ridpath, J. F., and S. R. Bolin.** 1991. Hybridization analysis of genomic variability among isolates of bovine viral diarrhoea virus using cDNA probes. *Mol. Cell. Probes* **5**:291–298.

141. **Ridpath, J. F., T. L. Lewis, S. R. Bolin, and E. S. Berry.** 1991. Antigenic and genomic comparison between non-cytopathic and cytopathic bovine viral diarrhoea viruses isolated from cattle that had spontaneous mucosal disease. *J. Gen. Virol.* **72**:725–729.

142. **Roeder, P. L., and T. W. Drew.** 1984. Mucosal disease of cattle: a late sequel to fetal infection. *Vet. Rec.* **114**:309–313.

143. **Rosenquist, B. D., J. E. English, D. W. Johnson, and R. W. Loan.** 1970. Mixed viral etiology of a shipping fever epizootic in cattle. *Am. J. Vet. Res.* **31**:989–994.

144. **Rosner, S. F.** 1968. Complications following vaccination of cattle against infectious bovine rhinotracheitis, bovine viral diarrhea-mucosal disease, and parainfluenza type 3. *J. Am. Vet. Med. Assoc.* **152**:898–902.

145. **Rossi, C. R., and G. K. Kiesel.** 1977. Susceptibility of bovine macrophage and tracheal-ring cultures to bovine viruses. *Am. J. Vet. Res.* **38**:1705–1708.

146. **Roth, J. A., S. R. Bolin, and D. E. Frank.** 1986. Lymphocyte blastogenesis and neutrophil function in cattle persistently infected with bovine viral diarrhea virus. *Am. J. Vet. Res.* **47**:1139–1141.

147. **Roth, J. A., and M. L. Kaeberle.** 1983. Suppression of neutrophil and lymphocyte function induced by a vaccinal strain of bovine viral diarrhea virus with and without the admin-

istration of ACTH. *Am. J. Vet. Res.* **44:**2366–2372.

148. **Roth, J. A., M. L. Kaeberle, and R. W. Griffith.** 1981. Effects of bovine viral diarrhea virus infection on bovine polymorphonuclear leukocyte function. *Am. J. Vet. Res.* **42:**244–250.

149. **Schweizer, M., and E. Peterhans.** 2001. Noncytopathic bovine viral diarrhea virus inhibits double-stranded RNA-induced apoptosis and interferon synthesis. *J. Virol.* **75:**4692–4698.

150. **Schweizer, M., and E. Peterhans.** 1999. Oxidative stress in cells infected with bovine viral diarrhoea virus: a crucial step in the induction of apoptosis. *J. Gen. Virol.* **80:**1147–1155.

151. **Sentsui, H., T. Nishimori, R. Kirisawa, and A. Morooka.** 2001. Mucosal disease induced in cattle persistently infected with bovine viral diarrhea virus by antigenically different cytopathic virus. *Arch. Virol.* **146:**993–1006.

152. **Shimizu, M., K. Satou, N. Nishioka, T. Yoshino, E. Momotani, and Y. Ishikawa.** 1989. Serological characterization of viruses isolated from experimental mucosal disease. *Vet. Microbiol.* **19:**13–21.

153. **Sopp, P., L. B. Hooper, M. C. Clarke, C. J. Howard, and J. Brownlie.** 1994. Detection of bovine viral diarrhoea virus p80 protein in subpopulations of bovine leukocytes. *J. Gen. Virol.* **75:**1189–1194.

154. **Steck, F., S. Lazary, H. Fey, A. Wandeler, C. Huggler, G. Oppliger, H. Baumberger, R. Kaderli, and J. Martig.** 1980. Immune responsiveness in cattle fatally affected by bovine virus diarrhea-mucosal disease. *Zentrbl. Vetmed. Reine B* **27:**429–445.

155. **Taylor, L. F., J. Van Donkersgoed, E. J. Dubovi, R. J. Harland, J. V. van den Hurk, C. S. Ribble, and E. D. Janzen.** 1995. The prevalence of bovine viral diarrhea virus infection in a population of feedlot calves in western Canada. *Can. J. Vet. Res.* **59:**87–93.

156. **Taylor, L. F., J. Van Donkersgoed, O. M. Radostits, C. W. Booker, E. J. Dubovi, J. V. van den Hurk, and E. D. Janzen.** 1994. Investigation of an outbreak of mucosal disease in a beef cattle herd in southwestern Saskatchewan. *Can. Vet. J.* **35:**425–432.

157. **Teichmann, U., E. M. Liebler-Tenorio, and J. F. Pohlenz.** 2000. Ultrastructural changes in follicles of small-intestinal aggregated lymphoid nodules in early and advanced phases of experimentally induced mucosal diseases in calves. *Am. J. Vet. Res.* **61:**174–182.

158. **Thoen, C. O., and K. J. Waite.** 1990. Some immune responses in cattle exposed to My-cobacterium paratuberculosis after injection with modified-live bovine viral diarrhea virus vaccine. *J. Vet. Diagn. Investig.* **2:**176–179.

159. **Underdahl, N. R., O. D. Grace, and A. B. Horlein.** 1957. Cultivation of a cytopathogenic agent from bovine mucosal disease. *Proc. Soc. Exp. Biol. Med.* **94:**795–797.

160. **van Regenmortel, M. H. V., C. M. Fauquet, D. H. L. Bishop, E. B. Carstens, M. K. Estes, S. M. Lemon, J. Maniloff, M. A. Mayo, D. J. McGeoch, C. R. Pringle, and R. B. Wickner (ed.).** 2000. *Virus Taxonomy: Classification and Nomenclature of Viruses. Seventh Report of the International Committee on Taxonomy of Viruses.* Academic Press, San Diego, Calif.

161. **Vassilev, V. B., and R. O. Donis.** 2000. Bovine viral diarrhea virus induced apoptosis correlates with increased intracellular viral RNA accumulation. *Virus Res.* **69:**95–107.

162. **Vilcek, S., I. Greiser-Wilke, P. Nettleton, and D. J. Paton.** 2000. Cellular insertions in the NS2-3 genome region of cytopathic bovine viral diarrhoea virus (BVDV) isolates. *Vet. Microbiol.* **77:**129–136.

163. **Walz, P. H., T. G. Bell, J. L. Wells, D. L. Grooms, L. Kaiser, R. K. Maes, and J. C. Baker.** 2001. Relationship between degree of viremia and disease manifestation in calves with experimentally induced bovine viral diarrhea virus infection. *Am. J. Vet. Res.* **62:**1095–1103.

164. **Welsh, M. D., B. M. Adair, and J. C. Foster.** 1995. Effect of BVD virus infection on alveolar macrophage functions. *Vet. Immunol. Immunopathol.* **46:**195–210.

165. **Westenbrink, F., P. J. Straver, T. G. Kimman, and P. W. de Leeuw.** 1989. Development of a neutralising antibody response to an inoculated cytopathic strain of bovine virus diarrhoea virus. *Vet. Rec.* **125:**262–265.

166. **Wilhelmsen, C. L., S. R. Bolin, J. F. Ridpath, N. F. Cheville, and J. P. Kluge.** 1990. Experimental primary postnatal bovine viral diarrhea viral infections in six-month-old calves. *Vet. Pathol.* **27:**235–243.

167. **Wilhelmsen, C. L., S. R. Bolin, J. F. Ridpath, N. F. Cheville, and J. P. Kluge.** 1991. Lesions and localization of viral antigen in tissues of cattle with experimentally induced or naturally acquired mucosal disease, or with naturally acquired chronic bovine viral diarrhea. *Am. J. Vet. Res.* **52:**269–275.

168. **Wittum, T. E., D. M. Grotelueschen, K. V. Brock, W. G. Kvasnicka, J. G. Floyd, C. L. Kelling, and K. G. Odde.** 2001. Persistent

bovine viral diarrhoea virus infection in US beef herds. *Prev. Vet. Med.* **49:**83–94.

169. **Woods, R. D., R. A. Kunkle, J. F. Ridpath, and S. R. Bolin.** 1999. Bovine viral diarrhea virus isolated from fetal calf serum enhances pathogenicity of attenuated transmissible gastroenteritis virus in neonatal pigs. *J. Vet. Diagn. Investig.* **11:**400–407.

170. **Wray, C., and P. L. Roeder.** 1987. Effect of bovine virus diarrhoea-mucosal disease virus infection on salmonella infection in calves. *Res. Vet. Sci.* **42:**213–218.

171. **Zhang, G., S. Aldridge, M. C. Clarke, and J. W. McCauley.** 1996. Cell death induced by cytopathic bovine viral diarrhoea virus is mediated by apoptosis. *J. Gen. Virol.* **77:**1677–1681.

INFECTIONS WITH MULTIPLE HEPATOTROPIC VIRUSES

Robert P. Myers, Vlad Ratziu, Yves Benhamou,
Vincent Di Martino, Joseph Moussalli, Marie Hélène Tainturier,
and Thierry Poynard

4

The hepatotropic viruses are a major public health problem representing the most common cause of liver disease worldwide. Viral hepatitis accounts for more than 15,000 deaths annually in the United States alone (34). Chronic infection with hepatitis B virus (HBV) is estimated to affect 400 million individuals globally, and is the leading cause of hepatocellular carcinoma (HCC) (76). It is estimated that 5% of HBV carriers, or approximately 20 million individuals, are coinfected with hepatitis D virus (HDV) (26). Hepatitis C virus (HCV), originally termed "non-A, non-B (NANB) hepatitis virus" and implicated in outbreaks of posttransfusion hepatitis, is estimated to affect more than 170 million people worldwide, and is the leading indication for liver transplantation in most centers (68). Furthermore, hepatitis A virus (HAV) is the most common cause of acute viral hepatitis in many countries, including the United States, where at least 130,000 infections occur annually (5). Although not a cause of chronic hepatitis, HAV superinfection has been implicated in the deterioration of patients chronically infected

with other hepatotropic viruses (58, 133). Considering the sheer prevalence of these infections, it is not surprising that coinfections are frequently encountered in the clinical setting. Furthermore, their propensity for chronicity sets the stage for superinfection with other hepatotropic viruses. Finally, their shared routes of transmission further compound this problem. HBV, HDV, and HCV are all transmitted through exposure to contaminated blood products. Thus, patients with parenteral exposures, particularly injection drug users and those who received transfusions before the era of sensitive screening assays, are at a particularly high risk of being infected with multiple hepatotropic viruses.

In this chapter, we aim to highlight the clinical, histologic, and virologic aspects of multiple hepatotropic viral infections. Features differentiating these from single hepatotropic infections and the mechanisms of viral interactions are emphasized. Furthermore, the efficacy and limitations of current treatment options are discussed in addition to future treatment approaches. Finally, the important interaction between the hepatotropic viruses and human immunodeficiency virus (HIV), not a hepatotropic virus per se, but frequently encountered in these patients because of common routes of transmission, will be reviewed.

Robert P. Myers, Vlad Ratziu, Yves Benhamou, Vincent Di Martino, Joseph Moussalli, Marie Hélène Tainturier, and Thierry Poynard, Service d'Hépato-Gastroentérologie, Groupe Hospitalier, Hôpital Pitié-Salpêtrière, 75651 Paris, France.

Polymicrobial Diseases, Edited by Kim A. Brogden and Janet M. Guthmiller,
© 2002 ASM Press, Washington, D.C.

ETIOLOGIC AGENTS

HAV

HAV is a single-stranded RNA virus in the family *Picornaviridae*. For decades it has been associated with outbreaks of "infectious hepatitis" stemming from fecally contaminated food and water, in particular, in countries with poor sanitary conditions (34). However, infections in industrialized nations are not infrequent, and often occur in outbreaks related to unsanitary food handling in restaurants (5). The clinical course of HAV infection ranges from asymptomatic infection, particularly in children, to fulminant hepatic failure necessitating liver transplantation. Most adults are symptomatic, with jaundice occurring in 70%, but infections are usually mild and self-limited; no chronic carrier state has been identified (61). However, the elderly (5, 61) and those with preexisting liver disease, particularly chronic HBV and HCV infection (58, 133), apparently are at an increased risk for severe hepatitis and death if superinfected with HAV. No effective treatment, other than supportive measures, is available for HAV infection. Vaccines are commercially available, effective, and well tolerated (59). International travelers, military personnel, and certain high-risk populations, including homosexual males and patients with chronic liver disease, have been targeted for vaccination (5).

HBV

HBV is a relaxed, circular, partially double-stranded DNA virus from the family *Hepadnaviridae* (26). Since its discovery nearly 35 years ago as the "Australia antigen" by Blumberg et al. (16), its virologic and clinical features have been investigated extensively. HBV DNA has four partially overlapping, open reading frames that encode: (i) the viral envelope proteins [including hepatitis B surface antigen (HBsAg)]; (ii) the nucleocapsid including the hepatitis Be (HBeAg) and core antigens (HBcAg) from the precore and core regions; (iii) the polymerase that has reverse transcriptase, DNA polymerase, and RNase activities involved in HBV

replication; and (iv) the X protein that is a potent transactivator and may play a role in hepatocarcinogenesis (76). Like HAV, acute HBV infection may be entirely asymptomatic, but 30% of patients have icteric hepatitis and some develop acute liver failure (26). The clinical features of chronic HBV infection include an asymptomatic carrier state, chronic hepatitis, cirrhosis, and HCC (26). The natural history of chronic infection varies with the time course of infection and host factors including age, gender, and race (36). When acquired perinatally or during infancy and childhood, either from an infected mother or close contact who is infected, as occurs in high-prevalence areas such as Southeast Asia and Africa, chronic infection ensues in more than 90% of individuals (26). These patients have a high risk of progression to cirrhosis and complications such as liver failure and HCC (36). When acquired in adulthood, usually by way of injection drug use or high-risk sexual practices, as occurs most often in North America, less than 5% of patients progress to chronicity, the remainder clearing HBsAg and remaining free of complications (26). Patients with chronic hepatitis B, and markers of active viral replication (including HBeAg and HBV-DNA positivity) and hepatic damage (including elevated liver enzymes and active necroinflammatory lesions on liver biopsy) are candidates for antiviral therapy. Currently, two forms of therapy are available: interferon alpha and the nucleoside analog lamivudine. Unfortunately, neither treatment is perfect; long-term response rates are only in the range of 20 to 30% (76). Again, as in HAV infection, effective vaccines are available and have proven effective in reducing the incidence of acute and chronic hepatitis (76, 80), and the incidence of childhood HCC in Taiwan (27), a major medical advance.

HCV

HCV is a single-stranded RNA virus in the family *Flaviviridae*, transmitted via the parenteral route. The virus has six major genotypes (1 to 6) with heterogeneous genetic sequences, and major differences in responsiveness to antiviral therapy. In North America and Western Europe, for example, HCV genotype 1 is found in approximately 70% of individuals and is notoriously resistant to interferon therapy (68). HCV causes acute icteric hepatitis in roughly 25% of individuals. Its major feature, however, is its propensity to cause chronic hepatitis in more than 80% of those infected (4). The natural history of chronic hepatitis C is generally characterized by slow histologic progression (98). Most patients remain asymptomatic or have nonspecific symptoms, and ultimately die of an unrelated condition (109, 110). Approximately 10 to 20% of individuals, however, progress to cirrhosis during a 20-year time span, and are at risk for complications including end-stage liver disease and HCC (98). This progressive fibrotic process is accelerated by factors including older age at infection, male gender, and alcohol consumption (96, 99). Thus far, because of the lack of small animal models and an effective cell culture system for HCV, as well as the genetic heterogeneity of the virus, development of a vaccine has been unsuccessful (69). Effective treatment, however, is available; long-acting, pegylated interferon in combination with ribavirin led to sustained clearance of HCV RNA from serum in approximately 60% of individuals (46, 87, 97, 146).

HDV

HDV is a defective RNA-containing passenger virus of the family *Deltaviridae* that requires the helper functions of HBV, including provision of the HBsAg coat, for virion assembly and penetration into hepatocytes. Transmission is by the same routes as HBV, mainly parenteral contact. The prevalence of HDV varies worldwide in correlation with that of HBV (101). With declining rates of HBV infection related to vaccination, the prevalence of HDV has also declined (41). The complex interaction of these two viruses is discussed below. The natural history of chronic HDV infection varies widely, but it has been linked to rapidly progressive liver disease (35, 38, 100, 106). In endemic areas, most individuals contract HDV

in their teenage years or early adulthood. Although most develop cirrhosis within a few years, the majority remain stable for two to three decades until they present with features of decompensation including esophageal variceal bleeding, ascites, and HCC (38, 101). The only approved therapy for chronic HDV is interferon alpha, but this leads to sustained clearance of the virus in less than 20% of noncirrhotic individuals (77, 103).

HEV

Hepatitis E virus (HEV) is a nonenveloped RNA virus of the family *Caliciviridae*. It is transmitted via the fecal-oral route, usually by contaminated water, and has been implicated in outbreaks and occasional sporadic cases of acute hepatitis in Southeast and Central Asia, Africa, the Middle East, and Mexico (34). In most cases, the clinical illness is similar to that of other forms of acute viral hepatitis. In pregnant women, however, acute HEV infection has been linked to serious illness with a case-fatality rate of nearly 25%. No chronic carrier state exists (34). The impact of HEV superinfection in patients with other hepatotropic viruses has rarely been studied, but it is not known to cause severe illness in these patients. In an Israeli study of 188 hemophiliacs, the prevalence of antibodies to HEV was 9% (7). The anti-HEV-seropositive hemophiliacs had the same seroprevalence of antibodies to HBV, HCV, and HIV, and the same number of cases with chronic hepatitis, as among those negative for anti-HEV. Because HEV is rare in North America and Europe, and it seems to have little impact on the course of other hepatotropic infections, HEV infection is not discussed further.

HGV

Hepatitis G virus (HGV) is a recently discovered, positive-stranded RNA virus that is a member of the family *Flaviviridae* (2, 75). HGV is transmitted parenterally (3), sexually (57), and perinatally (134). The prevalence of HGV infection is 1.4% among American blood donors, and approximately 10% among recipients of blood transfusions from the seventies to nineties (3). Since its discovery, numerous reports have attempted to link HGV to acute and chronic hepatitis (3), cryptogenic cirrhosis (28), and even HCC (74), but none have been convincing. Furthermore, as discussed, HGV infection apparently does not alter the clinical features or course of other hepatotropic infections (22, 86, 115, 124). HGV RNA levels decrease in many individuals receiving interferon treatment for coexistent HBV or HCV infection, but the results are transient (22, 67, 86). Ribavirin appears to have only a minimal antiviral effect (67).

COINFECTIONS WITH HEPATOTROPIC VIRUSES

HBV-HCV Coinfection

Since the identification of HCV in 1989 and development of an accurate serologic screening test (29, 64), interactions between HBV and HCV in coinfected individuals have been investigated extensively. Coexistent HCV infection is estimated to occur in 10 to 15% of patients with chronic hepatitis B, depending on the risk factors of the population studied (40, 93). Conversely, the prevalence of chronic hepatitis B in patients with hepatitis C is lower because of the greater propensity of HBV to clear spontaneously. In our own series of 3,546 French HCV-infected patients, only 119 (3.4%) were HBsAg-positive. Among these 119 patients, 34 (29%) were HIV-positive (T. Poynard, unpublished observations).

HBV-HCV coinfection is characterized by "viral interference," whereby the replication of one virus is suppressed by another (56, 93–95, 104). Early on, Brotman and colleagues reported this phenomenon in an animal study of 19 chimpanzees administered infected serum (20). In this study, all the chimpanzees exposed to HBV alone developed HBsAg positivity and biochemical hepatitis within 4 to 9 weeks after inoculation. On the contrary, only three of the seven animals inoculated with NANB and HBV simultaneously developed

liver enzyme abnormalities, and only five became positive for HBsAg. The onset of antigenemia was significantly delayed, and the duration of antigenemia and the clinical illness was significantly shorter in coinfected chimpanzees. The authors concluded that concurrent NANB infection had likely interfered with HBV replication and accounted for the apparent amelioration of the serologic and clinical features of HBV infection (20). These studies have been duplicated in other laboratories (21, 53, 132).

In most cases observed clinically, one virus remains dormant while the other replicates actively (72, 112). Most often, HCV replication is dominant, such that HBV DNA levels in serum (31, 56, 62, 72, 93, 104, 107) and liver (71, 142) are lower in coinfected individuals than in those with HBV alone. HCV genotype 1 may be particularly efficient in this regard (93, 94), but results have been inconsistent (56, 81). Several studies have also shown a lower frequency of HBV precore mutant strains (those unable to express HBeAg) in patients with dual (and triple) infection (56, 143). This may relate to an HCV-induced reduction in HBV synthesis because mutagenesis is directly related to the rate of HBV replication. The failure, however, to find a lower prevalence of precore mutants in HDV coinfection (56), which is also associated with a reduction in HBV replication (56, 81, 141), does not support this hypothesis. An alternative hypothesis, supported by an immunologic study assessing the proliferative responses of peripheral blood mononuclear cells to viral antigens (131), suggests that host immune responses react more vigorously to HCV antigens than those of HBV (56). The hitherto reduction in "selective pressure" exerted on HBV may explain the lower prevalence of precore mutant strains.

With respect to the replication of HCV, RNA levels tend to be lower in coinfected patients than in those with isolated HCV infection, suggesting that HBV replication exerts a counteracting inhibitory effect on the replication of HCV (56, 62, 81, 93, 104, 145). In some cases, HCV RNA is at very low levels or undetectable, and HBV is the dominant replicating virus (62). Furthermore, in other cases, patients may show alternating appearance of HBV DNA or HCV RNA with concomitant disappearance of the other virus (72). The role of host immunocompetence (e.g., organ transplantation or HIV infection) in affecting these interactions is unclear, although a recent study showed that coinfection with HIV had no impact on nucleic acid levels in HBV-HCV or HBV-HDV-HCV-coinfected patients (56).

The precise mechanism for these interactions is unknown, although it appears that several mechanisms involved in viral processes and host humoral and cellular immune responses can be implicated. For example, possible alterations in the mechanisms responsible for virus absorption, penetration and/or replication have been suggested (21). The induction of soluble mediators, including interferon, has been considered, but this cytokine was not detected in the serial serum samples of chimpanzees infected with NANB hepatitis (23). Other potential mediators include tumor necrosis factor alpha and interleukin 6, which appear to activate certain intracellular pathways that can down-regulate HBV gene expression (44). Another hypothesis relates to the subcellular localization of the HBV core protein, which is regulated by the cell cycle. It has been suggested that liver injury and the subsequent cell renewal induced by coexistent HCV infection may increase the expression of HBV epitopes on the hepatocyte surface (72). Subsequent T-lymphocyte-mediated elimination of HBV-infected hepatocytes may thus account for the reduced HBV DNA levels observed in serum and liver tissue. Finally, in a cotransfection study using a human hepatoma cell line (HuH-7), Shih and colleagues implicated the HCV core protein specifically in the down-regulation of the processes of transcription and encapsidation of HBV pregenomic RNA (113). In this study, the secretion of HBV viral particles, including the nucleocapsid and mature virion, was suppressed 20-fold in the presence of HCV structural genes. The authors suggested that the HCV core protein

mediates these effects via gene-regulatory functions (113). Pontisso and colleagues showed that the core protein of HCV genotypes 1 and 3 (not genotypes 2 and 4) share sequence homology with the HBV core protein (95). This potentially explains reciprocal inhibition of these viruses and the observation in some studies that HCV genotype 1 is a more potent inhibitor of HBV replication than the other HCV genotypes (93, 94). In light of all the available evidence, it seems that no single process can explain viral interference.

The impact of coinfection has been examined in the acute and chronic settings, and from the perspectives of both HBV and HCV in isolation. As in the chimpanzee experiments, in patients with chronic hepatitis B, HCV superinfection apparently increases the rate of HBsAg seroconversion by inhibiting HBV replication (71, 111). In doing so, HCV usurps HBV as the predominant cause of liver disease in these patients, as evidenced by liver biopsies showing HCV RNA, not HBV DNA, and histologic features compatible with chronic hepatitis C (71). In the setting of acute HBV-HCV coinfection, which has been reported in injection drug users and transfused patients, results have been discordant. An increased risk of acute liver failure has been reported (39, 140); however, others have described an attenuating effect of acute HCV on HBV-mediated hepatic damage (88). In one study, acute HBV-HCV coinfection was associated with a delay in the onset and a shortened duration of HBsAg seropositivity, and with lower peak aminotransferase levels (88).

In the chronic setting, HBV-HCV-coinfected patients seem to have more severe liver disease than those with isolated HBV infection (31, 40, 93, 104). For example, in a study of 148 patients with chronic hepatitis B, of whom 16 (11%) had coexistent HCV infection, the incidence of cirrhosis (44 versus 21%) and hepatic decompensation (24 versus 6%) were significantly higher in coinfected patients (40).

Similar results have been reported in studies using controls with isolated HCV infection (81, 104, 136, 145). In one study, 23 patients with chronic HBV-HCV coinfection were compared with 69 age- and sex-matched patients with hepatitis C, but negative for HBsAg (145). Although epidemiological, biochemical, and virologic parameters were the same between the groups, the prevalence of cirrhosis was significantly higher in those with dual infection. Among coinfected patients, HCV RNA levels were significantly lower in HBV DNA-positive patients, and histologic lesions (including piecemeal necrosis, fibrosis, and presence of cirrhosis) were more severe (145). We found similar results in a case-control study of 34 HBV-HCV-infected patients and 34 patients with isolated HCV infection matched on the basis of age, gender, alcohol consumption, and duration of HCV infection (81). In this study, serum HCV RNA levels were lower and more frequently undetectable [particularly in patients with serological markers of active HBV infection (HBeAg and/or HBV DNA)], fibrosis was greater, and a trend toward an increased prevalence of cirrhosis occurred in coinfected patients. Thus, it appears that HBV exerts an inhibitory effect on HCV replication, but contributes to accelerated liver injury in coinfected patients.

Because both viruses have been implicated in hepatocarcinogenesis, the influence of dual infection on the development of HCC has also been studied. HBV and HCV apparently act synergistically in this regard (13, 19, 144), in particular, with respect to the infiltrating variant of HCC (14). In a prospective study of 290 consecutive Italian patients with cirrhosis of varying etiologies, the cumulative incidence of HCC was 11% in HBsAg-positive cases, 9% in HCV-infected patients, and 36% in those with HBV-HCV coinfection (13). The significant effect of coinfection on the progression to HCC persisted in multivariate analysis in addition to the consistently identified risk factors of age and male gender. In another study from South Africa involving 231 black patients with HCC and matched controls, HBsAg positivity was associated with a 23-fold increase in the risk of HCC, whereas anti-HCV positivity was associated with a 6.6-fold risk (60). When both

markers were present, the relative risk rose to 82.5; dual infection was estimated to be the cause of 20% of HCC in this population. The mechanisms behind this synergism are unclear as are those underlying the hepatocarcinogenic potential of these viruses in isolation. It has been hypothesized that the oncogenic effects of HBV and HCV are related to chronic liver injury, which sets up a cascade of events including the increased rates of DNA synthesis necessary for cellular repair. This may set the scene for acquired DNA mutations that predispose to the development of HCC. If this is the case, HBV-HCV coinfection may exert its carcinogenic effect simply through enhanced hepatocellular injury as evidenced by the histologic studies. We also know that HCC is much more common in individuals with cirrhosis than those without cirrhosis. The synergism of HBV and HCV in causing HCC may occur via the propensity of coinfection to accelerate progression of fibrosis. Alternatively, the "hit" may occur after the development of cirrhosis, in the transition from cirrhosis to HCC. Whether the temporal course of HBV-HCV coinfection (i.e., simultaneous acquisition of both viruses, or superinfection of HBV in a patient with chronic hepatitis C, or vice versa) is a factor is also unclear.

HBV-HDV Coinfection

As described previously, HDV infection occurs only in the setting of coexistent HBV infection, acquired either simultaneously (coinfection) or through superinfection of a HBsAg-positive patient. The clinical course and virologic features differ markedly between these scenarios, but both are characterized by a complicated interplay between the two viruses. In HBV-HDV coinfection, acute hepatitis is usually icteric and often fulminant, likely more so than in HDV superinfection. Both viruses seem to replicate actively, but often in a transient manner (101). In fact, acute coinfection may have a biphasic nature with peaks of serum aminotransferases separated by several weeks; the first peak is typically related to active HBV replication, and the second to HDV replication (6). In milder cases of acute coinfection, HDV replication is lower and replication of HBV is suppressed by HDV (101). In fact, early suppression of HBV replication may be associated with a reduction in the synthesis of HBsAg. In such cases, the acute illness may be diagnosed as "non-A-E hepatitis" unless serologic markers for HDV are tested specifically (24). Most cases of coinfection resolve spontaneously; in fact, only 2% of coinfections evolve to chronic disease (102).

Cases of HDV superinfection are usually symptomatic and often lead to liver failure in patients with significant preexisting chronic hepatitis B (101). In general, HBV replication is suppressed markedly by superinfection with HDV, often to the point that HBV DNA is undetectable even by sensitive PCR-based assays. In a few fortunate patients, HBV replication is suppressed to the point of HBsAg clearance; that is, the HBV infection (and, therefore, the HDV infection) is aborted. In some, this inhibition is transient and accompanied by rising titers of antibody to HBsAg (anti-HBs), simulating resolution of HBV infection, only to 'relapse' when HDV replication diminishes after the acute illness. Unlike HDV coinfection, progression to chronicity occurs in approximately 90% of patients with HDV superinfection (101).

Most of the available literature suggests that chronic hepatitis D is a rapidly progressive disease, more so than isolated HBV infection (35, 38). Approximately 80% of individuals develop cirrhosis within 5 to 10 years of infection (35, 100, 101). Patients in whom both viruses are actively replicating seem to be at a particularly high risk of progression (106). Most patients with cirrhosis, however, remain stable until their fourth or fifth decade at which time they may show evidence of hepatic decompensation—one to two decades earlier than the typical patient with isolated HBV or HCV infection (35, 100, 101). Wu and colleagues investigated the virologic correlates of disease progression in 185 HBV-HDV-coinfected patient with use of sensitive PCR-based assays (141). As described above, acute HDV super-

infection was generally characterized by active HDV replication and HBV suppression with high alanine aminotransferase levels; during the chronic phase, HDV replication decreased and HBV synthesis reactivated with moderate alanine aminotransferase levels; and in the late phase, development of cirrhosis or HCC was associated with the replication of either virus, and disease remission with quiescence of both viruses (141).

HBV-HCV-HDV Coinfection

The relationship between the hepatotropic viruses in cases of triple infection is interesting; as in other hepatotropic coinfections, viral interference is prominent. We addressed this issue in a study of 16 patients with triple infection and 16 matched controls with isolated HCV infection (81). In patients with triple coinfection, HDV emerged as the dominant virus; 88% had markers of active HDV infection (HDV RNA, hepatitis D antigen, or IgM anti-HDV positivity). HCV RNA, on the other hand, was detectable in only 2 of 16 (12.5%) coinfected patients versus all the HCV-infected controls. Consequently, mean HCV RNA levels were significantly lower in the former group. Likewise, HBV replication, as indicated by the presence of HBeAg or detectable HBV DNA, was observed in only 27% of coinfected patients. A similar study from Spain confirmed the suppressive effect of HDV on HCV replication (56). In addition, using a control group of patients with isolated HBV infection, these authors documented suppression of HBV replication in patients with triple infection. In this study, the inhibitory influence of HDV was stronger on the replication of HCV than that of HBV (56). In terms of liver histology, necroinflammatory activity and fibrosis scores were significantly higher in the triple infection group, and the prevalence of cirrhosis was higher (58 versus 6%; $P = 0.004$) in our study (81).

Similar results have been reported in the post-liver transplantation setting (125). In a retrospective analysis of 13 HBV-HCV-co-infected patients undergoing transplantation for end-stage liver disease, 5 patients were also infected with HDV. After liver transplantation, HCV RNA was positive in all of the dually infected patients, but none of the patients with triple infection. With respect to liver damage, however, serum aminotransferases (admittedly a surrogate marker) were elevated in 88% of dually infected patients, but only 20% of those with triple infection. The authors concluded that HDV suppresses HCV replication and modulates the liver inflammatory process after liver transplantation in patients with HBV-HDV-HCV coinfection (125).

These results disagree with those of a Taiwanese group who reported that HCV, not HDV, dominates in patients with triple infection (73). In this study of 60 coinfected patients, HCV RNA was detectable in 70% of patients, HDV RNA in 23%, and HBV DNA in 13%. The reason for the discrepancy between these studies may relate to the study populations in terms of the timing of infection. Whereas the Taiwanese patients presumably acquired their infections perinatally or during early childhood, most of the patients in our study were infected as adults after blood transfusion or injection drug use. Differences in host immune responses and viral strains must also be considered. Whereas HDV genotype 1 predominates in Western Europe, HDV genotype 2 is more common in East Asia (56).

Coinfection with HGV in Chronic Hepatitis B and C

Coinfection with HGV apparently exists in 10 to 20% of patients with chronic hepatitis C (22, 86, 115, 124). Both agents are transfusion-transmissable, accounting for their high rate of association (3). Most reports suggest that HGV has a minimal impact, if any, on the virologic, biochemical, and histologic features, as well as clinical course, of HCV infection (22, 67, 115). In the largest such study thus far reported examining 671 patients with chronic hepatitis C, 65 patients (9.7%) were coinfected with HGV (115). In this study, no significant differences occurred in liver biochemistry, hepatic necroinflammation or fibrosis, or HCV geno-

type and viral load in HGV-infected versus uninfected controls. In this and other studies (22), patients with HGV had a shorter mean duration of infection with HCV, suggesting that HGV is a relatively recently introduced infection, at least in North American patients. Because most studies have shown no overall effect of HGV on liver fibrosis, this latter finding suggests that the rate of fibrosis in chronic hepatitis C may actually be increased by concurrent HGV infection. No studies, however, have carefully examined this issue by controlling for other factors, such as age, gender, and alcohol consumption, which influence the rate of fibrosis progression in this disease (96, 99).

The response to treatment, including antiviral therapy and liver transplantation, has also been examined in HCV-HGV-coinfected patients. Again, the impact of HGV coinfection apparently is minimal. The response to interferon therapy is unchanged (22, 67), and HGV status has no impact on patient or graft survival, or the recurrence of histological hepatitis in HCV-infected patients after liver transplantation (15, 22). In one study (22), HGV RNA levels decreased in all patients after transplantation. One possible explanation for this is that HCV may inhibit HGV replication, as observed in other forms of coinfection, because HCV RNA levels are know to climb substantially after transplantion (128). The failure to find any significant correlation between HGV and HCV RNA levels before transplantation, however, argues against this hypothesis and suggests that perhaps immunosuppressive therapy may play a role (22).

Not surprisingly, given their common modes of transmission, HGV infection is also frequent in patients with chronic hepatitis B, particularly those with HCV and/or HDV coinfection (mainly injection drug users) (37). In a study of 125 patients with chronic hepatitis B, 82 asymptomatic HBsAg carriers, and 103 healthy controls, the seroprevalence of HGV was 17, 16, and 17% (P = not significant) respectively (37). HGV coinfection apparently had no effect on the clinical course of the patients with chronic hepatitis B.

Superinfection with HAV in Chronic Hepatitis B and C

As discussed previously, the spectrum of illness caused by acute HAV is highly variable. Acute liver failure caused by HAV is uncommon, but often fatal, particularly in the elderly (61) and patients with a history of chronic hepatitis B or C (58, 133). In general, these individuals do not seem to be at an increased risk of acquiring HAV infection, although outbreaks of HAV have been reported in populations of injection drug users, a large proportion of whom are infected with HBV and HCV (49). Such epidemics presumably are related to the use of contaminated drug paraphernalia onto other behaviors such as high-risk sexual practices (49). The risk of HAV superinfection in patients with chronic hepatitis B is highlighted by the Shanghai epidemic of 1988 during which more than 300,000 individuals acquired HAV through the consumption of contaminated, raw shellfish (58). A retrospective analysis of this epidemic reported that the risk of death was 5.6-fold higher in patients with chronic HBV infection than in the general population (58). In the same study, 115,551 cases of HAV infection reported to the Centers for Disease Control between 1983 and 1988 were reviewed (58). In this analysis, the case-fatality rate was 58.5-fold greater in those with chronic HBV infection than in those without preexisting liver dysfunction.

Evidence linking acute HAV to more severe clinical outcomes in those with chronic hepatitis C is more controversial. In an alarming study from Italy, Vento and colleagues reported the course of 17 patients with chronic hepatitis C who acquired acute HAV infection (133). In this study, 41% of those infected developed acute liver failure and 86% of these individuals died, representing a case-fatality rate of 35%, approximately 45 times greater than the general population. These findings, however, have not been duplicated in other studies including several describing epidemics of HAV infection among intravenous drug abusers (49). Furthermore, retrospective analyses of cases of severe HAV infection have not revealed an increased prevalence of hepatitis C in affected patients (51).

In view of the potential severity of acute HAV in patients with preexisting liver disease, it is now recommended that all persons with chronic liver disease be vaccinated against HAV (5). Several HAV vaccines are commercially available and have been effective and well tolerated in patients with chronic hepatitis B and C (59). Indeed, vaccination has become the standard of care in these patients. In light of the relative rarity of acute HAV and the frequency of chronic hepatitis C in North America, and the high cost of available vaccines, we examined the cost-effectiveness of this recommendation in patients with chronic hepatitis C by using a decision analysis model (91). In this relatively low-prevalence area, routine vaccination of HCV-infected patients cost more than $21,000,000 (in 1998 Canadian dollars) per HAV-related death prevented. This expense is clearly in excess of traditional measures of cost-effectiveness particularly in today's era of finite healthcare resources. The feasibility of this approach in high-prevalence areas remains to be determined.

Coinfection with HIV in Chronic Hepatitis B and C

Although HIV is not a hepatotropic virus per se, coinfection with HIV and the hepatitis B and C viruses deserves mention for several reasons. First, coinfection occurs frequently because of common routes of transmission. In a French cohort study examining 1,935 HIV-positive patients, the prevalence of antibodies to HCV was 42.5%; this rose to 86.1% in patients with parenterally acquired HIV infection (predominantly injection drug users) (105). In the same cohort, the prevalence of antibodies to HBcAg, signifying prior exposure to HBV, was 56.4%; 6.9% had residual, chronic hepatitis B as evidenced by HBsAg positivity. Conversely, in our own cohort of 3,546 consecutive patients with chronic hepatitis C, 396 (11%) were positive for anti-HIV antibodies (Poynard, unpublished). Second, with the introduction of highly active antiretroviral therapy (HAART) in the nineties, the prognosis for HIV infection has improved significantly (90), such that chronic liver disease has emerged as an important cause of morbidity and mortality in these patients (89, 121). For example, in a retrospective analysis from an HIV/AIDS institution in Madrid, 9% of 1,670 consecutive admissions were attributable to end-stage liver disease (121). HCV, alone or in combination with other hepatotropic viruses, was responsible for 89% of these admissions; and liver-related deaths occurred in 15 individuals, representing 5% of all cases of in-hospital mortality. Finally, emerging evidence suggests that HIV and the hepatotropic viruses exert reciprocal effects that have negative implications for the respective diseases (45, 48, 92, 120, 123). The impact of the hepatotropic viruses on the progression of HIV-related disease is beyond the scope of this chapter, but the interested reader is referred elsewhere (45, 48, 92).

The Impact of HIV on HCV Infection

Most studies linking HIV infection to more severe disease in patients with hepatitis C have assessed virologic and histologic parameters. With respect to HCV virology, although results are conflicting, several studies suggest that HCV viremia is increased in the presence of HIV coinfection (8, 32, 83, 123, 127). Furthermore, HCV viral load seems to increase as HIV progresses (43, 83). It has been hypothesized that these findings relate to faulty cytotoxic (CD8$^+$) lymphocyte responses directed against HCV-infected hepatocytes and the HCV itself in patients with HIV coinfection (122). Paradoxically, although HAART leads to substantial reductions in HIV viral load and reciprocal increases in CD4$^+$ lymphocyte counts, this therapy apparently does not have an impact on HCV viremia (82). The explanation for this discordance in associations has yet to be elucidated.

Somewhat less controversial is the impact of HIV coinfection on hepatic histology in HCV-coinfected patients. HIV infection clearly intensifies the degree of hepatic necrosis and inflammation and accelerates the fibrotic process

that ultimately leads to cirrhosis and complications such as HCC, liver failure, and death (1, 9, 42, 123). We have studied the effect of HIV coinfection on hepatic pathology in a cohort of patients with chronic hepatitis C monitored at our institution (1, 9). HIV-HCV-coinfected patients were matched with HCV-infected controls for risk factors known to have an impact on liver fibrosis progression in hepatitis C (including age at infection, duration of infection, alcohol consumption, and gender) (96, 99). In a study of 58 HIV-HCV-coinfected patients and 58 HCV-infected controls, we found significantly higher scores for overall necroinflammatory activity, piecemeal necrosis, and a trend toward an increased frequency of cirrhosis in coinfected patients (1). When patients with advanced HIV disease (as defined by a CD4$^+$ count below 200 cells/μl) were compared with HIV-negative patients, the prevalence of cirrhosis was significantly higher in coinfected patients (10 versus 45%; $P = 0.003$). Other authors have duplicated these findings; in a Spanish series of injection drug users, the incidence of cirrhosis after 10 years of HCV infection was 14.9% in coinfected patients versus only 2.6% in those who were HIV negative (123).

In another study, we examined more rigorously hepatic fibrosis in a cohort of 244 coinfected patients in an attempt to identify risk factors for fibrosis progression in this population (9). In this study, the mean rate of fibrosis progression was significantly greater in coinfected patients than in well-matched, HCV-infected controls (0.181 versus 0.135 Metavir fibrosis units/year; $P < 0.0001$). At these rates of fibrosis progression, the median duration from HCV infection to cirrhosis was 26 years in HIV-infected patients versus 38 years in non-HIV-infected patients. With use of multivariate analysis, we identified alcohol consumption (>50 g/day), CD4$^+$ lymphocyte count (≤200 cells/μl), and age at infection (>25 years) as being independently associated with fibrosis progression in this population. As an example, an HIV-infected patient who has less than 200 CD4$^+$ cells/μl at the time of liver biopsy and drinks more than 50 g of alcohol daily could be expected to develop cirrhosis in only 16 years, whereas an HIV-infected patient with more than 200 CD4$^+$ cells/μl and drinking less alcohol would have an expected time to cirrhosis of 36 years (9). These results obviously have important implications for HIV-HCV-coinfected patients; alcohol consumption should be strongly discouraged, and antiviral therapy against HIV should be maximized in an attempt to maintain, and hopefully restore, the immune system.

With respect to the impact of antiviral therapy, per se, we recently investigated the role of protease inhibitors (PI) in the prevention of fibrosis progression in HIV-HCV-coinfected patients (12). In this study, PI therapy was associated with reduced necroinflammatory activity and a 4.7-fold reduction in the rate of progression to cirrhosis. After 15 years of follow-up, the actuarial rate of cirrhosis was 18% in PI-naïve patients versus only 5% in those who had received a PI. This protective effect was independent of CD4$^+$ lymphocyte count and HIV viral load, and not seen with other agents known to be effective against HIV, such as the nucleoside reverse transcriptase inhibitors (12).

Several explanations have been proposed for the damaging effects that HIV infection has in HCV-coinfected patients. First, as alluded to previously, HCV viremia may be increased in HIV-infected patients, particularly those with an advanced stage of HIV disease (8, 32, 83, 123, 127). Greater HCV replication may enhance the cytopathic effect of this virus on hepatocytes. It is most frequently suggested that the immunodeficiency associated with HIV infection is responsible for this phenomenon because of blunted T-lymphocyte responses (122). However, the failure to document a consistent relationship between HCV and HIV viral loads and CD4$^+$ lymphocyte counts, the absence of an association between HCV viral load and hepatic damage in the non-HIV-infected population, and our own observations with respect to HAART, would argue against this hypothesis. Alternatively, HIV and HCV may interact directly within lymphocytes or hepatocytes,

perhaps through the expression of various cytokines or adhesion molecules, which serve to alter the pathogenicity of HCV (1). Finally, it is known that HIV infects Kupffer cells and sinusoidal endothelial cells, but the importance of this interaction is unclear (54, 108). Kupffer cells are involved in the activation of hepatic stellate cells which are responsible for hepatic fibrosis. Likewise, an interaction between HIV and endothelial cells lining the sinusoids may be involved in perisinusoidal fibrosis, which is more frequent in coinfected patients (1).

Studies examining the impact of HIV coinfection on clinical outcomes in patients with chronic hepatitis C have revealed conclusions similar to those described above for virologic and histologic endpoints; HIV apparently has a negative impact on the morbidity and mortality of coinfected patients (33, 47, 126). In the largest reported study to our knowledge, which examined a cohort of 4,865 British hemophiliac males exposed to blood products at high risk of HCV contamination monitored between 1969 and 1993, the risk of death from liver-related causes was nearly fivefold higher in HIV-infected versus noninfected patients (33). Compared with the general population, liver-related deaths were nearly 94 times higher among male hemophiliacs with HIV (33). In another study of 255 hemophiliacs, liver failure was reported in 10.8% of HCV-infected patients 20 years after first exposure; the risk in HIV-HCV-coinfected patients was 21-fold higher than in those with HCV alone (126). Finally, a recent meta-analysis confirmed the detrimental effect of HIV infection on the clinical course of hepatitis C (47). In this review, the relative risks of progression to cirrhosis and hepatic decompensation were 2.07 (95% confidence interval, 1.40 to 3.07) and 6.14 (95% confidence interval, 2.86 to 13.20), respectively, in HIV-infected versus uninfected patients with chronic hepatitis C.

The Impact of HIV on HBV Infection

The outcome of chronic hepatitis B depends on the interaction between HBV, which is not directly cytopathic, and the immunologic response of the host to this virus (26). Not surprisingly, then, coinfection with HIV, which has a profound effect on host immunity, modifies the phenotype of chronic HBV infection. Most studies suggest that HIV has a permissive effect on HBV replication, that is, chronic hepatitis B patients with HIV have higher levels of HBV DNA (30, 45) and a greater proportion of hepatocyte nuclei which stain positive for HBcAg (30). Enhanced HBV replication may relate to decreased cytotoxic T (CD8$^+$) lymphocyte activity because of impairment of helper (CD4$^+$) T lymphocytes and monocyte function (30). Reports of exacerbations of chronic hepatitis B in HIV patients with immune reconstitution after the introduction of HAART lend further support to the importance of the immune system in this disease (25). Furthermore, patients with serologic markers of remote HBV infection may reactivate their disease as their immune system deteriorates because of advancing HIV infection (102).

Other features observed in HIV-HBV-coinfected patients deserve mention. In patients acutely infected with HBV, prior infection with HIV predisposes them to the development of the chronic HBV-carrier state (18, 114). These patients are more likely to express HBeAg (17), which has important implications for infectivity, and are less likely to have spontaneous seroconversion of HBeAg to anti-HBe (45, 63), an event that usually heralds clearance of the virus.

In the presence of HIV coinfection, serum aminotransferase concentrations tend to be lower, an effect that may increase with the progression of immunosuppression (17, 30, 45). Paradoxically, despite similar liver biochemistry, and liver biopsies that generally show no difference in the intensity of necroinflammation, those with HIV-HBV coinfection appear more likely to progress to cirrhosis (30). In fact, in one study of 132 homosexual men with chronic hepatitis B, the risk of cirrhosis was increased 4.2-fold in the presence of HIV infection, after controlling for confounders such as age, duration of HBV infection, HBeAg status, and alcohol consumption (30).

It is possible that some patients progress to advanced fibrosis or cirrhosis with only minimal hepatic inflammation, as seen in other immunosuppressed populations such as transplant recipients (128).

TREATMENT

Treatment of the patient infected with multiple hepatotropic viruses is largely empiric. Because patients with hepatic coinfections are typically excluded from randomized controlled trials, the existing literature consists predominantly of uncontrolled studies. The following review briefly describes the efficacy and difficulties associated with current approaches to treatment, and makes recommendations for therapy of this difficult population of patients.

HBV-HCV Coinfection

As discussed earlier, in most cases of HBV-HCV coinfection, one virus is dominant and the other is dormant with low or undetectable serum nucleic acid levels. In these situations, it is recommended that treatment be directed against the dominant virus with standard antiviral regimens (112). That being said, reports describing the efficacy of treatment in dually infected patients are limited. In one study of eight coinfected patients treated with interferon alpha (3 million units [MU] thrice weekly [TIW] for 6 months), liver enzymes normalized in only two patients, and HBsAg was lost in one (137). Long-term responses, including clearance of HBV DNA and HCV RNA, were not reported. In another study, 14 patients with detectable HBV DNA and HCV RNA were treated with interferon alpha 6 MU TIW for 6 months (50). Six months after the end of treatment, ten patients (71%) lost HBV DNA and four patients (29%) lost HCV RNA. In addition, all three HBeAg-positive patients cleared HBeAg after a flare at an average of 45 days into treatment. This report suggests that interferon therapy is effective in coinfected patients, particularly with respect to HBV clearance. On the contrary, Liaw retrospectively analyzed the responses to interferon of 15 patients with chronic HBV who were subsequently shown by serologic testing of stored serum to have dual infection with HCV (72). Only one of these patients cleared HBeAg and HBV DNA. Interferon therapy in patients with dual infection may successfully clear one virus, only to lead to symptomatic reactivation of the persistent virus at a later date (72, 135). Clearly, on the basis of the divergent results reported, randomized controlled trials of antiviral therapy are needed in this patient population.

HBV-HDV Coinfection

Numerous therapies have been tested in the treatment of chronic HDV infection, but most have been ineffective or downright detrimental. Interferon alpha is most widely used, but results have generally been disappointing (101). In a meta-analysis of five randomized, controlled trials in a total of 87 treated patients, Malaguarnera et al. reported a complete response (defined as sustained normalization of alanine aminotransferase, loss of HDV viremia, and improved histology during short-term follow-up) in 18.4% of interferon-treated patients versus only 1.5% of controls (77). Unfortunately, at standard doses and durations of therapy, prolonged responses are rare because relapses commonly occur after cessation of treatment. As a result, long-term therapy with high doses of interferon remains the recommended approach (66). Unfortunately, although useful in isolated HBV infection, the addition of lamivudine has not proven helpful for the eradication of HDV (138). In the future, long-acting, pegylated interferons, which are administered once weekly, may prove useful, particularly with respect to patient compliance during longer courses of therapy.

HBV-HCV-HDV Coinfection

Reports describing treatment in patients with triple hepatitis virus infection are sparse. In a single study of seven HBV-HDV-HCV-coinfected patients, interferon therapy at a dosage of 3 MU TIW for 6 months led to sustained liver enzyme normalization in only one patient (137). Virologic responses were not reported. On the basis of this single study, no firm recommendations can be made for the treatment of these coinfected patients.

HCV-HIV Coinfection

No randomized controlled trials of anti-HCV therapy have been reported in HIV-infected populations. Several small, uncontrolled studies of interferon alpha monotherapy have been published (20, 79, 84, 118), however. In the largest of these trials, 90 HIV-HCV-coinfected patients with $CD4^+$ lymphocyte counts above 200 cells/μl were treated with 5 MU of interferon TIW for 3 months (118). Responders were then treated for an additional 9 months with 3 MU TIW. Twelve months after treatment, a sustained response (defined as normalization of alanine aminotransferase and disappearance of HCV RNA from serum) was seen in 18 of the 80 patients (22.5%) who completed the study. This rate of response was no different from that observed in a control population of 27 HIV-negative patients (25.9%, P = not significant), and is consistent with those reported in HIV-negative patients (130). Two factors were independently associated with a response in HIV-positive patients: a $CD4^+$ lymphocyte count above 500 cells/μl, and a baseline HCV viral load below 10^7 copies/ml (118). The impact of baseline fibrosis on liver biopsy, which has an important impact on antiviral therapy in HIV-negative patients (87, 97), was not assessed in this trial. Because HIV-HCV-coinfected patients tend to have more advanced hepatic fibrosis, this may prove to be an important factor in determining the efficacy of antiviral therapy in this population.

More recently, an uncontrolled pilot study of interferon and ribavirin combination therapy, currently the standard of care in hepatitis C treatment, was reported in 20 HIV-HCV-coinfected patients (65). Treatment consisted of interferon alpha-2b 3 MU TIW and ribavirin 1,000 to 1,200 mg daily for 6 months. At the end of treatment, serum HCV RNA was no longer detectable in 50% of patients

(65). This rate is nearly identical with that observed in HIV-negative subjects treated for a similar duration in two large, randomized, controlled trials (87, 97). Although the rate of sustained virologic response was not reported, a recent report has suggested that the rate of relapse after cessation of treatment is similar in HIV-positive and -negative patients (119). Currently, several randomized controlled trials of combination therapy are ongoing in this patient population (Poynard, unpublished).

Treatment in both of the cited studies was well tolerated and seemed to have no effect on the progression of HIV infection (65, 117). This is an important point because previous reports have highlighted a rapid decline in $CD4^+$ lymphocyte counts following the introduction of interferon therapy in 10 to 15% of HIV-infected patients (116). Furthermore, HIV-positive patients frequently have cytopenias related to HIV and its therapies which may be exacerbated by both interferon and ribavirin. Finally, recent in vitro studies have highlighted important interactions between ribavirin and anti-HIV medications including zidovudine and stavudine (52). These interactions may predispose to adverse drug reactions and/or an insufficient anti-HIV effect. The significance of these effects in vivo has yet to be realized (55).

We recommend that HIV-HCV-co-infected patients be treated in expert centers, preferably in the setting of randomized, controlled trials. On the basis of the existing literature, combination therapy with interferon and ribavirin apparently is the treatment of choice. Pegylated interferons, which are being evaluated in ongoing studies and have shown positive preliminary results, may prove to be more efficacious in the future. Such therapy requires the close monitoring of $CD4^+$ lymphocyte counts and HIV viral loads, and the occurrence of treatment-related side effects. Alcohol consumption should be restricted in these patients because of its potent effect on the progression of hepatic fibrosis. Furthermore, because of the risk for severe hepatitis caused by superinfection with other hepatotropic viruses, and the frequent presence of risk factors that predispose to superinfection, these patients should receive HAV and HBV vaccination if they are susceptible. This vaccination preferably should be completed early in the course of HIV infection when immune responses to vaccination are maximal.

HBV-HIV Coinfection

The response to interferon therapy in HBV-HIV-coinfected patients is somewhat less promising than that reported in patients with HIV and HCV. Thus far, five uncontrolled studies of interferon therapy in dually infected patients have been published (78, 85, 129, 139, 147). In all, response rates have been modest with loss of HBeAg reported in fewer than 10% of patients. This rate is considerably lower than that reported in the HIV-negative patients enrolled in the same studies whose average response rate was 31% (76). Therefore, interferon seems to be a poor choice for therapy of HBV in the HIV-infected individual.

Another antiviral drug, lamivudine, has potent inhibitory effects on both HIV and HBV and has been tested in coinfected patients. In HIV-negative patients, lamivudine leads to rapid HBV DNA suppression to undetectable levels within a few weeks in most patients, and to HBeAg loss in 15 to 20% of patients after 1 year and nearly 40% after 3 years (70). The responses seen in HIV-positive patients seem lower, but prognostic factors and the duration of follow-up have not been taken into account. In a study of 57 patients treated with lamivudine for 1 to 5 years at our institution, HBV DNA suppression was observed in 47% of patients at 2 years, but this response dropped off dramatically to only 9% at 4 years with a 91% actuarial incidence of lamivudine resistance (10).

Trials of other nucleoside analogs, including adefovir dipivoxil in isolation and in combination, are currently underway and may hold promise for these patients who are at serious risk of morbidity and mortality (11). We evaluated the safety and efficacy of adefovir dipivoxil (10 mg daily) in an open-label trial for the treatment of lamivudine-resistant HBV infection in 35 HIV-infected patients (11). All patients had detectable serum HBV DNA despite lamivudine therapy, and mutations (M550V or M550I) in the HBV polymerase gene. Patients were treated for 48 weeks while continuing their existing anti-HIV therapy, including lamivudine. HIV disease in all patients was well controlled at screening, as assessed by HIV RNA levels (≤ 2.60 $\log_{10}$ copies/ml). Mean decreases in HBV DNA serum levels from baseline (8.64 $\pm$ 0.08 [standard error] $\log_{10}$ copies/ml) were 3.40 $\pm$ 0.12 $\log_{10}$ copies/ml at week 24 ($n = 31$) and 4.0 $\pm$ 0.17 $\log_{10}$ copies/ml at week 48 ($n = 29$) ($P <$ 0.0001), respectively. Two patients underwent HBeAg seroconversion at weeks 32 and 36, respectively. Adefovir dipivoxil was generally well tolerated; no significant changes in either HIV viral load or CD4$^+$ cell count were observed.

CONCLUSIONS

Multiple hepatotropic infections are common because of the high prevalence of these viruses in isolation, and their shared modes of transmission. In general, coinfections are associated with "viral interference," whereby one virus inhibits the replication of another. The mechanisms behind this phenomenon are poorly understood; however, it appears that a complex interplay between specific viral replicative processes and host humoral and cellular immunity are involved. In general, liver injury is more severe, the progression of fibrosis is more rapid, and clinical outcomes are worse in those coinfected with multiple hepatotropic viruses compared with patients with isolated infection. This highlights the importance of the development of effective vaccines and antiviral therapies, because current treatment options are clearly suboptimal.

ACKNOWLEDGMENTS

R.P.M. is supported by the Dr. V. Feinman Hepatology Fellowship from the Canadian Association for the Study of the Liver and Schering Canada and the Detweiler Traveling Fellowship from the Royal College of Physicians and Surgeons of Canada.

REFERENCES

1. **Allory, Y., F. Charlotte, Y. Benhamou, P. Opolon, Y. Le Charpentier, T. Poynard, and the MULTIVIRC Group.** 2000. Impact of human immunodeficiency virus infection on the histological features of chronic hepatitis C: a case-control study. *Hum. Pathol.* **31:**69–74.
2. **Alter, H. J.** 1996. The cloning and clinical implications of HGV and HGBV-C. *N. Engl. J. Med.* **334:**1536–1537.
3. **Alter, H. J., Y. Nakatsuji, J. Melpolder, J. Wages, R. Wesley, J. W. Shih, and J. P. Kim.** 1997. The incidence of transfusion-associated hepatitis G virus infection and its relation to liver disease. *N. Engl. J. Med.* **336:**747–754.
4. **Anonymous.** 1997. Management of hepatitis C: NIH Consensus Statement. *Hepatology* **15:**1–41.
5. **Anonymous.** 1999. Prevention of hepatitis A through active or passive immunization: recommendations of the Advisory Committee on Immunization Practices (ACIP). *Morb. Mortal. Wkly. Rep.* **48:**1–37.
6. **Balik, I., M. Onul, E. Tekeli, and F. Caredda.** 1991. Epidemiology and clinical outcome of hepatitis D virus infection in Turkey. *Eur. J. Epidemiol.* **7:**48–54.
7. **Barzilai, A., S. Schulman, Y. V. Karetnyi, M. O. Favorov, E. Levin, E. Mendelson, P. Weiss, H. A. Fields, D. Varon, and U. Martinowitz.** 1995. Hepatitis E virus infection in hemophiliacs. *J. Med. Virol.* **46:**153–156.
8. **Beld, M., M. Penning, V. Lukashov, M. McMorrow, M. Roos, N. Pakker, A. van den Hoek, and J. Goudsmit.** 1998. Evidence that both HIV and HIV-induced immunodeficiency enhance HCV replication among HCV seroconverters. *Virology* **244:**504–512.
9. **Benhamou, Y., M. Bochet, V. Di Martino, F. Charlotte, F. Azria, A. Coutellier, M. Vidaud, F. Bricaire, P. Opolon, C. Katlama, T. Poynard, and the Multivirc Group.** 1999. Liver fibrosis progression in human immunodeficiency virus and hepatitis C virus coinfected patients. *Hepatology* **30:**1054–1058.
10. **Benhamou, Y., M. Bochet, V. Thibault, V. Di Martino, E. Caumes, F. Bricaire, P. Opolon, C. Katlama, and T. Poynard.** 1999. Long-term incidence of hepatitis B virus resistance to lamivudine in human immunodeficiency virus-infected patients. *Hepatology* **30:**1302–1306.
11. **Benhamou, Y., M. Bochet, V. Thibault, V. Calvez, M. H. Fievet, C. Brosgart, J. Fry, C. S. Gibbs, P. Opolon, and T. Poynard.** 2001. An open-label pilot study of adefovir dipivoxil in HIV/HBV co-infected patients with lamivudine resistant HBV. *Lancet* **358:**718–723.

12. **Benhamou, Y., V. Di Martino, M. Bochet, G. Colombet, V. Thibault, A. Liou, C. Katlama, and T. Poynard.** 2001. Factors affecting liver fibrosis in human immunodeficiency virus and hepatitis C virus-coinfected patients: Impact of protease inhibitor therapy. *Hepatology* **34:**283–287.

13. **Benvegnu, L., G. Fattovich, F. Noventa, F. Tremolada, L. Chemello, A. Cecchetto, and A. Alberti.** 1994. Concurrent hepatitis B and C virus infection and risk of hepatocellular carcinoma in cirrhosis. A prospective study. *Cancer* **74:**2442–2448.

14. **Benvegnu, L., F. Noventa, E. Bernardinello, P. Pontisso, A. Gatta, and A. Alberti.** 2001. Evidence for an association between the aetiology of cirrhosis and pattern of hepatocellular carcinoma development. *Gut* **48:**110–115.

15. **Berenguer, M., N. A. Terrault, M. Piatak, A. Yun, J. P. Kim, J. Y. Lau, J. R. Lake, J. R. Roberts, N. L. Ascher, L. Ferrell, and T. L. Wright.** 1996. Hepatitis G virus infection in patients with hepatitis C virus infection undergoing liver transplantation. *Gastroenterology* **111:**1569–1575.

16. **Blumberg, B. S., B. J. Gerstley, D. A. Hungerford, W. T. London, and A. I. Sutnick.** 1967. A serum antigen (Australia antigen) in Down's syndrome, leukemia, and hepatitis. *Ann. Intern. Med.* **66:**924–931.

17. **Bodsworth, N., B. Donovan, and B. N. Nightingale.** 1989. The effect of concurrent human immunodeficiency virus infection on chronic hepatitis B: a study of 150 homosexual men. *J. Infect. Dis.* **160:**577–582.

18. **Bodsworth, N. J., D. A. Cooper, and B. Donovan.** 1991. The influence of human immunodeficiency virus type 1 infection on the development of the hepatitis B virus carrier state. *J. Infect. Dis.* **163:**1138–1140.

19. **Bonino, F., F. Oliveri, P. Colombatto, and M. R. Brunetto.** 1997. Impact of interferon-alpha therapy on the development of hepatocellular carcinoma in patients with liver cirrhosis: results of an international survey. *J. Viral. Hepat.* **4:**79–82.

20. **Boyer, N., P. Marcellin, C. Degott, F. Degos, A. G. Saimot, S. Erlinger, J. P. Benhamou, and the Comité des Anti-Viraux.** 1992. Recombinant interferon-alpha for chronic hepatitis C in patients positive for antibody to human immunodeficiency virus. *J. Infect. Dis.* **165:**723–726.

21. **Bradley, D. W., J. E. Maynard, K. A. McCaustland, B. L. Murphy, E. H. Cook, and J. W. Ebert.** 1983. Non-A, non-B hepatitis in chimpanzees: interference with acute hepatitis A virus and chronic hepatitis B virus infections. *J. Med. Virol.* **11:**207–213.

22. **Brandhagen, D. J., J. B. Gross, Jr., J. J. Poterucha, M. R. Charlton, J. Detmer, J. Kolberg, A. A. Gossard, K. P. Batts, W. R. Kim, J. J. Germer, R. H. Wiesner, and D. H. Persing.** 1999. The clinical significance of simultaneous infection with hepatitis G virus in patients with chronic hepatitis C. *Am. J. Gastroenterol.* **94:**1000–1005.

23. **Brotman, B., A. M. Prince, T. Huima, L. Richardson, M. C. van den Ende, and U. Pfeifer.** 1983. Interference between non-A, non-B and hepatitis B virus infection in chimpanzees. *J. Med. Virol.* **11:**191–205.

24. **Caredda, F., S. Antinori, C. Pastecchia, P. Coppin, M. Palla, A. Ponzetto, M. Rizzetto, and M. Moroni.** 1989. Incidence of hepatitis delta virus infection in acute HBsAg-negative hepatitis. *J. Infect. Dis.* **159:**977–979.

25. **Carr, A., and D. A. Cooper.** 1997. Restoration of immunity to chronic hepatitis B infection in HIV-infected patient on protease inhibitor. *Lancet* **349:**995–996.

26. **Chan, H. L., M. G. Ghany, and A. S. F. Lok.** 1999. Hepatitis B. *In* E. R. Schiff, M. F. Sorrell, and W. C. Maddrey (ed.), *Schiff's Diseases of the Liver,* 8th ed. [CD-ROM.] Lippincott Williams & Wilkins Publishers, Philadelphia, Pa.

27. **Chang, M. H., C. J. Chen, M. S. Lai, H. M. Hsu, T. C. Wu, M. S. Kong, D. C. Liang, W. Y. Shau, D. S. Chen, and the Taiwan Childhood Hepatoma Study Group.** 1997. Universal hepatitis B vaccination in Taiwan and the incidence of hepatocellular carcinoma in children. *N. Engl. J. Med.* **336:**1855–1859.

28. **Charlton, M. R., D. Brandhagen, R. H. Wiesner, J. B. Gross, Jr., J. Detmer, M. Collins, J. Kolberg, R. A. Krom, and D. H. Persing.** 1998. Hepatitis G virus infection in patients transplanted for cryptogenic cirrhosis: red flag or red herring? *Transplantation* **65:**73–76.

29. **Choo, Q. L., G. Kuo, A. J. Weiner, L. R. Overby, D. W. Bradley, and M. Houghton.** 1989. Isolation of a cDNA clone derived from a blood-borne non-A, non-B viral hepatitis genome. *Science* **244:**359–362.

30. **Colin, J. F., D. Cazals-Hatem, M. A. Loriot, M. Martinot-Peignoux, B. N. Pham, A. Auperin, C. Degott, J. P. Benhamou, S. Erlinger, D. Valla, and P. Marcellin.** 1999. Influence of human immunodeficiency virus infection on chronic hepatitis B in homosexual men. *Hepatology* **29:**1306–1310.

31. Crespo, J., J. L. Lozano, F. de la Cruz, L. Rodrigo, M. Rodriguez, G. San Miguel, E. Artinano, and F. Pons-Romero. 1994. Prevalence and significance of hepatitis C viremia in chronic active hepatitis B. *Am. J. Gastroenterol.* **89:** 1147–1151.

32. Daar, E. S., H. Lynn, S. Donfield, E. Gomperts, M. W. Hilgartner, W. K. Hoots, D. Chernoff, S. Arkin, W. Y. Wong, and C. A. Winkler. 2001. Relation between HIV-1 and hepatitis C viral load in patients with hemophilia. *J. Acquir. Immune Defic. Syndr.* **26:**466–472.

33. Darby, S. C., D. W. Ewart, P. L. Giangrande, R. J. Spooner, C. R. Rizza, G. M. Dusheiko, C. A. Lee, C. A. Ludlam, and F. E. Preston for the UK Haemophilia Centre Directors' Organisation. 1997. Mortality from liver cancer and liver disease in haemophilic men and boys in UK given blood products contaminated with hepatitis C. *Lancet* **350:**1425–1431.

34. Doo, E. C., and J. T. Liang. 1999. The hepatitis viruses. *In* E. R. Schiff, M. F. Sorrell, and W. C. Maddrey (ed.), *Schiff's Diseases of the Liver,* 8th ed. [CD-ROM.] Lippincott Williams & Wilkins Publishers, Philadelphia, Pa.

35. Fattovich, G., S. Boscaro, F. Noventa, E. Pornaro, D. Stenico, A. Alberti, A. Ruol, and G. Realdi. 1987. Influence of hepatitis delta virus infection on progression to cirrhosis in chronic hepatitis type B. *J. Infect. Dis.* **155:**931–935.

36. Fattovich, G., L. Brollo, G. Giustina, F. Noventa, P. Pontisso, A. Alberti, G. Realdi, and A. Ruol. 1991. Natural history and prognostic factors for chronic hepatitis type B. *Gut* **32:** 294–298.

37. Fattovich, G., M. L. Ribero, S. Favarato, F. Azzario, F. Donato, G. Giustina, M. Fasola, M. Pantalena, G. Portera, and A. Tagger. 1998. Influence of GB virus-C/hepatitis G virus infection on the long-term course of chronic hepatitis B. *Liver* **18:**360–365.

38. Fattovich, G., G. Giustina, E. Christensen, M. Pantalena, I. Zagni, G. Realdi, and S. W. Schalm for the European Concerted Action on Viral Hepatitis (Eurohep). 2000. Influence of hepatitis delta virus infection on morbidity and mortality in compensated cirrhosis type B. *Gut* **46:**420–426.

39. Feray, C., M. Gigou, D. Samuel, G. Reyes, J. Bernuau, M. Reynes, H. Bismuth, and C. Brechot. 1993. Hepatitis C virus RNA and hepatitis B virus DNA in serum and liver of patients with fulminant hepatitis. *Gastroenterology* **104:** 549–555.

40. Fong, T. L., A. M. Di Bisceglie, J. G. Waggoner, S. M. Banks, and J. H. Hoofnagle. 1991. The significance of antibody to hepatitis C virus in patients with chronic hepatitis B. *Hepatology* **14:**64–67.

41. Gaeta, G. B., T. Stroffolini, M. Chiaramonte, T. Ascione, G. Stornaiuolo, S. Lobello, E. Sagnelli, M. R. Brunetto, and M. Rizzetto. 2000. Chronic hepatitis D: a vanishing disease? An Italian multicenter study. *Hepatology* **32:**824–827.

42. Garcia-Samaniego, J., V. Soriano, J. Castilla, R. Bravo, A. Moreno, J. Carbo, A. Iniguez, J. Gonzalez, F. Munoz, and the Hepatitis/HIV Spanish Study Group. 1997. Influence of hepatitis C virus genotypes and HIV infection on histological severity of chronic hepatitis C. *Am. J. Gastroenterol.* **92:**1130–1134.

43. Ghany, M. G., C. Leissinger, R. Lagier, R. Sanchez-Pescador, and A. S. Lok. 1996. Effect of human immunodeficiency virus infection on hepatitis C virus infection in hemophiliacs. *Dig. Dis. Sci.* **41:**1265–1272.

44. Gilles, P. N., G. Fey, and F. V. Chisari. 1992. Tumor necrosis factor alpha negatively regulates hepatitis B virus gene expression in transgenic mice. *J. Virol.* **66:**3955–3960.

45. Gilson, R. J., A. E. Hawkins, M. R. Beecham, E. Ross, J. Waite, M. Briggs, T. McNally, G. E. Kelly, R. S. Tedder, and I. V. Weller. 1997. Interactions between HIV and hepatitis B virus in homosexual men: effects on the natural history of infection. *AIDS* **11:**597–606.

46. Glue, P., R. Rouzier-Panis, C. Raffanel, R. Sabo, S. K. Gupta, M. Salfi, S. Jacobs, R. P. Clement, and the Hepatitis C Intervention Therapy Group. 2000. A dose-ranging study of pegylated interferon alfa-2b and ribavirin in chronic hepatitis C. *Hepatology* **32:**647–653.

47. Graham, C. S., L. R. Baden, E. Yu, J. M. Mrus, J. Carnie, T. Heeren, and M. J. Koziel. 2001. Influence of human immunodeficiency virus infection on the course of hepatitis c virus infection: a meta-analysis. *Clin. Infect. Dis.* **33:**562–569.

48. Greub, G., B. Ledergerber, M. Battegay, P. Grob, L. Perrin, H. Furrer, P. Burgisser, P. Erb, K. Bogglan, J. C. Piffaretti, B. Hirschel, P. Janin, P. Francioli, M. Flepp, and A. Telenti. 2000. Clinical progression, survival, and immune recovery during antiretroviral therapy in patients with HIV-1 and hepatitis C virus coinfection: the Swiss HIV Cohort Study. *Lancet* **356:**1800–1805.

49. **Grinde, B., K. Stene-Johansen, B. Sharma, T. Hoel, M. Jensenius, and K. Skaug.** 1997. Characterisation of an epidemic of hepatitis A virus involving intravenous drug abusers—infection by needle sharing? *J. Med. Virol.* **53:**69–75.

50. **Guptan, R. C., V. Thakur, V. Raina, and S. K. Sarin.** 1999. Alpha-interferon therapy in chronic hepatitis due to active dual infection with hepatitis B and C viruses. *J. Gastroenterol. Hepatol.* **14:**893–898.

51. **Helbling, B., R. Kammerlander, and E. L. Renner.** 1998. Acute hepatitis A (AHA) in patients with chronic hepatitis C (CHC): no increased case-fatality rate. *Hepatology* **28:**276A. (Abstract.)

52. **Hoggard, P. G., S. Kewn, M. G. Barry, S. H. Khoo, and D. J. Back.** 1997. Effects of drugs on 2′,3′-dideoxy-2′,3′-didehydrothymidine phosphorylation in vitro. *Antimicrob. Agents Chemother.* **41:**1231–1236.

53. **Hollinger, F. B., G. Dolana, W. Thomas, and F. Gyorkey.** 1984. Reduction in risk of hepatitis transmission by heat-treatment of a human Factor VIII concentrate. *J. Infect. Dis.* **150:**250–262.

54. **Housset, C., E. Lamas, V. Courgnaud, O. Boucher, P. M. Girard, C. Marche, and C. Brechot.** 1993. Presence of HIV-1 in human parenchymal and non-parenchymal liver cells in vivo. *J. Hepatol.* **19:**252–258.

55. **Japour, A. J., J. J. Lertora, P. M. Meehan, J. Erice, J. D. Connor, B. P. Griffith, P. A. Clax, J. Holden-Wiltse, S. Hussey, M. Walesky, E. Cooney, R. Pollard, J. Timpone, C. McLaren, N. Johanneson, K. Wood, D. Booth, Y. Bassiakos, and C. S. Crumpacker.** 1996. A phase-I study of the safety, pharmacokinetics, and antiviral activity of combination didanosine and ribavirin in patients with HIV-1 disease. AIDS Clinical Trials Group 231 Protocol Team. *J. Acquir. Immune Defic. Syndr. Hum. Retrovirol.* **13:**235–246.

56. **Jardi, R., F. Rodriguez, M. Buti, X. Costa, M. Cotrina, R. Galimany, R. Esteban, and J. Guardia.** 2001. Role of hepatitis B, C, and D viruses in dual and triple infection: influence of viral genotypes and hepatitis B precore and basal core promoter mutations on viral replicative interference. *Hepatology* **34:**404–410.

57. **Kao, J. H., C. J. Liu, P. J. Chen, W. Chen, S. C. Hsiang, M. Y. Lai, and D. S. Chen.** 1997. Interspousal transmission of GB virus-C/hepatitis G virus: a comparison with hepatitis C virus. *J. Med. Virol.* **53:**348–353.

58. **Keeffe, E. B.** 1995. Is hepatitis A more severe in patients with chronic hepatitis B and other chronic liver diseases? *Am. J. Gastroenterol.* **90:**201–205.

59. **Keeffe, E. B., S. Iwarson, B. J. McMahon, K. L. Lindsay, R. S. Koff, M. Manns, R. Baumgarten, M. Wiese, M. Fourneau, A. Safary, R. Clemens, and D. S. Krause.** 1998. Safety and immunogenicity of hepatitis A vaccine in patients with chronic liver disease. *Hepatology* **27:**881–886.

60. **Kew, M. C., M. C. Yu, M. A. Kedda, A. Coppin, A. Sarkin, and J. Hodkinson.** 1997. The relative roles of hepatitis B and C viruses in the etiology of hepatocellular carcinoma in southern African blacks. *Gastroenterology* **112:**184–187.

61. **Koff, R. S.** 1992. Clinical manifestations and diagnosis of hepatitis A virus infection. *Vaccine* **10:**S15–S17.

62. **Koike, K., K. Yasuda, H. Yotsuyanagi, K. Moriya, K. Hino, K. Kurokawa, and S. Iino.** 1995. Dominant replication of either virus in dual infection with hepatitis viruses B and C. *J. Med. Virol.* **45:**236–239.

63. **Krogsgaard, K., B. O. Lindhardt, J. O. Nielson, P. Andersson, P. Kryger, J. Aldershvile, J. Gerstoft, and C. Pedersen.** 1987. The influence of HTLV-III infection on the natural history of hepatitis B virus infection in male homosexual HBsAg carriers. *Hepatology* **7:**37–41.

64. **Kuo, G., Q. L. Choo, H. J. Alter, G. L. Gitnick, A. G. Redeker, R. H. Purcell, T. Miyamura, J. L. Dienstag, M. J. Alter, C. E. Stevens, et al.** 1989. An assay for circulating antibodies to a major etiologic virus of human non-A, non-B hepatitis. *Science* **244:**362–364.

65. **Landau, A., D. Batisse, J. P. Van Huyen, C. Piketty, F. Bloch, G. Pialoux, L. Belec, J. P. Petite, L. Weiss, and M. D. Kazatchkine.** 2000. Efficacy and safety of combination therapy with interferon-alpha2b and ribavirin for chronic hepatitis C in HIV-infected patients. *AIDS* **14:**839–844.

66. **Lau, D. T., D. E. Kleiner, Y. Park, A. M. Di Bisceglie, and J. H. Hoofnagle.** 1999. Resolution of chronic delta hepatitis after 12 years of interferon alfa therapy. *Gastroenterology* **117:**1229–1233.

67. **Lau, J. Y., K. Qian, J. Detmer, M. L. Collins, E. Orito, J. A. Kolberg, M. S. Urdea, M. Mizokami, and G. L. Davis.** 1997. Effect of interferon-alpha and ribavirin therapy on serum GB virus C/hepatitis G virus (GBV-C/HGV) RNA levels in patients chronically infected with hepatitis C virus and GBV-C/HGV. *J. Infect. Dis.* **176:**421–426.

68. **Lauer, G. M., and B. D. Walker.** 2001. Hepatitis C virus infection. *N. Engl. J. Med.* **345:**41–52.

69. **Lechmann, M., and T. J. Liang.** 2000. Vaccine development for hepatitis C. *Semin. Liver Dis.* **20:**211–226.

70. **Leung, N. W., C. L. Lai, T. T. Chang, R. Guan, C. M. Lee, K. Y. Ng, S. G. Lim, P. C. Wu, J. C. Dent, S. Edmundson, L. D. Condreay, and R. N. Chien.** 2001. Extended lamivudine treatment in patients with chronic hepatitis B enhances hepatitis B e antigen seroconversion rates: results after 3 years of therapy. *Hepatology* **33:**1527–1532.

71. **Liaw, Y. F., S. L. Tsai, J. J. Chang, I. S. Sheen, R. N. Chien, D. Y. Lin, and C. M. Chu.** 1994. Displacement of hepatitis B virus by hepatitis C virus as the cause of continuing chronic hepatitis. *Gastroenterology* **106:**1048–1053.

72. **Liaw, Y. F.** 1995. Role of hepatitis C virus in dual and triple hepatitis virus infection. *Hepatology* **22:**1101–1108.

73. **Liaw, Y. F., S. L. Tsai, I. S. Sheen, M. Chao, C. T. Yeh, S. Y. Hsieh, and C. M. Chu.** 1998. Clinical and virological course of chronic hepatitis B virus infection with hepatitis C and D virus markers. *Am. J. Gastroenterol.* **93:**354–359.

74. **Lightfoot, K., M. Skelton, M. C. Kew, M. C. Yu, M. A. Kedda, A. Coppin, and J. Hodkinson.** 1997. Does hepatitis GB virus-C infection cause hepatocellular carcinoma in black Africans? *Hepatology* **26:**740–742.

75. **Linnen, J., J. Wages, Jr., Z. Y. Zhang-Keck, K. E. Fry, K. Z. Krawczynski, H. Alter, E. Koonin, M. Gallagher, M. Alter, S. Hadziyannis, P. Karayiannis, K. Fung, Y. Nakatsuji, J. W. Shih, L. Young, M. Piatak, Jr., C. Hoover, J. Fernandez, S. Chen, J. C. Zou, T. Morris, K. C. Hyams, S. Ismay, J. D. Lifson, J. P. Kim, et al.** 1996. Molecular cloning and disease association of hepatitis G virus: a transfusion-transmissible agent. *Science* **271:**505–508.

76. **Lok, A. S., E. J. Heathcote, and J. H. Hoofnagle.** 2001. Management of hepatitis B: 2000—summary of a workshop. *Gastroenterology* **120:**1828–1853.

77. **Malaguarnera, M., S. Restuccia, G. Pistone, P. Ruello, I. Giugno, and B. A. Trovato.** 1996. A meta-analysis of interferon-alpha treatment of hepatitis D virus infection. *Pharmacotherapy* **16:**609–614.

78. **Marcellin, P., N. Boyer, J. F. Colin, M. Martinot-Peignoux, V. Lefort, S. Matheron, S. Erlinger, and J. P. Benhamou.** 1993. Recombinant alpha interferon for chronic hepatitis B in anti-HIV positive patients receiving zidovudine. *Gut* **34:**S106.

79. **Marriott, E., S. Navas, J. del Romero, S. Garcia, I. Castillo, J. A. Quiroga, and V. Carreno.** 1993. Treatment with recombinant alpha-interferon of chronic hepatitis C in anti-HIV-positive patients. *J. Med. Virol.* **40:**107–111.

80. **Mast, E. E., F. J. Mahoney, M. J. Alter, and H. S. Margolis.** 1998. Progress toward elimination of hepatitis B virus transmission in the United States. *Vaccine* **16**(Suppl.):S48–S51.

81. **Mathurin, P., V. Thibault, K. Kadidja, N. Ganne-Carrie, J. Moussalli, M. El Younsi, V. Di Martino, F. Lunel, F. Charlotte, M. Vidaud, P. Opolon, and T. Poynard.** 2000. Replication status and histological features of patients with triple (B, C, D) and dual (B, C) hepatic infections. *J. Viral Hepat.* **7:**15–22.

82. **Matsiota-Bernard, P., G. Vrioni, C. Onody, L. Bernard, P. de Truchis, and C. Peronne.** 2001. Human immunodeficiency virus (HIV) protease inhibitors have no effect on hepatitis C virus (HCV) serum levels of HIV-HCV co-infected patients. *Int. J. Antimicrob. Agents* **17:**155–157.

83. **Matthews-Greer, J. M., G. C. Caldito, S. D. Adley, R. Willis, A. C. Mire, R. M. Jamison, K. L. McRae, J. W. King, and W. L. Chang.** 2001. Comparison of hepatitis C viral loads in patients with or without human immunodeficiency virus. *Clin. Diagn. Lab. Immunol.* **8:**690–694.

84. **Mauss, S., H. Klinker, A. Ulmer, R. Willers, B. Weissbrich, H. Albrecht, D. Haussinger, and H. Jablonowski.** 1998. Response to treatment of chronic hepatitis C with interferon alpha in patients infected with HIV-1 is associated with higher CD4+ cell count. *Infection* **26:**16–19.

85. **McDonald, J. A., L. Caruso, P. Karayiannis, L. J. Scully, J. R. Harris, G. E. Forster, and H. C. Thomas.** 1987. Diminished responsiveness of male homosexual chronic hepatitis B virus carriers with HTLV-III antibodies to recombinant alpha-interferon. *Hepatology* **7:**719–723.

86. **McHutchison, J. G., O. V. Nainan, M. J. Alter, A. Sedghi-Vaziri, J. Detmer, M. Collins, and J. Kolberg.** 1997. Hepatitis C and G co-infection: response to interferon therapy and quantitative changes in serum HGV-RNA. *Hepatology* **26:**1322–1327.

87. **McHutchison, J. G., S. C. Gordon, E. R. Schiff, M. L. Shiffman, W. M. Lee, V. K. Rustgi, Z. D. Goodman, M. H. Ling, S. Cort, J. K. Albrecht, and the Hepatitis Interventional Therapy Group.** 1998. Interferon alfa-2b alone or in combination with ribavirin as initial treatment for chronic hepatitis C. *N. Engl. J. Med.* **339:**1485–1492.

88. Mimms, L. T., J. W. Mosley, F. B. Hollinger, R. D. Aach, C. E. Stevens, M. Cunningham, D. V. Vallari, L. H. Barbosa, and G. J. Nemo. 1993. Effect of concurrent acute infection with hepatitis C virus on acute hepatitis B virus infection. *BMJ* **307**:1095–1097.

89. Monga, H. K., M. C. Rodriguez-Barradas, K. Breaux, K. Khattak, C. L. Troisi, M. Velez, and B. Yoffe. 2001. Hepatitis C virus infection-related morbidity and mortality among patients with human immunodeficiency virus infection. *Clin. Infect. Dis.* **33**:240–247.

90. Murphy, E. L., A. C. Collier, L. A. Kalish, S. F. Assmann, M. F. Para, T. P. Flanigan, P. N. Kumar, L. Mintz, F. R. Wallach, and G. J. Nemo. 2001. Highly active antiretroviral therapy decreases mortality and morbidity in patients with advanced HIV disease. *Ann. Intern. Med.* **135**:17–26.

91. Myers, R. P., J. C. Gregor, and P. J. Marotta. 2000. The cost-effectiveness of hepatitis A vaccination in patients with chronic hepatitis C. *Hepatology* **31**:834–839.

92. Piroth, L., M. Duong, C. Quantin, M. Abrahamowicz, R. Michardiere, L. S. Aho, M. Grappin, M. Buisson, A. Waldner, H. Portier, and P. Chavanet. 1998. Does hepatitis C virus co-infection accelerate clinical and immunological evolution of HIV-infected patients? *AIDS* **12**:381–388.

93. Pontisso, P., M. G. Ruvoletto, G. Fattovich, L. Chemello, A. Gallorini, A. Ruol, and A. Alberti. 1993. Clinical and virological profiles in patients with multiple hepatitis virus infections. *Gastroenterology* **105**:1529–1533.

94. Pontisso, P., M. Gerotto, M. G. Ruvoletto, G. Fattovich, L. Chemello, S. Tisminetzky, F. Baralle, and A. Alberti. 1996. Hepatitis C genotypes in patients with dual hepatitis B and C virus infection. *J. Med. Virol.* **48**:157–160.

95. Pontisso, P., M. Gerotto, L. Benvegnu, L. Chemello, and A. Alberti. 1998. Coinfection by hepatitis B virus and hepatitis C virus. *Antivir. Ther.* **3**:137–142.

96. Poynard, T., P. Bedossa, and P. Opolon. 1997. Natural history of liver fibrosis progression in patients with chronic hepatitis C. The OBSVIRC, METAVIR, CLINIVIR, and DOSVIRC groups. *Lancet* **349**:825–832.

97. Poynard, T., P. Marcellin, S. S. Lee, C. Niederau, G. S. Minuk, G. Ideo, V. Bain, J. Heathcote, S. Zeuzem, C. Trepo, J. Albrecht, and the International Hepatitis Interventional Therapy Group (IHIT). 1998. Randomised trial of interferon alpha2b plus ribavirin for 48 weeks or for 24 weeks versus interferon alpha2b plus placebo for 48 weeks for treatment of chronic infection with hepatitis C virus. *Lancet* **352**:1426–1432.

98. Poynard, T., V. Ratziu, Y. Benhamou, P. Opolon, P. Cacoub, and P. Bedossa. 2000. Natural history of HCV infection. *Bailliere's Best Pract. Res. Clin. Gastroenterol.* **14**:211–228.

99. Poynard, T., V. Ratziu, F. Charlotte, Z. Goodman, J. McHutchison, and J. Albrecht. 2001. Rates and risk factors of liver fibrosis progression in patients with chronic hepatitis C. *J. Hepatol.* **34**:730–739.

100. Rizzetto, M., G. Verme, S. Recchia, F. Bonino, P. Farci, S. Arico, R. Calzia, A. Picciotto, M. Colombo, and H. Popper. 1983. Chronic hepatitis in carriers of hepatitis B surface antigen, with intrahepatic expression of the delta antigen. An active and progressive disease unresponsive to immunosuppressive treatment. *Ann. Intern. Med.* **98**:437–441.

101. Rizzetto, M., and A. Smedile. 1999. Hepatitis D. *In* E. R. Schiff, M. F. Sorrell, and W. C. Maddrey (ed.), *Schiff's Diseases of the Liver,* 8th ed. [CD-ROM.] Lippincott Williams & Wilkins Publishers, Philadelphia, Pa.

102. Rodriguez-Mendez, M. L., A. Gonzalez-Quintela, A. Aguilera, and E. Barrio. 2000. Prevalence, patterns, and course of past hepatitis B virus infection in intravenous drug users with HIV-1 infection. *Am. J. Gastroenterol.* **95**:1316–1322.

103. Rosina, F., and M. Rizzetto. 1989. Treatment of chronic type D (delta) hepatitis with alpha interferon. *Semin. Liver Dis.* **9**:264–266.

104. Sagnelli, E., N. Coppola, C. Scolastico, P. Filippini, T. Santantonio, T. Stroffolini, and F. Piccinino. 2000. Virologic and clinical expressions of reciprocal inhibitory effect of hepatitis B, C, and delta viruses in patients with chronic hepatitis. *Hepatology* **32**:1106–1110.

105. Saillour, F., F. Dabis, M. Dupon, D. Lacoste, P. Trimoulet, P. Rispal E. Monlun, J. M. Ragnaud, P. Morlat, J. L. Pellegrin, H. Fleury, P. Couzigou, and the Groupe d'Épidémiologie Clinique du SIDA. 1996. Prevalence and determinants of antibodies to hepatitis C virus and markers for hepatitis B virus infection in patients with HIV infection in Aquitaine. *Br. Med. J.* **313**:461–464.

106. Saracco, G., F. Rosina, M. R. Brunetto, P. Amoroso, F. Caredda, P. Farci, P. Piantino, F. Bonino, and M. Rizzetto. 1987. Rapidly progressive HBsAg-positive hepatitis in Italy. The role of hepatitis delta virus infection. *J. Hepatol.* **5**:274–281.

107. Sato, S., S. Fujiyama, M. Tanaka, K. Yamasaki, I. Kuramoto, S. Kawano, T. Sato,

K. Mizuno, and S. Nonaka. 1994. Coinfection of hepatitis C virus in patients with chronic hepatitis B infection. *J. Hepatol.* **21:**159–166.

108. Scoazec, J. Y., and G. Feldmann. 1990. Both macrophages and endothelial cells of the human hepatic sinusoid express the CD4 molecule, a receptor for the human immunodeficiency virus. *Hepatology* **12:**505–510.

109. Seeff, L. B., Z. Buskell-Bales, E. C. Wright, S. J. Durako, H. J. Alter, F. L. Iber, F. B. Hollinger, G. Gitnick, R. G. Knodell, R. P. Perrillo, and the National Heart, Lung, and Blood Institute Study Group. 1992. Long-term mortality after transfusion-associated non-A, non-B hepatitis. *N. Engl. J. Med.* **327:**1906–1911.

110. Seeff, L. B., R. N. Miller, C. S. Rabkin, Z. Buskell-Bales, K. D. Straley-Eason, B. L. Smoak, L. D. Johnson, S. R. Lee, and E. L. Kaplan. 2000. 45-year follow-up of hepatitis C virus infection in healthy young adults. *Ann. Intern. Med.* **132:**105–111.

111. Sheen, I. S., Y. F. Liaw, D. Y. Lin, and C. M. Chu. 1994. Role of hepatitis C and delta viruses in the termination of chronic hepatitis B surface antigen carrier state: a multivariate analysis in a longitudinal follow-up study. *J. Infect. Dis.* **170:**358–361.

112. Sherman, M., for the CASL Hepatitis Consensus Group, Canadian Association for Study of the Liver. 1997. Management of viral hepatitis: clinical and public health perspectives—a consensus statement. *Can. J. Gastroenterol.* **11:**407–416.

113. Shih, C. M., S. J. Lo, T. Miyamura, S. Y. Chen, and Y. H. Lee. 1993. Suppression of hepatitis B virus expression and replication by hepatitis C virus core protein in HuH-7 cells. *J. Virol.* **67:**5823–5832.

114. Sinicco, A., R. Ralteri, M. Sciandra, C. Bertone, A. Lingua, B. Salassa, and P. Gioannini. 1997. Coinfection and superinfection of hepatitis B virus in patients infected with human immunodeficiency virus: no evidence of faster progression to AIDS. *Scand. J. Infect. Dis.* **29:**111–115.

115. Slimane, S. B., J. K. Albrecht, J. W. Fang, Z. Goodman, M. Mizokami, K. Qian, and J. Y. Lau. 2000. Clinical, virological and histological implications of GB virus-C/hepatitis G virus infection in patients with chronic hepatitis C virus infection: a multicentre study based on 671 patients. *J. Viral Hepat.* **7:**51–55.

116. Soriano, V., R. Bravo, J. G. Samaniego, J. Gonzalez, P. M. Odriozola, E. Arroyo, J. L. Vicario, A. Castro, M. Colmenero, E. Carballo, and the HIV-Hepatitis Spanish Study Group. 1994. CD4+ T-lymphocytopenia in HIV-infected patients receiving interferon therapy for chronic hepatitis C. *AIDS* **8:**1621–1622.

117. Soriano, V., J. Garcia-Samaniego, R. Bravo, J. Gonzalez, A. Castro, J. Castilla, P. Martinez-Odriozola, M. Colmenero, E. Carballo, D. Suarez, F. J. Rodriguez-Pinero, A. Moreno, J. del Romero, J. Pedreira, J. Gonzalez-Lahoz, and the Hepatitis-HIV Spanish Study Group. 1996. Interferon alpha for the treatment of chronic hepatitis C in patients infected with human immunodeficiency virus. *Clin. Infect. Dis.* **23:**585–591.

118. Soriano, V., J. Garcia-Samaniego, R. Bravo, J. Gonzalez, A. Castro, P. Martnez-Odriozola, M. Colmenero, E. Carballo, D. Suarez, J. Castilla, F. J. Rodriguez-Pinero, A. Moreno, J. del Romero, J. Pedreira, J. Gonzalez-Lahoz, and the Spanish Group for the Study of Viral Hepatitis in HIV+ Patients. 1986. The treatment of chronic hepatitis C with interferon in patients infected with the human immunodeficiency virus. *Med. Clin.* (Barcelona) **106:**486–490. (In Spanish.)

119. Soriano, V., R. Bravo, J. Garcia-Samaniego, J. Castilla, J. Gonzalez, A. Castro, J. M. Llibre, and the Hepatitis/HIV Spanish Study Group. 1997. Relapses of chronic hepatitis C in HIV-infected patients who responded to interferon therapy. *AIDS* **11:**400–401.

120. Soriano, V., J. Garcia-Samaniego, R. Rodriguez-Rosado, J. Gonzalez, and J. Pedreira. 1999. Hepatitis C and HIV infection: biological, clinical, and therapeutic implications. *J. Hepatol.* **31:**119–123.

121. Soriano, V., J. Garcia-Samaniego, E. Valencia, R. Rodriguez-Rosado, F. Munoz, and J. Gonzalez-Lahoz. 1999. Impact of chronic liver disease due to hepatitis viruses as cause of hospital admission and death in HIV-infected drug users. *Eur. J. Epidemiol.* **15:**1–4.

122. Soriano, V., R. Rodriguez-Rosado, and J. Garcia-Samaniego. 1999. Management of chronic hepatitis C in HIV-infected patients. *AIDS* **13:**539–546.

123. Soto, B., A. Sanchez-Quijano, L. Rodrigo, J. A. del Olmo, M. Garcia-Bengoechea, J. Hernandez-Quero, C. Rey, M. A. Abad, M. Rodriguez, M. Sales Gilabert, F. Gonzalez, P. Miron, A. Caruz, F. Relimpio, R. Torronteras, M. Leal, and E. Lissen. 1997. Human immunodeficiency virus infection modifies the natural history of chronic parenterally-

acquired hepatitis C with an unusually rapid progression to cirrhosis. *J. Hepatol.* **26**:1–5.

124. **Tanaka, E., H. J. Alter, Y. Nakatsuji, J. W. Shih, J. P. Kim, A. Matsumoto, M. Kobayashi, and K. Kiyosawa.** 1996. Effect of hepatitis G virus infection on chronic hepatitis C. *Ann. Intern. Med.* **125**:740–743.

125. **Taniguchi, M., A. O. Shakil, H. E. Vargas, T. Laskus, A. J. Demetris, T. Gayowski, S. F. Dodson, J. J. Fung, and J. Rakela.** 2000. Clinical and virologic outcomes of hepatitis B and C viral coinfection after liver transplantation: effect of viral hepatitis D. *Liver Transplant.* **6**:92–96.

126. **Telfer, P., C. Sabin, H. Devereux, F. Scott, G. Dusheiko, and C. Lee.** 1994. The progression of HCV-associated liver disease in a cohort of haemophilic patients. *Br. J. Haematol.* **87**:555–561.

127. **Telfer, P. T., D. Brown, H. Devereux, C. A. Lee, and G. M. DuSheiko.** 1994. HCV RNA levels and HIV infection: evidence for a viral interaction in haemophilic patients. *Br. J. Haematol.* **88**:397–399.

128. **Terrault, N. A.** 2000. Hepatitis C virus and liver transplantation. *Semin. Gastrointest. Dis.* **11**:96–114.

129. **Thevenot, T., V. Di Martino, J. F. Colin, F. Degos, S. Erlinger, J. P. Benhamou, and P. Marcellin.** 1998. Detrimental influence of HIV on the natural history and the interferon response rate in patients with chronic hepatitis B. *Gastroenterology* **114**:A1354. (Abstract.)

130. **Thevenot, T., C. Regimbeau, V. Ratziu, V. Leroy, P. Opolon, and T. Poynard.** 2001. Meta-analysis of interferon randomized trials in the treatment of viral hepatitis C in naive patients: 1999 update. *J. Viral Hepat.* **8**:48–62.

131. **Tsai, S. L., Y. F. Liaw, C. T. Yeh, C. M. Chu, and G. C. Kuo.** 1995. Cellular immune responses in patients with dual infection of hepatitis B and C viruses: dominant role of hepatitis C virus. *Hepatology* **21**:908–912.

132. **Tsiquaye, K. N., B. Portmann, G. Tovey, H. Kessler, S. Hu, X. Z. Lu, A. J. Zuckerman, J. Craske, and R. Williams.** 1983. Non-A, non-B hepatitis in persistent carriers of hepatitis B virus. *J. Med. Virol.* **11**:179–189.

133. **Vento, S., T. Garofano, C. Renzini, F. Cainelli, F. Casali, G. Ghironzi, T. Ferraro, and E. Concia.** 1998. Fulminant hepatitis associated with hepatitis A virus superinfection in patients with chronic hepatitis C. *N. Engl. J. Med.* **338**:286–290.

134. **Viazov, S., M. Riffelmann, S. Sarr, A. Ballauff, H. Meisel, and M. Roggendorf.** 1997.

Transmission of GBV-C/HGV from drug-addicted mothers to their babies. *J. Hepatol.* **27**:85–90.

135. **Villa, E., A. Grottola, P. Trande, Y. Selum, A. M. Rebecchi, A. Dugani, and F. Manenti.** 1993. Reactivation of hepatitis B virus infection induced by interferon (IFN) in HBsAg-positive, antiHCV-positive patients. *Lancet* **341**:1413.

136. **Villa, E., A. Grottola, P. Buttafoco, P. Trande, A. Merighi, N. Fratti, Y. Seium, G. Cioni, and F. Manenti.** 1995. Evidence for hepatitis B virus infection in patients with chronic hepatitis C with and without serological markers of hepatitis B. *Dig. Dis. Sci.* **40**:8–13.

137. **Weltman, M. D., A. Brotodihardjo, E. B. Crewe, G. C. Farrell, M. Bilous, J. M. Grierson, and C. Liddle.** 1995. Coinfection with hepatitis B and C or B, C and delta viruses results in severe chronic liver disease and responds poorly to interferon-alpha treatment. *J. Viral. Hepat.* **2**:39–45.

138. **Wolters, L. M., A. B. van Nunen, P. Honkoop, A. C. Vossen, H. G. Niesters, P. E. Zondervan, and R. A. de Man.** 2000. Lamivudine-high dose interferon combination therapy for chronic hepatitis B patients co-infected with the hepatitis D virus. *J. Viral. Hepat.* **7**:428–434.

139. **Wong, D. K., C. Yim, C. D. Naylor, E. Chen, M. Sherman, S. Vas, I. R. Wanless, S. Read, H. Li, and E. J. Heathcote.** 1995. Interferon alfa treatment of chronic hepatitis B: randomized trial in a predominantly homosexual male population. *Gastroenterology* **108**:165–171.

140. **Wu, J. C., C. L. Chen, M. C. Hou, T. Z. Chen, S. D. Lee, and K. J. Lo.** 1994. Multiple viral infection as the most common cause of fulminant and subfulminant viral hepatitis in an area endemic for hepatitis B: application and limitations of the polymerase chain reaction. *Hepatology* **19**:836–840.

141. **Wu, J. C., T. Z. Chen, Y. S. Huang, F. S. Yen, L. T. Ting, W. Y. Sheng, S. H. Tsay, and S. D. Lee.** 1995. Natural history of hepatitis D viral superinfection: significance of viremia detected by polymerase chain reaction. *Gastroenterology* **108**:796–802.

142. **Yap, S. H., J. A. Hellings, P. J. Rijntjes, A. M. van Loon, W. Duermeyer, and R. Stute.** 1985. Absence of detectable hepatitis B virus DNA in sera and liver of chimpanzees with non-A, non-B hepatitis. *J. Med. Virol.* **15**:343–350.

143. **Yeh, C. T., C. T. Chiu, S. L. Tsai, S. T. Hong, C. M. Chu, and Y. F. Liaw.**

1994. Absence of precore stop mutant in chronic dual (B and C) and triple (B, C, and D) hepatitis virus infection. *J. Infect. Dis.* **170:**1582–1585.

144. **Yu, M. C., M. J. Tong, P. Coursaget, R. K. Ross, S. Govindarajan, and B. E. Henderson.** 1990. Prevalence of hepatitis B and C viral markers in black and white patients with hepatocellular carcinoma in the United States. *J. Natl. Cancer Inst.* **82:**1038–1041.

145. **Zarski, J. P., B. Bohn, A. Bastie, J. M. Pawlotsky, M. Baud, F. Bost-Bezeaux, J. Tran van Nhieu, J. M. Seigneurin, C. Buffet, and D. Dhumeaux.** 1998. Characteristics of patients with dual infection by hepatitis B and C viruses. *J. Hepatol.* **28:**27–33.

146. **Zeuzem, S., S. V. Feinman, J. Rasenack, E. J. Heathcote, M. Y. Lai, E. Gane, J. O'-Grady, J. Reichen, M. Diago, A. Lin, J. Hoffman, and M. J. Brunda.** 2000. Peginterferon alfa-2a in patients with chronic hepatitis C. *N. Engl. J. Med.* **343:**1666–1672.

147. **Zylberberg, H., J. Jiang, G. Pialoux, F. Driss, F. Carnot, F. Dubois, C. Brechot, P. Berthelot, and S. Pol.** 1996. Alpha-interferon for chronic active hepatitis B in human immunodeficiency virus-infected patients. *Gastroenterol. Clin. Biol.* **20:**968–971.

CONCOMITANT INFECTIONS WITH HUMAN IMMUNODEFICIENCY VIRUS TYPE 1 AND HUMAN T-LYMPHOTROPIC VIRUS TYPES 1 AND 2

Abelardo Araujo, Noreen Sheehy, Hidehiro Takahashi, and William W. Hall

5

Two distinct families of human retroviruses, the human immunodeficiency viruses (HIVs) and human T-lymphotropic viruses (HTLVs), cause significant infections worldwide. The viruses have common modes of transmission, both vertically and horizontally, and share an in vivo tropism for cells of the immune system, and in particular, T lymphocytes. As a result a significant number of individuals worldwide have coinfection. At present, it is unclear if coinfection influences the natural history of infection or alters the pathogenicity of an individual virus and/or if this results in the development of unique clinical features. In this article, we summarize our current understanding of these issues with a specific focus on the influence of the HTLVs on the progression and outcome of HIV type 1 (HIV-1) infection.

EPIDEMIOLOGY AND MODES OF TRANSMISSION

It has now been established that HIV-1 and HIV-2 have arisen from cross-species transmis-

Abelardo Araujo, Centro de Pesquisa Hospital Evandro Changas, Ministerio da Saude, Av. Brasil, 4365, Manguinhos, Cep., Rio de Janeiro 21045-900, Brazil. *Noreen Sheehy and William W. Hall,* Department of Medical Microbiology, Conway Institute of Biomolecular and Biomedical Research, University College Dublin, Belfield, Dublin 4, Ireland. *Hidehiro Takahashi,* Department of Pathology, National Institute of Infectious Diseases, Tokyo, Japan.

sion from chimpanzees and sooty mangabeys, respectively, within the past century (189). HIV-1 and HIV-2 are members of a family of primate lentiviruses and have the characteristic properties of being cytopathic with high levels of replication and cell death at all stages of infection. HIV-2 appears to be less pathogenic than HIV-1 with a much slower progression of disease, and infection is relatively geographically restricted. In contrast, in the 20 years since the first description of AIDS, the HIV-1 pandemic remains unchecked, and it has been estimated that to date the cumulative number of individuals infected may be more than 56 million (147). Sexual transmission, predominantly heterosexual, is clearly the primary mode of infection worldwide. Horizontal transmission through contaminated blood products remains significant, and whereas donor screening in many countries has essentially eliminated transmission by blood transfusion, infection in intravenous drug users (IDUs) remains unabated in many areas of the world. The significance of HIV-2/HTLV coinfections remains poorly understood, and although individual reports have been made (121), these seem to occur much less frequently than with HIV-1. As such, this article primarily focuses on coinfections with HIV-1 and the HTLVs.

HTLV type 1 (HTLV-1) and type 2 (HTLV-2) are closely related members of a

Polymicrobial Diseases, Edited by Kim A. Brogden and Janet M. Guthmiller,
© 2002 ASM Press, Washington, D.C.

family of mammalian retroviruses having a similar genomic organization, sharing 65 to 70% nucleotide homology, and belonging to the HTLV/bovine leukemia virus (BLV) group of the subfamily *Oncovirinae* (49, 70). In contrast to the cytopathic effects of HIV-1, these viruses are relatively noncytopathic and instead often cause proliferation or expansion of infected cell populations. These viruses preferentially infect mature T lymphocytes, with HTLV-1 having a preferential tropism for $CD4^+$ and HTLV-2 having a preferential tropism for $CD8^+$ T lymphocytes (85, 152). In addition, in settings of high proviral loads, infection has been found to extend to non-T-cell populations, including monocytes and B lymphocytes (28, 85, 102, 152). As discussed in detail below, infection is lifelong; it is transmissible vertically by breast-feeding and horizontally by sexual intercourse and contaminated blood products through transfusion of blood and intravenous drug usage. Despite having similar modes of transmission, the efficiencies of transmission of HTLV-1 and -2 are much less than the efficiencies of HIV-1 transmission, because the former are cell-associated and require transfer of infected cells in contrast to the cell-free nature of HIV-1.

HTLV-1 is endemic in many well-defined geographic areas including Japan, the Caribbean, sub-Saharan Africa, South and North America, and Melanesia (49, 70); at present, approximately 20 million individuals are infected worldwide. Most infected individuals are clinically asymptomatic (asymptomatic carriers) but remain infectious throughout their lifetimes. HTLV-2 infection has been prevalent in blood donors and can be considered epidemic among IDUs in the United States, Europe, South America, and Asia (10, 18, 28, 40–42, 45, 47, 52, 53, 69, 71, 72, 97, 98, 105–107, 113, 114, 129, 153, 158, 159, 181, 198). Infection rates vary widely in different geographic areas ranging from less than 1% in certain European countries to as high as 60% in parts of Vietnam. In many countries HTLV-2 infection is more prevalent in IDUs with HIV-1 infection than in those who are not infected (40). The virus has also been endemic in numerous native American Indian

groups (1, 11, 12, 14, 22, 31, 39, 42, 48, 51, 62, 83, 86, 87, 100, 110, 111, 113, 118, 122, 144, 146, 176). At present, no estimates are available for the global number of HTLV-2 infections. Molecular analysis of HTLV-2 isolates from both IDUs and the endemically infected populations noted above have shown the existence of three distinct subtypes, 2a, 2b, and 2c, which can be differentiated on the basis of a combination of genetic and phenotypic analyses (42, 72, 113). At present, there is no evidence that there are differences in the pathogenic properties of these subtypes. HTLV-2a is the predominant infection in urban areas and particularly in IDUs in North America (38, 72). HTLV-2b infection also occurs in IDUs both in North America and Southern Europe and is also the predominant infection in native Amerindian groups in the Americas with the exception of Brazil (38, 42, 72, 113). HTLV-2c is unique, because to date it has been found exclusively in Brazil both in native Amerindian groups and in urban areas, particularly in IDUs (42, 113). HTLV-2 infection in the African continent, specifically among African pygmies, has also been reported (32, 33, 50, 57, 64, 65, 180), and an African origin of HTLV-2 is suggested by the discovery of a fourth and quite divergent HTLV-2d subtype in Efe pygmies and of related simian viruses isolated from African bonobos (*Pan paniscus*) (66, 185). The origin of HTLV-2 among native Amerindians is unclear, but it is likely that this virus was introduced to the American continent some 15,000 to 35,000 years ago during migrations across the Bering land bridge of HTLV-2-infected Asian groups, which were the ancestors of present-day American Indians. The spread of HTLV-2 among IDUs is almost certainly a recent occurrence, and it is most probable that American IDUs initially acquired the infection from native American Indians. After this introduction, which probably occurred within the past 50 years (159), the virus has successively spread among IDUs through sharing of needles and other drug paraphernalia. Finally, there may have been at least two separate introductions of HTLV-2 into European IDUs from the United States, perhaps at different times, at least one for the 2b subtype in Southern Europe and a second for the 2a subtype in Northern Europe (40). The introduction of HTLV-2 to Southeast Asia almost certainly originated from U.S. military personnel during the Vietnam War, probably through drug use and contaminated blood products (52).

HTLV-1-related simian viruses, termed simian T-lymphotropic virus type 1 (STLV-1), have been discovered in many nonhuman primates in Africa and in Asia (84, 172, 187). HTLV-1 and STLV-1 cannot be separated into distinct phylogenetic groups according to their species of origin but instead are related or grouped on the basis of geographic origin (183), suggesting frequent interspecies transmission (160, 161). As noted above, a simian relative of HTLV-2, termed STLV-2, has been identified in *P. paniscus* in Africa (60, 115, 184). STLV-2 clusters distinctly from HTLV-2 in phylogenetic analysis, indicating that either there has been ancient interspecies transmission in Africa, or possibly that there has been a coevolution of STLV-2 and HTLV-2 within their respective hosts (182, 185).

As noted above, HIV-1 and HTLV-1 and -2 have common modes of transmission. With HTLV-1 and -2, horizontal infection via contaminated cellular blood products is an important route of transmission (35, 82, 140, 175). As for HIV-1, the introduction of donor screening in many countries has markedly reduced transmission by blood transfusion but this remains a major mode of transmission in IDUs. Whereas HTLV-2 transmission in IDUs occurs worldwide, HTLV-1 transmission in this population is essentially restricted to a small number areas of endemic HTLV-1 infection and notably Brazil (19, 69). It seems certain that the high rates of infection of HTLV-2 in IDUs are caused by the exchange of contaminated blood in shared syringes and other drug-using equipment. However, it remains unclear why the prevalence of HTLV-2 infection in IDUs in the majority of countries is so much higher than that of HTLV-1.

Sexual transmission also seems to be an important means of HTLV-1 and HTLV-2 infec-

tion (81, 92, 95). Studies in areas where HTLV-1 is endemic have shown that heterosexual transmission seems to be more efficient from male to female, and the chance of transmission of HTLV-1 to wives of infected men is approximately 60% (92). In contrast transmission from seropositive women to their uninfected husbands is 0.4%, and this adequately accounts for the much higher seropositivity rates in older women in areas in which HTLV-1 is endemic (16). A similar increase in the prevalence of antibodies to HTLV-2 in women compared with men has also been observed in several of the South American Indian groups (87). This with the extremely high infection rates, which have been reported in elderly women in these populations, supports the importance of sexual transmission of the virus. Indirect support for heterosexual transmission comes also from the observation that among female blood donors who have been shown to have HTLV-2 infection, the most important documented risk factor was sexual contact with an IDU.

Vertical transmission also appears to be extremely important in the maintenance of infection in areas of endemicity. In areas where HTLV-1 is endemic, mother-to-child transmission occurs primarily through breast-feeding (79, 99, 174), and as many as 25% of breast-fed infants become infected. Perinatal infection occurs much less frequently with less than 5% of children born to infected mothers who did not breast-feed becoming infected. A study of Kayapo Indian groups in Brazil, where HTLV-2 infection is endemic, provided strong evidence that vertical transmission is extremely important, with high rates of seropositivity (in some instances, over 20% in children under the age of 9). In addition, familial studies demonstrated that the chance of infection in a child born to an infected mother could be as high as 50% (87). Although the routes of vertical transmission are unknown, these and other studies (101) have suggested that vertical transmission occurs primarily through breast-feeding. It is unclear if HTLV-2 infection may also occur in utero.

However, one study has reported that of 20 children born to 19 HTLV-2-infected mothers who did not breast-feed, none became infected, suggesting that this route may be of much less importance (94).

HTLV-1 CLINICAL FEATURES AND INFLUENCE OF HIV-1 INFECTION

The spectrum of HTLV-1-related illness ranges from lymphoproliferative malignancies to several inflammatory disorders. The former, adult T-cell leukemia/lymphoma (ATLL), is a group of CD4$^+$ T-cell malignancies with distinct clinical subtypes (178). ATLL generally occurs in individuals infected early in life, often shortly after birth, which suggests that infection of an immature or developing immune system may be important in pathogenesis. ATLL develops after some 20 to 50 years, and the lifetime risk in asymptomatic carriers is between 1 and 5%. The distinct clinical subtypes include the acute, smoldering, chronic, and lymphomatous forms of disease (169). The acute and lymphomatotus forms are clinically the most aggressive and present with extensive lymphadenopathy, hepatosplenomegaly, lytic bone lesions with an associated hypercalcemia, and visceral involvement with skin, gastrointestinal tract, and lung infiltration (178). In addition, these patients are functionally immunocompromised and may develop a variety of opportunistic infections similar to that observed in HIV-1 infection and AIDS. Acute ATLL is characterized by an aggressive CD4$^+$ T-cell leukemia, whereas in the lymphomatous form less than 1% of leukemic cells are present in peripheral blood. Both forms of ATLL have an extremely poor prognosis, with a median survival of approximately 6 and 10 months, respectively. Smoldering ATLL is characterized by skin or lung infiltration without any other visceral involvement, and an absence or only a low number of leukemic cells in peripheral blood. In chronic ATLL, a higher leukocyte count is observed, and this is associated with a lymphadenopathy and hepatosplenomegaly. However, in both of these forms there is no hypercalcemia and no visceral involvement.

The pathogenetic mechanisms involved in the development of ATLL are incompletely understood, but the viral regulatory protein Tax is believed to play a central role. This is related specifically to the ability of Tax to deregulate several normal cellular processes including intracellular protein signalling, transcription of genes involved in cellular proliferation, cell cycle control, and apoptosis (49, 193).

HTLV-1 Tax is a potent transcriptional transactivator not only of viral genes but also of cellular gene expression (49, 193). Tax does not bind DNA directly but physically interacts with many cellular transcription factors that include cyclic AMP (cAMP) response element/activating transcription factor (CREB/ATF) family members, components of the NF-κB/Rel signalling complex, and serum response factors. In many cases this results in the upregulation of a range of cellular genes involved in cell proliferation. These include the genes for interleukin-2 (IL-2) and the IL-2 receptor. The activities of such gene products are believed to contribute to the expansion of infected and possibly transformed cell populations. Although upregulation of these cellular genes may be important in the transformation process, this is also certainly related to the ability of Tax to also disrupt cell-cycle control and apoptosis. Tax upregulates cyclic D2 expression and stimulates G$_1$-to-S-phase transition through upregulated CD4/C4 and CDK6 activities (162, 164). Tax also directly binds and affects the activity of several cell-cycle regulatory proteins, including p15, p16, and cyclin D3 (117, 138).

In addition to disruption of normal G$_1$-to-S-phase transition, Tax interacts with an M-phase regulator HsMADI (91), the human homologue of the yeast mitotic checkpoint MADI protein. Overexpression of Tax and HsMADI results in multinucleated cells, which could explain the karyotypic abnormalities seen in ATLL. The tumor suppressor protein p53 plays a key role in cell cycle control, and Tax has also been shown to disrupt the normal function of this protein. In the presence of Tax, p53 is unable to maintain G_1 arrest in response to DNA damage and is also unable to trigger apoptosis when overexpressed. Several recent studies have shown that wild-type p53 protein is stabilized and functionally impaired in HTLV-1-transformed cultured cells, resulting in reduced induction of p53-responsive genes (25, 148, 149). However, HTLV-1 Tax does not seem to interact directly with p53 but instead is thought to alter posttranslational modification of the protein, thus abrogating its function.

It has also been reported (17, 162) that Tax expression induces IL-2-independent proliferation and resistance to apoptosis in IL-2-dependent cutaneous T-cell leukemia/lymphoma type 2 (CTLL-2) cells. In addition, a number of other in vitro studies have shown that Tax alone can induce bcl-2 and bcl-XL expression and apoptosis resistance (68, 139); it is believed that the poor responses of ATLL to conventional chemotherapeutic regimens (169, 178) may be caused by Tax-related apoptosis resistance.

At present, effective treatment of the aggressive forms of ATLL remains poor, and standard combination chemotherapy regimens as used in other lymphoid malignancies have been largely unsuccessful. Survival is directly related to the subtype of ATLL. In a large study of ATLL in Japan (169), the median survival time of ATLL and the projected 4-year survival rate were 6.2 months and 5%, respectively, for the acute type; 10.2 months and 5.7%, respectively, for the lymphomatous type; and 24.3 months and 26.9%, respectively, for the chronic type. In the smoldering type, the median survival was not reached after a median follow-up of 13.3 months, but the projected 4-year survival rate was only about 60%. Recently, there have been reports of the treatment of ATLL with a combination of the reverse transcriptase (RT) inhibitor zidovudine (AZT) and alpha interferon (IFN-α) with good response rates and little toxicity (59, 77, 125). The success of directed antiretroviral therapy in the treatment of ATLL suggests that active virus replication in vivo exists; it also indicates that the use of higher doses of AZT possibly with other antiretroviral agents combined with IFN-α and/or other immune modulators might also prove effective (4). Other agents which also might have a role include biological mediators such as retinoic acid, which induces apoptosis of ATL cells in vitro (4, 43). The recent demonstration that the combination of arsenic trioxide and IFN-α induces specific degradation of the viral transactivator Tax in HTLV-1-transformed cells in vitro, followed by cell cycle arrest and apoptosis of HTLV-1-positive cells, indicates that this could also be effective in vivo (4).

It is unclear if HIV-1 coinfection can influence the development of ATLL or its response to treatment. Although individual cases of the development of ATLL (168) in the setting of HTLV-1 and HIV-1 coinfection have been reported, these have not been of sufficient number to investigate this in detail.

Inflammatory diseases associated with HTLV-1 include the neurological disorder HTLV-1-associated myelopathy/tropical spastic paraparesis (HAM/TSP) (56, 142). The onset of HAM/TSP generally occurs in the 3rd and 4th decades of life, although it has been described to occur in children as young as 6 years. HAM/TSP occurs more frequently in women than in men, and the onset is usually subacute and insidious. Initial symptoms generally include stiffness, with weakness of the lower extremities, and urgency and frequency of urination. Physical findings are weakness of the legs with spasticity, hyperreflexia, and extensor plantar responses. Although strength in the arms is usually preserved, deep tendon reflexes tend to be brisk in the upper extremities, and sensory findings are usually minimal. The lifetime risk of developing HAM/TSP is similar to that of ATLL, and although the pathogenesis is understood incompletely, this disorder is associated with high HTLV-1 proviral loads ranging from 10- to 100-fold greater than that seen in asymptomatic carriers (136). Similarly, high levels of specific antiviral cytotoxic T-cell responses, which correlate with high viral loads, seem to be important, and the frequency of such responses is also significantly higher in individuals with HAM/TSP than in asymptomatic carriers (135). HAM is characterized by a perivascular lymphocytic infiltration in the central nervous system, notably in the thoracic region of the spinal cord and mainly in the early phases of the disease. Investigations in the pathogenesis of HAM have focused on the potential role of HTLV-1 Tax-specific CD8$^+$ cytotoxic T lymphocytes (CTL), and it has been suggested that during cytotoxic T-cell killing, cytokines and lymphokines released may produce local parenchymal damage (9). It is unclear why certain individuals develop HAM/TSP and others develop ATLL; however, genetic factors seem to be important (89, 90, 192), and in relation to HAM/TSP, several have been identified that seem either to be protective or to predispose to the development of this disorder (89, 90). It is unclear if concomitant HIV-1 infection might influence the development of HAM/TSP or if HTLV-1 might influence the development of HIV-1-associated neurological disease (6). In this regard one report from Brazil compared the development of myelopathy in individuals coinfected versus those infected with HIV-1 alone. A statistically significant higher proportion of coinfected individuals developed not only myelopathy but also peripheral neuropathy (75). However, the relative contribution of each virus to the development of myelopathy could not be determined. In addition, it is unclear if all patients who developed myelopathy would fully satisfy the clinical criteria for HAM/TSP.

To date, no consistently effective treatments for HAM/TSP have been reported. Interventions with corticosteroids, plasmapheresis, interferon, and, more recently, with antiretroviral drugs have been attempted, but with mixed and generally poor results. Early reports on the use of AZT produced conflicting results (67, 166).

Recently, virological improvement has been reported for HAM/TSP patients receiving the RT inhibitor lamivudine (3TC). Specifically, treatment resulted in a 10-fold re-duction in levels of proviral DNA in five patients with HAM/TSP, and in one of these there was a concomitant fall in the frequency of HTLV-1-specific CTL responses (179). This also suggests that active RT activity and virus replication are important in HTLV-1 infection and in patients with HAM/TSP. The observation that lamivudine can reduce HTLV-1 proviral loads in vivo contrasts with in vitro susceptibility studies of RT inhibitors. Garcia-Lerma and coworkers (54) studied five HTLV-1 isolates and found that, although they were susceptible to AZT, dideoxycytosine, dideoxyinosine, and stavudine, all had inherent high-level resistance to 3TC, suggesting that the latter may not be useful in treatment of HTLV-1 infections. The development of resistance apparently is not a problem at present, because no mutations developed in the RT region of the HTLV-1 provirus, whereas resistance was present in HIV-1 in five HIV-1/HTLV-1-coinfected patients who had been treated with AZT (55). More recently, a study of two TSP/HAM patients treated with AZT plus 3TC showed that whereas one patient had a 2-log-unit decrease in HTLV-1 proviral load, an increase of 1 log unit was observed in the second after several months of treatment (120). The reasons for these conflicting data are unclear, but it is possible that the RT inhibitors used may have other effects perhaps involving normal cellular processes in addition to inhibition of reverse transcription. Little experience has taken place in the use of protease inhibitors in treating HTLV-1 infections. However, a comparison of the substrate specificities of HTLV-1 and HIV-1 suggests that the substrate binding site of the HTLV-1 protease is more extended than that of the HIV-1. It remains unclear, however, if these differences will be reflected in vivo both in terms of susceptibility to protease inhibitors and of the range of inhibitors available for effective treatment.

Other inflammatory processes associated with HTLV-1 include uveitis, arthritis, thyroiditis, alveolitis, and in children an infective dermatitis (49). The pathogenesis of these disorders remains unknown, but their development also seems to be associated with high proviral loads. At present, it is unclear if concomitant HIV-1 infection may alter the natural history or development of these disorders.

HTLV-2 CLINICAL FEATURES AND INFLUENCE OF HIV-1 INFECTION

In contrast to HTLV-1, the role of HTLV-2 in human disease remains poorly defined; however, increasing evidence shows that the infection may also be associated with rare lymphoproliferative and a spectrum of neurological disorders (70). In addition, several epidemiological studies have suggested that underlying HTLV-2 infection may predispose to the development of a wide range of bacterial infections. The major limitations of many these studies are that they have often been based on individual case reports and that many patients have also had concomitant HIV-1 infection. As a result, in some instances it has been difficult to accurately assess the exact role of HTLV-2 and to confidently define and establish contributing factors that might have arisen from HIV-1 coinfection. Moreover, because numerous HTLV-2-infected patients have a history of intravenous drug use, it is unclear if this activity or related activities could also have confounded the analysis and interpretation of the clinical studies. In this section the clinical disorders that have been associated with HTLV-2 infection are summarized, and where possible the role and impact of HIV-1 coinfection is discussed.

Lymphoproliferative Disorders

The first two isolations of HTLV-2 were from cultures of peripheral blood lymphocytes of patients with hairy cell leukemia (93, 155). Although subsequent studies using both serological and molecular methods have failed to support the involvement of HTLV-2 in this disorder, reevaluation of one of these patients showed that, in addition to hairy cell leukemia, a coexisting $CD8^+$ T-lymphoproliferative process occurred (154). Molecular studies showed integration of the HTLV-2 provirus in

the $CD8^+$ T lymphocytes but not in the malignant hairy cell population (154). This was the first direct demonstration of the potential of HTLV-2 to cause lymphoproliferative disorders, and in contrast to HTLV-1, this involved $CD8^+$ T lymphocytes. Subsequently, several reports described HTLV-2 infection in patients with disorders of large granular lymphocytes (116, 123). Specifically, two patients with large granular lymphocytic leukemia and one with a large granular lymphocytosis were shown to have HTLV-2 infection. However, as noted in the patient with hairy cell leukemia, it could be shown that in the latter patient the provirus was not present in the abnormal large granular lymphocytes but instead was found primarily in the $CD8^+$ T-lymphocyte population. In addition, serological evaluation of numerous additional patients did not support a role for HTLV-2 infection in disorders involving large granular lymphocytes. It is thus unclear if infection of $CD8^+$ T lymphocytes in these patients was merely coincidental or if it contributed in any way to the development of their lymphoproliferative disorders. The observation that HTLV-2 had infected $CD8^+$ T lymphocytes in two such diverse clinical conditions is consistent with the direct studies of Ijichi and colleagues (85), who demonstrated that the virus has a preferential in vivo tropism for this lymphocyte population in both HTLV-2-infected and HTLV-2/HIV-coinfected individuals.

In the setting of HIV-1 and HTLV-2 coinfection we observed the development of a syndrome of severe exfoliative erythroderma with prominent dermal infiltration with $CD8^+$ T lymphocytes, lymphadenopathy, and eosinophilia in two IDUs (96). Although this disorder clinically resembled a cutaneous T-cell leukemia/lymphoma, no attempts were made to determine whether the infiltrating $CD8^+$ T-cell populations were clonal or represented a malignant expansion. However, subsequently Poiesz et al. (150) described a patient also infected with HIV-1 and HTLV-2 with a closely similar if not identical clinical presentation in whom a clonal $CD3^+$ $CD8^+$

CD4$^-$ cutaneous T-cell lymphoma was diagnosed. Taken together, these studies have clearly demonstrated that HTLV-2 infection can result in proliferation of infected CD8$^+$ T-lymphocyte populations, which seem in most instances to be clinically benign. However, in the setting of HIV-1 infection it seems possible that malignant CD8$^+$ T-lymphoproliferative disorders can develop. It remains unclear if HIV-1 infection directly contributes to the development of these disorders or if this may be secondary to a state of generalized immunosuppression. Because an intact immune system would be essential in controlling the expansion of HTLV-2-infected T lymphocytes, HIV-1 coinfection could alter this and, as a result, coinfected individuals might be expected to develop a higher incidence of HTLV-2-associated T-cell malignant disorders. It is also possible that after HTLV-2 infection alone, additional intracellular events could occur which could also lead to transformation as in ATLL.

Neurological Disorders

By analogy with HTLV-1, HTLV-2 infection might also be expected to be associated with neurological disorders. The first descriptions of such disorders were from two patients who were dually infected with HIV-1 and HTLV-2 and who presented with a myelopathy indistinguishable from HAM/TSP (7, 156). Subsequently, a report (80) described two sisters only infected with HTLV-2, who had developed a chronic neurodegenerative process characterized by spasticity, paraparesis, and prominent ataxia. Overall, the clinical features were suggestive of a syndrome of the olivopontocerebellar atrophy variant of multiple system atrophy. Although these two patients had spasticity as a prominent component of their illness, this disorder did not remotely resemble HAM/TSP. The association of HTLV-2 with spastic ataxia was supported by two studies in Miami, which described two and four females, respectively (73, 167), with a distinctive picture of ataxia, spasticity, and variable alterations in mental status. Although it is unclear if these two studies may have included some of the same patients, these reports strongly support an association of HTLV-2 and neurological disorders where ataxia is a prominent feature. Subsequently, at least five other reports (13, 88, 109, 131, 132) described patients with single HTLV-2 infection who presented with symptoms identical with classical HAM/TSP. In addition to myelopathy, a single report told of the development of a spinocerebellar syndrome in a HTLV-2-infected Guaymi Indian from Panama (23). Similar syndromes have been described in several patients with HTLV-1 infection, and it has been suggested that this may represent a unique neurological manifestation of either HTLV-1 or HTLV-2 infection (23). In a recent study of a cohort of HIV-1-coinfected individuals, the prevalence of antibodies to HTLV-2 was significantly higher in those with a predominantly sensory polyneuropathy (PSP) than in asymptomatic controls (196). Moreover, patients with PSP have higher proviral loads than those without PSP (197), which is similar to that in individuals with HAM/TSP compared with asymptomatic carriers (136). To date, all cases of neurological disease, with only one exception that was singly infected with HTLV-2, were female, which is similar to HTLV-1 where females have also been found to be more likely to develop HAM/TSP. In addition to specific disease entities epidemiological studies have suggested that HTLV-2 may cause a form of generalized neurological dysfunction. In a cohort of IDUs, HTLV-2 infection was independently associated with the development of global neurological disability (36).

Thus, although support is now increasing for the existence of HTLV-2-associated neurological syndromes, the real frequency of each of these syndromes is unknown. As already noted, confounding elements exist, which often make it difficult to definitely attribute infection to the clinical outcome. HIV-1 can cause a variety of neurological disorders, and this may have played a role in some of the disorders described above. Moreover, because many HTLV-2-infected individuals may be involved in drug usage, the effect of these compounds or adulterants used in their preparation may also confound any study involving such individuals (21, 137).

Prospective studies of endemically infected Amerindian groups, which would be relatively free of confounders such as HIV and intravenous drug usage, will help elucidate the exact role of HTLV-2 in neurological disease. However, it is possible that these studies might be confounded by other factors such as nutritional deficiencies. Similarly, it might be expected that unique neurological disorders or perhaps other related diseases (173) will present only in the setting of HIV-1 and HTLV-2 coinfection, and long-term prospective studies in this population will help to resolve this.

HTLV-2 and Infectious Disease

Murphy and coworkers in the Retrovirus Epidemiology Donor Study (REDS) have conducted prospective studies of HTLV-1- and HTLV-2-infected and seronegative individuals in five U.S. cities to determine whether HTLV-2 is associated with an increased incidence of infectious diseases. At the time of enrollment initial observations suggested that HTLV-2 infection was associated with a history of pneumonia and with urogenital and soft tissue infections within the previous 5 years (133, 134, 165, 188). Follow-up evaluation approximately 2 years after enrollment supported the view that HTLV-2 infection seemed to be associated with an increased incidence of bronchitis, bladder or kidney infection, and oral herpes infection, with the overall conclusion that there is an increased incidence of infectious diseases among otherwise healthy HTLV-2-infected individuals (133, 134). An independent study of HTLV-2-infected IDUs (126) also demonstrated the existence of an increased risk for the development of bacterial pneumonia, soft tissue abscess formation, and lymphadenopathy compared with noninfected IDUs. However, these findings were not confirmed by Safaeian and coworkers (157), who failed to demonstrate an association of HTLV-2 infection with the development of bacterial pneumonia, infective

endocarditis, and soft tissue abscess formation. Moreover, Murphy et al. (130), in a more detailed study of IDUs, failed to confirm their earlier findings that HTLV-2 infection was associated with abscess formation. The reasons for the conflicting findings are unclear, but confounding factors including race, sex, and frequency of intravenous drug use may have played a role. Recently, an investigation into cause-specific mortality in a large population of IDUs with HIV and HTLV-2 infections failed to demonstrate that HTLV-2 infection was significantly associated with mortality from any cause, and it was suggested that the virus was not a significant pathogen even in the setting of concomitant HIV infection (61).

To date, experience in the treatment of HTLV-2 infections has been extremely limited. Machucha et al. (120) evaluated the responses in two HTLV-2/HIV-1-coinfected patients receiving triple antiretroviral drug combinations including lamivudine and a protease inhibitor. The two HTLV-2/HIV-1-coinfected patients showed an initial increase in HTLV-2 proviral load after beginning treatment, followed by a slight decline several months later. As expected, plasma HIV-1 RNA declined to <50 copies/ml in both patients during therapy. Thus, it is unclear if antiretroviral therapy will prove to be of benefit. However, in the setting of increased viral loads with myelopathy or another neurological disorder, empiric treatment might be warranted and might prove beneficial.

INFLUENCE OF HTLV-1 AND HTLV-2 INFECTION ON HIV-1 INFECTION

Concomitant infections with HIV-1 and HTLV-2 are common in urban areas worldwide primarily as a result of intravenous drug use. In contrast, infections with HTLV-1 and HIV-1 are relatively restricted to geographical regions endemic for HTLV-1. Coinfection with HTLV-1 and HIV-1 infection in IDUs is comparatively rare, although recent reports have suggested that it may be as significant as that involving HTLV-2 in certain urban areas of Brazil. Information on the influence of

HTLV-1 and HTLV-2 infections on the progression of HIV-1 infection is conflicting. Although many have suggested an acceleration of HIV-1 infection (3, 44, 58, 63, 76, 108, 143, 163), others showed little or no influence (78, 186) and one study even suggested the possibility of a slowing of HIV-1 progression (190). Unfortunately, most of these studies have been limited by small numbers of patients, by the inability to determine exactly the relationship between the origins and relative timing of the HIV-1 and HTLV-1/2 infections, and in some cases, by the fact that in several studies no attempts were made to differentiate between HTLV-1 and -2 (108, 143). One exception was an international study specifically designed to determine whether HTLV-2 infection may influence the progression of HIV-1 infection (78). In all, a total of 370 IDUs from three urban areas in the United States and one in Italy, all of whom had seroconverted to HIV-1 positivity within 2 years, were enrolled. Of these, 61 (16%) were coinfected with HTLV-2 and patient follow-up times ranged from 5 to 10 years. With use of the development of an AIDS-defining illness and death as end points, it could be clearly shown that HTLV-2 coinfection was associated neither with progression to AIDS nor with mortality. Analysis of CD4$^+$ T-lymphocyte levels also showed similar declines over time in both groups. Whereas there appeared to be a more rapid fall in the percentage of CD4 cells in the first year in the HTLV-2-infected individuals after seroconversion, this difference was not found to be significant in regression analysis, and overall the study demonstrated that HTLV-2 infection did not affect this immunological marker of HIV-1 progression. In contrast, Brites et al. in a Brazilian study (20) evaluated 895 HIV-1-infected individuals, of whom 16.3% were coinfected with either HTLV-1 or HTLV-2 and although this study was not as strictly controlled, it was reported that women coinfected with HTLV-1 or HTLV-2 had a higher risk of developing AIDS than those infected with HIV-1 alone.

A cross-sectional study (163) suggested that persons with HTLV-1 infection were more likely to be in late clinical stages of HIV infection than those with HIV alone. It could also be shown that coinfected individuals had higher levels of CD4$^+$ lymphocytes (46), suggesting that HTLV-1 infection may produce proliferation of CD4 lymphocytes. Similarly, a study of CD4$^+$ and CD8$^+$ T-lymphocyte counts in HIV and HTLV-1 coinfected patients also showed that these were both higher in the setting of coinfection (8). In the former study it was not possible to determine whether HTLV-1 infection actually contributed to the development of their presenting clinical conditions. Sobesky et al. (171), in a study of a cohort of adults in French Guiana, of whom about 12% were coinfected with HIV-1 and HTLV-1, reported that coinfection could be strongly correlated with decreased survival and also noted an increase in CD4$^+$ T-lymphocyte levels.

In a comparative analysis of virus loads, a study of 23 patients with HIV-1/HTLV-1 coinfection and 92 with single HIV-1 infection in Brazil reported no significant differences in HIV-1 viral load (74). Moreover, these results were not influenced by AZT treatment or adjustment of CD4 levels. Although this study did not report on the influence of HIV-1 on HTLV-1 proviral loads, a subsequent report (26) compared HTLV-1 proviral loads in asymptomatic HTLV-1-infected individuals, singly infected patients with HAM/TSP, and 25 HIV-1/HTLV-1-coinfected patients from Martinique. Whereas proviral loads were higher in HAM/TSP patients, there was no significant difference in HTLV-1 and HTLV-1/HIV-1 coinfections. In contrast to previous studies, this study showed no differences in CD4 counts between singly infected and coinfected individuals. In view of reports that the development of neurological and inflammatory disorders is associated with higher HTLV-1 proviral loads, this would suggest indirectly that HIV-1 coinfection would not be expected to influence or accelerate the development of such processes. Similarly, Woods et al. (191) found no influence of HIV-1 on HTLV-2 proviral loads.

Although the influence of HTLV-1 and HTLV-2 infection on HIV-1 progression remains unclear, and is limited by factors alluded to above, numerous in vitro studies have provided compelling evidence for potential interactions, both direct and indirect, between the viruses and have established a theoretical basis for how the former may influence the progression of HIV-1 infection. Specifically, several studies have demonstrated that both HTLV-1 virions and envelope proteins are mitogenic and can activate $CD4^+$ T cells and upregulate HIV-1 replication (127, 170, 194, 197). The two viruses can activate each other in vitro (34), and there is increased antigen production in peripheral blood mononuclear cell (PBMC) cultures and higher levels of expression of HTLV-1 mRNA-expressing cells in peripheral blood after HIV-1 coinfection (5). Coinfection of cultured macrophages by T-cell-tropic HIV-1 and HTLV-1 enhances HIV-1 replication, whereas coinfection with macrophage-tropic (M-tropic) HIV-1 and HTLV-1 upregulates HTLV-1 infection (177). It has also been proposed that coinfection might lead to the development of "pseudoviruses" that might have an extended in vivo tropism and as a result an increase in pathogenicity (104, 119, 151). The HTLV-1 regulatory protein Tax can influence HIV-1 replication in many ways. Tax has been shown to increase HIV transcription by activation of the HIV-1 long terminal repeat (15). Although this seems inherently weak, this effect can be enhanced dramatically by the presence of low levels of HIV-1 Tat and is apparently mediated through cooperation of Tat and NF-κB (27). In addition one study demonstrated that HTLV-1 Tax can interact with the p21 cyclin-dependent kinase to activate HIV-1 replication, and it has also been reported that soluble Tax can increase the susceptibility of CD4 T cells to both M- and T-tropic HIV by an as yet unknown mechanism (128).

More recently, several studies have provided evidence for important indirect effects of HTLV-1 and HTLV-2 on HIV-1 replication via the production of CC-chemokines. Stud-

ies conducted several years ago showed that HTLV-1 and HTLV-2 infections are associated with the spontaneous proliferation of PBMCs in vitro, and this has been associated with the production of a range of cytokines and lymphokines (103, 124). More recently, investigations with infected cell lines or PBMC cultures have shown that HTLV-1 infection was associated with the production of the CC-chemokines MIP-1α, MIP-1β, and RANTES and that these in turn could influence HIV-1 replication (2, 29, 30, 37, 127, 141). The CC-chemokines are the natural ligands for the coreceptors required for HIV-1 entry, and it could be shown that these could suppress in vitro infection by M-tropic HIV-1 strains and enhance infection by T-cell-tropic HIV-1 strains (127). Moreover, it has also been suggested that overproduction of CC-chemokines may actually protect individuals from infection by M-tropic HIV-1 strains, on the basis of observations that individuals who have been repeatedly exposed to HIV-1 yet remain uninfected produce high levels of CC-chemokines (145, 195).

These observations have been supported by two studies (24, 112) that investigated CC-chemokine production in cell lines from HTLV-2- and HIV-1-coinfected individuals. Casoli et al. (24) demonstrated that cultured PBMCs from coinfected individuals produced high levels of these CC-chemokines and that the kinetics of production and concentrations were inversely related to those of HIV-1 replication. With cocultures of PBMCs or isolated $CD8^+$ T lymphocytes from singly infected HTLV-2 individuals, and with $CD4^+$ T lymphocytes from singly infected HIV-1 individuals separated by a semipermeable membrane, it could be demonstrated directly that CC-chemokines produced by the former could inhibit HIV-1, and that MIP-1α played the predominant inhibitory role. These studies were supported and extended in an independent study (112) by using short-term cultures of PBMCs from HTLV-2-infected and HIV-1-coinfected individuals where it could be demonstrated that there was spontaneous production of significant levels of MIP-1α and -1β and, to a lesser extent, RANTES. In contrast, spontaneous CC-chemokine production was not observed in PBMCs from uninfected or HIV-1-infected individuals. Although HTLV-2 preferentially infects CD8$^+$ lymphocytes in vivo, it was also shown that whereas RANTES was produced exclusively by the CD8$^+$-enriched population, MIP-1α and MIP-1β were produced by both the CD8$^+$-enriched and CD8$^+$-depleted populations of HTLV-2-infected PBMCs. RT-PCR demonstrated active expression of the HTLV-2 regulatory protein Tax in the infected CD8$^+$ T-lymphocyte population, and it was also shown that Tax could transactivate the promoters of MIP-1β and RANTES. Therefore, it seems that HTLV-2 stimulates the production of CC-chemokines both directly at a transcriptional level via the viral transactivator Tax and also indirectly from noninfected CD4$^+$ T cells. These findings suggest that HTLV-2, via chemokine production, would be expected to alter the progression of HIV-1 infection in coinfected individuals, and specifically it could be anticipated that, depending on the time course and dynamics of coinfection, HTLV-2 infection could potentially inhibit or enhance the progression of HIV-1 infection. Specifically, it might be expected that, if HTLV-2 infection preceded that of HIV-1, inhibition of M-tropic HIV-1 by CC-chemokines early in infection could delay or prevent the progression of HIV-1 infection. In contrast, if infection occurred after or late in HIV-1 infection this could possibly enhance the pathogenicity of T-tropic strains. Moreover, it is possible these different influences may well account for the differences noted in the clinical outcomes in coinfected individuals.

CONCLUSIONS

HIV-1 and HTLV-2 coinfections are epidemic in many urban areas of the world where they are maintained primarily through practices associated with IDU. HIV-1 and HTLV-1 coinfections primarily occur in areas endemic for HTLV-1. Although IDU is important in maintaining coinfections in certain of these areas, it is not as significant as that involving HTLV-2. At present, no evidence suggests that HIV-1 may influence the natural history of HTLV-1 infection. However, several studies have suggested the possibility that HIV-1 may contribute to the development of HTLV-2 malignant lymphoproliferative processes. Whether HTLV-1 and HTLV-2 infection may influence the progression of HIV-1 infection is also unclear. However, compelling evidence shows that HTLV-2 may certainly influence this through CC-chemokine production, and this may have either a negative or positive influence depending on the temporal relationship of infection by the two viruses. Prospective clinical, immunological, and virological analyses will allow a clearer understanding of the interactions of these viruses in coinfected individuals, which in turn will allow the development of optimal therapeutic interventions.

ACKNOWLEDGMENTS

These studies were supported by the Japanese Foundation for AIDS Prevention (W.W.H.) and the Brazilian Research Council (CNPq) (A.A.).

REFERENCES

1. **Arango, C., E. Maloney, M. T. Rugeles, E. Bernal, C. Bernal, I. Borrero, S. Herrera, M. Restrepo, A. Espinal, and W. A. Blattner.** 1999. HTLV-I and HTLV-II coexist among the Embera and Inga Amerindians of Colombia. *J. Acquir. Immune Defic. Syndr. Hum. Retrovirol.* **20:**102–103.

2. **Baba, M., T. Imai, T. Yoshida, and O. Yoshie.** 1996. Constitutive expression of various chemokine genes in human T-cell lines infected with human T-cell leukemia virus type 1: role of the viral transactivator Tax. *Int. J. Cancer* **66:**124–129.

3. **Bartholomew, C., W. Blattner, and F. Cleghorn.** 1987. Progression to AIDS in homosexual men co-infected with HIV and HTLV-I in Trinidad. *Lancet* **ii:**1469.

4. **Bazarbachi, A., and O. Hermine.** 2001. Treatment of adult T-cell leukaemia/lymphoma: current strategy and future perspectives. *Virus Res.* **78:**79–92.

5. **Beilke, M. A., S. Japa, and D. G. Vinson.** 1998. HTLV-I and HTLV-II virus expression in-

crease with HIV-1 coinfection. *J. Acquir. Immune Defic. Syndr. Hum. Retrovir.* **15:**391–397.

6. **Berger, J. R., S. Raffanti, A. Svenningsson, M. McCarty, S. Snodgrass, and L. Resnick.** 1991. The role of HLTV in HIV-1 neurologic disease. *Neurology* **41:**197–202.

7. **Berger, J. R., A. Svenningsson, S. Raffanti, and L. Resnick.** 1991. Tropical spasticparaparesis-like illness occurring in a patient dually infected with HIV-1 and HTLV-II. *Neurology* **41:**85–87.

8. **Bessinger, R., M. Beilke, P. Kissinger, C. Jarrott, and O. F. Tabak.** 1997. Retroviral coinfections at a New Orleans HIV outpatient clinic. *J. Acquir. Immune Defic. Syndr. Hum. Retrovirol.* **14:**67–71.

9. **Biddison, W. E., R. Kubota, T. Kawanishi, D. D. Taub, W. W. Cruikshank, D. M. Center, E. W. Connor, U. Utz, and S. Jacobson.** 1997. Human T cell leukemia virus type I (HTLV-I)-specific DC8+ clones from patients with HTLV-I-associated neurologic disease secrete proinflammatory cytokines, chemokines, and matrix metalloproteinase. *J. Immunol.* **159:**2018–2025.

10. **Biggar, R. J., Z. Buskell-Bales, P. N. Yakshe, D. Caussy, G. Gridley, and L. Seeff.** 1991. Antibody to human retroviruses among drug users in three east coast American cities, 1972–1976. *J. Infect. Dis.* **16:**57–63.

11. **Biggar, R. J., M. E. Taylor, J. V. Neel, B. Hjelle, P. H. Levine, F. L. Black, G. M. Shaw, P. M. Sharp, and B. H. Hahn.** 1996. Genetic variants of human T-lymphotropic virus type II in American Indian groups. *Virology* **216:**165–173.

12. **Biglione, M., A. Gessain, S. Quiruelas, O. Fay, M. A. Taborda, E. Fernandez, S. Lupo, A. Panzita, and G. de The.** 1993. Endemic HTLV-II infection among Tobas and Matacos Amerindians from North Argentina. *J. Acquir. Immune Defic. Syndr.* **6:**631–633.

13. **Black, F. L., R. J. Biggar, R. B. Lal, A. A. Gabbai, and J. P. Filho.** 1996. Twenty-five years of HTLV type II follow-up with a possible case of tropical spastic paraparesis in the Kayapo, a Brazilian Indian tribe. *AIDS Res. Hum. Retrovir.* **12:**1623–1627.

14. **Black, F. L., R. J. Biggar, J. V. Neel, E. M. Maloney, and D. J. Waters.** 1994. Endemic transmission of HTLV type II among Kayapo Indans of Brazil. *AIDS Res. Hum. Retrovir.* **10:**1165–1171.

15. **Böhnlein, E., M. Siekevitz, D. W. Ballard, J. W. Lowenthal, L. Rimsky, H. Rogerd, J. Hoffman, Y. Wano, B. R. Franza, and W. C. Greene.** 1989. Stimulation of the human im-

munodeficiency virus type 1 enhancer by the human T-cell leukemia virus type I *tax* gene product involves the action of inducible cellular proteins. *J. Virol.* **63:**1578–1586.

16. **Brabin, L., B. J. Brabin, R. R. Doherty, I. D. Gust, M. P. Alpers, R. Fujino, J. Imai, and Y. Hinuma.** 1989. Patterns of migration indicate sexual transmission of HTLV-I infection in non-pregnant women in Papua New Guinea. *Int. J. Cancer* **44:**59–62.

17. **Brauweiler, A., J. E. Garrus, J. C. Reed, and J. K. Nyborg.** 1997. Repression of bax gene expression by the HTLV-1 Tax protein: implications for suppression of apoptosis in virally infected cells. *Virology* **231:**135–140.

18. **Briggs, N. C., R. J. Battjes, K. P. Cantor, W. A. Blattner, F. M. Yellin, S. Wilson, A. L. Ritz, S. H. Weiss, and J. J. Goedert.** 1995. Seroprevalence of human T cell lymphotropic virus type II infection, with or without human immunodeficiency virus type 1 coinfection, among US intravenous drug users. *J. Infect. Dis.* **172:**51–58.

19. **Brites, C., W. Harrington, Jr., C. Pedroso, E. Martins-Netto, and R. Badaro.** 1997. Epidemiological characteristics of HTLV-I and II coinfection in Brazilian subjects infected by HIV-1. *Braz. J. Infect. Dis.* **1:**42–47.

20. **Brites, C., C. Pedroso, E. Netto, W. Harrington, Jr., B. Galvao-Castro, J. C. Couto-Fernandez, D. Pedral-Sampaio, M. Morgado, R. Teixeira, and R. Badaro.** 1998. Co-infection by HTLV-I/II is associated with increased viral load in PBMC of HIV-1 infected patients in Bahia, Brazil. *Braz. J. Infect. Dis.* **2:**70–77.

21. **Buttner, A., G. Mall, R. Penning, and S. Weis.** 2000. The neuropathology of heroin abuse. *Forensic Sci. Int.* **113:**435–442.

22. **Cartier, L., F. Araya, J. L. Castillo, V. Zaninovic, M. Hayami, T. Miura, J. Imai, S. Sonoda, H. Shiraki, K. Miyamoto, and K. Tajima.** 1993. Southernmost carriers of HTLV-I/II in the world. *Jpn. J. Cancer Res.* **84:**1–3.

23. **Castillo, L. C., F. Gracia, G. C. Roman, P. Levine, W. C. Reeves, and J. Kaplan.** 2000. Spinocerebellar syndrome in patients infected with human T-lymphotropic virus types I and II (HTLV-I/HTLV-II): report of 3 cases from Panama. *Acta Neurol. Scand.* **101:**405–412.

24. **Casoli, C., E. Vicenzi, A. Cimarelli, G. Magnani, P. Ciancianaini, E. Cattaneo, P. Dall'Aglio, G. Poli, and U. Bertazzoni.** 2000. HTLV-II downregulates HIV-1 replication in IL-2-stimulated primary PBMC of coinfected individuals through expression of MIP-1alpha. *Blood* **95:**2760–2769.

25. Cereseto, A., F. Diella, J. C. Mulloy, A. Cara, P. Michieli, R. Grassmann, G. Franchini, and M. E. Klotman. 1996. p53 functional impairment and high p21waf1/cip1 expression in human T-cell lymphotropic/leukemia virus type I-transformed T cells. *Blood* **88**:1551–1560.

26. Cesaire, R., A. Dehee, A. Lezin, N. Desire, O. Bourdonne, F. Dantin, O. Bera, D. Smadja, S. Abel, A. Cabie, G. Sobesky, and J. C. Nicolas. 2001. Quantification of HTLV type I and HIV type 1 DNA load in coinfected patients: HIV type 1 infection does not alter HTLV type 1 proviral amount in the peripheral blood compartment. *AIDS Res. Hum. Retrovir.* **17**:799–805.

27. Cheng, H., J. Tarnok, and W. P. Parks. 1998. Human immunodeficiency virus type 1 genome activation induced by human T-cell leukemia virus type 1 Tax protein is through cooperation of NF-κB and Tat. *J. Virol.* **72**:6911–6916.

28. Cimarelli, A., C. A. Duclos, A. Gessain, E. Cattaneo, C. Casoli, M. Biglione, P. Mauclere, and U. Bertazzoni. 1995. Quantification of HTLV-II proviral copies by competitive polymerase chain reaction in peripheral blood mononuclear cells of Italian injecting drug users, central Africans, and Amerindians. *J. Acquir. Immune Defic. Syndr. Hum. Retrovirol.* **10**:198–204.

29. Cocchi, F., A. L. De Vico, A. Garzino-Demo, S. K. Arya, R. C. Gallo, and P. Lusso. 1995. Identification of RANTES, MIP-1 alpha, and MIP-1 beta as the major HIV-suppressive factors produced by CD8+ T cells. *Science* **270**:1811–1815.

30. Connor, R. I., K. E. Sheridan, D. Ceradini, S. Choe, and N. R. Landau. 1997. Change in coreceptor use coreceptor use correlates with disease progression in HIV-1-infected individuals. *J. Exp. Med.* **185**:621–628.

31. De Cabral, M. B., M. E. Vera, M. Samudio, A. R. Arias, A. Cabello, R. Moreno, I. Zapiola, M. B. Bouzas, and G. Muchinik. 1998. HTLV-I/II antibodies among three different Indian groups from Paraguay. *J. Acquir. Immune Defic. Syndr. Hum. Retrovirol.* **19**:548–549.

32. Delaporte, E., J. Louwagie, M. Peeters, N. Montplaisir, L. d'Auriol, Y. Ville, L. Bedjabaga, B. Larouze, G. Van der Groen, and P. Piot. 1991. Evidence of HTLV-II infection in central Africa. *AIDS* **6**:771–772.

33. Delaporte, E., N. Monplaisir, J. Louwagie, M. Peeters, Y. Martin-Prevel, J. P. Louis, A. Trebucq, L. Bedjabaga, S. Ossari, C. Honore, B. Larouze, L. Dauriol, G. Vandergroen, and P. Piot. 1991. Prevalence of HTLV-I and HTLV-II infection in Gabon, Africa: comparison of the serological and PCR results. *Int. J. Cancer* **49**:373–376.

34. De Rossi, A., D. Saggioro, M. L. Calabro, R. Cenzato, and L. Chieco-Bianchi. 1991. Reciprocal activation of human T-lymphotropic viruses in HTLV-I-transformed cells superinfected with HIV-1. *J. Acquir. Immune Defic. Syndr.* **4**:380–385.

35. Donegan, E., M. P. Busch, J. A. Galleshaw, G. M. Shaw, and J. W. Mosley. 1990. Transfusion of blood components from a donor with human T-lymphotropic virus type II (HTLV-II) infection. The Transfusion Safety Study Group. *Ann. Intern. Med.* **113**:555–556.

36. Dooneief, G., R. Marlink, K. Bell, K. Marder, B. Renjifo, Y. Stern, and R. Mayeux. 1996. Neurologic consequences of HTLV-II infection in injection-drug users. *Neurology* **46**:1556–1560.

37. Dragic, T., V. Litwin, G. P. Allaway, S. R. Martin, Y. Huang, K. A. Nagashima, C. Cayanan, P. J. Maddon, R. A. Koup, J. P. Moore, and W. A. Paxton. 1996. HIV-1 entry into CD4+ cells is mediated by the chemokine receptor CC-CKR-5. *Nature* **381**:667–673.

38. Dube, D. K., M. P. Sherman, N. K. Saksena, V. Bryz-Gornia, J. Mendelson, J. Love, C. B. Arnold, T. Spicer, S. Dube, J. B. Glaser, A. E. Williams, M. Nishimura, S. Jacobsen, J. F. Ferrer, N. Del Pino, S. Quiruelas, and B. J. Poiesz. 1993. Genetic heterogeneity in human T-cell leukemia/lymphoma virus type II. *J. Virol.* **67**:1175–1184.

39. Duenas-Barajas, E., J. E. Bernal, D. R. Vaught, I. Briceno, C. Duran, R. Yanagihara, and D. C. Gajdusek. 1992. Coexistence of human T-lymphotropic virus types I and II among the Wayuu Indians from the Guajira Region of Colombia. *AIDS Res. Hum. Retrovir.* **8**:1851–1855.

40. Egan, J. F., B. O'Leary, M. J. Lewis, F. Mulcahy, N. Sheehy, H. Hasegawa, F. Fitzpatrick, J. J. O'Connor, J. O'Riordan, and W. W. Hall. 1999. High rate of human T lymphotropic virus type IIa infection in HIV type 1-infected intravenous drug abusers in Ireland. *AIDS Res. Hum. Retrovir.* **15**:699–705.

41. Ehrlich, G. D., J. B. Glaser, K. La Vigne, D. Quan, D. Mildvan, J. J. Sninsky, S. Kwok, L. Papsidero, and B. J. Poiesz. 1989. Prevalence of human T-cell leukemia/lymphoma virus (HTLV) type II infection among high-risk individuals: type-specific identification of HTLVs by polymerase chain reaction. *Blood* **74**:1658–1664.

42. Eiraku, N., P. Novoa, M. da Costa Ferreira, C. Monken, R. Ishak, O. da Costa Ferreira,

S. W. Zhu, R. Lorenco, M. Ishak, V. Azvedo, J. Guerreiro, M. P. de Oliveira, P. Loureiro, N. Hammerschlak, S. Ijichi, and W. W. Hall. 1996. Identification and characterization of a new and distinct molecular subtype of human T-cell lymphotropic virus type 2. *J. Virol.* **70:**1481–1492.

43. El-Sabban, M. E., R. Nasr, G. Dbaibo, O. Hermine, N. Abboushi, F. Quignon, J. C. Ameisen, F. Bex, H. de The, and A. Bazarbachi. 2000. Arsenic-interferon-alpha-triggered apoptosis in HTLV-I transformed cells is associated with tax down-regulation and reversal of NF-kappa B activation. *Blood* **96:**2849–2855.

44. Eskild, A., H. H. Samdal, and B. Heger. 1996. Co-infection with HIV-1/HTLV-II and the risk of progression to AIDS and death. The Oslo HIV Cohort Study Group. *APMIS* **104:** 666–672.

45. Etzel, A., G. Y. Shibata, M. Rozman, M. L. Jorge, C. D. Damas, and A. A. Segurado. 2001. HTLV-1 and HTLV-2 infections in HIV-infected individuals from Santos, Brazil: seroprevalence and risk factors. *J. Acquir. Immune Defic. Syndr.* **26:**185–190.

46. Fantry, L., E. De Jonge, P. G. Auwaerter, and H. M. Lederman. 1995. Immunodeficiency and elevated CD4 T lymphocyte counts in two patients coinfected with human immunodeficiency virus and human lymphotropic virus type I. *Clin. Infect. Dis.* **21:**1466–1468.

47. Feigal, E., E. Murphy, K. Vranizan, P. Bacchetti, R. Chaisson, J. E. Drummond, W. Blattner, M. McGrath, J. Greenspan, and A. Moss. 1991. Human T cell lymphotropic virus types I and II in intravenous drug users in San Francisco: risk factors associated with seropositivity. *J. Infect. Dis.* **164:**36–42.

48. Ferrer, J. F., N. Del Pino, E. Esteban, M. P. Sherman, S. Dube, D. K. Dube, M. A. Basombrio, E. Pimentel, A. Segovia, S. Quirulas, and B. J. Poiesz. 1993. High rate of infection with the human T-cell leukemia retrovirus type II in four Indian populations of Argentina. *Virology* **197:**576–584.

49. Franchini, G. 1995. Molecular mechanisms of human T-cell leukemia/lymphotropic virus type I infection. *Blood* **86:**3619–3639.

50. Froment, A., E. Delaporte, M. C. Dazza, and B. Larouze. 1993. HTLV-II among pygmies from Cameroon. *AIDS Res. Hum. Retrovir.* **9:**707.

51. Fujiyama, C., T. Fujiyoshi, T. Miura, S. Yashiki, D. Matsumoto, V. Zaninovic, O. Blanco, W. Harrington, Jr., J. J. Byrnes, M. Hayami, K. Tajima, and S. Sonoda. 1993. A new endemic focus of human T lymphotropic virus type II carriers among Orinoco natives in Colombia. *J. Infect. Dis.* **168:**1075–1077.

52. Fukushima, Y., M. J. Lewis, C. Monken, K. Komuro, S. Kusagawa, H. Sato, Y. Takebe, S. Yamazaki, T. H. Nguyen, A. Hoang, T. L. Hoang, M. Honda, and W. W. Hall. 1998. Identification and molecular characterization of human T lymphotropic virus type II infections in intravenous drug abusers in the former South Vietnam. *AIDS Res. Hum. Retrovir.* **14:**537–540.

53. Fukushima, Y., H. Takahashi, W. W. Hall, T. Nakasone, S. Nakata, P. Song, D. D. Duc, B. Hien, N. X. Quang, T. N. Trinh, K. Nishioka, K. Kitamura, K. Komuro, A. Vahlne, and M. Honda. 1995. Extraordinary high rate of HTLV type II seropositivity in intravenous drug abusers in south Vietnam. *AIDS Res. Hum. Retrovir.* **11:**637–645.

54. Garcia-Lerma, J. G., S. Nidtha, and W. Heneine. 2001. Susceptibility of human T cell leukemia virus type 1 to reverse-transcriptase inhibitors: evidence for resistance to lamivudine. *J. Infect. Dis.* **184:**507–510.

55. Gasmi, M., S. Fillon, K. Leriche, C. Neisson-Vernant, and C. Desgranges. 1997. Zidovudine treatment is not associated with HTLV-1 reverse transcriptase gene mutations in HTLV-I/HIV-1 co-infected patients. *Antivir. Ther.* **2:**91–97.

56. Gessain, A., F. Barin, J. C. Vernant, O. Gout, L. Maurs, A. Calender, and G. de The. 1985. Antibodies to human T-lymphotropic virus type-I in patients with tropical spastic paraparesis. *Lancet* **ii:**407–410.

57. Gessain, A., P. Mauclere, A. Froment, M. Biglione, J. Y. Le Hesran, F. Tekaia, J. Millan, and G. de The. 1995. Isolation and molecular characterization of a human T-cell lymphotropic virus type II (HTLV-II), subtype B, from a healthy Pygmy living in a remote area of Cameroon: an ancient origin for HTLV-II in Africa. *Proc. Natl. Acad. Sci. USA* **25:**4041–4045.

58. Giacomo, M., E. G. Franco, C. Claudio, C. Carlo, D. A. Anna, D. Anna, and F. Franco. 1995. Human T-cell leukemia virus type II infection among high risk groups and its influence on HIV-1 disease progression. *Eur. J. Epidemiol.* **11:**527–533.

59. Gill, P. S., W. Harrington, Jr., M. H. Kaplan, R. C. Ribeiro, J. M. Bennett, H. A. Liebman, M. Bernstein-Singer, B. M. Espina, L. Cabral, S. Allen, S. Kornblau, M. C. Pike, and A. M. Levine. 1995. Treatment of adult T-cell leukemia-lymphoma with a combination of interferon alfa and zidovudine. *N. Engl. J. Med.* **332:**1744–1748.

60. **Giri, A., P. Markham, L. Digilio, G. Hurteau, R. C. Gallo, and G. Franchini.** 1994. Isolation of a novel simian T-cell lymphotropic virus from *Pan paniscus* that is distantly related to the human T-cell leukemia/lymphotropic virus types I and II. *J. Virol.* **68:** 8392–8395.

61. **Goedert, J. J., M. W. Fung, S. Felton, R. J. Battjes, and E. A. Engels.** 2001. Cause-specific mortality associated with HIV AND HTLV-II infections among injecting drug users in the USA. *AIDS* **15:**1295–1302.

62. **Gongora-Biachi, R. A., R. B. Lal, D. L. Rudolph, C. Castro-Sansores, P. Gonzalez-Martinez, and N. Pavia-Ruz.** 1997. Low prevalence of HTLV-II in Mayan Indians in the Yucatan Peninsula, Mexico. *Arch. Med. Res.* **28:**555–558.

63. **Gotuzzo, E., J. Escamilla, I. A. Phillips, J. Sanchez, F. S. Wignall, and J. Antigoni.** 1992. The impact of human T-lymphotrophic virus type I/II infection on the prognosis of sexually acquired cases of acquired immunodeficiency syndrome. *Arch. Intern. Med.* **152:**1429–1432.

64. **Goubau, P., J. Desmyter, J. Ghesquiere, and B. Kasereka.** 1992. HTLV-II among pygmies. *Nature* **359:**201.

65. **Goubau, P., H. F. Liu, G. G. De Lange, A. M. Vandamme, and J. Desmyter.** 1993. HTLV-II seroprevalence in pygmies across Africa since 1970. *AIDS Res. Hum. Retrovir.* **9:**709–713.

66. **Goubau, P., A. Vandamme, K. Beuselinck, and J. Desmyter.** 1996. Proviral HTLV-I and HTLV-II in the Efe pygmies of northeastern Zaire. *J. Acquir. Immune Defic. Syndr. Hum. Retrovirol.* **12:**208–209.

67. **Gout, O., A. Gessain, M. Iba-Zizen, S. Kouzan, F. Bolgert, G. de The, and O. Lyon-Caen.** 1991. The effect of zidovudine on chronic myelopathy associated with HTLV-1. *J. Neurol.* **238:**108–109.

68. **Grassmann, R., C. Dengler, I. Muller-Fleckenstein, B. Fleckenstein, K. McGuire, M. C. Dokhelar, J. G. Sodroski, and W. A. Haseltine.** 1989. Transformation to continuous growth of primary human T lymphocytes by human T-cell leukemia virus type I X-region genes transduced by a Herpesvirus saimiri vector. *Proc. Natl. Acad. Sci. USA* **86:**3351–3355.

69. **Guimaraes, M. L., F. I. Bastos, P. R. Telles, B. Galvao-Castro, R. S. Diaz, V. Bongertz, and M. G. Morgado.** 2001. Retrovirus infections in a sample of injecting drug users in Rio de Janeiro City, Brazil: prevalence of HIV-1 subtypes, and co-infection with HTLV-I/II. *J. Clin. Virol.* **21:**143–151.

70. **Hall, W. W., R. Ishak, S. W. Zhu, P. Novoa, N. Eiraku, H. Takahashi, M. D. Ferreira, V. Azevedo, M. O. Ishak, O. D. Ferreira, C. Monken, and T. Kurata.** 1996. Human T lymphotropic virus type II (HTLV-II): epidemiology, molecular properties, and clinical features of infection. *J. Acquir. Immune Defic. Syndr. Hum. Retrovirol.* **13:**204–214.

71. **Hall, W. W., M. H. Kaplan, S. Z. Salahuddin, N. Oyaizu, C. Gurgo, M. Coronesi, K. Nagashima, and R. C. Gallo.** 1990. Concomitant infections with human T-cell leukemia viruses (HTLVs) and human immunodeficiency virus (HIV): identification of HTLV-II infection in intravenous drug abusers (IVDUs), p. 115–127. *In* W. A. Blattner (ed.), *Human Retrovirology: HTLV.* Raven Press, New York, N.Y.

72. **Hall, W. W., H. Takahashi, C. Liu, M. H. Kaplan, O. Scheewind, S. Ijichi, K. Nagashima, and R. C. Gallo.** 1992. Multiple isolates and characteristics of human T-cell leukemia virus type II. *J. Virol.* **66:**2456–2463.

73. **Harrington, W. Jr., W. Sheremata, B. Hjelle, D. K. Dube, P. Bradshaw, S. K. H. Foung, S. Snodgrass, A. Towdter, L. Cabral, and B. Poiesz.** 1993. Spastic ataxia associated with human T-cell lymphotropic virus type II infection. *Ann. Neurol.* **33:**411–414.

74. **Harrison, L. H., T. C. Quinn, and M. Schechter.** 1997. Human T cell lymphotropic virus type I does not increase human immunodeficiency virus viral load in vivo. *J. Infect. Dis.* **175:**438–440.

75. **Harrison, L. H., B. Vaz, D. M. Taveira, T. C. Quinn, C. J. Gibbs, S. H. de Souza, J. C. McArthur, and M. Schechter.** 1997. Myelopathy among Brazilians coinfected with human T-cell lymphotropic virus type I and HIV. *Neurology* **48:**13–18.

76. **Hattori, T., A. Koito, K. Takatsuki, S. Ikematsu, J. Matsuda, H. Mori, M. Fukui, K. Akashi, and K. Matsumoto.** 1989. Frequent infection with human T-cell lymphotropic virus type I in patients with AIDS but not in carriers of human immunodeficiency virus type 1. *J. Acquir. Immune Defic. Syndr.* **2:**272–276.

77. **Hermine, O., D. Bouscary, A. Gessain, P. Turlure, V. Leblond, N. Franck, A. Buzyn-Veil, B. Rio, E. Macintyre, F. Dreyfus, and A. Bazarbachi.** 1995. Brief report: treatment of adult T-cell leukemia-lymphoma with zidovudine and interferon alfa. *N. Engl. J. Med.* **332:**1749–1751.

78. **Hershow, R. C., N. Galai, K. Fukuda, J. Graber, D. Vlahov, G. Rezza, R. S. Klein, D. C. Des Jarlais, C. Vitek, R. Khabbaz, S. Freels, R. Zuckerman, P. Pezzotti, and J. E.**

Kaplan. 1996. An international collaborative study of the effects of coinfection with human T-lymphotropic virus type II on human immuno-deficiency virus type 1 disease progression in in-jection drug users. *J. Infect. Dis.* **174:**309–317.

79. **Hino, S., K. Yamaguchi, S. Katamine, H. Sugiyama, T. Amagasaki, K. Kinoshita, Y. Yoshida, H. Doi, Y. Tsuji, and T. Miyamoto.** 1985. Mother-to-child transmission of human T-cell leukemia virus type-I. *Jpn. J. Cancer Res.* **76:**474–480.

80. **Hjelle, B., O. Appenzeller, R. Mills, S. Alexander, N. Torrez-Martinez, R. Jahnke, and G. Ross.** 1992. Chronic neurodegenerative disease associated with HTLV-II infection. *Lancet* **339:**645–646.

81. **Hjelle, B., S. Cyrus, and S. G. Swenson.** 1992. Evidence for sexual transmission of human T lymphotropic virus type II. *Ann. Intern. Med.* **116:**90–91.

82. **Hjelle, B., R. Mills, G. Mertz, and S. Swenson.** 1990. Transmission of HTLV-II via blood transfusion. *Vox Sang.* **59:**119–122.

83. **Hjelle, B., S. W. Zhu, H. Takahashi, S. Ijichi, and W. W. Hall.** 1993. Endemic human T cell leukemia virus type II infection in south-western US Indians involves two prototype vari-ants of virus. *J. Infect. Dis.* **168:**737–740.

84. **Ibrahim, F., G. de The, and A. Gessain.** 1995. Isolation and characterization of a new simian T-cell leukemia virus type 1 from naturally infected Celebes macaques (*Macaca tonkeana*): complete nucleotide sequence and phylogenetic relation-ship with the Australo-Melanesian human T-cell leukemia virus type 1. *J. Virol.* **69:**6980–6993.

85. **Ijichi, S., M. B. Ramundo, H. Takahashi, and W. W. Hall.** 1992. In vivo cellular tropism of human T cell leukemia virus type II (HTLV-II). *J. Exp. Med.* **176:**293–296.

86. **Ijichi, S., K. Tajima, V. Zaninovic, F. E. Leon, Y. Katahira, S. Sonoda, T. Miura, M. Hayami, and W. W. Hall.** 1993. Identification of human T cell leukemia virus type IIb infection in the Wayu, an aboriginal population of Colom-bia. *Jpn. J. Cancer Res.* **84:**1215–1218.

87. **Ishak, R., W. J. Harrington, V. N. Azevedo, N. Eiraku, M. O. G. Ishak, J. F. Guerreiro, S. B. Santos, T. Kubo, C. Monken, S. Alexan-der, and W. W. Hall.** 1995. Identification of hu-man T cell lymphotropic virus type IIa infection in the Kayapo, an indigenous population of Brazil. *AIDS Res. Hum. Retrovir.* **11:**813–821.

88. **Jacobson, S., T. Lehky, M. Nishimura, S. Robinson, and D. E. McFarlin.** 1993. Isola-tion of HTLV-II from a patient with chronic pro-gressive neurological disease indistinguishable from HTLV-I associated myelopathy/tropical spastic paraparesis. *Ann. Neurol.* **33:**392–395.

89. **Jeffery, K. J., A. A. Siddiqui, M. Bunce, A. L. Lloyd, A. M. Vine, A. D. Witkover, S. Izumo, K. Usuku, K. I. Welsh, M. Osame, and C. R. Bangham.** 2000. The influence of HLA class I alleles and heterozygosity on the out-come of human T cell lymphotropic virus type I infection. *J. Immunol.* **165:**7278–7284.

90. **Jeffery, K. J., K. Usuku, S. E. Hall, W. Mat-sumoto, G. P. Taylor, J. Procter, M. Bunce, G. S. Ogg, K. I. Welsh, J. N. Weber, A. L. Lloyd, M. A. Nowak, M. Nagai, M. D. Ko-dama, S. Izumo, M. Osame, and C. R. Bangham.** 1999. HLA alleles determine human T-lymphotropic virus-I (HTLV-I) proviral load and the risk of HTLV-I-associated myelopathy. *Proc. Natl. Acad. Sci. USA* **96:**3848–3853.

91. **Jin, D. Y., F. Spencer, and K. T. Jeang.** 1998. Human T cell leukemia virus type 1 onco-protein Tax targets in human mitotic checkpoint protein MAD1. *Cell* **93:**81–91.

92. **Kajiyama, W., S. Kashiwagi, J. Hayashi, H. Nomura, H. Ikematsu, and K. Okochi.** 1986. Intrafamilial clustering of anti-ATLA-posi-tive persons. *Am. J. Epidemiol.* **124:**800–806.

93. **Kalyanaraman, V. S., M. G. Sarngadharan, M. Robert-Guroff, I. Miyoshi, D. Golde, and R. C. Gallo.** 1982. A new subtype of hu-man T-cell leukemia virus (HTLV-II) associated with a T-cell variant of hairy cell leukemia. *Science* **218:**571–573.

94. **Kaplan, J. E., E. Abrams, N. Shaffer, R. O. Cannon, A. Kaul, K. Krasinski, M. Bamji, T. M. Hartley, B. Roberts, B. Kilbourne, P. Thomas, M. Rogers, W. Heneine, and The NYC Perinatal HIV Transmission Collabo-rative Study.** 1992. Low risk of mother-to-child transmission of human T lymphotropic virus type II in non-breast-fed infants. *J. Infect. Dis.* **166:** 892–895.

95. **Kaplan, J. E., R. F. Khabbaz, E. L. Murphy, S. Hermansen, C. Roberts, R. Lal, W. Heneine, D. Wright, L. Matijas, R. Thom-son, D. Rudolph, W. M. Switzer, S. Klein-man, M. Busch, and G. B. Schreiber.** 1996. Male-to-female transmission of human T-cell lymphotropic virus types I and II: association with viral load. The Retrovirus Epidemiology Donor Study Group. *J. Acquir. Immune Defic. Syndr. Hum. Retrovirol.* **12:**193–201.

96. **Kaplan, M. H., W. W. Hall, M. Susin, S. Pahwa, S. Z. Salahuddin, C. Heilman, J. Fetten, M. Coronesi, B. F. Farber, and S. Smith.** 1991. Syndrome of severe skin disease, eosinophilia, and dermatopathic lymphadenopa-thy in patients with HTLV-II complicating hu-man immunodeficiency virus infection. *Am. J. Med.* **91:**300–309.

97. Khabbaz, R. F., D. Hartel, M. Lairmore, C. R. Horsburgh, E. E. Schoenbaum, B. Roberts, T. M. Hartley, and G. Friedland. 1991. Human T lymphotropic virus type II (HTLV-II) infection in a cohort of New York intravenous drug users: an old infection? *J. Infect. Dis.* **163**:252–256.

98. Khabbaz, R. F., I. M. Onorato, R. O. Cannon, T. M. Hartley, B. Roberts, B. Hosein, and J. E. Kaplan. 1992. Seroprevalence of HTLV-1 and HTLV-2 among intravenous drug users and persons in clinics for sexually transmitted diseases. *N. Engl. J. Med.* **326**:375–380.

99. Kusuhara, K., S. Sonoda, K. Takahashi, K. Tokugawa, J. Fukushige, and K. Ueda. 1987. Mother-to-child transmission of human T-cell leukemia virus type I (HTLV-I): a fifteen-year follow-up study in Okinawa, Japan. *Int. J. Cancer.* **40**:755–757.

100. Lairmore, M. D., S. Jacobson, F. Gracia, B. K. De, L. Castillo, M. Arreategui, B. D. Roberts, P. H. Levine, W. A. Blattner, and J. E. Kaplan. 1990. Isolation of human T-cell lymphotropic virus type 2 from Guaymi Indians in Panama. *Proc. Natl. Acad. Sci. USA* **87**:8840–8844.

101. Lal, R. B., R. A. Gongora-Biachi, D. Pardi, W. M. Switzer, I. Goldman, and A. F. Lal. 1993. Evidence for mother-to-child transmission of human T lymphotropic virus type II. *J. Infect. Dis.* **168**:586–591.

102. Lal, R. B., S. M. Owen, D. L. Rudolph, C. Dawson, and H. Prince. 1995. In vivo cellular tropism of human T-lymphotropic virus type II is not restricted to CD8^{+} cells. *Virology* **210**:441–447.

103. Lal, R. B., D. Rudolph, C. Buckner, D. Pardi, and W. C. Hooper. 1993. Infection with human T-lymphotropic viruses leads to constitutive expression of leukemia inhibitory factor and interleukin-6. *Blood* **81**:1827–1832.

104. Lawson, V. A., J. Y. Lee, J. C. Doultree, J. A. Marshall, and D. A. Mc Phee. 2000. Visualisation of phenotypically mixed HIV-1 and HTLV-I virus particles by electron microscopy. *J. Biomed. Sci.* **7**:71–74.

105. Lee, H., K. B. Idler, P. Swanson, J. J. Aparicio, K. K. Chin, J. P. Lax, M. Nguyen, T. Mann, G. Leckie, A. Zanetti, G. Marinucci, I. S. Y. Chen, and J. D. Rosenblatt. 1993. Complete nucleotide sequence of HTLV-II isolate NRA: comparison of envelope sequence variation of HTLV-II isolates from U.S. blood donors and U.S. and Italian i.v. drug users. *Virology* **196**:57–69.

106. Lee, H. H., P. Swanson, J. D. Rosenblatt, I. S. Y. Chen, W. C. Sherwood, D. E. Smith, G. E. Tegtmeier, L. P. Fernando, C. T. Fang, M. Osame, and S. H. Kleinman. 1991. Relative prevalence and risk factors of HTLV-I and HTLV-II infection in US blood donors. *Lancet* **337**:1435–1439.

107. Lee, H., P. Swanson, V. S. Shorty, J. A. Zack, J. D. Rosenblatt, and I. S. Chen. 1989. High rate of HTLV-II infection in seropositive i.v. drug abusers in New Orleans. *Science* **244**:471–475.

108. Lefrere, J. J., A. M. Courouce, M. Mariotti, E. Wattel, O. Prou, F. Bouchardeau, and P. Lambin. 1990. Rapid progression to AIDS in dual HIV-1/HTLV-I infection. *Lancet* **336**:509.

109. Lehky, T. J., N. Flerlage, D. Katz, S. Houff, W. W. Hall, K. Ishii, C. Monken, S. Dhib-Jalbut, H. F. McFarland, and S. Jacobson. 1996. Human T-cell lymphotropic virus type II-associated myelopathy: clinical and immunologic profiles. *Ann. Neurol.* **40**:714–723.

110. Leon-Ponte, M., O. Noya, N. Bianco, and G. Echeverria de Perez. 1996. Highly endemic human T-lymphotropic virus type II (HTLV-II) infection in a Venezuelan Guahibo Amerindian group. *J. Acquir. Immune Defic. Syndr. Hum. Retrovirol.* **13**:281–286.

111. Levine, P. H., S. Jacobson, R. Elliott, A. Cavallero, G. Colclough, C. Dorry, C. Stephenson, R. M. Knigge, J. Drummond, M. Nishimura, M. E. Taylor, S. Wiktor, and G. M. Shaw. 1993. HTLV-II infection in Florida Indians. *AIDS Res. Hum. Retrovir.* **9**:123–127.

112. Lewis, M. J., V. W. Gautier, X. P. Wang, M. H. Kaplan, and W. W. Hall. 2000. Spontaneous production of C-C chemokines by individuals infected with human T lymphotropic virus type II (HTLV-II) alone and HTLV-II/HIV-1 co-infected individuals. *J. Immunol.* **165**:4127–4132.

113. Lewis, M. J., P. Novoa, R. Ishak, M. Ishak, M. Salemi, A. M. Vandamme, M. H. Kaplan, and W. W. Hall. 2000. Isolation, cloning, and complete nucleotide sequence of a phenotypically distinct Brazilian isolate of human T-lymphotropic virus type II (HTLV-II). *Virology* **271**:142–154.

114. Lin, M. T., B. T. Nguyen, T. V. Binh, T. V. Be, T. Y. Chiang, L. H. Tseng, Y. C. Yang, K. H. Lin, and Y. C. Chen. 1997. Human T-lymphotropic virus type II infection in Vietnamese thalassemic patients. *Arch. Virol.* **142**:1429–1440.

115. Liu, H. F., A. M. Vandamme, M. Van Brussel, J. Desmyter, and P. Goubau. 1994. New retroviruses in human and simian T-lymphotropic viruses. *Lancet* **344**:265–266.

116. Loughran, T. P. Jr., T. Coyle, M. P. Sherman, G. Starkebaum, G. D. Ehrlich, F. W. Ruscetti, and B. J. Poiesz. 1992. Detection of human T-cell leukemia/lymphoma virus, type II, in a patient with large granular lymphocyte leukemia. *Blood* **80:**1116–1119.

117. Low, K. G., L. F. Dorner, D. B. Fernando, J. Grossman, K. T. Jeang, and M. J. Comb. 1997. Human T-cell leukemia virus type 1 Tax releases cell cycle arrest induced by p16INK4a. *J. Virol.* **71:**1956–1962.

118. Lowis, G. W., W. A. Sheremata, P. R. Wickman, D. Dube, K. Dube, and B. J. Poiesz. 1999. HTLV-II risk factors in Native Americans in Florida. *Neuroepidemiology* **18:**37–47.

119. Lusso, P., F. Lori, and R. C. Gallo. 1990. CD4-independent infection by human immunodeficiency virus type 1 after phenotypic mixing with human T-cell leukemia viruses. *J. Virol.* **64:**6341–6344.

120. Machuca, A., B. Rodes, and V. Soriano. 2001. The effect of antiretroviral therapy on HTLV infection. *Virus Res.* **78:**93–100.

121. Mahe, A., A. Gessain, M. Huerre, F. Valensi, S. Keita, and P. Bobin. 1994. Adult T-cell leukemia associated with HTLV-1 in a HIV-2 seropositive African. *Ann. Dermatol. Venereol.* **121:**704–709.

122. Maloney, E. M., R. J. Biggar, J. V. Neel, M. E. Taylor, B. H. Hahn, G. M. Shaw, and W. A. Blattner. 1992. Endemic human T cell lymphotropic virus type II infection among isolated Brazilian Amerindians. *J. Infect. Dis.* **166:**100–107.

123. Martin, M. P., R. J. Biggar, G. Hamlin-Green, S. Staal, and D. Mann. 1993. Large granular lymphocytosis in a patient infected with HTLV-II. *AIDS Res. Hum. Retrovir.* **9:**715–719.

124. Masataka, B., T. Imai, T. Yoshida, and O. Yoshie. 1996. Constitutive expression of various chemokine genes in human T-cell lines infected with human T-cell leukemia virus type 1: role of the viral transactivator tax. *Int. J. Cancer* **66:**124–129.

125. Matutes, E., G. P. Taylor, J. Cavenagh, A. Pagliuca, D. Bareford, A. Domingo, M. Hamblin, S. Kelsey, N. Mir, and J. T. Reilly. 2001. Interferon alpha and zitlovudine therapy in adult T-cell leukaemia lymphoma: response and outcome in 15 patients. *Br. J. Haematol.* **113:**779–784.

126. Modahl, L. E., K. C. Young, K. F. Varney, H. Khayam-Bashi, and E. L. Murphy. 1997. Are HTLV-II-seropositive injection drug users at increased risk of bacterial pneumonia, abscess, and lymphadenopathy? *J. Acquir. Immune Defic. Syndr. Hum. Retrovirol.* **16:**169–175.

127. Moriuchi, H., and M. Moriuchi. 2000. In vitro induction of HIV-1 replication in resting CD4(+) T cells derived from individuals with undetectable plasma viremia upon stimulation with human T-cell leukemia virus type I. *Virology* **278:**514–519.

128. Moriuchi, H., M. Moriuchi, and A. S. Fauci. 1998. Factors secreted by human T lymphotropic virus type I (HTLV-I)-infected cells can enhance or inhibit replication of HIV-1 in HTLV-I uninfected cells: implications for in vivo coinfection with HTLV-I and HIV-1. *J. Exp. Med.* **187:**1689–1697.

129. Murphy, E. L. 1996. The clinical epidemiology of human T-lymphotropic virus type II (HTLV-II). *J. Acquir. Immune Defic. Syndr. Hum. Retrovirol.* **13:**S215–S219.

130. Murphy, E. L., D. DeVita, H. Liu, E. Vittinghoff, P. Leung, D. H. Ciccarone, and B. R. Edlin. 2001. Risk factors for skin and soft-tissue abscesses among injection drug users: a case-control study. *Clin. Infect. Dis.* **33:**35–40.

131. Murphy, E. L., J. W. Engstrom, K. Miller, R. A. Sacher, M. P. Busch, and C. G. Hollingsworth. 1993. HTLV-II associated myelopathy in a 43 year old woman. *Lancet.* **371:**757–758.

132. Murphy, E. L., J. Fridey, J. W. Smith, J. Engstrom, R. A. Sacher, K. Miller, J. Gibble, J. Stevens, R. Thomson, D. Hansma, J. Kaplan, R. Khabbaz, G. Nemo, and the REDS Investigators. 1997. HTLV-associated myelopathy in a cohort of HTLV-I and HTLV-II infected blood donors. *Neurology* **48:**315–320.

133. Murphy, E. L., S. A. Glynn, J. Fridey, R. A. Sacher, J. W. Smith, D. J. Wright, B. Newman, J. W., Gibble, D. I. Ameti, C. C. Nass, G. B. Schreiber, G. J. Nemo, and the Retrovirus Epidemiology Donor Study (REDS) Study Group. 1997. Increased prevelance of infectious disease and other adverse outcomes in human T lymphotropic virus types I- and II-infected blood donors. *J. Infect. Dis.* **176:**1468–1475.

134. Murphy, E. L., S. A. Glynn, J. Fridey, J. W. Smith, R. A. Sacher, C. C. Nass, H. E. Ownby, D. J. Wright, and G. J. Nemo. 1999. Increased incidence of infectious diseases during prospective follow-up of human T-lymphotropic virus type II- and I-infected blood donors. Retrovirus Epidemiology Donor Study. *Arch. Intern. Med.* **159:**1485–1491.

135. Nagal, M., and S. Jacobson. 2001. Immunopathogenesis of human T cell lym-

photropic virus type I-associated myelopathy. *Curr. Opin. Neurol.* **14:**381–386.

136. **Nagal, M., K. Usuku, W. Matsumoto, D. Kodama, N. Takenouchi, T. Moritoyo, S. Hashiguchi, M. Ichinose, C. R. Bangham, S. Izumo, and M. Osame.** 1998 Analysis of HTLV-I proviral load in 202 HAM/TSP patients and 243 asymptomatic HTLV-I carriers: high proviral load strongly predisposes to HAM/TSP. *J. Neurovirol.* **4:**586–593.

137. **Neiman, J., H. M. Haapaniemi, and M. Hillbom.** 2000. Neurological complications of drug abuse: pathophysiological mechanisms. *Eur. J. Neurol.* **7:**595–606.

138. **Neuveut, C., K. G. Low, F. Maldarelli, I. Schmitt, F. Majone, R. Grassmann, and K. T. Jeang.** 1998. Human T-cell leukemia virus type 1 Tax and cell cycle progression: role of cyclin D-cdk and p110Rb. *Mol. Cell. Biol.* **18:**3620–3632.

139. **Nicot, C., T. Astier-Gin, and B. Guillemain.** 1997. Activation of Bcl-2 expression in human endothelial cells chronically expressing the human T-cell lymphotropic virus type I. *Virology* **236:**47–53.

140. **Okochi, K., H. Sato, and Y. Hinuma.** 1984. A retrospective study on transmission of adult T cell leukemia virus by blood transfusion: seroconversion in recipients. *Vox Sang.* **46:**245–253.

141. **Oravecz, T., M. Pall, and M. A. Norcross.** 1996. Beta-chemokine inhibition of monocytotropic HIV-1 infection. Interference with a postbinding fusion step. *J. Immunol.* **157:**1329–1332.

142. **Osame, M., K. Usuku, S. Izumo, N. Ijichi, H. Amitani, A. Igata, M. Matsumoto, and M. Tara.** 1986. HTLV-I associated myelopathy, a new clinical entity. *Lancet* **i:**1031–1032.

143. **Page, J. B., S. H. Lai, D. D. Chitwood, N. G. Klimas, P. C. Smith, and M. A. Fletcher.** 1990. HTLV-I/II seropositivity and death from AIDS among HIV-1 seropositive intravenous drug users. *Lancet* **335:**1439–1441.

144. **Pardi, D., W. M. Switzer, K. G. Hadlock, J. E. Kaplan, R. B. Lal, and T. M. Folks.** 1993. Complete nucleotide sequence of an Amerindian human T-cell lymphotropic virus type II (HTLV-II) isolate: identification of a variant HTLV-II subtype b from a Guaymi Indian. *J. Virol.* **67:**4659–4664.

145. **Paxton, W. A., S. R. Martin, D. Tse, T. R. O'Brien, J. Skurnick, N. L. VanDevanter, N. Padian, J. F. Braun, D. P. Kotler, S. M. Wolinsky, and R. A. Koup.** 1996. Relative resistance to HIV-1 infection of CD4 lymphocytes from persons who remain uninfected despite multiple high-risk sexual exposure. *Nat. Med.* **2:**412–417.

146. **Peters, A. A., M. B. Coulthart, J. J. Oger, D. J. Waters, K. A. Crandall, A. A. Baumgartner, R. H. Ward, and G. A. Dekaban.** 2000. HTLV type I/II in British Columbia Amerindians: a seroprevalence study and sequence characterization of an HTLV type IIa isolate. *AIDS Res. Hum. Retrovir.* **16:**883–892.

147. **Piot, P., M. Bartos, P. D. Ghys, N. Walker, and B. Schwartlander.** 2001. The global impact of HIV/AIDS. *Nature* **410:**968–973.

148. **Pise-Masison, C. A., M. Radonovich, K. Sakaguchi, E. Appella, and J. N. Brady.** 1998. Phosphorylation of p53: a novel pathway for p53 inactivation in human T-cell lymphotropic virus type 1-transformed cells. *J. Virol.* **72:**6348–6355.

149. **Pise-Masison, C. A., K. S. Choi, M. Radonovich, J. Dittmer, S. J. Kim, and J. N. Brady.** 1998. Inhibition of p53 transactivation function by the human T-cell lymphotropic virus type 1 Tax protein. *J. Virol.* **72:**1165–1170.

150. **Poiesz, B., D. Dube, S. Dube, J. Love, L. Papsidero, A. Uner, and R. Hutchinson.** 2000. HTLV-II associated cutaneous T-cell lymphoma in a patient with HIV-1 infection. *N. Engl. J. Med.* **342:**930–936.

151. **Raffanti, A., A. Svenningsson, and L. Resnick.** 1991. HIV-1 infection of CD4-negative cells via HTLV pseudovirions. *AIDS* **5:**769–783.

152. **Richardson, J. H., A. J. Edwards, J. K. Cruickshank, P. Rudge, and A. G. Dalgleish.** 1990. In vivo cellular tropism of human T-cell leukemia virus type 1. *J. Virol.* **64:**5682–5687.

153. **Robert-Guroff, M., S. H. Weiss, J. A. Giron, A. M. Jennings, H. M. Ginzburg, I. B. Margolis, W. A. Blattner, and R. C. Gallo.** 1986. Prevalence of antibodies to HTLV-I, -II, and -III in intravenous drug abusers from an AIDS endemic region. *JAMA* **255:**3133–3137.

154. **Rosenblatt, J. D., J. V. Giorgi, D. W. Golde, J. B. Ezra, A. Wu, C. D. Winberg, J. Glaspy, W. Wachsman, and I. S. Chen.** 1988. Integrated human T-cell leukemia virus II genome in CD8 + T cells from a patient with "atypical" hairy cell leukemia: evidence for distinct T and B cell lymphoproliferative disorders. *Blood.* **71:**363–369.

155. **Rosenblatt, J. D., D. W. Golde, W. Wachsman, J. V. Giorgi, A. Jacobs, G. M. Schmidt, S. Quan, J. C. Gasson, and I. S. Chen.** 1986 A second isolate of HTLV-II asso-

ciated with atypical hairy-cell leukemia. *N. Engl. J. Med.* **315:**372–377.

156. **Rosenblatt, J. D., P. Tomkins, M. Rosenthal, A. Kacena, G. Chan, R. Valderama, W. Harrington, Jr., E. Saxton, A. Diagne, J. Q. Zhao, R. T. Mitsuyasu, and R. H. Weisbart.** 1992. Progressive spastic myelopathy in a patient co-infected with HIV-1 and HTLV-II: autoantibodies to the human homologue of rig in blood and cerebrospinal fluid. *AIDS* **6:**1151–1158.

157. **Safaelan, M., L. E. Wilson, E. Taylor, D. L. Thomas, and D. Vlahov.** 2000. HTLV-II and bacterial infections among injection drug users. *J. Acquir. Immune Defic. Syndr.* **24:**483–487.

158. **Salemi, M., E. Cattaneo, C. Casoli, and U. Bertazzoni.** 1995. Identification of IIa and IIb molecular subtypes of human T-cell lymphotropic virus type II among Italian injecting drug users. *J. Acquir. Immune Defic. Syndr. Hum. Retrovirol.* **8:**516–520.

159. **Salemi, M., M. Lewis, J. F. Egan, W. W. Hall, J. Desmyter, and A. M. Vandamme.** 1999. Different population dynamics of human T cell lymphotropic virus type II in intravenous drug users compared with endemically infected tribes. *Proc. Natl. Acad. Sci. USA* **96:**13253–13258.

160. **Salemi, M., A. M. Vandamme, J. Desmyter, C. Casoli, and U. Bertazzoni.** 1999. The origin and evolution of human T-cell lymphotropic virus type II (HTLV-II) and the relationship with its replication strategy. *Gene* **234:**11–21.

161. **Salemi, M., S. Van Dooren, E. Audenaert, E. Delaporte, P. Goubau, J. Desmyter, and A. M. Vandamme.** 1998. Two new human T-lymphotropic virus type I phylogenetic subtypes in seroindeterminates, a Mbuti pygmy and a Gabonese, have closest relatives among African STLV-I strains. *Virology* **246:**277–287.

162. **Santiago, F., E. Clark, S. Chong, C. Molina, F. Mozafari, R. Mahieux, M. Fujii, N. Azimi, and F. Kashanchi.** 1999. Transcriptional up-regulation of the cyclin D2 gene and acquisition of new cyclin-dependent kinase partners in human T-cell leukemia virus type 1-infected cells. *J. Virol.* **73:**9917–9927.

163. **Schechter, M., L. H. Moulton, and L. H. Harrison.** 1997. HIV viral load and CD4+ lymphocyte counts in subjects coinfected with HTLV-I and HIV-1. *J. Acquir. Immune Defic. Syndr. Hum. Retrovirol.* **15:**308–311.

164. **Schmitt, I., O. Rosin, P. Rohwer, M. Gossen, and R. Grassmann.** 1998. Stimulation of cyclin-dependent kinase activity and G_1-to S-phase transition in human lymphocytes by the human T-cell leukemia/lymphotropic virus type 1 Tax protein. *J. Virol.* **72:**633–640.

165. **Schreiber, G. B., E. L. Murphy, J. A. Horton, D. J. Wright, R. Garfein, H. C. Chien, and C. C. Nass.** 1997. Risk factors for human T-cell lymphotropic virus types I and II (HTLV-I and II) in blood donors: the Retrovirus Epidemiology Donor Study. *J. Acquir. Immune Defic. Syndr. Hum. Retrovirol.* **14:**263–271.

166. **Sheremata, W. A., D. Benedict, D. C. Squilacote, A. Sazant, and E. DeFreitas.** 1993. High-dose zidovudine induction in HTLV-I-associated myelopathy: safety and possible efficacy. *Neurology* **43:**2125–2129.

167. **Sheremata, W., W. J. Harrington, Jr., P. A. Bradshaw, S. K. H. Foung, J. R. Berger, L. Resnick, and B. J. Poiesz.** 1993. Association of '(tropical) ataxic neuropathy' with HTLV-II. *Virus Res.* **29:**71–77.

168. **Shibata, D., R. K. Brynes, A. Rabinowitz, C. A. Hanson, M. L. Slovak, T. J. Spira, and P. Gill.** 1989. Human T-cell lymphotropic virus type I (HTLV-I)-associated adult T-cell leukemia-lymphoma in a patient infected with human immunodeficiency virus type 1 (HIV-1). *Ann. Intern. Med.* **111:**871–875.

169. **Shimoyama, M.** 1991. Diagnostic criteria and classification of clinical subtypes of adult T-cell leukaemia-lymphoma. A report from the Lymphoma Study Group (1984–87). *Br. J. Haematol.* **79:**428–437.

170. **Siekewitz, M., S. F. Josephs, M. Dukovitch, N. Peffer, F. Wong-Staal, and W. C. Greene.** 1987. Activation of the HIV-1 LTR by T-cell mitogens and the trans-activator protein of HTLV-I. *Science* **238:**1557–1559.

171. **Sobesky, M., P. Couppie, R. Pradinaud, M. C. Godard, F. Alvarez, B. Benoit, B. Carme, P. Lebeux, and GECVIG (Clinical HIV Study Group in Guiana).** 2000. Coinfection with HIV and HTLV-I infection and survival in AIDS stage. French Guiana Study. *Presse Med.* **29:**413–416.

172. **Song, K. J., V. R. Nerurkar, N. Saitou, A. Lazo, J. R. Blakeslee, I. Miyoshi, and R. Yanagihara.** 1994. Genetic analysis and molecular phylogeny of simian T-cell lymphotropic virus type I: evidence for independent virus evolution in Asia and Africa. *Virology* **199:**56–66.

173. **Soriano, V., M. Gutierrez, R. Bravo, F. Diaz, J. Olivan, and J. Gonzalez-Lahoz.** 1994. Severe myopathy in an injection drug user coinfected with human immunodeficiency virus type 1 and human T cell leukemia virus type II. *Clin. Infect. Dis.* **19:**350–351.

174. **Sugiyama, H., H. Doi, K. Yamaguchi, Y. Tsuji, T. Miyamoto, and S. Hino.** 1986. Significance of postnatal mother-to-child transmission of human T-lymphotropic virus type-I on the development of adult T-cell leukemia/lymphoma. *J. Med. Virol.* **20:**253–260.

175. **Sullivan, M. T., A. E. Williams, C. T. Fang, T. Grandinetti, B. J. Poiesz, G. D. Ehrlich, and the American Red Cross HTLV-I/II Collaborative Study Group.** 1991. Transmission of human T-lymphotropic virus types I and II by blood transfusion. A retrospective study of recipients of blood components (1983 through 1988). *Arch. Intern. Med.* **151:**2043–2048.

176. **Switzer, W. M., S. M. Owen, D. A. Pieniazek, V. R. Nerurkar, E. Duenas-Barajas, W. Heneine, and R. B. Lal.** 1995. Molecular analysis of human T-cell lymphotropic virus type II from Wayuu Indians of Colombia demonstrates two subtypes of HTLV-IIb. *Virus Genes* **10:**153–162.

177. **Szabo, J., Z. Beck, E. Csoman, X. Liu, I. Andriko, J. Kiss, A. Basci, P. Ebbesen, and F. D. Toth.** 1999. Differential patterns of interaction between HIV type 1 and HTLV type I in monocyte-derived macrophages cultured in vitro: implications for in vivo coinfection with HIV type 1 and HTLV type I. *AIDS Res. Hum. Retrovir.* **15:**1653–1666.

178. **Takatsuki, K., K. Yamaguchi, F. Kawano, T. Hattori, H. Nishimura, H. Tsuda, I. Sanada, K. Nakada, and Y. Itai.** 1985. Clinical diversity in adult T-cell leukemia-lymphoma. *Cancer Res.* **45:**4644s–4645s.

179. **Taylor, G. P., S. E. Hall, S. Navarrete, C. A. Michie, R. Davis, A. D. Witkover, M. Rossor, M. A. Nowak, P. Rudge, E. Matutes, C. R. Bangham, and J. N. Weber.** 1999. Effect of lamivudine on human T-cell leukemia virus type 1 (HTLV-1) DNA copy number, T-cell phenotype, and anti-tax cytotoxic T-cell frequency in patients with HTLV-1-associated myelopathy. *J. Virol.* **73:**10289–10295.

180. **Tuppin, P., A. Gessain, M. Kazanji, R. Mahieux, J. Y. Cosnefroy, F. Tekaia, M. C. Georges-Courbot, A. Georges, and G. de The.** 1996. Evidence in Gabon for an intrafamilial clustering with mother-to-child and sexual transmission of a new molecular variant of human T-lymphotropic virus type-II subtype B. *J. Med. Virol.* **48:**22–32.

181. **Vallejo, A., and A. Garcia-Saiz.** 1994. Isolation and nucleotide sequence analysis of human T-cell lymphotropic virus type II in Spain. *J. Acquir. Immune Defic. Syndr.* **7:**517–519.

182. **Van Brussel, M., M. Salemi, H. F. Liu, P. Goubau, J. Desmyter, and A. M. Vandamme.** 1999. The discovery of two new divergent STLVs has implications for the evolution and epidemiology of HTLVs. *Rev. Med. Virol.* **9:**155–170.

183. **Vandamme, A. M., H. F. Liu, P. Goubau, and J. Desmyter.** 1994. Primate T-lymphotropic virus type I LTR sequence variation and its phylogenetic analysis: compatibility with an African origin of PTLV-I. *Virology* **202:**212–223.

184. **Vandamme, A. M., H. F. Liu, M. Van Brussel, W. De Meurichy, J. Desmyter, and P. Goubau.** 1996. The presence of a divergent T-lymphotropic virus in a wild-caught pygmy chimpanzee (Pan paniscus) supports an African origin for the human T-lymphotropic/simian T-lymphotropic group of viruses. *J. Gen. Virol.* **77:**1089–1099.

185. **Vandamme, A.-M., M. Salemi, M. Van Brussel, H.-F. Liu, K. Van Laethem, M. Van Ranst, L. Michels, J. Desmyter, and P. Goubau.** 1998. African origin of human T-lymphotropic virus type 2 (HTLV-2) supported by a potential new HTLV-2d subtype in Congolese Bambuti Efe Pygmies. *J. Virol.* **72:**4327–4340.

186. **Visconti, A., L. Visconti, R. Bellocco, N. Binkin, G. Colluci, L. Vernocchi, M. Amendola, and D. Ciaci.** 1993. HTLV-II/HIV-I coinfection and risk for progression to AIDS among intravenous drug users. *J. Acquir. Immune Defic. Syndr.* **6:**1228–1237.

187. **Watanabe, T., M. Seiki, Y. Hirayama, and M. Yoshida.** 1986. Human T-cell leukemia virus type I is a member of the African subtype of simian viruses (STLV). *Virology* **148:**385–388.

188. **Watanabe, K. K., A. E. Williams, G. B. Schreiber, and H. E. Ownby.** 2000. Infectious disease markers in young blood donors. Retrovirus Epidemiology Donor Study. *Transfusion* **40:**954–960.

189. **Weiss, R. A.** 2001. Gulliver's travels in HIV-land. *Nature* **410:**963–967.

190. **Willy, R. J., C. M. Salas, G. E. Macalino, and J. D. Rich.** 1999. Long-term non-progression of HIV-1 in a patient coinfected with HTLV-II. *Diagn. Microbiol. Infect. Dis.* **35:**269–270.

191. **Woods, T. C., J. M. Graber, R. C. Hershow, R. F. Khabbaz, J. E. Kaplan, and W. Heneine.** 1995. Investigation of proviral load in individuals infected with human T-lymphotropic virus type II. *AIDS Res. Hum. Retrovir.* **11:**1235–1239.

192. **Yashiki, S., T. Fujiyoshi, N. Arima, M. Osame, M. Yoshinaga, Y. Nagata, M. Tara, K.**

Nomura, A. Utsunomiya, S. Hanada, K. Tajima, and S. Sonoda. 2001. HLA-a*26, HLA-b*4002, HLA-b*4006, and HLA-b*4801 alleles predispose to adult T cell leukemia: the limited recognition of HTLV type 1 tax peptide anchor motifs and epitopes to generate anti-HTLV type 1 tax CD8+ cytotoxic T lymphocytes. *AIDS Res. Hum. Retrovir.* **17:**1047–1061.

193. **Yoshida, M.** 2001. Multiple viral strategies of HTLV-1 for dysregulation of cell growth control. *Annu. Rev. Immunol.* **19:**475–496.

194. **Zack, J. A., A. J. Cann, J. D. Lugo, and I. S. Y. Chen.** 1988. HIV-I production from peripheral blood cells after HTLV-I induced mitogenic stimulation. *Science* **240:**1026–1029.

195. **Zagury, D., A. Lachgar, V. Chams, L. S. Fall, J. Bernard, J. F. Zagury, B. Bizzini, A. Gringeri, E. Santagostino, J. Rappaport, M. Feldman, S. J. O'Brien, A. Burny, and R. C. Gallo.** 1998. C-C chemokines, pivotal in protection against HIV type 1 infection. *Proc. Natl. Acad. Sci. USA* **95:**3857–3861.

196. **Zehender, G., C. De Maddalena, M. Osio, B. Cavalli, C. Parravicini, M. Moroni, and M. Galli.** 1995. High prevalence of human T cell lymphotropic virus type II infection in patients affected by human immunodeficiency virus type 1-associated predominantly sensory polyneuropathy. *J. Infect. Dis.* **172:**1595–1598.

197. **Zehender, G., L. Meroni, S. Varchetta, C. De Maddalena, B. Cavalli, M. Gianotto, A. B. Bosisio, C. Colasante, G. Rizzardini, M. Moroni, and M. Galli.** 1998. Human T-lymphotropic virus type 2 (HTLV-2) provirus in circulating cells of the monocyte/macrophage lineage in patients dually infected with human immunodeficiency virus type 1 and HTLV-2 and having predominantly sensory polyneuropathy. *J. Virol.* **72:**7664–7668.

198. **Zella, D., L. Mori, M. Sala, P. Ferrante, C. Casoli, G. Magnani, G. Achilli, E. Cattaneo, F. Lori, and U. Bertazzoni.** 1990. HTLV-II infection in Italian drug abusers. *Lancet* **336:**575–576.

VIRUSES AND MULTIPLE SCLEROSIS

Donatella Donati and Steven Jacobson

6

Multiple sclerosis (MS) is a complex demyelinating disease of the central nervous system (CNS) affecting mostly young adults. Its first description by Charcot and colleagues dates back more than 100 years. However, despite the abundance of research and the plethora of reports regarding MS in the literature, many aspects of its etiology and pathophysiology remain unclear. In part, this is due to the difficulty in diagnosis and the variability in the course and prognosis of this disease. Several non-mutually exclusive factors are believed to contribute to the etiology of MS. A widely accepted view of MS is that it is an inflammatory disease with autoimmune characteristics influenced by environmental or infectious factors in genetically susceptible individuals. Therefore, the etiology of MS is likely to involve multiple factors that interact with each other, ultimately resulting in this chronic, progressive neurologic disease.

The role of infectious and viral agents in MS etiology and pathogenesis is still under debate. The epidemiology of MS suggests that infectious agents might affect the development and clinical course of MS, and the list of viruses studied as candidate etiologic agents is rather long. A clear association with a particular viral pathogen has not been found. However, a few viruses, including human herpesvirus 6 (HHV-6), are accumulating considerable and consistent support for a role in MS. It is also possible that one or more viruses or infectious agents can interact synergistically and trigger an autoimmune response.

CLINICAL FEATURES

The clinical course of MS tends to result in progressive neurological impairment. The symptoms at presentation, as well as during the course of the disease, may vary greatly among patients, depending on the localization of lesions, which may theoretically affect any myelinated tract in the white matter. However, some preferential sites for plaque formation exist, making symptoms such as optic neuritis, paresthesia, limb weakness, and spasticity more common at onset. Cortical signs, such as aphasia, apraxia, seizures, or extrapyramidal signs (chorea or rigidity), are observed more rarely. Following the first attack, MS pa-

Donatella Donati, Viral Immunology Section, Neuroimmunology Branch, National Institute of Neurological Disorders and Stroke, National Institutes of Health, Bethesda, MD 20892, and Dipartimento di Biologia Molecolare, Sezione di Microbiologia, Università di Siena, via Laterina 8, 53100 Siena, Italy. *Steven Jacobson,* Viral Immunology Section, Neuroimmunology Branch, National Institute of Neurological Disorders and Stroke, National Institutes of Health, Bethesda, MD 20892.

Polymicrobial Diseases, Edited by Kim A. Brogden and Janet M. Guthmiller,
© 2002 ASM Press, Washington, D.C.

tients will experience one of four clinical courses, which have been standardized and classified (93). A relapsing-remitting course is characterized by a sequence of relapses with full or partial recovery between clinical relapse events. About 80 to 90% of patients present this form of the disease at onset. Approximately 40% of patients with relapsing-remitting MS will eventually develop a secondary progressive course. Secondary progressive MS is marked by a gradual progression of symptoms with or without occasional relapses and minor remissions. Eventually, other signs of CNS dysfunction (cognitive impairment, progressive motor and sensory loss) accumulate. Alternatively, a primary progressive form may develop from onset, with progressive worsening of symptoms with occasional minor remissions. Patients with this form often have a slowly progressive upper motor neuron syndrome affecting primarily the legs. A relapsing progressive form of MS, a rare progressive disease from onset with clear acute relapses, has also been defined.

NEUROPATHOLOGY

The complexity and diversity of MS pathologic features in relation to the history of the disease have made the identification of a single pathogenic pathway unsuccessful and are now contributing to a new approach to the study of the disease pathogenesis.

Myelin sheaths in the CNS are provided by oligodendrocytes, whose cell membrane wraps in layers around axons. Serial sheaths along axons are separated by the nodes of Ranvier, which are responsible for the saltatory conduction and ensure a fast conduction of stimuli. Additionally, myelin sheaths have a trophic function on nerves. Thus, demyelination subsequently leads to slowing of nerve conduction and finally neuronal death. The typical MS lesions are perivascular white matter plaques of primary demyelination associated with various degrees of inflammatory cells according to the stage of the plaque (115).

Though there are reports of early axonal loss in MS independent from oligodendrocyte damage (13), the hallmark of the disease is demyelination. Different plaques at various stages can be present in the same patient. A plaque is considered active if infiltrating macrophages contain myelin degradation products. Conversely, plaques with some degree of remyelination (shadow plaques) can be observed in acute and early MS.

The recent detection of different patterns of demyelination (48, 95, 96) suggests a possible heterogeneity in the mechanisms involved in lesion development. In particular, a study by Lucchinetti et al. (96) described a number of active MS plaques closely resembling autoimmune encephalitis, such as that seen in myelin oligodendrocyte glycoprotein (MOG)-induced experimental autoimmune encephalomyelitis (EAE). This pattern of demyelination was characterized by perivascular inflammation, infiltrating T lymphocytes, macrophages with deposition of immunoglobulin Gs (IgGs), and increased complement at sites of active myelin breakdown. However, other lesions described in the same study showed prominent signs of oligodendrocyte dystrophy without IgG and complement deposition, suggesting primary oligodendrocyte damage. The latter pattern of demyelination, observed mostly at early stages of MS, was reminiscent of a primary injury of oligodendrocytes, possibly resulting from viral or toxic damage. The authors concluded that, at least in a subset of MS patients, a direct and possibly virus-induced oligodendrocyte disturbance might be the starting point for a subsequent switch to autoimmune demyelination. This finding confirmed a previous study (48) showing that, at least in some patients, demyelination appeared to occur prior to T-cell inflammation, suggesting a possible initiation of a pathogenic mechanism within the CNS.

Studies on oligodendrocyte pathology also demonstrated a great variability (95), ranging from extensive loss to normal or increased oligodendrocyte density in active plaques. Interestingly, the pattern of oligodendrocyte loss was heterogeneous among MS patients but homogeneous within individual patients.

Collectively, recent pathological studies of MS strongly support the view of different pathogenetic mechanisms as a first trigger of disease. One possible pattern might rely on a primary inflammatory process in which demyelinating antibodies and complement activation play a relevant role. In other cases, a primary myelin, oligodendrocyte, or precursor cell damage might occur. Therefore, a new concept of MS as a group of syndromes with different initial pathogenetic mechanisms has emerged.

MECHANISM OF MS PATHOGENESIS

There has been a strong contribution to MS research by use of the murine EAE model and the demonstration of myelin-reactive T cells that has focused considerable attention on cellular immunity. MS has been typically considered a Th1-driven disease. Th1 (inflammatory) cells produce cytokines involved in T-cell mediated immunity such as interleukin-2 (IL-2), gamma interferon (IFN-γ), and tumor necrosis factor alpha (TNF-α) and induce antibody switching from IgM to IgG2a and IgG3. Th2 (anti-inflammatory) cells are those secreting IL-4, IL-5, IL-10, and transforming growth factor β1 and are important stimulators of antibody production (132). Most of the studies on the role of T cells in MS have focused on myelin-activated peripheral T cells restricted by major histocompatibility complex (MHC) class II molecules. Myelin basic protein (MBP) has been the first and most extensively studied myelin protein involved in MS. Other myelin proteins, such as proteolipid protein (PLP), MOG, myelin-associated glycoprotein (MAG), and myelin-associated oligodendrocytic basic protein, have also been suggested to play a role as potential autoantigens in MS (62, 72, 171).

It was widely accepted that, in normal conditions, there is an immune tolerance to myelin antigens sequestered in the CNS and protected by the blood-brain barrier (BBB). However, the finding that healthy individuals may also have myelin-reactive peripheral T cells has challenged this assumption (20, 88,

123). These findings suggest that the presence of myelin-reactive T cells *per se* does not appear to be sufficient for a pathogenetic role for such cells. However, similar frequencies of MBP-specific T cells were observed in families of patients with MS and those of healthy individuals, in agreement with the immunogenetic susceptibility to the disease (66). Furthermore, MBP and PLP-reactive T cells from MS patients were found to be significantly more responsive to IL-2 stimulation than those from control subjects (179). Therefore, myelin-reactive T cells appear to be in a different state of activation in patients with MS than in healthy subjects.

Myelin T–cell activation in the periphery could also result from a mechanism of molecular mimicry, which implies a potent cross–reactive autoimmune response due to sequence or conformational homology between self (i.e., myelin) and foreign antigens. Activated T cells might then cross the BBB and establish an inflammatory response to myelin antigens. Consistent with this process is perivascular inflammatory infiltration observed in MS plaques. Moreover, focal BBB breakdown seems to precede the development of most lesions (94). The entry of activated T cells across the BBB may be due to a selective leakage, involving a multistep interaction between T cells and endothelial cells and specific secretion of adhesion molecules (21). This theory is supported by the finding of increased expression of adhesion molecules ICAM-I, VCAM-I, and E-selectin in cerebrospinal fluid (CSF) and sera from MS patients (38).

Another aspect associated with a Th1 response in MS is related to cytokine production. An overexpression of Th1-dependent cytokines such as IFN-γ and TNF-α in MS plaques has been observed. Moreover, treatment of MS patients with IFN-γ resulted in increased exacerbations (118). Th1 cytokines therefore can sustain a chronic state of inflammation by either mediating a continuous recruitment of activated T cells or directly inducing myelin breakdown, as demonstrated for TNF-α (144). Additionally, an active expression of TNF-α in peripheral blood mononuclear cells (PBMCs) has been demonstrated to be associated with MS activity (131).

An increasing body of evidence is now supporting a crucial role for B-cell-mediated immunity and antibodies in MS (5, 35). Antibodies directed to myelin components such as MBP, PLP, MAG, and MOG have been observed in the serum (113) and in the CSF (107, 168) of MS patients. However, the trend of antibody response appears to differ when specific antigens are considered. Anti-MBP antibodies seem to increase over time during the course of MS, whereas anti-MOG antibodies have been demonstrated to arise early in the course of the disease and constantly persist over time (129). As described above, antibody deposition is present in subsets of MS plaques (96, 155). Antibody-mediated demyelinating EAE (ADEAE) is a variant of EAE obtained by addition of antimyelin antibodies at the beginning of the disease, and its pathological characteristics are more similar to those observed in MS than those of EAE (125).

A laboratory hallmark of MS is the presence of immunoglobulins (Igs) in a restricted spectrotype pattern, i.e., oligoclonal bands (OCBs) in the CSF, due to an intrathecal synthesis of Igs. OCB levels are stable and do not vary with changes in clinical stages of the disease and are used in support of the laboratory diagnosis of MS. MS patients have a specific individual OCB pattern of CSF antibody titer. OCBs are not specific for MS and are also observed in other chronic inflammatory CNS diseases, such as CNS Lyme disease, chronic meningitis, and CNS lupus erythematosus. OCBs are also found in subacute sclerosing panencephalitis (SSPE), where antibodies are directed specifically to measles virus components. Conversely, the search for OCB specificity in MS has been unsuccessful, and only a small portion of OCBs can be accounted for by known antiviral antibodies.

Intrathecal synthesis of viral antibodies can be also observed following primary infection with viruses such as mumps or measles virus. What is particular to MS is the persistent and consistent production of antibodies directed against a few specific antigens. It is not clear whether the source of the OCBs is resident or passively recruited plasma cells crossing the BBB. However, it might be indicative of one or more persisting factors stimulating continuing IgG synthesis.

The role of complement in the pathogenesis of MS is not fully understood. The presence of IgGs in the active border of MS plaques can be accompanied by deposition of C9neo, a marker of complement cascade activation (155). Serum complement-related proteins might leak through an altered BBB into the CNS and damage susceptible cells with subsequent demyelination. Rat and human myelin membranes are able to activate complement either with or without complement-activating antibodies (162). Activated complement factors can disregulate cytokine and adhesion molecule production with cell lysis. To prevent autologous complement-mediated lysis, most cells normally express a wide range of complement regulatory proteins on their surface. In MOG-induced EAE, the potential demyelinating activity of antibodies has been demonstrated to be due to their ability to fix complement (124). Similarly, MBP-induced ADEAE was reduced in severity in Lewis rats treated with soluble complement regulatory molecule complement receptor 1, and demyelination was prevented in the majority of treated animals (125).

ANIMAL MODELS

EAE

EAE is a T-cell-mediated autoimmune demyelinating disease induced by the peripheral injection of whole white matter or peptides of myelin proteins such as MBP, PLP, and MOG in complete Freund's adjuvant or by passive transfer of autoreactive T cells in susceptible inbred rodent or monkey strains (172). The initial autoreactivity appears to be CD4$^+$ Th1 dependent, with the exception of MOG-induced EAE, in which a Th2 response inducing demyelinating antibodies seems to have an important role (89). Mice deficient in the IL-12 p40 gene, which is expressed in a Th1 response, are not susceptible to EAE (143), and anti-IL-12 antibodies are able to prevent EAE (86). However, Th2 cells might also have a role in the autoimmune process. Th2 cells from MBP-specific T-cell receptor transgenic mice were able to induce EAE in immunodeficient mice (84). Moreover, marmoset EAE induction using MOG can drive a Th2 response resulting in fatal demyelination (49).

Once they have entered the CNS, $CD4^+$ T cells interact with antigen-presenting cells (APCs) in an MHC class II-restricted manner (43), with a local inflammatory lesion leading to a subsequent antigen-independent recruitment of inflammatory cells into the CNS and BBB alteration. EAE can have an acute or chronically relapsing course, depending on the susceptibility of the species and strains of animals used (92).

EAE in humanized animal models has also been described. Of particular interest are triple transgenic mice expressing HLA-DR2, a T-cell receptor specific for the encephalitogenic MBP epitope 84-102, and the human CD4 coreceptor (99). These mice were able to spontaneously develop EAE, suggesting a necessary and sufficient role of the trimolecular complex for the disease in this system.

Virally Induced Demyelinating Diseases

Not only can viruses induce direct damage of the infected cells, but they can also trigger autoimmune reactions leading to demyelination. Virus-induced demyelinating autoimmunity is strongly supportive for an infectious etiology of MS and can help to shed light on the role of a possible microbial agent(s) in the pathogenesis of this disease. Such models have been extensively studied and are thought to develop by either bystander activation or molecular mimicry.

Bystander activation implies that once a viral infection has been established, a wide sequence of different events can occur (175). Infection can elicit cytokine and chemokine production, or expression of a host's otherwise quiescent genes, or unveiling of hidden self-antigens. This cascade of events induces a self-generating inflammation with continuous cell damage and subsequent release of host antigens and activation of bystander T cells. Inflammatory cytokines, such as TNF-α, have been demonstrated to directly induce demyelination (19). Bystander effects are a common pathway suggested to play a role in many autoimmune disorders, such as for diabetes in mice infected with coxsackie B4 virus (57).

Molecular mimicry is an alternative mechanism by which a viral component can induce an immune cross-reaction with myelin proteins. The involvement of such mechanisms has been demonstrated in the induction of EAE in rabbits by hepatitis B virus polymerase peptides showing homology with MBP (46). MBP-specific T-cell clones have also been demonstrated to be reactive to mimicry peptides from a group of herpesviruses (Epstein-Barr virus [EBV], herpes simplex virus [HSV], and cytomegalovirus [CMV]), influenza viruses, and papillomaviruses (177).

A process known as epitope spreading can also perpetuate an autoimmune reaction. Such a mechanism was first described by Lehman et al. (85) and implies that an initial inflammatory reaction to an MBP epitope can give rise to additional recognition of further epitopes of the same protein in time. This phenomenon can be explained by the self-sustained breakdown of myelin, whose epitopes are continuously unveiled during the inflammatory reaction. Interestingly, epitope spreading in both EAE and MS has been described in a study showing that the initial autoreactivity to a primary self-antigen waned and disappeared, being replaced by secondary autoreactivity to new antigens during the progression of the disease. Though this finding was described for only three patients, it might indicate a possible temporal interplay among different antigenic determinants leading to MS disease progression (160).

Among the various murine models of demyelinating diseases, three have been particularly useful in understanding the mechanisms of acute and chronic demyelination: Semliki Forest virus (SFV), mouse hepatitis virus (MHV), and Theiler's murine encephalomyelitis virus (TMEV). SFV induces an acute infection with viral clearance followed by secondary demyelination. After peripheral injection into B6 mice, SFV establishes a transient infection in the brain followed by secondary demyelination after the virus has been cleared. Demyelination due to SFV appears to be T cell mediated (105). Recent findings demonstrated that the initial lesion is possibly induced by molecular mimicry between the viral surface glycoprotein E2 and MOG peptide 18–32, with a contribution of antipeptide antibody production, possibly crossing the BBB (106).

The coronavirus MHV is a common enteric pathogen of laboratory mice. The JHM strain of the virus (JHMV) was first isolated from a mouse with hind limb paralysis (6). Several JHM variants with different neurotropisms have been developed; however, all parental strains induce an acute encephalomyelitis with primary demyelination in mice, rats, and nonhuman primates (154). After intracerebral injection, an early demyelinating phase takes place, preferentially located in the ependymal cells with viral replication in astrocytes, microglia, and oligodendroglia, which appear to undergo apoptosis (8). As the disease progresses, demyelination declines, but new foci of demyelination appear (41). Though the virus is hardly detected in the CNS, it may establish a latent infection in astroglial and microglial cell (157). $CD4^+$ as well as $CD8^+$ T cells are associated with viral clearance after the early demyelinating phase (173), while humoral immunity is associated with prevention of viral reactivation during the latent phase.

An immune component seems to actively support JHMV demyelination. There is evidence that myelin might be degraded by infiltrating macrophages (176), though a recent report suggested that demyelination could be ascribed to microglial cells (178). Another intriguing finding is the possibility of EAE induction by adoptive transfer of T cells from

JHMV subacute encephalomyelitis (170), while T cells have been demonstrated to be reactive to peripheral self-antigen and not to CNS self-antigen during JHMV infection (83). Therefore, the JHMV model seems to be due to an interaction between viral persistence and immune reaction.

The demyelination disease induced by TMEV probably can be considered the most relevant virus-induced animal model of MS, and the mechanisms underlying the progression of the disease have been widely studied (154). TMEV-induced demyelination has some interesting similarities to MS, since the virus establishes a persistent infection resembling the chronically progressive form of MS, with myelin-reactive T cells as well as antimyelin antibodies. Furthermore, mice with TMEV-induced chronic disease can undergo spontaneous remyelination with partial restoration of neurological function, as observed also in the relapsing-remitting or chronically relapsing forms of MS (110).

TMEV belongs to the family *Picornaviridae* (158) and in susceptible SJL mice causes first an acute and then a chronic progressive disease similarly to the secondary chronic progressive form of MS. Strains of mice not susceptible to TMEV infection go through only the first phase, with no neurological symptoms after the clearance of the virus. After intracerebral inoculation, TMEV replicates in the CNS, and ensuing symptoms such as paralysis seem to be due to a cytolytic infection of motor neurons, similar to that caused by poliovirus, another neurotropic picornavirus. During this early phase, there is little or no inflammation. The second phase is characterized by an increase in inflammation, consisting of $CD4^+$ T cells and macrophages, and demyelination. Like JHMV, the virus cannot be detected in the peripheral circulation during this phase but persists in the CNS, mostly infecting macrophages or microglial cells (90). Oligodendrocytes are rarely infected, despite demyelination. The subsequent immune reaction does not eliminate the virus but leads to a chronic inflammation. $CD8^+$ T cells may be critical in preventing disease progression during the first phase, while their role does not seem to be relevant during the chronic phase (16, 154).

The progression of TMEV-induced disease does not appear to be due to direct or CD8$^+$-T-cell-mediated damage of TMEV-infected oligodendrocytes. Rather, a bystander demyelination might result from the chronic virus-specific T-cell-mediated demyelination, thus triggering the release and recognition of multiple host neuroantigen epitopes (i.e., epitope spreading) (104). A Th1 response seems to be critical for TMEV demyelination, as suggested by an increase in IgG2a during infection (122). The Th1 response appears to be achieved by virus-specific chronic CD4$^+$-T-cell activation, which is also consistent with a delayed-type hypersensitivity (DTH) mechanism (29). Furthermore, tolerance induction in SJL mice was demonstrated to prevent clinical disease as well as CNS inflammation and DTH and T-cell responses (67). Therefore, a virus-specific Th1 response may initiate and maintain a chronic inflammation with sustained release of otherwise hidden antigens. Astrocytes have recently been demonstrated to harbor most of the replicating virus and are considered to be a main site of persistent infection (180). The same study showed a great amount of viral antigen in macrophages or microglial cells, which are CNS-resident local APCs and are thought to play a key role in TMEV-induced demyelination (70). Indeed, APCs were demonstrated to process and present not only viral epitopes, but also a variety of proteolipid protein epitopes during the course of the disease. Katz-Levy et al. (70) also showed that antigen presentation occurs in the context of MHC class II molecules with B7-1, and to a minor extent B7-2, antigen expression. Moreover, only APCs from TMEV-infected mice, and not those from naïve mice, were able to activate Th1 cells.

An interesting set of results comes from a recent study using a nonpathogenic genetically engineered TMEV variant encoding a mimic PLP epitope (116). The intracerebral injection of this modified virus resulted in a demyelinating disease due to PLP-specific Th1 cells, thus demonstrating the development of an autoimmune demyelinating disease supported by a molecular mimicry mechanism.

Collectively, these findings can be of great help in understanding MS pathogenesis, due to the similarity between the mouse and human diseases. MS plaques also contain cells expressing MHC class II molecules, B7-1, and IL-12 (174) as well as products of activated T cells such as IFN-γ and IL-2 (56). Therefore, a virus-initiated event, at least in a subset of MS patients, with a temporal interplay between viral and myelin epitopes represents a viable model for disease pathogenesis in MS.

HUMAN MODELS OF VIRUS-INDUCED DEMYELINATION

Virus-induced demyelination can also occur in humans. By definition of specific virus-induced pathways leading to demyelination, these syndromes can be of great help in adding knowledge on how similar mechanisms may play a role in MS. There are a number of demyelinating diseases following systemic infections with viruses such as mumps, varicella-zoster, influenza, and measles viruses, termed postinfectious encephalomyelitis (PIE) (64). Other demyelinating diseases with well-defined viral etiologies are progressive multifocal leukoencephalopathy (PML), SSPE, and human T-cell leukemia virus type 1 (HTLV-1)-associated myelopathy/tropical spastic paraparesis (HAM/TSP).

PIE

The pathogenesis of PIE is not clear, but some possible autoimmune mechanisms have been suggested by the inability to detect the respective virus in the CNS. The most common form is associated with measles virus infection. It occurs in 1 case per 1,000 infected children and is coincident with the onset of the immune response. Clinically, there are multifocal neurological symptoms with fever and seizures. The disease is fatal in 20% of cases, and survivors usually have sequelae. Neuropathological findings include perivenular lesions with mononuclear infiltration and demyelination. Interestingly, these lesions are similar to those observed in EAE, and the loss of myelin proteins in the two syndromes has similar patterns (50). Thus, PIE could be considered an autoimmune disease triggered by a viral infection. Measles virus is not usually detected in the CNS of post-measles encephalomyelitis, nor has intrathecal synthesis of antimeasles antibody been observed (65). Measles infection is known to induce leukopenia and altered lymphocyte function (64) with activation of lymphocyte clusters. Lymphocytes from PIE patients were found to respond to MBP at a significantly higher percentage than those from patients with non-complicated measles (65). Therefore, evidence is consistent with an initial peripheral proliferation of measles virus in lymphoid organs with lymphocyte activation. PIE appears to result from a homing of these activated lymphocytes to the CNS, similar to EAE in animals.

SSPE

SSPE is a very rare disease of children and young adults occurring in 1 case per million children 5 to 10 years after primary measles virus infection. The clinical course may range from months to years, but it invariably results in death. Histopathological findings include patches of perivascular cuffings with lymphocytes and plasma cells. In contrast to post-measles encephalomyelitis, which appears to be due to an autoimmune mechanism, the onset of SSPE seems to be related to a direct viral infection of the CNS. Measles virus is a highly lymphotropic virus and might transiently gain access to the CNS during primary infection by activated peripheral white blood cells entering the BBB. However, the type of cells harboring the virus during the latent phase has yet to be identified. Measles virus inclusions are found in neurons and oligodendroglia, but there is absence of viral budding from the plasma membrane. It has been hypothesized that defective measles virus replication occurs in the CNS and the virus is passed by cell-to-cell spread. As a result, SSPE can be considered a chronic defective viral infection, with a defect in viral assembly. This was suggested to be re-

lated to a defect in M-protein synthesis, which is important for viral assembly (54). Alternatively, it could be due to multiple mutations in genomic RNA. Indeed, it was demonstrated that measles virus in SSPE has deletions in genes involved in the assembly of infectious virus (23).

A typical characteristic of SSPE is an extremely high titer of antimeasles antibody in the CSF (32). Investigations of SSPE models in rats suggested that the antimeasles antibody titer is essential for viral persistence, since the antibodies can alter the viral envelope proteins expressed on the cell surface (45). Additionally, a role for a cell-mediated contribution to the disease has also been claimed, due to the expression of IFN-γ and TNF-α in SSPE lesions (111). However, the switch from wild-type to defective virus during latency, being so rare in occurrence, might also be due to host factors which still have to be defined.

PML

Like SSPE, PML is a rare, fatal demyelinating disease, but it is typically found in immuno-compromised subjects. Clinically, neurological symptoms such as ataxia, paralysis, and dementia develop and subsequently worsen, resulting in death within 6 months, although a few stabilized cases have been described (10). Neuropathological findings include focal areas of demyelination, with enlarged oligodendrocytes containing intranuclear inclusions and atypical astrocytes (64, 154). Characteristically, there is no inflammation. The etiologic agent of PML is JC virus, a ubiquitous papovavirus which commonly infects humans early in life, and no typical symptoms are associated with such primary infections (117). The virus is supposed to remain latent throughout life unless an immunosuppressive condition disrupts the host's immune response. The site of latency is not known, but in contrast to SSPE, in which measles virus can establish latency within the CNS, JC virus might persist in the periphery. This assumption is suggested by the lack of recovery of the virus from the brains of healthy or immunosuppressed subjects with no evidence of PML (27). PML could result from a peripheral viral reactivation during immunosuppression, with further hematogenous entry into the CNS. Human immunodeficiency virus type 1-induced immunosuppression seems to particularly affect JC virus reactivation, and a possible synergism between the two viruses has been hypothesized (9). Distribution of demyelinating foci could account for the hematogenous viral spread, though PML lesions are not perivascular. The selective infection of oligodendrocytes and, to a lesser extent, of astrocytes may suggest selection of a neurotropic variant. The occurrence of the disease on a background of immune deficiency again supports an interaction between viral infection and host-related factors.

HAM/TSP

HTLV-1 is the causative agent of a demyelinating disease in humans (HAM/TSP) with some clinical, pathological, and epidemiological characteristics closely resembling those of MS. HTLV-1 has a definite geographical distribution, with high-incidence areas such as Japan, the Caribbean, Central and South America, and Africa. Between 15 million and 25 million people are infected worldwide, but less than 5% will ever develop HAM/TSP. The demyelinating disease affects mostly the thoracic spinal cord, and the resulting symptoms are muscle weakness, hyperreflexia, and spastic paraparesis. The spinal cord shows demyelinating lesions with perivascular T cells in which $CD8^+$ cells predominate. It has been suggested that recognition of HTLV-1 gene products in the CNS may result in the lysis of glial cells and cytokine release (58). This model is based on the observation that extraordinarily high frequencies of HTLV-1-specific cytotoxic T lymphocytes (CTLs) restricted to HTLV-1 Tax immunodominant epitopes have been demonstrated in the peripheral blood lymphocytes and CSF of HAM/TSP patients, while the frequency of HTLV-1-specific CTLs is lower or absent in asymptomatic HTLV-1 carriers. The target of the HTLV-1-specific CTLs in the CNS could be either a resident glial cell (oligodendrocyte, astrocyte, or resident microglia) infected with HTLV-1 or an infiltrating $CD4^+$ cell. While HLA classes I and II are not normally expressed in the CNS, which would prevent antigen presentation necessary for CTL activity, HLA class I and class II expression can be upregulated by several cytokines, including IFN-γ and TNF-α, which can be induced by HTLV-1 and are also known to be upregulated in HAM/TSP patients. The release of cytokine and chemokine by HTLV-1 is potentially destructive to cells of the CNS. A similar mechanism could explain the virus induction of demyelinating disease in MS.

GENETIC AND ENVIRONMENTAL FACTORS IN MS SUSCEPTIBILITY

Epidemiological Considerations

The prevalence of MS varies greatly worldwide, ranging from 30 cases per 100,000 individuals in northern Europe and North America to fewer than 5 cases per 100,000. The prevalence of MS follows a north-south gradient in both hemispheres, with higher prevalences occurring in the north. Isolated areas of high prevalence are also observed in southern Europe (137). Different MS rates have been reported for clusters of genetically disparate populations in the same geographic areas, underscoring the importance of genetic background for susceptibility to MS. MS, like most autoimmune disorders, is more common in women than in men, with a ratio of 1.5:1. MS has age-specific incidence rates, with a peak age of onset of 27. Studies of MS in migrants have also been performed to evaluate the combined influence of genetic and environmental factors. Immigrants from high- or medium-risk areas tend to retain the risk of their birthplaces, while immigrants who move from low- to high-risk areas may increase their risk (80). Additional studies have reported that individuals who immigrate after age 15 retain the risk of their birthplace, while those who immigrate before they are 15 acquire the risk of their new country. This finding suggests that an infectious agent acquired before age 15 may influence an individual's likelihood of developing MS. Also, four MS epidemic outbreaks in the Faroe Islands occurred after the occupation by British troops during the Second World War (81), supporting the view of MS as a rare and delayed result of an infection acquired during adolescence.

Genetic Factors

Though genetic inheritance alone is not sufficient to cause the disease, genetic factors play a significant role in predisposition to MS. The absolute risk of developing the disease for biological relatives of individuals with MS is 20- to 40-fold higher than for the general population. The risk is greater for siblings, especially sisters, and decreases for second and third relatives (136). Additionally, the MS concordance rate is 31% in monozygotic twins and only 5% in dizygotic twins (137). This rate of MS disease discordance in twins has been used to support the view that genetics alone cannot explain this disorder and that other factors, such as environmental effects, must also be associated with disease pathogenesis. It is known that an increased risk is related to the presence of the MHC alleles HLA-DR2 and DQw1 on chromosome 6 (30). HLA-DR and DQw1 polymorphism seems to be associated with only MS susceptibility, not with the severity and course of the disease. However, the roles of other genes putatively linked to the disease are being evaluated (26, 115). The pattern of transmission of genetic susceptibility is not clear. The difficulty in establishing an inheritance pattern for MS may be due to several factors, including the inability to characterize specific polymorphisms of the HLA region, the difficulty in diagnosing MS, and the relatively large age range of high risk (from late teens to late 50s).

VIRUSES ASSOCIATED WITH MS

A considerable body of MS research has focused on the search for a viral etiology in MS and is reviewed by Cermelli and Jacobson (24). Although no specific virus has been definitely associated with MS, investigation in this area has continued based on several compelling lines of evidence. Epidemiological data, as described above, suggest either an association of MS with a viral infection acquired during adolescence or the distribution of MS as a form of epidemic with a definite point source (52, 81). Furthermore, in several studies, upper respiratory tract infections have been demonstrated to be related to an increased risk of both onset and exacerbations of MS (40, 100, 145). A possible explanation for this association might be linked to the virus-induced secretion of IFN-γ, a proinflammatory cytokine that has been demonstrated to enhance MS exacerbations (118).

Additional support for an association of MS and viral infections relies on the well-known occurrence of persistent viral infections in animal models and humans resulting in CNS damage and demyelination with either a chronically progressive or a relapsing–remitting course after a long incubation period (64). Moreover, viral agents have been isolated from the CNS and plaques from MS patients, and immunological studies have demonstrated an altered immune response to a number of viruses in peripheral lymphocytes of MS patients (61, 112).

Over the years, a large number of different viruses have been associated with MS, and yet attempts to detect a specific "MS virus" have not been successful. Nonetheless, all interpretations of evidence implicating infectious agents in the pathogenesis of MS have to be taken with great caution. Attempts to establish a clear-cut association between MS and viral infections have been hampered by several factors. A given viral infection detected at the time of diagnosis might not be related to the disease, and demyelination might occur after the possible causative virus has been cleared. Another possible hypothesis is that a ubiquitous virus is associated with this disorder in a subset of genetically or immunologically susceptible individuals (60). Additionally, rather than a single specific virus, multiple agents might be involved in MS. These viruses may trigger disease through different mechanisms in individuals with different genetic backgrounds, resulting in the different forms of the disorder. This theory is supported by clinical and pathological data showing different patterns of demyelination in MS patients, as described below.

Measles Virus

The association of measles virus infection and MS was extensively studied due to the ability of measles virus to induce PIE as well as a chronic, progressive neurologic disease, SSPE. Circulating anti-measles virus antibodies may persist for decades after primary infection, suggesting a continuous low-grade viral persistence or a cross-reactive immune response. CSF samples from MS patients were found to have high anti-measles virus antibody indices, suggesting an intrathecal synthesis of measles virus-specific antibodies (114). However, the CTL response to measles virus was unexpectedly found to be impaired in MS patients compared to that in healthy subjects (61). Although research has waned with regard to measles virus as a possible etiologic agent in MS, the similarities between MS, PIE, and SSPE warrant further investigation as to the role of this agent in MS.

HHV-6

A number of reports have suggested that several members of the family *Herpesviridae* may be involved in MS pathogenesis (11). Indeed, herpesviruses establish persistent lifelong infections, are highly neurotropic, and can disregulate the immune response. Among the herpesviruses, HHV-6 has received serious consideration as a possible etiological agent in MS. HHV-6 is a β-herpesvirus that was first isolated from PBMCs in 1986 by Salahuddin et al. (138). Despite its high tropism for B and mostly T cells, HHV-6 is a pleiotropic virus and has been demonstrated to infect a wide spectrum of cell lines, including all types of glial cells (97). HHV-6 has a worldwide distribution, with seroprevalence rates ranging around 90% (28). Primary infection is acquired usually in infancy. The early acquisition of

HHV-6 is consistent with the epidemiology of MS suggesting that one component of disease pathogenesis may be exposure to an environmental agent early in life (82). Furthermore, neurological complications, such as meningitis and meningoencephalitis, may develop during primary HHV-6 infection (59). HHV-6 establishes latency without symptomatic reactivations in immunocompetent hosts, whereas in immunocompromised patients, such as bone marrow and organ transplant recipients or AIDS patients, clinically evident reactivations have been observed and are associated with severe pneumonia and CNS disease (31, 39, 76).

Two distinct HHV-6 variants are known (HHV-6A and HHV-6B) and differ in their genomic and antigenic compositions (1). Although they are closely related, the two variants have unique properties and features, so as to fulfil the criteria for classification into two distinct viral species (37). Their biological properties appear to differ substantially, with HHV-6B accounting for most symptomatic infections during infancy, including exanthem subitum (36). In contrast, HHV-6A has not been associated with a well-defined pathology, but recent evidence suggests that this variant may preferentially persist and cause viral reactivations in the CNS (53).

One of the first reports of HHV-6 as a possible causative agent of MS came from the detection of viral DNA in MS plaques (25) by means of a nonbiased search using representational difference analysis. This technology allowed the selection and amplification of previously unknown DNA sequences present in the brains of MS patients but absent in control DNA by means of successive cycles of subtracting hybridization and subsequent PCR amplification. Among the resulting DNA fragments, one was found to be virtually identical to the MDBP gene of the Z29 isolate of HHV-6B. Consistent with data demonstrating the CNS as a site of HHV-6 latency (22), the percentage of HHV-6 DNA-positive brains of MS patients was not significantly different from that of control brains (78 versus 74%, respectively). However, monoclonal antibodies against the virion proteins 101K and p41 were able to detect HHV-6 antigen expression in MS plaques and not in control brain tissues. This study had a significant impact and opened the way for a new line of research on HHV-6 as an etiologic agent in MS.

Another study suggesting a possible association between HHV-6 and MS demonstrated a significant increase of anti-p41/38 early antigen IgM in relapsing-remitting MS patients with respect to healthy controls and controls with other neurological disease (148). The same study also revealed the presence of HHV-6 DNA in the sera of MS patients (15 of 50). Free viral DNA in serum was shown previously to correlate with active HHV-6 infection (142) and was also confirmed by the demonstration of the absence of HHV-6 DNA in the sera of controls without MS (0 of 47) (148). Further attempts to support these results have given equivocal results (2, 51, 103, 134). A recent study by Blumberg et al. (15), using a two-step in situ PCR technique, demonstrated the presence of HHV-6 DNA in oligodendrocytes and neurons of white matter plaques from chronic MS patients. HHV-6 DNA was also unexpectedly detected in white matter lesions from the brains of PML patients in greater amounts than JC virus, the etiologic agent of PML. Such findings were paralleled by the detection of HHV-6 p41 and gp101 protein gene expression in PML tissues, whereas the same antigens were not detected in MS plaques. These findings have added to the debate of whether HHV-6 can be considered a commensal agent in the brain or a potentially active virus in MS. Another investigation performed on brain tissues from patients having either secondary progressive or relapsing-remitting MS demonstrated the presence of HHV-6 DNA in 17 of 19 diseased tissue sections and in 3 of 23 uninvolved regions (75). The presence of viral DNA was statistically significant in tissues from MS patients (8 of 11) with respect to control CNS tissues, which were positive in 2 of 28 cases. Furthermore, 54% of total blood samples from MS patients were positive for active HHV-6 infec-

tion, as demonstrated by a rapid culture assay (75). Interestingly, the incidence of active HHV-6 viremia decreased in patients with longer duration of the disease, possibly reflecting a shift in pathogenic mechanisms.

Contrasting results obtained by investigators might be due to several factors, including the ability to distinguish between latent and active infection, differences in the populations studied, different sensitivities in the technologies used, and the DNA template sequences used for PCR amplification (60). In confirmation of this theory, it is worth noting that a recent study using the TaqMan quantitative PCR assay for the detection of the HHV-6 U67 open reading frame (91) showed a higher degree of accuracy and reproducibility than the nested PCR assay for the detection of the sequence encoding the HHV-6 major capsid protein (142).

The presence of two different HHV-6 variants may also account for contrasting results. Greater lymphoproliferative responses to HHV-6B than to HHV-6A in healthy subjects have been described (167). Additionally, the HHV-6B variant has been detected in saliva and PBMCs from healthy donors, while the HHV-6A variant has been demonstrated in serum and urine from MS patients but not from controls (3). Ablashi et al. (2) have also demonstrated that PBMCs from MS patients were mostly variant B (87%), similar to isolates from healthy donors (67%). These data are in agreement with the higher frequency of HHB-6B variant infection in the healthy population. Conversely, since HHV-6A appears to be a more neurotropic variant, it is reasonable to hypothesize that the association of HHV-6 and MS might be variant specific. Indeed, some studies have supported this suggestion (3, 73, 151), demonstrating a significantly greater lymphoproliferative response to HHV-6A in MS patients than in control subjects. No difference was observed in the lymphoproliferative responses of MS patients and controls to HHV-6B or HHV-7.

HHV-6 has been reported to use CD46 as its receptor (140). CD46 is a member of a family of glycoproteins described as regulators of complement activation (RCA) which is distributed on all nucleated cells and has a protective role in preventing spontaneous activation of complement on cells, which appears to have a crucial role in demyelination. The ubiquitous distribution of such receptors is consistent with the pleiotropism of HHV-6. Intriguingly, adult oligodendrocytes have been demonstrated to lack all RCA proteins except CD55, which appears to be much weaker than other RCA family members in its ability to protect cells from complement-mediated lysis (141). This finding would account for an increased susceptibility of these cells to complement-mediated damage but suggests that HHV-6 would not use CD46 as a receptor for infection of oligodendrocytes, as CD46 is not present on the surface of these cells. However, HHV-6 has been reported to infect oligodendrocytes and actively replicate both in vivo (15, 25, 75) and in vitro (4). Therefore, how does HHV-6 infect oligodendrocytes? One possibility might be that HHV-6 receptors other than CD46 are used on oligodendrocytes. Another possibility might involve cell-to-cell viral spread. Indeed, HHV-6 is a highly cell-associated virus, and HHV-6B infection has been demonstrated to cause cell-to-cell fusion in isolated adult oligodendrocytes with very little extracellular release of infectious virus (4).

EBV

Among gammaherpesviruses, EBV has been the most extensively studied as a potential agent in the pathogenesis of MS. EBV is ubiquitous, with seropositivity rates ranging from 85 to 95%. A prevalence rate of almost 100% in MS patients has been described (156). EBV infection can induce neurological complications such as demyelination (33). A history of infectious mononucleosis has been associated with a higher prevalence of MS (100). Moreover, an oligoclonal CSF banding pattern specific for anti-EBV nuclear antigen EBNA-1 was found for a subset of MS patients (5 of 15) but not for control CSF samples (0 of 12) (128). Since similar intrathecal synthesis of antibodies against viral capsid antigen was not de-

tected, active replication of EBV in the CNS is unlikely. Possible explanations for the presence of anti-EBNA-1 antibodies in OCBs are cross-reactivity with host cell components; a mechanism known as molecular mimicry, since EBNA-1 and MBP share two different pentapeptide sequences (18); or a chronic release of EBNA-1 due to apoptosis of latently infected B cells infiltrating MS plaques. Interestingly, despite these findings, EBV has been rarely observed in MS lesions (139), and EBV mRNA has not been detected in plaques (55). Such contrasting findings might suggest that EBV infection, and possibly reactivation, could act as a peripheral trigger for the pathogenesis of MS. Indeed, EBV reactivation measured either by serology or by EBV DNA in serum was demonstrated to parallel disease activity in MS patients (166).

Other Herpesviruses

Anti-HSV type 1 (anti-HSV-1) antibodies (12) as well as HSV-1-coupled immune complexes (34) have been detected in CSF from MS patients. The viral strain isolated by Bergström et al. (12) from a patient having her first MS attack was not detected later in the course of the disease. This strain was less neurovirulent in vivo and replicated in cell cultures at lower titers than other strains. This finding might suggest that only specific viral strains would be involved in the disease, but further attempts to isolate an HSV from MS samples, including those from patients during acute attacks, have failed (102).

In a mouse model, HSV-1 was able to induce a demyelinating disease showing some similarities with MS (161). Different HSV-1 susceptibility to multifocal demyelination was demonstrated in different mouse strains (68). The same group also demonstrated that an increased viral spread was associated with a lack of demyelination in immunosuppressed mice (69). This finding is consistent with a demyelinating mechanism dependent on combined immunity- and genetics-related factors.

The association between MS and another alphaherpesvirus, varicella-zoster virus (VZV), has been investigated on the basis of epidemiological data showing similar dual spread of VZV infection and MS in a north-south prevalence gradient (133), with the exception of the North American Hutterite population, which lives relatively isolated in a high-risk area, whose people have lower incidence of both MS and VZV infection. Moreover, VZV encephalitis is characterized by focal white matter demyelination (74). Intrathecal synthesis of anti-VZV antibodies in the CSF of MS patients has been described (146).

Apart from HHV-6, there is little evidence supporting a role for the other β-herpesviruses in MS. CMV has been described as one possible causative factor in Guillain-Barré syndrome (87), and CMV DNA has been detected in the brains of healthy subjects as well as MS patients by PCR (139). A role for CMV in MS pathogenesis has not been documented. Similarly, HHV-7 has not yet been associated clearly either with a specific disease or with demyelination. Further, the lymphoproliferative response to HHV-7 in MS patients was not found to be different from that of controls (151).

Retroviruses

Retroviruses have been investigated as potential etiological agents in MS, mostly due to the similarities between the HTLV-1-associated neurologic disease termed HAM/TSP and MS. After the discovery of HTLV-1 as the etiologic agent of HAM/TSP, the possibility that MS and HAM/TSP might be two forms of the same disease was considered (77).

Anti-HTLV-1 Gag (p24) protein antibodies were detected in the serum and CSF of MS patients (78). The same study revealed HTLV-1 genomic sequences in cell cultures inoculated with CSF from one-third of MS patients. Further, HTLV-1 sequences were detected in PBMCs and CSF T cells from either HTLV-1-seropositive or -seronegative MS patients (77), but these findings were not confirmed by others (130). The hypothesis that MS and HAM/TSP could have the same etiology has subsequently been abandoned, but HAM/TSP is still considered of interest and one of the closest human models for our understanding of MS pathogenesis, as described above.

The interest in retroviruses led in 1989 to the detection of extracellular virions with reverse transcriptase activity produced by leptomeningeal cells from an MS patient (119). Eight years later, the same group characterized this putative retrovirus, which was named MS-associated retrovirus (MSRV) (120). MSRV *pol* sequences were detected in the serum and in the CSF of MS patients at significantly higher percentages than in those of controls (50 versus 0%), and viral RNA was detected in 9 of 17 MS patients and in 3 of 44 control subjects (47). MSRV *pol* gene sequencing revealed a high degree of homology with the respective gene of the well-characterized endogenous retrovirus 9 (ERV-9), which had been detected in brains and tissues from MS patients as well as control subjects (17). Endogenous retroviruses are widely present in humans and represent a substantial part of human genomes. These endogenous retroviruses are vertically transmitted and are normally quiescent, being stably integrated within cellular DNA. However, endogenous retroviruses might become replication competent under particular conditions and are thought to play a role in autoimmune diseases (79). The results of an extensive characterization of a new family of endogenous retroviruses, named HERV-W, suggested that MSRV could be considered a member of the HERV-W family (14, 44). However, endogenous retroviral mRNA was found only in placental and fetal liver tissues, while brain and lymphoid tissues were negative. Therefore, the hypothesis that MSRV might be a replication-competent human endogenous retrovirus has not yet been confirmed, nor is it clear whether MSRV is definitely involved in the disease. Further studies are needed to fully understand the role, if any, that MSRV may play in MS.

Multiple Viral Infections

In addition to the numerous reports focused on single viral infections in MS, there are also some studies suggesting that multiple viruses might be involved in the disease and act as triggers at least in a subset of patients.

Epidemiological findings suggest that common viral infections parallel MS disease exacerbations (40, 145). It is possible that common viral infections might have a stimulatory activity on persistent infections or reactivate latent viruses. These possibilities have been suggested by Wandinger et al. (166) in the case of EBV infection. A rise in anti-EBV early antigen has been demonstrated during exacerbations. Therefore, an EBV reactivation might lead to autoreactive T-cell activation by mechanisms such as molecular mimicry. Indeed, MBP-reactive T-cell clones from MS patients have been demonstrated to be highly reactive to EBV as well as to influenza A virus (177).

Alternatively, EBV might coactivate a putative retrovirus. A lymphoblastoid cell line from an MS patient was established by Munch et al. (109) and was demonstrated to actively produce both retroviruslike particles and EBV particles. However, a further characterization of these retroviruslike particles has yet to be reported. Additionally, it is unknown if the retrovirus had an exogenous or endogenous origin. Moreover, a study on relapsing MS patients reported the presence of EBV DNA in 6 of 14 PBMC samples on the first day of relapse, with subsequent detection of HTLV-1 *tax-rex* DNA up to day 10 in 5 patients (42), suggesting a possible interaction between the two agents. However, further confirmation of this finding based on a larger cohort of patients is lacking.

Perron and colleagues (121) also suggested that interactions between multiple viruses may contribute to the pathogenesis of MS. It was demonstrated that HSV-1 proteins were able to transactivate MSRV in vitro. However, additional evidence about the interactions between MSRV and HSV-1 in MS patients is required.

To date, HHV-6 has not been reported to be in association with other viruses in MS, but possible mechanisms involving interaction with other viruses such as EBV might be hypothesized (166). Two different viruses might trigger MS-specific events by a synergistic action in which one virus transactivates genes of the other. In addition, different families of viruses may have some common mechanisms or pathways. For example, both HHV-6 and measles virus (two highly divergent viruses, one containing DNA and the other containing RNA) use CD46 as a cellular receptor (140). As discussed above, both measles virus and HHV-6 have been strongly implicated in the pathogenesis of MS. CD46 is a member of a family of glycoproteins, described as RCA, which is widely distributed on cell surfaces and has a protective action, preventing spontaneous activation of complement on cells. Of interest is the observation that EBV, another virus that has been suggested to play a role in MS, also uses a member of the RCA family as its receptor, CD21. It is possible that a number of ubiquitous and neurotropic viruses may be may be associated with MS, acting by a common mechanism (i.e., a common receptor or family of receptors) that manifests in clinical disease. This may help to explain why no single viral agent has ever been shown definitively to be associated with all MS patients.

POSSIBLE LINKS BETWEEN VIRAL INFECTIONS AND AUTOIMMUNITY

Despite the great effort focused on etiological, pathological, and pathogenetic aspects of MS, most of these issues have yet to be fully defined. Epidemiological data and clinical and laboratory findings, as well as the documentation of virus-induced demyelinating diseases closely resembling MS in animals and humans, are consistent with a role for viral infections in the etiology and pathogenesis of the disease but strongly suggest that two or more ubiquitous microbial agents may interact with each other in genetically susceptible individuals (150). A wide variety of viruses, including HHV-6, MSRV, measles virus, and EBV, have been associated with MS. However, recent evidence suggests that the association between MS and viruses might not be restricted to a single causal agent but, rather, multiple agents might be involved. Consistent with this hypothesis, MS could be considered as a group of different diseases, each with specific pathological, clinical, and possibly pathogenetic mechanisms, sharing autoimmune characteristics.

In addition to the search for an association between viral infection and MS, other lines of research have focused on peripheral T-cell antimyelin autoimmunity. Animal models of the disease parallel this dual approach, and the respective lines of research have independently developed over time. A clear-cut association between one or more viruses and MS has not yet been demonstrated. Similarly, the hypothesized autoimmunity in MS is far from universally accepted as the sole mechanism that causes clinical disease.

Recent findings and approaches are now suggesting a possible link between microbial infections and myelin-specific autoimmunity. Again, the demonstration of complement regulatory protein CD46 as an HHV-6 cellular receptor (140) has fueled much interest in the possible effects of a viral infection in MS. As mentioned above, complement seems to play a key role in demyelination, and oligodendrocytes might be particularly susceptible to its effects. Complement-mediated oligodendrocyte lysis might be the first step of a cascade of events resulting in myelin breakdown with subsequent release of myelin antigens and an autoimmune response. Soluble forms of CD46 have been detected in patients with autoimmune diseases such as lupus erythematosus (71) and recently also in the serum and CSF of patients with MS (149). Additionally, anti-CD46 autoantibodies in MS patients have been described (126). The latter finding might be explained by the possible incorporation of the receptor into the viral envelope during replication. While this hypothesis has yet to be formally proven for HHV-6, other viruses such as CMV, human immunodeficiency virus, and HTLV-1 have been found to incorporate host proteins, including CD46, CD55, and CD59 (101, 108, 153). Once incorporated, the viruses might be protected from complement-mediated virolysis (101) or, alternatively, the immune system would recognize these host proteins incorporated into virion membranes as "non-self" (147).

Another possibility for a link between viral infection and autoimmunity is suggested by studies on αB-crystallin, a protein belonging to the family of small stress proteins which, in contrast to other stress proteins, has a very restricted tissue distribution (163, 165). For example, αB-crystallin is not present in lymphoid cells but is normally expressed only intracellularly in a few tissues, such as the eye lens, cardiac and skeletal muscles, and, most notably, astrocytes and oligodendrocytes. Thus, in the absence of constitutive expression of this protein, a condition of immune tolerance to αB-crystallin can occur. In contrast, αB-crystallin is present in lymphoid cells from other mammalian species. Oligodendrocytes and astrocytes from MS-affected white matter have been demonstrated to express αB-crystallin, which was not detectable in unaffected white matter (164). A number of viruses, such as HHV-6 (strain U1102, a clinical isolate of the HHV-6A variant), EBV, and measles virus, have been demonstrated in vitro to induce αB-crystallin expression in human B cells in an HLA-restricted manner (165). Thus, the appearance and presentation of such a protein may induce a proinflammatory Th1 response. According to this hypothesis, the subsequent stress-induced production of this self-antigen in oligodendrocytes would trigger a self-sustaining myelin breakdown, with unveiling of other myelin antigens (163). In agreement with this suggestion, the subdominant epitope of αB-crystallin was demonstrated to induce EAE in mice (159), and the expression of αB-crystallin was related to the early active stages of MS plaques (7).

Thus, HHV-6 and/or measles virus and EBV infection might trigger the generation of an anti-αB-crystallin immune response leading to myelin destruction. This theory would gain further support if virus-induced αB-crystallin expression were to be demonstrated in oligodendrocytes.

MS THERAPY

Patients with MS are usually treated with corticosteroids during clinical relapses, with the specific aim of reducing inflammation. Although corticosteroid therapy can generally achieve transient recovery, it is far from being an optimal treatment and is not able to affect the course of the disease. For this reason, several clinical trials with immunomodulatory drugs have been performed. Among these substances, IFN-β has been shown to be successful in reducing clinical relapses and delaying the development of new lesions as determined by magnetic resonance imaging (MRI) (115). Although the mechanism of action is not completely understood, treatment with IFN-β appears to have an immunomodulatory effect by inducing a shift from a Th1 to a Th2 T-cell response, with upregulation of IL-4 and IL-10 and downregulation of IFN-γ (135). Additionally, IFN-β can reduce the leakage of immune cells through the BBB by acting on adhesion molecules, chemokines, and proteases. However, IFN-β has also been reported to have an antiviral activity on a number of viruses, including HSV (127), and at least a part of its beneficial effect might be due to this effect. Glatiramer acetate, known also as copolymer-1, is a mixture of the amino acids alanine, lysine, glutamic acid, and tyrosine and is thought to act as an altered peptide ligand for MBP. Copolymer-1 is able to bind competitively to MHC class II-restricted binding sites and has been demonstrated to be effective in early-remitting MS patients (63). These results support an autoimmune component in MS pathogenesis and development.

The possibility of a direct viral involvement in MS can be tested by controlled trials using antiviral drugs. However, the only controlled trial using an antiviral compound was undertaken by Lycke et al. (98) with acyclovir. This drug is effective only on alphaherpesviruses in vitro. The specific antialphaherpesvirus activity of acyclovir was confirmed by a significant decrease in anti-HSV antibodies, while the titers of antibody to other herpesviruses did not change. The study reported a decrease in exacerbation rate, though there were no clear signs of reduction of neurological deterioration in the MS patients studied.

Another type of experimental therapy which is gathering much interest is based on the use of polyclonal Igs (IVIg), which has been shown to have some beneficial effects in controlled trials. Similarly to IFN-β, IVIg has been reported to reduce the rate of relapse and the number of lesions detected by gadolinium-enhanced MRI (152). The mechanism of action of IVIg is not fully understood. However, it has been observed that human monoclonal antibodies can induce remyelination in TMEV-induced encephalomyelitis (169). Myelin-reactive antibodies, which are present in the normal human Ig repertoire, might then have a nonpathogenic role.

CONCLUSION

As illustrated above, many issues concerning virtually all aspects of MS still require further investigation. MS is a multifactorial disease, and the extent of overlap or interaction among candidate etiologic agents is unclear. With regard to the etiology and pathogenesis of MS, many questions remain. Is there a role for viral agents in the disease? If so, why has there been such difficulty in supporting such a hypothesis? How can microbial agent infections be linked to autoimmunity? This chapter has tried to address some of these questions.

New sets of data are contributing to a new view of MS. Contrasting reports about MS pathology might be explained by considering MS as not only one disorder but a group of diseases with possible different subsets of pathogenetic factors variably interacting with each other. Therefore, a specific pathogenesis may be present in each subset of patients. A final common pathway resulting in demyelination would then characterize and unify these syndromes. In the context of such a dynamic view, a role for infectious agents is undoubtedly important. Mechanisms responsible for MS induction might be different from those related to progression.

The study of this unique, multifaceted disorder represents a challenging opportunity not only to better define the disease itself, but also to understand how the CNS, which once was considered an immune privileged site, reacts to infections and how one or more viral agents can cause aberrant autoimmunity.

REFERENCES

1. **Ablashi, D. V., N. Balachandran, S. F. Josephs, C. L. Hun, G. R. F. Krueger, B. Kramarsky, S. Z. Salahuddin, and R. C. Gallo.** 1991. Genomic polymorphism, growth properties, and immunologic variations in human herpesvirus-6 isolates. *Virology* **184**:545–552.

2. **Ablashi, D. V., H. B. Eastman, C. B. Owen, M. M. Roman, J. Friedman, J. B. Zabriskie, D. L. Peterson, G. R. Pearson, and J. E. Whitman.** 2000. Frequent HHV-6 reactivation in multiple sclerosis (MS) and chronic fatigue syndrome (CFS) patients. *J. Clin. Virol.* **16**:179–191.

3. **Akhyani, N., R. Berti, M. B. Brennan, S. S. Soldan, J. M. Eaton, H. F. McFarland, and S. Jacobson.** 2000. Tissue distribution and variant characterization of human herpesvirus (HHV)-6: increased prevalence of HHV-6A in patients with multiple sclerosis. *J. Infect. Dis.* **182**:1321–1325.

4. **Albright, A. V., E. Lavi, J. B. Black, S. Goldberg, M. J. O'Connor, and F. González-Scarano.** 1998. The effect of human herpesvirus-6 (HHV-6) on cultured human neural cells: oligodendrocytes and microglia. *J. Neurovirol.* **4**:486–494.

5. **Archelos, J. J., M. K. Storch, and H. P. Hartung.** 2000. The role of B cells and autoantibodies in multiple sclerosis. *Ann. Neurol.* **47**:694–706.

6. **Bailey, O. T., A. M. Pappenheimer, F. S. Cheever, and J. B. Daniels.** 1949. A murine hepatitis virus (JHM) causing disseminated encephalomyelitis with extensive destruction of myelin. II. Pathology. *J. Exp. Med.* **90**:195–212.

7. **Bajramovic, J. J., H. Lassmann, and J. M. van Noort.** 1997. Expression of alphaB-crystallin in glia cells during lesional development in multiple sclerosis. *J. Neuroimmunol.* **78**:143–151.

8. **Barac-Latas, V., G. Suchanek, H. Breitschopf, A. Stuehler, H. Wege, and H. Lassmann.** 1997. Patterns of oligodendrocyte pathology in coronavirus-induced subacute demyelinating encephalomyelitis in the Lewis rat. *Glia* **19**:1–12.

9. **Berger, J. R., B. Kaszovitz, M. J. Post, and G. Dickinson.** 1987. Progressive multifocal leukoencephalopathy associated with human immunodeficiency virus infection. A review of the literature with a report of sixteen cases. *Ann. Intern. Med.* **107**:78–87.

10. **Berger, J. R., and L. Mucke.** 1988. Prolonged survival and partial recovery in AIDS-associated progressive multifocal leukoencephalopathy. *Neurology* **38**:1060–1065.

11. **Bergström, T.** 1999. Herpesviruses—a rationale for antiviral treatment in multiple sclerosis. *Antiviral Res.* **41**:1–19.

12. **Bergström, T., O. Andersen, and A. Vahlne.** 1989. Isolation of herpes simplex type 1 during first attack of multiple sclerosis. *Ann. Neurol.* **26**:283–285.

13. **Bitsch, A., J. Schuchardt, S. Bunkowski, T. Kuhlmann, and W. Brück.** 2000. Acute axonal injury in multiple sclerosis. Correlation with demyelination and inflammation. *Brain* **123**:1174–1183.

14. **Blond, J. L., F. Beseme, L. Duret, O. Bouton, F. Bedin, H. Perron, B. Mandrand, and F. Mallet.** 1999. Molecular characterization and placental expression of HERV-W, a new human endogenous retrovirus family. *J. Virol.* **73**:1175–1185.

15. **Blumberg, B. M., D. J. Mock, J. M. Powers, M. Ito, J. G. Assouline, J. V. Backer, B. Chen, and A. D. Goodman.** 2000. The HHV6 paradox: ubiquitous commensal or insidious pathogen? A two-step in situ PCR approach. *J. Clin. Virol.* **16**:159–178.

16. **Borrow, P., P. Tonks, C. J. R. Welsh, and A. A. Nash.** 1992. The role of CD8⁺ T cells in the acute and chronic phases of Theiler's virus-induced disease in mice. *J. Gen. Virol.* **73**:1861–1865.

17. **Brahic, M., and J.-F. Bureau.** 1997. Multiple sclerosis and retroviruses. *Ann. Neurol.* **42**:984–985.

18. **Bray, P. F., J. Luka, P. F. Bray, K. W. Culp, and J. P. Schlight.** 1992. Antibodies against Epstein-Barr nuclear antigen (EBNA) in multiple sclerosis CSF, and two pentapeptide sequence identities between EBNA and myelin basic protein. *Neurology* **42**:1798–1804.

19. **Brosnan, C. F., M. K. Racke, and K. Selmaj.** 1988. Hypothesis: a role of tumor necrosis factor in immune-mediated demyelination and its relevance to multiple sclerosis. *J. Neuroimmunol.* **18**:87–94.

20. **Burns, J., A. Rosenzweig, B. Zweiman, and R. P. Lisak.** 1983. Isolation of myelin basic protein-reactive T-cell lines from normal human blood. *Cell. Immunol.* **81**:435–440.

21. **Butcher, E. C.** 1991. Leukocyte-endothelial cell recognition: three (or more) steps to specificity and diversity. *Cell* **67**:1033–1036.

22. Caserta, M. T., C. Breese-Hall, K. Schnabel, K. McIntyre, C. Long, M. Costanzo, S. Dewhurst, R. Insel, and L. G. Epstein. 1994. Neuroinvasion and persistence of human herpesvirus 6 in children. *J. Infect. Dis.* **170:**1586–1589.

23. Cattaneo, R., A. Schmid, M. A. Billeter, R. D. Sheppard, and S. A. Udem. 1988. Multiple viral mutations rather than host factors cause defective measles virus gene expression in a subacute sclerosing panencephalitis cell line. *J. Virol.* **62:**1388–1397.

24. Cermelli, C., and S. Jacobson. 2000. Viruses and multiple sclerosis. *Viral Immunol.* **13:**255–267.

25. Challoner, P. B., K. T. Smith, J. D. Parker, D. L. MacLeod, S. N. Coulter, T. M. Rose, E. R. Schultz, J. L. Bennett, R. L. Garber, M. Chang, P. A. Schad, P. M. Stewart, R. C. Nowinski, J. P. Brown, and G. C. Burmer. 1995. Plaque-associated expression of human herpesvirus 6 in multiple sclerosis. *Proc. Natl. Acad. Sci. USA* **92:**7440–7444.

26. Chataway, J., R. Feakes, F. Coraddu, J. Gray, J. Deans, M. Fraser, N. Robertson, S. Broadley, H. Jones, D. Clayton, P. Goodfellow, S. Sawcer, and A. Compston. 1998. The genetics of multiple sclerosis: principles, background and updated results of the United Kingdom systematic region screen. *Brain* **121:**1869–1887.

27. Chesters, P. M., J. Heritage, and D. McCance. 1983. Persistence of DNA sequences of BK virus and JC virus in normal human tissues and in diseased tissues. *J. Infect. Dis.* **147:**676–682.

28. Clark, D. A. 2000. Human herpesvirus 6. *Rev. Med. Virol.* **10:**155–173.

29. Clatch, R. J., H. L. Lipton, and S. D. Miller. 1986. Characterization of Theiler's murine encephalomyelitis virus (TMEV)-specific delayed type hypersensitivity responses in TMEV-induced demyelinating disease: correlation with clinical signs. *J. Immunol.* **136:**920–927.

30. Compston, A. 1994. The epidemiology of multiple sclerosis: principles, achievements, and recommendations. *Ann. Neurol.* **36**(Suppl. 2):S211–217.

31. Cone, R. W., R. C. Hackman, M. L. Huang, R. A. Bowden, J. D. Meyers, M. Metcalf, J. Zeh, R. Ashley, and L. Corey. 1993. Human herpesvirus 6 in lung tissue from patients with pneumonitis after bone marrow transplantation. *N. Engl. J. Med.* **329:**156–161.

32. Connolly, J. H., I. V. Allen, L. J. Hurwitz, and J. H. Millar. 1967. Measles-virus antibody and antigen in subacute sclerosing panencephalitis. *Lancet* **i:**542–544.

33. Corssmit, E. P., M. A. Leverstein-van Hall, P. Portegies, and P. Bakker. 1997. Severe neurological complications in association with Epstein-Barr virus infection. *J. Neurovirol.* **3:**460–464.

34. Coyle, P. K. 1985. CSF immune complexes in multiple sclerosis. *Neurology* **35:**429–432.

35. Cross, A. H., J. L. Trotter, and J.-A. Lyons. 2001. B cells and antibodies in CNS demyelinating disease. *J. Neuroimmunol.* **112:**1–14.

36. Dewhurst, S., K. McIntyre, K. Schnabel, and C. B. Hall. 1993. Human herpesvirus-6 (HHV-6) variant accounts for the majority of symptomatic primary HHV-6 infections in a population of U.S. infants. *J. Clin. Microbiol.* **31:**416–418.

37. Dominguez, G., T. R. Dambaugh, F. R. Stamey, S. Dewhurst, N. Inoue, and P. E. Pellett. 1999. Human herpesvirus 6B genome sequence: coding content and comparison with human herpesvirus 6A. *J. Virol.* **73:**8040–8052.

38. Dore-Duffy, P., W. Newman, R. Balabanov, R. P. Lisak, E. Mainolfi, R. Rothlein, and M. Peterson. 1995. Circulating soluble adhesion proteins in cerebrospinal fluid and serum of patients with multiple sclerosis: correlation with clinical activity. *Ann. Neurol.* **37:**55–62.

39. Drobyski, W. R., K. K. Knox, D. Majewski, and D. R. Carrigan. 1994. Brief report: fatal encephalitis due to variant B human herpesvirus-6 infection in a bone marrow transplant recipient. *N. Engl. J. Med.* **330:**1356–1360.

40. Edwards, S., M. Zvartau, H. Clarke, W. Irving, and L. D. Blumhardt. 1998. Clinical relapses and disease activity on magnetic resonance imaging associated with viral upper respiratory tract infections in multiple sclerosis. *J. Neurol. Neurosurg. Psychiatry* **64:**736–741.

41. Erlich, S., J. Fleming, S. Stohlman, and L. Weiner. 1987. Experimental neuropathology of remote infection with a JHM virus variant (DS). *Arch. Neurol.* **44:**2483–2489.

42. Ferrante, P., E. Omodeo-Zorini, M. R. Zuffolato, R. Mancuso, R. Caldarelli-Stefano, S. Puricelli, M. Mediati, L. Losciale, and D. Caputo. 1997. Human T-cell lymphotropic virus *tax* and Epstein-Barr virus DNA in peripheral blood of multiple sclerosis patient during acute attack. *Acta Neurol. Scand.* **169** (Suppl.):79–85.

43. Fritz, R. B., M. J. Skeen, C. H.-J. Chen, M. Garcia, and I. K. Egorov. 1985. Major histocompatibility complex linked control of the immune response to myelin basic protein. *J. Immunol.* **134:**2328–2332.

44. Fujinami, R. B., and J. E. Libbey. 1999. Endogenous retroviruses: are they the cause of multiple sclerosis? *Trends Microbiol.* **7:**263–264.

45. Fujinami, R. S., and M. B. A. Oldstone. 1980. Alterations in expression of measles virus

polypeptides by antibody: molecular events in antibody-induced antigenic modulation. *J. Immunol.* **125**:78–85.

46. **Fujinami, R. S., and M. B. A. Oldstone.** 1985. Amino acid homology between the encephalitogenic site of myelin basic protein and virus: mechanism for autoimmunity. *Science* **230**:1043–1045.

47. **Garson, J. A., P. W. Tuke, P. Giraud, G. Paranhos-Baccala, and H. Perron.** 1998. Detection of virion-associated MSRV-RNA in serum of patients with multiple sclerosis. *Lancet* **351**:33.

48. **Gay, F. W., T. J. Drye, G. W. A. Dick, and M. M. Esiri.** 1997. The application of multifactorial cluster analysis in the staging of plaques in early multiple sclerosis. Identification and characterization of the primary demyelinating lesion. *Brain* **120**:1461–1483.

49. **Genain, C. P., M. H. Nguyen, N. L. Letvin, R. Pearl, R. L. Davis, M. Adelman, M. B. Lees, C. Linington, and S. L. Hauser.** 1995. Antibody facilitation of multiple sclerosis-like lesions in a nonhuman primate. *J. Clin. Investig.* **96**:2966–2974.

50. **Gendelman, H. E., G. H. Pezeshkpour, N. J. Pressman, J. S. Wolinsky, R. H. Quarles, M. J. Dobersen, B. D. Trapp, C. A. Kitt, A. Aksamit, and R. T. Johnson.** 1985. A quantitation of myelin-associated glycoprotein and myelin basic protein loss in different demyelinating diseases. *Ann. Neurol.* **18**:324–328.

51. **Goldberg, S. H., A. V. Albright, R. P. Lisak, and F. Gonzalez-Scarano.** 1999. Polymerase chain reaction analysis of human herpesvirus 6 sequences in the sera and cerebrospinal fluid of patients with multiple sclerosis. *J. Neurovirol.* **5**:134–139.

52. **Haar, S., M. Munch, T. Christensen, A. Meller-Larson, and J. Hvas.** 1997. Cluster of multiple sclerosis patients from Danish community. *Lancet* **349**:9056.

53. **Hall, C. B., M. T. Caserta, K. C. Schnabel, C. Long, L. G. Epstein, R. A. Insel, and S. Dewhurst.** 1998. Persistence of human herpesvirus 6 according to site and variant: possible greater neurotropism of variant A. *Clin. Infect. Dis.* **26**:132–137.

54. **Hall, W. W., and P. W. Choppin.** 1981. Measles virus proteins in the brain tissue of patients with subacute sclerosing panencephalitis. *N. Engl. J. Med.* **304**:1152–1155.

55. **Hilton, D. A., S. Love, A. Fletcher, and J. H. Pringle.** 1994. Absence of Epstein-Barr virus RNA in multiple sclerosis as assessed by in situ hybridization. *J. Neurol. Neurosurg. Psychiatry* **57**:975–976.

56. **Hofman, F. M., R. I. von Hanwehr, C. A. Dinarello, S. B. Mizel, D. Hinton, and J. E. Merrill.** 1986. Immunoregulatory molecules and IL 2 receptors identified in multiple sclerosis brain. *J. Immunol.* **136**:3239–3245.

57. **Horwitz, M. S., L. M. Bradley, J. Harbertson, T. Krahl, J. Lee, and N. Sarvetnick.** 1998. Diabetes induced by coxsackievirus: initiation by bystander damage and not molecular mimicry. *Nat. Med.* **4**:781–785.

58. **Ijichi, S., S. Izumo, N. Eiraku, K. Machigashira, R. Kubota, M. Nagai, N. Ikegami, N. Kashio, F. Umehara, and I. Maruyama.** 1993. An autoaggressive process against bystander tissues in HTLV-I infected individuals: a possible pathomechanism of HAM/TSP. *Med. Hypotheses* **41**:572–547.

59. **Ishiguro, M.** 1990. Meningo-encephalitis associated with HHV-6 related exanthem subitum. *Acta Paediatr. Scand.* **79**:987–989.

60. **Jacobson, S.** 1998. Association of human herpesvirus-6 and multiple sclerosis: here we go again? *J. Neurovirol.* **4**:471–473.

61. **Jacobson, S., M. L. Flerlage, and H. F. McFarland.** 1985. Impaired measles virus specific cytotoxic-T cell responses in multiple sclerosis. *J. Exp. Med.* **162**:839–850.

62. **Johns, T. G., and C. C. Bernard.** 1999. The structure and function of myelin oligodendrocyte glycoprotein. *J. Neurochem.* **71**:1–9.

63. **Johnson, K. P., B. R. Brooks, J. A. Cohen, C. C. Ford, J. Goldstein, R. P. Lisak, L. W. Myers, H. S. Panitch, J. W. Rose, R. B. Schiffer, et al.** 1995. Copolymer 1 reduces relapse rate and improves disability in relapsing-remitting multiple sclerosis: results of a phase III multicenter, double-blind placebo-controlled trial. *Neurology* **45**:1268–1276.

64. **Johnson, R. T.** 1994. The virology of demyelinating diseases. *Ann. Neurol.* **36**:S54–S60.

65. **Johnson, R. T., D. E. Griffin, R. L. Hirsch, J. S. Wolinsky, S. Roedenbeck, I. Lindo de Soriano, and A. Vaisberg.** 1984. Measles encephalomyelitis: clinical and immunological studies. *N. Engl. J. Med.* **310**:137–141.

66. **Joshi, N., K. Usuku, and S. L. Hauser.** 1993. The T-cell response to myelin basic protein in familial multiple sclerosis: diversity of fine specificity restricting elements, and T-cell receptor usage. *Ann. Neurol.* **34**:385–393.

67. **Karpus, W. J., J. G. Pope, J. D. Peterson, M. C. Dal Canto, and S. D. Miller.** 1995. Inhibition of Theiler's virus-mediated demyelination by peripheral immune tolerance induction. *J. Immunol.* **155**:947–957.

68. **Kastrukoff, L. F., A. S. Lau, and S. U. Kim.** 1987. Multifocal CNS demyelination following

peripheral inoculation with herpes simplex virus type I. *Ann. Neurol.* **22**:52–59.

69. **Kastrukoff, L. F., A. S. Lau, G. Y. Leung, and E. E. Thomas.** 1993. Contrasting effects of immunosuppression on herpes simplex virus type I (HSV I) induced central nervous system (CNS) demyelination in mice. *J. Neurol. Sci.* **117**:148–158.

70. **Katz-Levy, Y., K. L. Neville, A. M. Girvin, C. L. Vanderlugt, J. G. Pope, L. J. Tan, and S. D. Miller.** 1999. Endogenous presentation of self myelin epitopes by CNS-resident APCs in Theiler's virus-infected mice. *J. Clin. Investig.* **104**:599–610.

71. **Kawano, M., T. Seya, I. Koni, and H. Mabuchi.** 1999. Elevated serum levels of soluble membrane cofactor protein (CD46, MCP) in patients with systemic lupus erythematosus (SLE). *Clin. Exp. Immunol.* **116**:542–546.

72. **Kaye, J. F., N. Kerlero de Rosbo, I. Mendel, S. Fletcher, M. Hoffman, I. Yust, and A. Ben-Nun.** 2000. The central nervous system-specific myelin oligodendrocytic basic protein (MOBP) is encephalitogenic and a potential target antigen in multiple sclerosis (MS). *J. Neuroimmunol.* **102**:189–198.

73. **Kim, J., K. Lee, J. Park, M. Kim, and W. Shin.** 2000. Detection of human herpesvirus 6 variant A in peripheral blood mononuclear cells from multiple sclerosis patients. *Eur. Neurol.* **43**:170–173.

74. **Kleinschmidt-DeMasters, B. K., C. Amlie-Lefond, and D. H. Gilden.** 1996. The patterns of varicella-zoster virus encephalitis. *Hum. Pathol.* **27**:927–938.

75. **Knox, K. K., J. H. Brewer, J. M. Henry, D. J. Harrington, and D. R. Carrigan.** 2000. Human herpesvirus 6 and multiple sclerosis: systemic active infections in patients with early disease. *Clin. Infect. Dis.* **31**:894–903.

76. **Knox, K. K., and D. R. Carrigan.** 1995. Active human herpesvirus (HHV-6) infection in the central nervous system in patients with AIDS. *J. Acquir. Immune Defic. Syndr. Hum. Retrovirol.* **9**:69–73.

77. **Koprowski, H., and E. DeFreitas.** 1988. HTLV-I and chronic nervous diseases: present status and a look into the future. *Ann. Neurol.* **23**(Suppl.):166–170.

78. **Koprowski, H., E. C. DeFreitas, M. E. Harper, M. Sandberg-Wollheim, W. A. Sheremata, M. Robert-Guroff, C. W. Saxinger, M. B. Feinberg, F. Wong-Staal, and R. C. Gallo.** 1985. Multiple sclerosis and human T-cell lymphotropic retroviruses. *Nature* **318**:154–160.

79. **Krieg, A. M., M. F. Gourley, and A. Perl.** 1992. Endogenous retroviruses: potential etio-

logic agents in autoimmunity. *FASEB J.* **6**:2537–2544.

80. **Kurtzke, J. F.** 1993. Epidemiologic evidence for multiple sclerosis as an infection. *Clin. Microbiol. Rev.* **6**:382–427.

81. **Kurtzke, J. F.** 1995. MS epidemiology worldwide. One view of current status. *Acta Neurol. Scand.* **161**(Suppl.):23–33.

82. **Kurtzke, J. F., K. Hyllested, and A. Heltberg.** 1995. Multiple sclerosis in the Faroe islands: transmission across four epidemics. *Acta Neurol. Scand.* **91**:321–325.

83. **Kyuwa, S., K. Yamaguchi, Y. Toyoda, and K. Fujiwara.** 1991. Induction of self-reactive T cells after murine infection. *J. Virol.* **65**:1789–1795.

84. **Lafaille, J. J., F. V. Keere, A. L. Hsu, J. L. Baron, W. Haas, C. S. Raine, and S. Tonegawa.** 1997. Myelin basic protein specific T helper 2 (Th2) cells cause experimental autoimmune encephalomyelitis in immunodeficient hosts rather than protect them from the disease. *J. Exp. Med.* **186**:307–312.

85. **Lehman, P. V., T. Forsthuber, A. Miller, and E. E. Sercarz.** 1992. Spreading of T-cell autoimmunity to cryptic determinants of an autoantigen. *Nature* **358**:155–157.

86. **Leonard, J. P., K. E. Waldburger, and S. J. Goldman.** 1995. Prevention of experimental autoimmune encephalomyelitis by antibodies against interleukin 12. *J. Exp. Med.* **181**:381–386.

87. **Liedtke, W., K. Quabeck, D. W. Beelen, V. Straeten, and U. W. Schaefer.** 1994. Recurrent acute inflammatory demyelinating polyradiculitis after allogeneic bone marrow transplantation. *J. Neurol. Sci.* **125**:110–111.

88. **Lindert, R.-B., C. G. Haase, U. Brehm, C. Linington, H. Wekerle, and R. Hohfeld.** 1999. Multiple sclerosis: B- and T-cell responses to the extracellular domain of the myelin oligodendrocyte glycoprotein. *Brain* **122**:2089–2099.

89. **Linington, C., M. Bradl, H. Lassmann, C. Brunner, and K. Vass.** 1988. Augmentation of demyelination in rat acute allergic encephalomyelitis by circulating mouse monoclonal antibodies directed against a myelin/oligodendrocyte glycoprotein. *Am. J. Pathol.* **130**:443–454.

90. **Lipton, H. L., G. Twaddle, and M. L. Jelachich.** 1995. The predominant virus antigen burden is present in macrophages in Theiler's murine encephalomyelitis virus-induced demyelinating disease. *J. Virol.* **69**:2525–2533.

91. **Locatelli, G., F. Santoro, F. Veglia, A. Gobbi, P. Lusso, and M. S. Malnati.** 2000. Real-time quantitative PCR for human herpesvirus 6 DNA. *J. Clin. Microbiol.* **38**:4042–4048.

92. Lorentzen, J. C., S. Issazadeh, M. Storch, M. I. Mustafa, H. Lassmann, C. Linington, L. Klareskog, and T. Olsson. 1995. Protracted relapsing and demyelinating experimental autoimmune encephalomyelitis in DA rats immunized with syngeneic spinal cord and incomplete Freund's adjuvant. *J. Neuroimmunol.* **63:**193–205.

93. Lublin, F. D., and S. C. Reingold for the National Multiple Sclerosis Society (USA) Advisory Committee on Clinical Trials of New Agents in Multiple Sclerosis. 1996. Defining the clinical course of multiple sclerosis: results of an international survey. *Neurology* **46:**907–911.

94. Lucchinetti, C., W. Brück, and J. Noseworthy. 2001. Multiple sclerosis: recent developments in neuropathology, pathogenesis, magnetic resonance imaging studies and treatment. *Curr. Opin. Neurol.* **14:**259–269.

95. Lucchinetti, C., W. Brück, J. Parisi, B. Scheithauer, M. Rodriguez, and H. Lassmann. 1999. A quantitative analysis of oligodendrocytes in multiple sclerosis lesions. A study of 113 cases. *Brain* **122:**2279–2295.

96. Lucchinetti, C., W. Brück, J. Parisi, B. Scheithauer, M. Rodriguez, and H. Lassmann. 2000. Heterogeneity of multiple sclerosis lesions: implications for the pathogenesis of demyelination. *Ann. Neurol.* **47:**707–717.

97. Lusso, P., F. Di Marzo Veronese, S. Z. Salahuddin, D. V. Ablashi, S. Pahwa, K. Krohn, and R. C. Gallo. 1988. In vitro cellular tropism of human B-lymphotropic virus (human herpesvirus 6). *J. Exp. Med.* **167:**1659–1670.

98. Lycke, J., B. Svennerholm, E. Hjelmquist, L. Frisen, G. Badr, M. Andersson, A. Vahlne, and O. Andersen. 1996. Acyclovir treatment of relapsing-remitting multiple sclerosis. A randomized, placebo-controlled, double-blind study. *J. Neurol.* **243:**214–224.

99. Madsen, L. S., E. C. Andersson, L. Jansson, M. Krogsgaard, C. B. Andersen, J. Engberg, J. L. Strominger, A. Svejgaard, J. P. Hjorth, R. Holmdahl, K. W. Wucherpfennig, and L. Fugger. 1999. A humanized model for multiple sclerosis using HLA DR2 and a human T cell receptor. *Nat. Genet.* **23:**343–347.

100. Marrie, R. A., C. Wolfson, M. C. Sturkenboom, O. Gout, O. Heinzlef, E. Roullet, and L. Abenhaim. 2000. Multiple sclerosis and antecedent infections: a case-control study. *Neurology* **54:**2307–2310.

101. Marschang, P., J. Sodroski, R. Wurzner, and M. P. Dierich. 1995. Decay accelerating factor (CD55) protects human immunodeficiency virus type 1 from inactivation by human complement. *Eur. J. Immunol.* **25:**285–290.

102. Martin, C., M. Enbom, M. Söderström, S. Fredrikson, H. Dahl, J. Lycke, T. Bergström, and A. Linde. 1997. Absence of seven human herpesviruses, including HHV-6, by polymerase chain reaction in CSF and blood from patients with multiple sclerosis and optic neuritis. *Acta Neurol. Scand.* **95:**280–283.

103. Mayne, M., J. Krishnana, L. Metz, A. Nath, A. Auty, B. M. Sahai, and C. Power. 1998. Infrequent detection of human herpesvirus 6 DNA in peripheral mononuclear cells from multiple sclerosis patients. *Ann. Neurol.* **44:**391–394.

104. Miller, S. D., C. L. Vanderlugt, W. S. Begolka, W. Pao, R. L. Yauch, K. L. Neville, Y. Katz-Levy, A. Carrizosa, and B. S. Kim. 1997. Persistent infection with Theiler's virus leads to CNS autoimmunity via epitope spreading. *Nat. Med.* **3:**1133–1136.

105. Mokhtarian, F., and P. Swoveland. 1987. Predisposition to EAE induction in resistant mice by prior infection with Semliki Forest virus. *J. Immunol.* **138:**3264–3268.

106. Mokhtarian, F., Z. Zhang, Y. Shi, E. Gonzales, and R. A. Sobel. 1999. Molecular mimicry between a viral peptide and myelin oligodendrocyte glycoprotein induces autoimmune demyelinating disease in mice. *J. Neuroimmunol.* **95:**43–54.

107. Moller, J. R., D. Johnson, R. O. Brady, W. W. Tourtellotte, and R. H. Quarles. 1989. Antibodies to myelin-associated glycoprotein (MAG) in the cerebrospinal fluid of multiple sclerosis patients. *J. Neuroimmunol.* **22:**55–61.

108. Montefiori, D. C., R. J. Cornell, J. Y. Zhou, J. T. Zhou, V. M. Hirschand, and P. R. Johnson. 1994. Complement control proteins, CD46, CD55 and CD59, as common surface constituents of human and simian immunodeficiency viruses and possible targets for vaccine protection. *Virology* **205:**82–92.

109. Munch, M., A. Møller-Larsen, T. Christensen, N. Morling, H. J. Hansen, and S. Haar. 1997. Production of retrovirus and Epstein-Barr virus in cell lines from multiple sclerosis patients. *Acta Neurol. Scand.* **169**(Suppl.)**:**65–69.

110. Murray, P. D., D. B. McGavern, S. Sathornsumetee, and M. Rodriguez. 2001. Spontaneous remyelination following extensive demyelination is associated with improved neurological function in a viral model of multiple sclerosis. *Brain* **124:**1403–1416.

111. Nagano, I., S. Nakamura, M. Yoshioka, J. Onodera, K. Kogure, and Y. Itoyama. 1994. Expression of cytokines in brain lesions in subacute sclerosing panencephalitis. *Neurology* **44:**710–715.

112. **Neighbour, P. A., A. E. Miller, and B. R. Bloom.** 1981. Interferon responses of leukocytes in multiple sclerosis. *Neurology* **31:**561–566.

113. **Newcombe, J., S. Gahan, and M. L. Cuzner.** 1985. Serum antibodies against central nervous system proteins in human demyelinating disease. *Clin. Exp. Immunol.* **59:**383–390.

114. **Norrby, E., H. Link, and J. E. Olsson.** 1974. Measles virus antibodies in multiple sclerosis, comparison of antibody titres in cerebrospinal fluid and serum. *Arch. Neurol.* **30:**285–292.

115. **Noseworthy, J. H., C. Lucchinetti, M. Rodrigez, and B. G. Weinshenker.** 2000. Multiple sclerosis. *N. Engl. J. Med.* **343:**938–952.

116. **Olson, J. K., J. L. Croxford, M. A. Calenoff, M. C. Dal Canto, and S. D. Miller.** 2001. A virus-induced molecular mimicry model of multiple sclerosis. *J. Clin. Investig.* **108:**311–318.

117. **Padgett, B. L., and D. L. Walker.** 1973. Prevalence of antibodies in human sera against JC virus: an isolate from a case of progressive multifocal leukoencephalopathy. *J. Infect. Dis.* **127:**467–470.

118. **Panitch, H. S., R. L. Hirsch, J. Schindler, and K. P. Johnson.** 1987. Treatment of multiple sclerosis with gamma interferon: exacerbations associated with activation of the immune system. *Neurology* **37:**1097–1102.

119. **Perron, H., C. Geny, A. Laurent, C. Mouriquand, J. Pellat, J. Perret, and J. M. Seigneurin.** 1989. Leptomeningeal cell line from multiple sclerosis with reverse transcriptase activity and viral particles. *Res. Virol.* **140:**551–561.

120. **Perron, H., J. A. Garson, F. Bedin, F. Beseme, G. Paranhos-Baccala, F. Komurian-Pradel, F. Mallet, P. W. Tuke, C. Voisset, J. L. Blond, B. Lalande, J. M. Seigneurin, B. Mandrand, et al.** 1997. Molecular identification of a novel retrovirus repeatedly isolated from patients with multiple sclerosis. *Proc. Natl. Acad. Sci. USA* **94:**7583–7588.

121. **Perron, H., M. Suh, B. Lalande, B. Gratacap, A. Laurent, P. Stoebner, and J. M. Seigneurin.** 1993. Herpes simplex virus ICP0 and ICP4 immediate early proteins strongly enhance expression of a retrovirus harboured by a leptomeningeal cell line from a patient with multiple sclerosis. *J. Gen. Virol.* **74:**65–72.

122. **Peterson, J. D., C. Waltenbaugh, and S. D. Miller.** 1992. IgG subclass responses in Theiler's murine encephalomyelitis virus infection and immunization suggest a dominant role for Th1 cells in susceptible mouse strains. *Immunology* **75:**652–658.

123. **Pette, M., K. Fujita, B. Kitze, J. N. Whitaker, E. Albert, L. Kappos, and H. Wekerle.** 1990. Myelin basic protein-specific T lymphocyte lines from MS patients and healthy individuals. *Neurology* **40:**1770–1776.

124. **Piddlesden, S. J., H. Lassmann, F. Zimprich, B. P. Morgan, and C. Linington.** 1993. The demyelinating potential of antibodies to myelin oligodendrocyte glycoprotein is related to their ability to fix complement. *Am. J. Pathol.* **143:**555–564.

125. **Piddlesden, S. J., M. K. Storch, M. Hibbs, A. M. Freeman, H. Lassmann, and B. P. Morgan.** 1994. Soluble recombinant complement receptor 1 inhibits inflammation and demyelination in antibody-mediated demyelinating experimental allergic encephalomyelitis. *J. Immunol.* **152:**5477–5484.

126. **Pinter, C., S. Beltrami, D. Caputo, P. Ferrante, and A. Clivio.** 2000. Presence of autoantibodies against complement regulatory proteins in relapsing-remitting multiple sclerosis. *J. Neurovirol.* **6**(Suppl. 2)**:**S42–S46.

127. **Pinto, A. J., P. S. Morahan, M. Brinton, D. Stewart, and E. Gavin.** 1990. Comparative therapeutic efficacy of recombinant interferons-alpha, -beta, and -gamma against alphatogavirus, bunyavirus, flavivirus, and herpesvirus infections. *J. Interferon Res.* **10:**293–298.

128. **Rand, H. K., H. Houck, N. D. Denslow, and K. M. Heilman.** 2000. Epstein-Barr virus nuclear antigen-1 (EBNA-1) associated oligoclonal bands in patients with multiple sclerosis. *J. Neurol. Sci.* **173:**32–39.

129. **Reindl, M., C. Linington, U. Brehm, E. Dilitz, F. Deisenhammer, W. Poewe, and T. Berger.** 1999. Antibodies against the myelin oligodendrocyte glycoprotein and the myelin basic protein in multiple sclerosis and other neurological diseases: a comparative study. *Brain* **122:**2047–2056.

130. **Richardson, J. H., K. W. Wurcherpfennig, and N. Endo.** 1989. PCR analysis of DNA from multiple sclerosis patients for the presence of HTLV-I. *Science* **246:**821–824.

131. **Rieckmann, P., M. Albrecht, B. Kitze, T. Weber, H. Tumani, A. Brooks, W. Luer, A. Helwig, and S. Poser.** 1995. Tumor necrosis factor-alpha messenger RNA expression in patients with relapsing-remitting multiple sclerosis is associated with disease activity. *Ann. Neurol.* **37:**82–88.

132. **Romagnani, S.** 1997. The Th1/Th2 paradigm. *Immunol. Today* **18:**263–266.

133. **Ross, R. T., and M. Cheang.** 1995. Geographic similarities between varicella and multiple sclerosis: an hypothesis on the environmental factor of multiple sclerosis. *J. Clin. Epidemiol.* **48:**731–737.

134. **Rotola, A., E. Cassai, M. R. Tola, E. Granieri, and D. Di Luca.** 1999. Human herpesvirus 6 is latent in peripheral blood of patients with relapsing-remitting multiple sclerosis. *J. Neurol. Neurosurg. Psychiatry* **67:**529–531.

135. **Rudick, R. A., R. M. Ransohoff, J. C. Lee, R. Peppler, M. Yu, P. M. Mathisen, and V. K. Tuohy.** 1998. In vivo effects of interferon beta-1a on immunosuppressive cytokines in multiple sclerosis. *Neurology* **50:**1294–1300.

136. **Sadovnick, A. D., P. A. Baird, and R. H. Ward.** 1988. Multiple sclerosis: updated risks for relatives. *Am. J. Med. Genet.* **29:**533–541.

137. **Sadovnick, A. D., and G. C. Ebers.** 1993. Epidemiology of multiple sclerosis: a critical overview. *Can. J. Neurol. Sci.* **20:**17–29.

138. **Salahuddin, S. Z., D. V. Ablashi, P. D. Markham, S. F. Josephs, S. Sturzenegger, M. Kaplan, G. Halligan, P. Biberfeld, F. Wong-Staal, B. Kramarsky, and R. C. Gallo.** 1986. Isolation of a new virus, HBLV, in patients with lymphoproliferative disorders. *Science* **234:**596–601.

139. **Sanders, V. J., S. Felisan, A. Waddel, and W. W. Tourtellotte.** 1996. Detection of herpesviridae in postmortem multiple sclerosis brain tissue and controls by polymerase chain reaction. *J. Neurovirol.* **2:**249–258.

140. **Santoro, F., P. E. Kennedy, G. Locatelli, M. S. Malnati, E. A. Berger, and P. Lusso.** 1999. CD46 is a cellular receptor for human herpesvirus 6. *Cell* **99:**817–827.

141. **Scolding, N. J., B. P. Morgan, and D. A. S. Compston.** 1998. The expression of complement regulatory proteins by adult human oligodendrocytes. *J. Neuroimmunol.* **84:**69–75.

142. **Secchiero, P., D. R. Carrigan, Y. Asano, L. Benedetti, R. W. Crowley, A. L. Komaroff, R. C. Gallo, and P. Lusso.** 1995. Detection of human herpesvirus 6 in plasma of children with primary infection and immunosuppressed patients by polymerase chain reaction. *J. Infect. Dis.* **171:**273–280.

143. **Segal, B. M., B. K. Dwyer, E. M. Shevach.** 1998. An interleukin (IL)-10/IL-12 immunoregulatory circuit controls susceptibility to autoimmune disease. *J. Exp. Med.* **187:**537–546.

144. **Selmaj, K., and C. S. Raine.** 1988. Tumor necrosis factor mediates myelin and oligodendrocyte damage in vitro. *Ann. Neurol.* **23:**339–346.

145. **Sibley, W. A., C. R. Bamford, and K. Clark.** 1985. Clinical viral infections and multiple sclerosis. *Lancet* **i:**1313–1315.

146. **Sindic, C. J. M., P. Monteyne, and E. C. Laterre.** 1994. The intrathecal synthesis of virus-specific oligoclonal IgG in multiple sclerosis. *J. Neuroimmunol.* **54:**75–80.

147. **Soderberg-Naucler, C. S., S. Larsson, and E. Moller.** 1996. A novel mechanism for virus-induced autoimmunity in humans. *Immunol. Rev.* **152:**175–192.

148. **Soldan, S. S., R. Berti, N. Salem, P. Secchiero, L. Flamand, P. A. Calabresi, M. B. Brennan, H. W. Maloni, H. F. McFarland, H.-C. Lin, M. Patnaik, and S. Jacobson.** 1997. Association of human herpesvirus 6 (HHV-6) with multiple sclerosis: increased IgM response to HHV-6 early antigen and detection of serum HHV-6 DNA. *Nat. Med.* **3:**1394–1397.

149. **Soldan, S. S., A. Fogdell-Hahn, M. B. Brennan, B. B. Mittleman, C. Ballerini, L. Massacesi, T. Seya, H. F. McFarland, and S. Jacobson.** 2001. Elevated serum and CSF levels of soluble HHV-6 receptor, membrane cofactor protein, in patients with multiple sclerosis. *Ann. Neurol.* **50:**486–493.

150. **Soldan, S. S., and S. Jacobson.** 2001. Role of viruses in the etiology and pathogenesis of multiple sclerosis. *Adv. Virus Res.* **56:**513–551.

151. **Soldan, S. S., T. P. Leist, K. N. Juhng, H. F. McFarland, and S. Jacobson.** 2000. Increased lymphoproliferative response to human herpesvirus type 6A variant in multiple sclerosis patients. *Ann. Neurol.* **47:**306–316.

152. **Sorensen, P. S., B. Wanscher, C. V. Jensen, K. Schreiber, M. Blinkenberg, M. Ravnborg, H. Kirsmeier, V. A. Larsen, and M. L. Lee.** 1998. Intravenous immunoglobulin G reduces MRI activity in relapsing remitting multiple sclerosis. *Neurology* **50:**1273–1281.

153. **Spear, G. T., N. S. Lurain, C. J. Parker, M. Ghassemi, G. H. Payne, and M. Saifuddin.** 1995. Host cell-derived complement control proteins CD55 and CD59 are incorporated into the virions of two unrelated enveloped viruses, human T cell leukemia/lymphoma virus type I (HTLV-I) and human cytomegalovirus (HCMV). *J. Immunol.* **155:**4376–4381.

154. **Stohlman, S. A., and D. R. Hinton.** 2001. Viral induced demyelination. *Brain Pathol.* **11:**92–106.

155. **Storch, M. K., S. Piddlesden, M. Haltia, M. Iivainen, P. Morgan, and H. Lassmann.** 1998. Multiple sclerosis: in situ evidence for antibody- and complement-mediated demyelination. *Ann. Neurol.* **43:**465–471.

156. **Sumaya, C. V., L. W. Myers, G. W. Ellison, and Y. Ench.** 1985. Increased prevalence and titres of Epstein-Barr virus antibodies in patients with multiple sclerosis. *Ann. Neurol.* **17:**371–377.

157. **Sun, N., D. Grzybicki, R. Castro, S. Murphy, and S. Perlman.** 1995. Activation of astrocytes in the spinal cord of mice chronically infected with a neurotropic coronavirus. *Virology* **213:**482–493.

158. **Theiler, M.** 1937. Spontaneous encephalomyelitis of mice, a new virus disease. *J. Exp. Med.* **65:**705–719.

159. **Thoua, N.-M., J. M. van Noort, D. Baker, A. Bose, A. C. van Sechel, M. J. B. van Stipdonk, P. J. Travers, and S. Amor.** 2000. Encephalitogenic and immunogenic potential of the stress protein αB-crystallin in Biozzi ABH (H2A^{g7}) mice. *J. Neuroimmunol.* **104:**47–57.

160. **Thuoy, V. K., M. Yu, L. Yin, J. A. Kawczak, and P. Kinkel.** 1999. Spontaneous regression of primary autoreactivity during chronic progression of experimental autoimmune encephalomyelitis and multiple sclerosis. *J. Exp. Med.* **189:**1033–1042.

161. **Vahlne, A., S. Edström, P. Hanner, O. Andersen, B. Svennerholm, and E. Lycke.** 1985. Possible association of herpes simplex virus with demyelinating disease. *Scand. J. Infect. Dis.* **47:**16–21.

162. **Vanguri, P., B. Silverman, L. Koski, and M. L. Shin.** 1982. Complement activation by isolated myelin: activation of the classical pathway in the absence of myelin-specific antibodies. *Proc. Natl. Acad. Sci. USA* **79:**3290–3294.

163. **Van Noort, M. J., J. J. Bajramovic, A. C. Plomp, and M. J. B. Stipdonk.** 2000. Mistaken self, a novel model that links microbial infections with myelin-directed autoimmunity in multiple sclerosis. *J. Neuroimmunol.* **105:**46–57.

164. **van Noort, M. J., A. C. van Sechel, J. J. Bajramovic, M. El Ouagmiri, C. H. Polman, H. Lassmann, and R. Ravid.** 1995. The small heat-shock protein αB-crystallin as candidate autoantigen in multiple sclerosis. *Nature* **375:**798–801.

165. **Van Sechel, A. C., J. J. Bajramovic, M. J. B. van Stipdonk, C. Persoon-Deen, S. B. Geutskens, and J. M. van Noort.** 1999. EBV-induced expression and HLA-DR-restricted presentation by human B cells of αB-crystallin, a candidate autoantigen in multiple sclerosis. *J. Immunol.* **162:**129–135.

166. **Wandinger, K. P., W. Jabs, A. Siekhaus, S. Bubel, P. Trillenberg, H. J. Wagner, K. Wessel, H. Kirchner, and H. Hennig.** 2000. Association between clinical disease activity and Epstein-Barr virus reactivation in MS. *Neurology* **55:**178–184.

167. **Wang, F. Z., H. Dahl, P. Ljungman, and A. Linde.** 1999. Lymphoproliferative responses to human herpesvirus-6 variant A and variant B in healthy adults. *J. Med. Virol.* **57:**134–139.

168. **Warren, K. G., and I. Catz.** 1994. Relative frequency of autoantibodies to myelin basic protein and proteolipid protein in optic neuritis and multiple sclerosis cerebrospinal fluid. *J. Neurol. Sci.* **121:**66–73.

169. **Warrington, A. E., K. Asakura, A. J. Bieber, B. Ciric, V. Van Keulen, S. V. Kaveri, R. A. Kyle, L. R. Pease, and M. Rodriguez.** 2000. Human monoclonal antibodies reactive to oligodendrocytes promote remyelination in a model of multiple sclerosis. *Proc. Natl. Acad. Sci. USA* **97:**6820–6825.

170. **Watanabe, R., H. Wege, and V. ter Meulen.** 1987. Comparative analysis of coronavirus JHM-induced demyelinating encephalomyelitis in Lewis and Brown Norway rats. *Lab. Investig.* **57:**375–383.

171. **Weerth, S., T. Berger, H. Lassmann, and C. Linington.** 1999. Encephalitogenic and neuritogenic T cell responses to the myelin-associated glycoprotein (MAG) in the Lewis rat. *J. Neuroimmunol.* **95:**157–164.

172. **Wekerle, H., K. Kojima, J. Lannes-Vieira, H. Lassmann, and C. Linington.** 1994. Animal models. *Ann. Neurol.* **36**(Suppl.):S47–S53.

173. **Williamson, J. S. P., and S. A. Stohlman.** 1990. Effective clearance of mouse hepatitis virus from the central nervous system requires both CD4$^+$ and CD8$^+$ T cells. *J. Virol.* **64:**3817–3823.

174. **Windhangen, A., J. Newcombe, F. Dangond, C. Strand, M. N. Woodroofe, M. L. Cuzner, and D. A. Hafler.** 1995. Expression of costimulatory molecules B7-1 (CD80), B7-2 (CD86), and interleukin 12 cytokine in multiple sclerosis lesions. *J. Exp. Med.* **182:**1985–1996.

175. **Wisniewski, H. M., and B. R. Bloom.** 1975. Primary demyelination as a non-specific consequence of a cell-mediated immune reaction. *J. Exp. Med.* **141:**346–359.

176. **Wu, G. F., and S. Perlman.** 1999. Macrophage infiltration, but not apoptosis, is correlated with immune-mediated demyelination following murine infection with a neurotropic coronavirus. *J. Virol.* **73:**8771–8780.

177. **Wucherpfennig, K. W., and J. L. Strominger.** 1995. Molecular mimicry in T cell-mediated autoimmunity: viral peptides activate human T cell clones specific for myelin basic protein. *Cell* **80:**695–705.

178. **Xue, S., N. Sun, N. van Roijen, and S. Perlman.** 1999. Depletion of blood-borne macrophages does not reduce demyelination in mice infected with a neurotropic coronavirus. *J. Virol.* **73**:6327–6334.

179. **Zhang, J., S. Markovic-Plese, B. Lacet, J. Raus, H. L. Weiner, and D. A. Hafler.** 1994. Increased frequency of interleukin 2-responsive T cells specific for myelin basic protein and proteolipid protein in peripheral blood and cerebrospinal fluid of patients with multiple sclerosis. *J. Exp. Med.* **179**:973–984.

180. **Zheng, L., M. A. Calenoff, and M. C. Dal Canto.** 2001. Astrocytes, not microglia, are the main cells responsible for viral persistence in Theiler's murine encephalomyelitis virus infection leading to demyelination. *J. Neuroimmunol.* **118**:256–267.

POLYBACTERIAL
DISEASES

BACTERIAL VAGINOSIS AS A MIXED INFECTION

Phillip E. Hay

7

The vagina is a unique environment for bacterial colonization. It is subject to dramatic changes over the course of a lifetime, induced by developmental and hormonal changes. At birth, it is lined by stratified squamous epithelium, which regresses as the influence of maternal estrogen wanes. In childhood, the vaginal flora contains skin commensals and bowel organisms. At menarche, the pH falls from neutral to approximately 4, and the flora becomes dominated by lactobacilli. Many other organisms may be present in lower concentrations, including anaerobic and facultative anaerobic bacteria and *Candida* spp. The hormonal environment alters on a monthly basis, with additional disturbances to the ecosystem produced by menstruation, washing, and hygiene. Sexual activity can introduce a number of new species and pathogens, as well as alter the pH. Pregnancy and breast-feeding produce longer fluctuations in the hormonal balance. In the climacteric, the vaginal epithelium gradually atrophies, the pH rises, and a flora more similar to that of skin may become reestablished.

Bacterial vaginosis (BV) can be thought of as a disturbance in this vaginal ecosystem in which the lactobacilli are replaced by an overgrowth of vaginal commensal organisms. It may be transient or become persistent. It is recognized as the most common cause of abnormal vaginal discharge in women of childbearing age. The symptoms of a thin, white or yellow discharge accompanied by a fishy smell are so characteristic that it is surprising that BV was not widely recognized until described as nonspecific vaginitis by Gardner and Dukes in 1955 (11). In the 1920s, Schroder in Germany described three grades of vaginal flora and changes in the bacterial composition of the vagina, which broadly correspond to our current understanding of normal, intermediate, and BV flora (36).

PREVALENCE

The reported prevalence of BV varies widely, from 5 to 51% between different populations. In the United States, Bump and Buesching reported a prevalence of approximately 13% among adolescent girls (8). We reported a similar prevalence in a gynecology clinic (16) and antenatal clinic (14) in the United Kingdom. The incidence is higher in women undergoing termination of pregnancy (28%) (5) and in a group of women having in vitro fertilization treatment (24.6%) (31). In the United States, a high incidence was reported for some populations, e.g.,

Phillip E. Hay, Department of Genitourinary Medicine, St. George's Hospital Medical School, Cranmer Terrace, London SW17 0QT, United Kingdom.

Polymicrobial Diseases, Edited by Kim A. Brogden and Janet M. Guthmiller, inner-city pregnant women (32.5%) (21). The highest incidence, however, has been reported from Rakai in rural Uganda, where 50.9% of women had BV, along with a prevalence for *Trichomonas vaginalis* of 23.8% (27). Eighty percent of these women were asymptomatic.

Vaginal Physiology and BV

At menarche, under the influence of estrogen, stratified squamous epithelium develops in the vagina. Lactobacilli become the dominant organism. The source of the vaginal lactobacilli in an individual woman has not been determined. Lactic acid is produced by both bacterial metabolism and that of the epithelium, and the vaginal pH falls to a level usually between 4.0 and 4.5. Physiological discharge consists of mucus, desquamated epithelial cells, and lactobacilli. The pH may rise above 4.5 at the time of menstruation, when the concentration of lactobacilli is reduced. Cervical mucus and semen have pH between 7 and 8. In mice, exogenous treatment with progesterone alters the flora to one that resembles BV (40). How much do the hormonal changes of a menstrual cycle influence the flora in women?

If BV develops, the pH rises to a level between 4.5 and 7.0. The anaerobic or facultative anaerobic organisms which are usually present in low numbers increase by between 100- and 1,000-fold, to considerably outnumber the lactobacilli, which may eventually disappear. Trimethylamine and the polyamines putrescine and cadaverine are produced by anaerobic metabolism, and they are thought to be responsible for the fishy smell. Microscopy of vaginal fluid shows multiple small bacteria and epithelial cells with large numbers of adherent bacteria. Gardner and Dukes called these clue cells, as they gave a clue to the diagnosis of nonspecific vaginitis (11).

DIAGNOSIS

Nonspecific vaginitis was defined as a clinical entity recognizable from the symptoms of a fishy-smelling vaginal discharge confirmed by detecting thin homogenous vaginal fluid adherent to the walls of the vagina and confirmed

TABLE 1 The composite (Amsel) criteria used for the diagnosis of BV in clinical practice[a]

- Vaginal pH of >4.5
- Release of a fishy smell on addition of alkali (10% potassium hydroxide)
- Characteristic discharge on examination
- Presence of "clue cells" on microscopy

[a] The diagnosis of BV is established if at least three of the four criteria are present.

by finding clue cells on microscopy. Initially, it was thought to be a straightforward infection by one organism, now called *Gardnerella vaginalis*. Subsequently, other bacteria were identified as part of the BV flora. In 1983, the term BV was coined, with the recognition that there are many bacterial spp. contributing to the condition and that inflammation is usually absent. The KOH or "whiff" test was added as a fourth criterion for the diagnosis, as shown in Table 1 (2).

More recently, scoring systems for interpreting Gram-stained vaginal smears have been used to diagnose BV (14, 23). Self-administered vaginal swabs can be used, making noninvasive screening possible. They are smeared on a glass slide, which is air dried and subsequently read in a central laboratory. The composite criteria define a dichotomy of BV or normal flora. Scoring systems for interpreting Gram-stained smears allow a gradation to accommodate intermediate patterns.

TREATMENT AND COMPLICATIONS

The reason that some women get BV frequently and others either never get BV or get it infrequently has yet to be fully defined. This will be discussed below. Treatment with antibiotics to suppress the anaerobic overgrowth is usually successful in eradicating BV but not necessarily in eliminating the underlying disturbance which allowed it to develop in the first place. In some women, BV may relapse within 2 to 3 weeks of antibiotic treatment. Standard treatments are shown in Table 2.

Women with BV have an increased risk of many obstetric and gynecological complications. These include second-trimester miscar-

TABLE 2 Standard treatments for BV

Drug	Dose	Duration (days)
Oral metronidazole	400 mg twice a day	5–7
Metronidazole gel	1 applicator once a day	5
2% Clindamycin cream	1 applicator once a day	3–7
Oral clindamycin[a]	300 mg twice a day	5

[a] This is not a licensed indication.

riage and preterm birth, early failure of in vitro fertilization, an increased risk of upper genital tract infection following termination of pregnancy, and an increased risk of infective complications after hysterectomy. In addition, in prospective studies, BV has emerged as a risk factor for acquisition of sexually transmitted infection, including human immunodeficiency virus (HIV) infection (18).

NATURAL HISTORY AND EPIDEMIOLOGY

In many women, the vaginal ecosystem is in a state of flux, changing at different stages of the menstrual cycle. Four studies have looked at self-collected Gram-stained vaginal smears to examine the natural history of vaginal flora. Schwebke and colleagues monitored 51 women considered to be at low risk for sexually transmitted infection for up to 6 weeks (38). Only 11 of these women had normal flora throughout, with 25 having an intermediate pattern at some point and 13 developing BV. Five of the 13 reported symptoms. There were significant associations between developing BV and prior BV (44 versus 12%), mean number of lifetime partners (13.4 versus 7.15), and a higher mean number of episodes of receptive cunnilingus (3.6 versus 1.4). Of these, only cunnilingus remained significant in a multivariate analysis. Changes in flora were also associated with menses and use of vaginal medication or spermicide.

Increased abnormalities of vaginal flora occur during the first 9 days of the cycle, and studies have concluded that abnormal flora occur in most women at some time and that we might therefore need to revise our concept of what is normal. One study examined daily smears from 18 women with recurrent BV (17). Again, BV usually developed spontaneously early in the menstrual cycle and resolved spontaneously in the second half of the cycle, if it did resolve. Interestingly, in some women, the onset followed episodes of vaginal candidiasis and if anything, BV was more likely to resolve than to appear after unprotected sex with the regular partner. In some women, the onset in resolution of BV occurred within 2 or 3 days, usually after an intermediate stage. The association with resolution of candidiasis is interesting in light of an in vitro study which demonstrated inhibition of candidal growth by putrescine and cadaverine (33). These amines are produced by *Gardnerella* and other organisms found in BV. An earlier study also reported an association between *Candida* and recurrent BV (32). Changes in the vaginal flora over a period of 3 months in a woman with recurrent BV are shown in Fig. 1 (17). Another woman in the study had frequent symptomatic relapses of BV over a 10-month period (17). She received standard treatments for BV and one course of doxycycline and metronidazole for pelvic inflammatory disease during this time. She has had no relapses in the following 4 years. It is not clear what happened to prevent BV from recurring again.

For the results shown in Fig. 1, self-collected vaginal smears were prepared by the subject daily. They were subsequently Gram stained. The Nugent score is used, in which 0 to 3 is considered normal flora, 4 to 6 is intermediate, and 7 to 10 is considered BV. An arbitrary scoring system has been used for candidiasis, with 0 being no *Candida,* 2 being

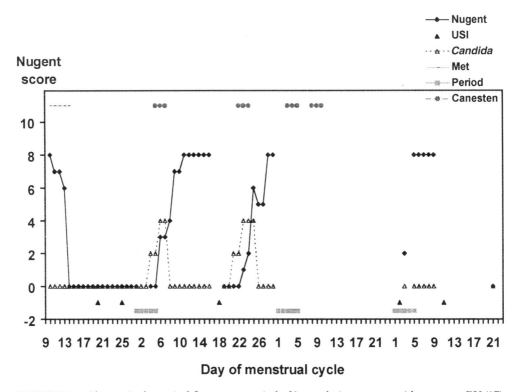

FIGURE 1   Changes in the vaginal flora over a period of 3 months in a woman with recurrent BV (17). The day of the menstrual cycle, treatment with metronidazole (Met) or clotrimazole pessaries (Canesten), menstruation (Period), and unprotected sexual intercourse (USI) (indicated by diary and the presence of sperm on the smear) are shown. Days on which no slide was collected are shown as interruptions in the graph. The subject presents with BV, which resolves with metronidazole treatment. During her next period, *Candida* develops. This resolves with treatment, to be followed by BV. The BV spontaneously resolves in midcycle, but candidiasis and BV recur shortly afterwards, and BV recurs again in the final month.

presence of spores, and 4 being presence of hyphae. Overall, the subject presented with BV, which resolved with metronidazole treatment. During her next period, candidiasis developed. This resolved with treatment, only to be followed by BV. The BV spontaneously resolved in midcycle, but candidiasis and BV recurred shortly afterwards, and BV recurred again in the final month.

During pregnancy, the vagina is not subjected to the frequent changes in hormone levels associated with menstrual cycles. Few observational studies have been performed during pregnancy, but it appears that BV resolves spontaneously in approximately 50% of women in whom it is present at around 16 weeks gestation

and may develop in 2 to 3% of those who did not have it at 16 weeks gestation (15).

EPIDEMIOLOGY

Most studies have found an increased prevalence of BV in women of black race compared to those of white race and in those who report cunnilingus, smoking, and use of an intrauterine contraceptive device. In community-based studies, BV is more common in women with chlamydial infection and also those undergoing termination of pregnancy. It has also been associated with changing sex partners and high-risk lifestyle (22). These associations suggest that it behaves as a sexually transmitted disease (STD), but the early study by Bump and Buesching found no difference in the prevalence between virgin and nonvirgin adolescent women, with clue cells detected in 9% of both groups (8). Thus, BV appears to be associated with sexual intercourse and risk of STDs but appears to not be an STD itself. Moreover, BV seems to be common in lesbians, a group at low risk for most STDs. In one study, there was a trend for both members of couples to have either normal flora or BV, suggesting transmission of an etiological agent (4).

A large prospective study of 1,248 women who did not have BV at baseline has recently been reported (M. A. Krohn et al., International Society for Sexually Transmitted Disease Research Meeting, presentation, June 2001). Development of BV was associated with smoking, douching, and no contraceptive use. In the multivariate analysis, independent risk factors were nonwhite race, intermediate flora on Gram stain, a lack of H_2O_2-producing lactobacilli, two or more sex partners in the previous 4 months, and intercourse more than 3 times/week.

Factors That Reduce Lactobacilli

Vaginal douching or other washing practices are frequently cited as a cause of disturbance of the vaginal flora leading to the onset of BV. In a prospective study, douching was associated with loss of protective H_2O_2-producing lactobacilli and acquisition of BV (13). A case-control study of 200 women attending a genitourinary medicine clinic in London, United Kingdom, investigated associations between vulval washing, vaginal washing, and douching and BV (30). BV was more common in black Caribbean women than in white women (odds ratio, 2.1; 95% confidence interval, 1.1 to 4.1). Use of bubble bath, antiseptic solution, and douching was more common in women with BV. Prior history of BV was the strongest predictor for current BV (odds ratio, 13.4; 95% confidence interval, 5.5 to 32.6). In the multivariate analysis, after controlling for washing practices, there was no ethnic difference in the incidence of BV. In contrast, in a study of 842 women early in the third trimester of pregnancy in North Carolina, it was reported that race remained associated with BV after controlling for many possible confounding variables, including douching (35). BV was found in 22.3% of black women compared to 8.5% of white women. Black women were also more likely to have the highest Nugent scores of 9 or 10, weighted by the presence of high counts of *Mobiluncus* morphotypes.

An elegant new hypothesis to explain the occurrence of BV is that lactobacilli are killed by a phage infection (6). *Lactobacillus* phages are known to affect yogurt cultures in the food industry. They can remain in a temperate (inactive) state or become lytic, when up to 99% of the lactobacillus population may be killed. These phages have now been isolated from human lactobacilli from the vagina (25) and gut and from lactobacilli in yogurt. The last were shown to inhibit vaginal lactobacilli (39). Blackwell hypothesizes that phages might be transmitted by sexual intercourse, dairy products, or feco-oral spread (6). Moreover, carcinogens such as benzo[*a*]pyrene diol epoxide (26), which is present in cigarette smoke, can induce lysogeny in cultures. If a male partner has triggered BV by transmitting a lactobacillus phage, it is not surprising that treatment with antibiotics makes no difference to the subsequent relapse rate for his partner. Clearly, further prospective studies are warranted.

MICROBIOLOGY

The organisms most commonly associated with BV are *G. vaginalis*, *Bacteroides* (*Prevotella*) spp., *Mobiluncus* spp., and *Mycoplasma hominis*. High concentrations of *Gardnerella*, >100-fold greater than normal, are found in up to 95% of women with BV, but *Gardnerella* was also found in more than 50% of women without BV, so culture has a poor specificity. Quantitative culture showing high concentrations correlates better with BV in research studies, but culture should not be used for routine diagnosis. The reported prevalence of other organisms often reflects the sensitivity of the culture method for the specific organism. For instance, *Fusobacter* spp., peptostreptococci, and non-viridans group streptococci have also been associated with BV.

One study looked at the changes in bacterial flora that occur as it passes from normal to intermediate and BV (34). At the intermediate stage, *Gardnerella* and *Bacteroides* were present in moderate concentrations, but high concentrations of those organisms and of *M. hominis* were not seen until full BV had developed. The presence of high concentrations of *Mobiluncus,* visible on a Gram stain, have been used to define the most abnormal flora, with a Nugent score of 9 or 10. Recently, by use of PCR, *Mobiluncus* spp. were detected in 84.5% of women with BV and 38% of those without BV (37).

Bacterial Interactions

After isolating *Haemophilus vaginalis* (now called *G. vaginalis*), Gardner and Dukes investigated its role in inoculation experiments (11). Thirteen volunteer subjects were inoculated with a pure culture of *H. vaginalis*. Ten of them failed to develop clinical evidence of the disease or positive cultures subsequently. Cultures were positive for two subjects for 2 or 3 months, but neither developed the disease. One patient developed the clinical manifestations and had the organism recovered in pure culture. A further 15 women, of whom 4 were pregnant, were inoculated directly with material obtained from infected patients. Eleven (73%) of these subjects developed clinical signs of "nonspecific vaginitis," and the organism was recovered from all of them. In eight of these women, the syndrome developed within 1 week of inoculation. This suggests that inoculation with the full cocktail of bacteria found in BV is more likely to induce the condition than is inoculation with a single organism. This is supported by in vitro studies.

Anaerobic metabolism produces succinic rather than lactic acid. One study looked at the symbiotic relationship between *Gardnerella,* a facultative aerobe, and *Prevotella bivia* (29). The former produces amino acids that are utilized by the latter. In turn, *Prevotella* produces ammonia, which is utilized by *Gardnerella* in a symbiotic fashion. The same group also demonstrated another symbiotic relationship in vitro, with *P. bivia* making amino acids available for *Peptostreptococcus anaerobius* (28).

A host of enzymes which break down mucus are produced by the different bacteria involved in BV. Thus, mucinases, sialidases, and neuraminidases are present. These break down cervical and vaginal mucus. This is probably the explanation for the thin homogenous discharge, which lacks the cohesion normally induced by mucus. Additional virulence factors cleave immunoglobulin A (IgA) and IgM, reducing the ability of the host to prevent infections (9). Other protective mediators, such as secretory leukocyte protease inhibitor (SLPI), are also reduced (10).

Lactobacilli

Lactobacilli produce a variety of substances, such as bacteriocins and lactocins, which are toxic to other bacterial species and lactobacilli, respectively. Acidification of the vagina is an important defense mechanism. H_2O_2 is also an important inhibitor of anaerobic growth, and it is thought that *Lactobacillus* spp. producing high levels of H_2O_2 provide protection against BV and acquisition of sexually transmitted infections. Thus, in vitro at a pH of <4.5, H_2O_2-producing lactobacilli inhibit the growth of BV-associated organisms effectively, but at higher pHs the effect wanes (20). The inhibition is also reduced by addition of myeloperoxidase, which breaks down H_2O_2.

Is a change in pH such as occurs at the time of menstruation and following unprotected intercourse sufficient to trigger BV? Alternatively, if sufficient numbers of bacteria are inoculated into the vagina from a partner, will BV develop? Another possible trigger is anything that reduces the number or quality of lactobacilli. Interestingly, broad-spectrum antibiotics that inhibit lactobacilli do not seem to trigger BV (1), possibly because they also inhibit some of the BV organisms.

An absence of healthy H_2O_2-producing lactobacilli might contribute to frequent recurrences of BV in some women. One approach under study is to recolonize the vagina with healthy lactobacilli. A recent study of 215 sexually active women used whole-chromosome DNA probes to determine the most common strains of vaginal lactobacilli. The most prevalent species was *Lactobacillus crispatus* (32%), followed by *L. jensenii* (23%) and a previously undescribed sp. designated *Lactobacillus* sp. strain 1086V (15%) (3). An in vitro study investigated the rate of acid production by *Lactobacillus* spp. (7). The growth medium was acidified to an asymptotic pH of 3.2 to 4.8. In contrast, BV-associated organisms such as *G. vaginalis, P. bivia,* and *Peptostreptococcus anaerobius* reached an asymptotic level at a pH of 4.7 to 6.0, consistent with the pH levels found in BV. The authors calculate that 3 ml of semen would be acidified at a rate of 0.56 to 0.75 pH units/h. Unfortunately, they do not speculate on whether a transient pH change induced by a single episode of unprotected intercourse is likely to favor the growth of BV organisms sufficiently to produce a change in the bacterial flora. However, repeated episodes of intercourse within 24 h might produce a longer period of favorable growth conditions.

In a small study from Belgium, 32 women with BV or intermediate flora were treated with vaginal tablets containing 50 mg of a lyophilisate of viable, H_2O_2-producing *L. acidophilus* and 0.03 mg of estriol for 6 days (24). There was a significant benefit, with a cure rate after 6 weeks of 88% in the treatment group compared to 22% in the placebo group.

COMPLICATIONS

A full discussion of the complications of BV is outside the scope of this chapter. The pregnancy complications of late miscarriage and preterm birth are mediated through the development of chorioamnionitis (12). Once again, this is a mixed infection with the various organisms associated with BV producing a mixture of enzymes which break down cervical mucus, invade the membranes, and produce enzymes which can weaken the membranes, increasing the risk of premature rupture. In vitro studies have assessed the levels of such

virulence factors caused by different bacteria. Although in many studies only one organism may be isolated from the membranes, it is likely that with improved means of detection a multiplicity of organisms would be found.

BV has also been associated with acquisition of HIV. H_2O_2 reduces the ability of HIV to infect cells in vitro (19), and its absence in BV is one putative mechanism. Cleavage of IgA, reduction in SLPI, and inhibition of leukocyte chemotaxis are other possible factors (18).

CONCLUSIONS

Our understanding of BV is improving through observational studies and study of the interactions between bacteria in the laboratory. The vaginal ecosystem is subjected to a variety of hormonal changes that affect the balance between lactobacilli and anaerobes. It is likely that the normal lactobacillus flora may be overwhelmed by factors such as a prolonged alteration in the pH of the vagina following vaginal douching or frequent sexual intercourse. Instillation of large numbers of organisms from a male or female sex partner might trigger BV. Alternative hypotheses include the introduction of a lytic bacteriophage infection, reducing the lactobacillus population. Once the BV organisms are allowed to flourish, they utilize each other's metabolites in a symbiotic manner and continue to maintain a pH of >4.5.

Possibly, the lack of H_2O_2-producing lactobacilli in the vagina makes it easier for sexually transmitted pathogens, including HIV, to gain a foothold, although it may be that the same risk factors for acquiring STDs are in fact precipitating BV. Failure to reestablish a H_2O_2-producing lactobacillus flora after antibiotics have suppressed anaerobic growth might account for frequent relapses in some women. There are still many women who are troubled by frequent symptomatic relapses of BV, and we need improved understanding of the triggers for it so that we can help them. There is an urgent need to determine how to effectively prevent the adverse outcomes of pregnancy associated with BV. If we could control BV, we might additionally be able to reduce the risk of HIV infection, for which BV is an important risk factor. A promising approach is to recolonize the vagina with lactobacilli that are high-level H_2O_2 producers and may be better able to inhibit the growth of anaerobes than the native lactobacillus flora.

REFERENCES

1. **Agnew, K. J., and S. L. Hillier.** 1995. The effect of treatment regimens for vaginitis and cervicitis on vaginal colonization by lactobacilli. *Sex. Transm. Dis.* **22:**269–273.

2. **Amsel, R., P. A. Totten, C. A. Spiegel, K. C. Chen, D. Eschenbach, and K. K. Holmes.** 1983. Nonspecific vaginitis. Diagnostic criteria and microbial and epidemiologic associations. *Am. J. Med.* **74:**14–22.

3. **Antonio, M. A., S. E. Hawes, and S. L. Hillier.** 1999. The identification of vaginal *Lactobacillus* species and the demographic and microbiologic characteristics of women colonized by these species. *J. Infect. Dis.* **180:**1950–1956.

4. **Berger, B. J., S. Kolton, J. M. Zenilman, M. C. Cummings, J. Feldman, and W. M. McCormack.** 1995. Bacterial vaginosis in lesbians: a sexually transmitted disease. *Clin. Infect. Dis.* **21:**1402–1405.

5. **Blackwell, A. L., P. D. Thomas, K. Wareham, and S. J. Emery.** 1993. Health gains from screening for infection of the lower genital tract in women attending for termination of pregnancy. *Lancet* **342:**206–210.

6. **Blackwell, A. L.** 1999. Vaginal bacterial phaginosis? *Sex. Transm. Infect.* **75:**352–353.

7. **Boskey, E. R., K. M. Telsch, K. J. Whaley, T. R. Moench, and R. A. Cone.** 1999. Acid production by vaginal flora in vitro is consistent with the rate and extent of vaginal acidification. *Infect. Immun.* **67:**5170–5175.

8. **Bump, R. C., and W. J. Buesching.** 1988. Bacterial vaginosis in virginal and sexually active adolescent females: evidence against exclusive sexual transmission. *Am. J. Obstet. Gynecol.* **158:**935–939.

9. **Cauci, S., R. Monte, S. Driussi, P. Lanzafame, and F. Quadrifoglio.** 1998. Impairment of the mucosal immune system: IgA and IgM cleavage detected in vaginal washings of a subgroup of patients with bacterial vaginosis. *J. Infect. Dis.* **178:**1698–1706.

10. **Draper, D. L., D. V. Landers, M. A. Krohn, S. L. Hillier, H. C. Wiesenfeld, and R. P. Heine.** 2000. Levels of vaginal secretory leukocyte protease inhibitor are decreased in women with lower reproductive tract infections. *Am. J. Obstet. Gynecol.* **183:**1243–1248.

11. **Gardner, H. L., and C. D. Dukes.** 1955. *Haemophilus vaginalis* vaginitis. A newly defined specific infection previously classified "nonspecific" vaginitis. *Am. J. Obstet. Gynecol.* **69:**962–976.

12. **Goldenberg, R. L., J. C. Hauth, and W. W. Andrews.** 2000. Intrauterine infection and preterm delivery. *N. Engl. J. Med.* **342:**1500–1507.

13. **Hawes, S. E., S. L. Hillier, J. Benedetti, C. E. Stevens, L. A. Koutsky, P. Wolner-Hanssen, and K. K. Holmes.** 1996. Hydrogen peroxide-producing lactobacilli and acquisition of vaginal infections. *J. Infect. Dis.* **174:**1058–1063.

14. **Hay, P. E., R. F. Lamont, D. Taylor-Robinson, D. J. Morgan, C. Ison, and J. Pearson.** 1994. Abnormal bacterial colonisation of the genital tract and subsequent preterm delivery and late miscarriage. *Br. Med. J.* **308:**295–298.

15. **Hay, P. E., D. J. Morgan, C. A. Ison, S. A. Bhide, M. Romney, P. McKenzie, et al.** 1994. A longitudinal study of bacterial vaginosis during pregnancy. *Br. J. Obstet. Gynaecol.* **101:**1048–1053.

16. **Hay, P. E., D. Taylor-Robinson, and R. F. Lamont.** 1992. Diagnosis of bacterial vaginosis in a gynaecology clinic. *Br. J. Obstet. Gynaecol.* **99:**63–66.

17. **Hay, P. E., A. Ugwumadu, and J. Chowns.** 1997. Sex, thrush and bacterial vaginosis. *Int. J. STD AIDS* **8:**603–608.

18. **Hillier, S. L.** 1998. The vaginal microbial ecosystem and resistance to HIV. *AIDS Res. Hum. Retrovir.* **14**(Suppl. 1)**:**S17–S21.

19. **Klebanoff, S. J., and R. W. Coombs.** 1991. Viricidal effect of *Lactobacillus acidophilus* on human immunodeficiency virus type 1: possible role in heterosexual transmission. *J. Exp. Med.* **174:**289–292.

20. **Klebanoff, S. J., S. L. Hillier, D. A. Eschenbach, and A. M. Waltersdorph.** 1991. Control of the microbial flora of the vagina by H_2O_2-generating lactobacilli. *J. Infect. Dis.* **164:**94–100.

21. **McGregor, J. A., J. I. French, R. Parker, D. Draper, E. Patterson, W. Jones, K. Thorsgard, and J. McFee.** 1995. Prevention of premature birth by screening and treatment for common genital tract infections: results of a prospective controlled evaluation. *Am. J. Obstet. Gynecol.* **173:**157–167.

22. **Nilsson, U., D. Hellberg, M. Shoubnikova, S. Nilsson, and P. A. Mardh.** 1997. Sexual behavior risk factors associated with bacterial vaginosis and *Chlamydia trachomatis* infection. *Sex. Transm. Dis.* **24:**241–246.

23. **Nugent, R. P., M. A. Krohn, and S. L. Hillier.** 1991. Reliability of diagnosing bacterial vaginosis is improved by a standardized method of Gram stain interpretation. *J. Clin. Microbiol.* **29:**297–301.

24. **Parent, D., M. Bossens, D. Bayot, C. Kirk-patrick, F. Graf, F. E. Wilkinson, and R. R. Kaiser.** 1996. Therapy of bacterial vaginosis using exogenously-applied Lactobacilli acidophili and a low dose of estriol: a placebo-controlled multicentric clinical trial. *Arzneimittel-Forschung* **46:**68–73.

25. **Pavlova, S. I., A. O. Kilic, S. M. Mou, and L. Tao.** 1997. Phage infection in vaginal lactobacilli: an in vitro study. *Infect. Dis. Obstet. Gynecol.* **5:**36–44.

26. **Pavlova, S. I., and L. Tao.** 2000. Induction of vaginal *Lactobacillus* phages by the cigarette smoke chemical benzo[a]pyrene diol epoxide. *Mutat. Res.* **466:**57–62.

27. **Paxton, L. A., N. Sewankambo, R. Gray, D. Serwadda, D. McNairn, C. Li, and M. J. Wawer.** 1998. Asymptomatic non-ulcerative genital tract infections in a rural Ugandan population. *Sex. Transm. Infect.* **74:**421–425.

28. **Pybus, V., and A. B. Onderdonk.** 1998. A commensal symbiosis between *Prevotella bivia* and *Peptostreptococcus anaerobius* involves amino acids: potential significance to the pathogenesis of bacterial vaginosis. *FEMS Immunol. Med. Microbiol.* **22:**317–327.

29. **Pybus, V., and A. B. Onderdonk.** 1997. Evidence for a commensal, symbiotic relationship between *Gardnerella vaginalis* and *Prevotella bivia* involving ammonia: potential significance for bacterial vaginosis. *J. Infect. Dis.* **175:**406–413.

30. **Rajamanoharan, S., N. Low, S. B. Jones, and A. L. Pozniak.** 1999. Bacterial vaginosis, ethnicity, and the use of genital cleaning agents: a case control study. *Sex. Transm. Dis.* **26:**404–409.

31. **Ralph, S. G., A. J. Rutherford, and J. D. Wilson.** 1999. Influence of bacterial vaginosis on conception and miscarriage in the first trimester: cohort study. *Br. Med. J.* **319:**220–223.

32. **Redondo-Lopez, V., C. Meriwether, C. Schmitt, M. Opitz, R. Cook, and J. D. So-**bel. 1990. Vulvovaginal candidiasis complicating recurrent bacterial vaginosis. *Sex. Transm. Dis.* **17:**51–53.

33. **Rodrigues, A. G., P. A. Mardh, C. Pina-Vaz, J. Martinez-de-Oliveira, and A. F. da Fonseca.** 1999. Is the lack of concurrence of bacterial vaginosis and vaginal candidosis explained by the presence of bacterial amines? *Am. J. Obstet. Gynecol.* **181:**367–370.

34. **Rosenstein, I. J., D. J. Morgan, M. Sheehan, R. F. Lamont, and D. Taylor-Robinson.** 1996. Bacterial vaginosis in pregnancy: distribution of bacterial species in different Gram-stain categories of the vaginal flora. *J. Med. Microbiol.* **45:**120–126.

35. **Royce, R. A., T. P. Jackson, J. M. Thorp, Jr., S. L. Hillier, L. K. Rabe, L. M. Pastore, and D. A. Savitz.** 1999. Race/ethnicity, vaginal flora patterns, and pH during pregnancy. *Sex. Transm. Dis.* **26:**96–102.

36. **Schroder, R.** 1921. Zur Pathogenese und Klinik des vaginalen Fluors. *Zentbl. Gynakol.* **38:**1350–1361.

37. **Schwebke, J. R., and L. F. Lawing.** 2001. Prevalence of *Mobiluncus* spp. among women with and without bacterial vaginosis as detected by polymerase chain reaction. *Sex. Transm. Dis.* **28:**195–199.

38. **Schwebke, J. R., S. C. Morgan, and H. L. Weiss.** 1997. The use of sequential self-obtained vaginal smears for detecting changes in the vaginal flora. *Sex. Transm. Dis.* **24:**236–239.

39. **Tao, L., S. I. Pavlova, S. M. Mou, W. G. Ma, and A. O. Kilic.** 1997. Analysis of *Lactobacillus* products for phages and bacteriocins that inhibit vaginal lactobacilli. *Infect. Dis. Obstet. Gynecol.* **5:**244–251.

40. **Taylor-Robinson, D., and P. E. Hay.** 1997. The pathogenesis of the clinical signs of bacterial vaginosis and possible reasons for its occurrence. *Int. J. STD AIDS* **8**(Suppl. 1):35–37.

PERIODONTAL DISEASES

Janet M. Guthmiller and Karen F. Novak

8

The periodontal diseases are a diverse group of clinical entities in which induction of an inflammatory process results in destruction of the attachment apparatus, loss of supporting alveolar bone, and, if untreated, tooth loss. Periodontal disease is one of the most common diseases of the oral cavity and is the major cause of tooth loss in adults. Recently, there has been increasing interest in the relationship of periodontal disease to important systemic diseases, such as cardiovascular disease and complications in pregnancy (97).

Historically, the etiology of periodontal diseases has focused on bacterial plaque, microbial by-products, and the host immune response. Although recent studies have suggested a role for environmental (39), behavioral (50, 51), and genetic (71) risk factors in periodontal disease progression, most, if not all, forms of periodontitis should be viewed as infectious diseases. Bacteria are the primary etiologic factor of periodontal diseases, however, recent evidence also lists yeast and herpesviruses as putative pathogens (21, 122). Meanwhile, our understanding of the pathogenic process has been

hindered by the fact that it is usually the result of a polymicrobial infection including indigenous organisms with little pathogenic potential.

There are two main categories of periodontal disease in which loss of supporting structures around the tooth occurs: chronic periodontitis and aggressive periodontitis (6). The diseases can be further characterized by the extent of bone loss (localized or generalized) and the severity of the disease (slight, moderate, or advanced). Most patients suffer from chronic periodontitis, an insidious disease in which the destruction is consistent with the presence of bacterial plaque and mineralized plaque or calculus (Color Plate 1 [see color insert]). Chronic periodontitis is the result of a polymicrobial infection with variable microbial patterns. In contrast, aggressive periodontitis involves rapid attachment loss and bone destruction, and the destruction seen is usually not commensurate with the amount of microbial deposits. The localized form of aggressive periodontitis is an unusually unique disease relative to other forms of periodontitis in that it usually occurs during adolescence (a group traditionally exhibiting a low incidence of periodontal disease); the subgingival microbiota demonstrate an unusually high association (96.5%) with a single bacterium, *Actinobacillus actinomycetemcomitans* (141); bone resorption

Janet M. Guthmiller, Department of Periodontics and Dows Institute for Dental Research, College of Dentistry, University of Iowa, Iowa City, IA 52242. *Karen F. Novak,* Center for Oral Health Research, Division of Periodontics, College of Dentistry, University of Kentucky, Lexington, KY 40536.

Polymicrobial Diseases, Edited by Kim A. Brogden and Janet M. Guthmiller,
© 2002 ASM Press, Washington, D.C.

progresses at a rate three to four times faster than that observed for chronic periodontitis (106), may spontaneously arrest (11), and is localized to very specific teeth (first molars and incisors); finally, the disease tends to cluster in families suggesting that predisposition to the disease may be genetically regulated (12, 13, 56, 64, 89, 110, 111).

More than 500 different bacterial species have been estimated to reside in the subgingival plaque (95). However, studies from the 1930s to 1970s focused on the nonspecific plaque hypothesis which implicated the overall mass of the microbiota as the key factor in the initiation of tissue destruction rather than stressing the significance of specific bacterial species (132). This theory was subsequently challenged when different bacterial species were seen to play a pivotal role in the initiation and progression of periodontal disease, which supported the specific plaque hypothesis (83, 104, 119, 120, 124, 125).

A persistent concern with the specific plaque hypothesis is the fact that all of the potentially pathogenic organisms can be isolated from healthy as well as diseased subjects (54). This suggests that different strains of the same species may demonstrate varying pathogenicity. Molecular biological techniques have enabled us to examine associations between specific strains of a bacterial species with distinct diseases. For example, recent data imply that strains of *A. actinomycetemcomitans* associated with localized aggressive periodontitis differ from strains of the bacterium found in other forms of periodontal disease or in health (14, 57, 142). For the first time, evidence further delineates the role of virulent bacteria to include certain pathogenic strains or clones of bacterial species in the initiation and progression of particular periodontal diseases (53).

OVERVIEW OF DENTAL PLAQUE DEVELOPMENT

As previously stated, more than 500 different bacterial species can be found in the oral cavity (95). The sites colonized by these different microorganisms are diverse, ranging from the nonshedding tooth surface to the continually shedding epithelium covering the mucosal surfaces. The microorganisms colonizing these surfaces are not present in a free-floating planktonic state. Rather, they are present as a biofilm—a "community of microorganisms attached to a surface" (98). While the communities found on soft tissues often comprise a single microbial species, the most prevalent oral biofilm, dental plaque, exists as a complex multispecies entity attached to the tooth surface.

Within this multispecies biofilm are grampositive, gram-negative, aerobic, facultative, and anaerobic microorganisms that are deposited on the tooth surface in a sequential fashion. This sequential deposition begins with the adherence of early colonizers, streptococci and actinomycetes spp., to host-derived glycoproteins, mucins, and other proteins coating the tooth surface (41). These salivary proteins are deposited within minutes on a clean tooth surface and are called the "acquired pellicle." Bacterial surface structures, such as pili and outer membrane proteins, as well as proteins and enzymes in the acquired pellicle, are important mediators of this initial attachment (19, 37, 42).

Continued development of the plaque biofilm relies on physical interaction of bacteria of the same or different genera through coaggregation and coadhesion (68). Lectin-like receptors appear to be involved in coaggregation among streptococci, and lipoproteins and pili play a role in cell-cell interactions among other early colonizers. The biofilm continues to develop as late colonizers, such as veillonellae, prevotellae, propionibacteria, and certain streptococci, begin to colonize the tooth surface (98). Many of these bacteria would not usually interact with each other in a way that results in aggregation. However, certain bacteria, such as *Fusobacterium nucleatum,* serve as important bridges between these noncoaggregating, early colonizing bacteria and the late colonizers (68).

As the biofilm begins to mature, there is a progressive shift from a gram-positive, facultative flora to one predominated by gram-negative, anaerobic species. This shift is associated with the development of the biofilm beneath the gingival surface. The supragingival (above the gingival surface) and subgingival (beneath the gingival surface) habitats differ in terms of pH, redox potential, and nutrient availability. In addition, salivary and masticatory influences that have an impact on the supragingival microflora do not have the same influence on subgingival bacteria (7). Subgingival plaque is either designated as tooth-associated or tissue-associated. The tooth-associated plaque primarily comprises gram-positive rods and cocci, whereas the plaque associated with the epithelial tissue lining the gingival crevice is predominated by gram-negative rods, filaments, and spirochetes. Increased prevalence of several genera of proposed importance in the development of periodontitis may be seen as the subgingival plaque matures. These genera include, but are not limited to, *Treponema, Bacteroides, Porphyromonas, Prevotella, Capnocytophaga, Peptostreptococcus, Fusobacterium, Actinobacillus,* and *Eikenella.*

Certain periodontal bacteria are often found together in subgingival plaque samples. Cluster analysis and community ordination techniques were used to further define these relationships and to determine whether there were correlations between certain clusters and clinical parameters of disease (128). Results of these studies demonstrated that the bacteria could be sorted into five major groups that were given color designations. The designated "red" complex (*Treponema denticola, Porphyromonas gingivalis,* and *Bacteroides forsythus*) and the "orange" complex (*Prevotella intermedia, Prevotella nigrescens, Peptostreptococcus micros, F. nucleatum* subspecies, *Eubacterium nodatum, Streptococcus constellatus,* and three *Campylobacter* species) were generally found together, and evidence showed that colonization by the red complex was preceded by colonization by orange complex species. Both complexes could be associated with clinical parameters of disease supporting the polymicrobial nature of periodontitis.

Although it is clear that periodontal disease is a polymicrobial infection, there has historically been an interest in identifying specific microorganisms that contribute to the disease process. Attempts to apply Koch's postulates to specific bacteria have been hampered because these pathogens often cannot be grown in pure culture (e.g., large spirochetes), they may have long incubation times, they can occur in an asymptomatic carrier state, and they may exhibit a limited host range (121). Socransky (126) proposed a modified series of criteria for microbial causation for periodontitis which included (i) association of the microorganism with periodontitis, (ii) demonstration that elimination of the bacteria reduced the disease, (iii) evidence of a host response to the pathogen, (iv) demonstration of ability of the pathogen to cause disease in an animal model, and (v) evidence that the pathogen produces virulence factors that contribute to the disease process (126). Following this approach, three bacteria have been recognized as causative agents of periodontitis: *P. gingivalis, A. actinomycetemcomitans,* and *B. forsythus* (40). Although not completely supported by these criteria for causation, there is also evidence that *E. nodatum, Campylobacter rectus, P. intermedia/nigrescens, P. micros,* and *T. denticola* are etiologic factors in periodontitis (40).

PATHOGENIC POTENTIAL OF PERIODONTAL PATHOGENS
Pathogenic bacteria must be able to (i) colonize the host, (ii) evade host defense mechanisms, and (iii) damage host tissues. Mechanisms for each of these required steps for pathogenesis have been identified for many of the periodontal pathogens. The purpose of this section is not to provide an exhaustive evaluation of each of these mechanisms. Rather, examples of pathogenic processes used by selected periodontal pathogens are presented with appropriate review articles listed for further reference.

ADHERENCE, COLONIZATION, AND GROWTH
As discussed in the section on development of the biofilm, adhesion is a necessary element in the colonization of subgingival bacteria, either

directly to the periodontal tissues or through the association with other organisms by coaggregation and coadhesion. As the biofilm develops, there are areas of high and low bacterial biomass interlaced with aqueous channels which will provide for movement of essential nutrients (derived primarily from the gingival crevicular fluid) for the growth of the organisms and removal of metabolic waste products (24). While the space limitations of the subgingival environment (pocket) attempt to limit the expansion of the subgingival microbial complex, the apical migration of the epithelium and destruction of the attachment apparatus adjacent to the tooth (deeper periodontal pockets) allows for expansion of the subgingival biomass. As a result of the polymicrobial infection, the bacteria act in concert supporting nutrition and aggregation factors necessary for the biofilm development. For example, bacterial derived proteinases destroy tissue providing polypeptides utilized for growth by other organisms (62).

Although primarily a subgingival microorganism, *P. gingivalis* can adhere to many of the early plaque formers (80). For example, adherence between *P. gingivalis* and *Actinomyces naeslundii* is mediated by fimbrillin and a 40-kDa membrane protein of *P. gingivalis* and a high molecular weight carbohydrate on *A. naeslundii*. *P. gingivalis* can also interact with later colonizers such as *F. nucleatum, T. denticola, Treponema medium,* and *B. forsythus.* These interactions promote *P. gingivalis* colonization of the plaque biofilm. On the host side, *P. gingivalis* also can bind to epithelial cells, fibroblasts, and erythrocytes, and to components of the extracellular matrix. These interactions are mediated by *P. gingivalis* fimbriae and may be facilitated by proteolytic enzymes (80).

T. denticola attaches to human gingival fibroblasts, possibly through a lectin-mediated mechanism. Most strains adhere well to extracellular and basement membrane proteins, such as fibronectin and laminin (17). *T. denticola* coaggregates with *F. nucleatum* and *P. gingivalis,* which may be an important factor in colonization and development of the plaque biofilm (61).

Other important periodontal pathogens are also known for their ability to aggregate and/or adhere. For example, *A. actinomycetemcomitans* adheres to the tooth or epithelium via surface proteins, microvesicles, and fimbrae (139). *P. micros* adherence to epithelial cells has been shown to vary with morphologic characteristics of particular strains (74). And *Eikenella corrodens* demonstrates an aggregating factor, which is believed to play an important role in the accumulation of plaque (32).

INTERFERENCE WITH HOST DEFENSES

Periodontal pathogens use a variety of means to interfere with host defense mechanisms, thereby prolonging their presence in the periodontal pocket. One of the best-studied virulence factors is the leukotoxin produced by *A. actinomycetemcomitans.* This cytotoxic protein specifically kills a subset of leukocytes in vitro that includes polymorphonuclear leukocytes and peripheral blood monocytes (10, 134). The leukotoxin gene was cloned and sequenced (69, 73, 76, 77) and, on the basis of sequence homology, was found to be a member of the RTX (repeats in toxin) family of pore-forming bacterial toxins including toxins from such other species as *Pasteurella haemolytica* and *Actinobacillus pleuropneumoniae,* producing devastating infections in cattle and swine, respectively. The members of the RTX family all share a common gene organization, and the toxins contain tandemly repeated nonapeptides that have the consensus sequence GGXGXDX(L/I/V/W/Y/F)X.

A. actinomycetemcomitans elaborates many other factors that may allow the organism to evade detection/destruction by the host's immune system. These include inhibition of polymorphonuclear chemotaxis, production of immunosuppressive factors, secretion of proteases, which cleave immunoglobulin G (IgG), and production of Fc binding proteins (139). Recently, the organism was also shown to produce a cytolethal distending toxin (CDT) (88, 117, 130). The CDT of *A. actinomycetemcomitans* (previously described as the immunosuppressive factor) (115, 117, 118) induces cell cycle arrest in lymphocytes. The biological effects of the CDT, however, extend beyond immunosuppression and could play a role in other phenomena associated with *A. actinomycetemcomitans* including cell invasion (90, 91, 93).

P. gingivalis produces proteinases that cleave IgA1, IgA2, and IgG (36, 66, 67), including hydrolysis of immunoglobulin already bound to the bacterial surface (48). The lipopolysaccharide (LPS) produced by *P. gingivalis* does not stimulate E-selectin expression on endothelial cells and therefore hinders leukocyte extravasation (26). *P. gingivalis* LPS also is a poor activator of the release of tumor necrosis factor by mononuclear cells (22). *P. gingivalis* produces a capsule that inhibits phagocytosis and decreases interactions with bacterial serum proteins (131); this resistance to phagocytosis varies between strains (20). Other proteinases produced by *P. gingivalis* render polymorphonuclear leukocytes inactive (102).

TISSUE PENETRATION AND INVASION

One of the hallmarks of pathogenesis is the ability of the pathogenic microorganism to invade surrounding tissues, yet another mechanism to evade the host defense. Here, the bacteria may survive, replicate, and eventually be released back into the extracellular environment. Currently, evidence of host cell invasion exists for *A. actinomycetemcomitans, P. gingivalis, P. intermedia,* and *F. nucleatum.*

The invasive ability of *A. actinomycetemcomitans* has been demonstrated in vitro using a human epidermoid carcinoma cell line (KB) that is of oral origin (34, 35). The efficiency of invasion varies among the clinical and laboratory isolates examined. *A. actinomycetemcomitans* is taken up in a host-derived membrane-bound vacuole by an active process involving signaling between the bacterium and KB cell microvilli (129). Primary and secondary receptors for uptake may be the transferrin receptor and integrins, respectively (92, 107). Following uptake, *A. actinomycetemcomitans* subsequently escapes from the vacuole, replicates rapidly in the cytoplasm, and is transmitted to adjacent cells through bacteria-induced protrusions of the host cell membrane. Through these processes, *A. actinomycetemcomitans* may not only evade host defenses but also gain access to underlying periodontal tissues.

As seen with *A. actinomycetemcomitans,* invasion of primary cultures of gingival epithelial cells by *P. gingivalis* is an active process that requires energy production by both the epithelial cell and the bacterium (58, 79). While clinical and laboratory strains have the ability to invade epithelial cells, considerable variation occurs in the invasive potential among the various strains (109). Internalization of *P. gingivalis* involves a receptor-mediated endocytosis pathway (108). Protease inhibitors can inhibit invasion, suggesting a role for *P. gingivalis* proteases in the invasion process. Invasion of epithelial cells by *P. gingivalis* results in an interleukin-1β (IL-1β) mRNA response, decreased IL-8 accumulation (25), and inhibition of neutrophil migration through the epithelium (84), all factors that have an impact on the host defense system. *P. gingivalis* also can replicate and persist within KB cells (85). Additional evidence has shown that *P. gingivalis* can invade human endothelial cells by a mechanism that involves fimbriae, cytoskeletal rearrangements, protein phosphorylation, energy metabolism, and *P. gingivalis* proteases (28).

Invasive capabilities have been evaluated for other periodontal pathogens. For example, a single clinical isolate of *P. intermedia* was shown to invade a KB cell line. The type C fimbriae and a cytoskeletal rearrangement were required for this invasion. However, neither a different clinical isolate nor the type strain was able to invade the cell line (29). *F. nucleatum* also adheres to and invades primary cultures of human gingival epithelial cells (55). Invasion is via a "zipping" mechanism and requires the involvement of actins, microtubules, signal transduction, protein synthesis, and energy metabolism of the epithelial cell and protein synthesis by *F. nucleatum. F. nucleatum* invasion of epithelial cells is accompanied by high levels of IL-8 secretion. In this same study, *B. forsythus, Campylobacter curvus,* and *E. corrodens* were shown to be noninvasive.

In addition to invasion of the surrounding soft tissues, a recent study demonstrated the invasion of *P. intermedia, P. gingivalis, F. nucleatum, B. forsythus, P. micros,* and *S. intermedius* in radicular dentin (43). Thus, the tooth itself may serve as a reservoir for bacterial colonization.

DAMAGE TO THE HOST

Although the primary cause for connective tissue destruction is the result of proteolytic activity of host cells, bacteria produce several enzymes that damage the extracellular matrix proteins, including collagenase.

P. gingivalis produces numerous hydrolytic, proteolytic, and lipolytic enzymes (58). Among the proteolytic enzymes are two cysteine proteases (gingipains). There are indications that these proteases are involved in several functions including adherence to host cells, inhibition of host defenses, and damage to host cells. They appear to contribute to the local generation of the proinflammatory molecules, bradykinin and thrombin, ultimately having an indirect effect on bone resorption (102).

Human gingival fibroblasts incubated with *T. denticola* demonstrate a variety of pathologic responses, including cell detachment, reduced cell proliferation, and cell death (33). This pathogen also can agglutinate and lyse red blood cells (47) and induce membrane blebbing of epithelial cells (17). In addition, it has been proposed that *T. denticola* outer sheath components, such as surface proteases, membrane lipids, and lipoproteins, may contribute to the induction of an inflammatory reaction in the periodontal tissues that can contribute to tissue damage (61).

A. actinomycetemcomitans LPS and acid and alkaline phosphatases induce bone resorption (60), and collagenolytic activity has been observed in both media and cell sonicates of the organism (105). *A. actinomycetemcomitans* also produces a factor that inhibits fibroblast proliferation in cell cultures and their production of substances of the extracellular matrix, thus modulating tissue turnover (116).

In addition to the independent virulence mechanisms by individual species and strains,

complex, interdependent interactions also exist that occur among the different genera in the plaque biofilm, which can affect their pathogenic potential. For example, it has been suggested that *F. nucleatum* may have a synergistic interaction with *P. gingivalis. F. nucleatum* binds plasminogen that can be converted by protease activity to plasmin (23). The conversion of the cell-bound plasminogen to plasmin may allow *F. nucleatum* to evade host defenses and to invade tissues. *P. gingivalis,* a coaggregation partner with *F. nucleatum,* may provide the proteolytic activity needed for this conversion (68). A synergistic effect is also seen with *A. actinomycetemcomitans* and *P. gingivalis* where a coinfection with these organisms showed enhanced induction of the humoral and cell-mediated response (18). In contrast, the mixed microbial milieu may be beneficial in suppressing growth of various species, inhibiting expression of various virulence factors or neutralizing virulence factors. For instance, H_2O_2 production by *Streptococcus sanguis* is lethal to *A. actinomycetemcomitans* (127), and the leukotoxicity of *A. actinomycetemcomitans* was recently shown to be inhibited by other subgingival inhabitants (*P. gingivalis, P. intermedia, P. nigrescens, Prevotella melaninogenica,* and *Prevotella loeschii*) (63).

In summary, many proposed virulence factors have been identified for specific periodontal pathogens. Development of dental plaque and subsequent tissue destruction, however, rely on complex interactions among these bacteria in the biofilm environment. Although the nature of these interactions in biofilm development is currently being investigated in in vivo model systems, many of the previous studies were based on in vitro assays on either planktonic cells or in vitro-generated biofilms. It is becoming clear that, while these assays do provide important information on specific pathogenic properties, they may not accurately mimic the in vivo environment. Therefore, additional studies are necessary to better define the roles of proposed periodontal pathogens and their virulence factors in vivo in the destructive processes of periodontal disease.

INNATE HOST RESPONSE

Despite the importance of infection and colonization by bacteria in periodontal infections, the immune status of the host and effectiveness of the host response are key determinants of disease susceptibility.

In periodontal disease, bacterial colonization of the subgingival area results in both an innate host response and an acquired immune response. Even in the presence of such immune responses, the bacterial challenge may be too severe to overcome. The result is the initiation and progression of periodontitis. Alternatively, periodontal disease may be found in individuals with defects in either their innate or acquired immunity which limits their ability to mount an adequate response. Evidence is accumulating supporting the host response as a major determinant of disease susceptibility.

Innate immunity plays a significant role in the response to microbial colonization seen in periodontal diseases. As a part of the innate response, secretory IgA and numerous enzymes and antimicrobial factors present in the saliva neutralize microbial components. These factors include lysozyme, lactoferrin, peroxidases, antimicrobial peptides, histatins, defensins, and cathelicidins (78, 113). All these factors attempt to minimize the effect of the offending biofilm complex and may function synergistically.

As plaque extends subgingivally, the flora becomes more complex and exists in a more protected environment. The immune response also changes. Salivary components no longer have access to the bacteria colonizing the subgingival environment. However, the crevicular fluid bathing the gingival sulcus or pocket contains many factors capable of resisting bacterial progression such as lysozyme, bradykinin, thrombin, fibrinogen, complement, antibodies, and neutrophil-derived components (24).

Recent investigations have looked toward defensins (innate immune peptides with antimicrobial properties) and their role in periodontal and other oral infections. The α (classical)-defensins are found in the primary granules of neutrophils and are believed to produce their antimicrobial activity by forming channels in the bacterial or fungal membranes. These channels increase membrane permeability in a charge- or voltage-dependent manner, ultimately resulting in cell lysis or cell death (65).

The cationic β-defensins produced by epithelial cells represent a local defense mechanism in contrast to the more systemic response seen with the neutrophil-derived α-defensins. Three β-defensins, HBD-1, HBD-2, and HBD-3, are expressed in the gingival epithelial tissue, which makes them excellent candidate peptides contributing to the defenses at mucosal surfaces, including the periodontium (75, 87). In addition, β-defensin expression on other mucosal surfaces, such as buccal mucosa, tongue, and salivary derived defensins, may limit initial bacterial colonization by certain periodontal pathogens (75, 87, 114). In vitro, β-defensins exhibit broad-spectrum antimicrobial activity against gram-positive and gram-negative bacteria and fungi (38). Although the specific antimicrobial mechanism for the β-defensins is not known, they are believed to act similarly to the α-defensins.

The neutrophil response is the host's first innate cellular response and probably the most significant in limiting the subgingival biofilm accumulation (24). As reviewed by Dennison and Van Dyke (27), the pivotal role of these cells in protection from periodontal diseases has been proven, because individuals with a decreased number or function demonstrate a marked increase in susceptibility to rapid and severe periodontal destruction.

ADAPTIVE HOST RESPONSE

The importance and correlation of adaptive/acquired immunity in periodontal diseases is proven by several factors. First, there is an elevation in the cell-mediated (both CD4$^+$ and CD8$^+$ cellular response) or humoral response (a composite of antibodies) with the presence of periodontitis and increasing severity of periodontitis. Second, both systemic and local antibody formation have been demonstrated following mechanical periodontal therapy most likely as a result of a treatment-induced bacteremia. Third, antibody formation is specific for specific periodontal organisms, i.e., *A. actinomycetemcomitans, P. gingivalis, P. intermedia, F. nucleatum, Capnocytophaga gingivalis, Capnocytophaga ochracea, Capnocytophaga sputigena, E. corrodens, C. rectus,* oral spirochetes, and is specific for certain virulence factors such as the leukotoxin and other components of *A. actinomycetemcomitans* and the capsule of *P. gingivalis* (30). However, the protective role of the adaptive immune response is not fully understood. This may be because both antibody titers and function (avidity) may vary with the patient's age and disease, making some individuals more or less susceptible to tissue breakdown (30). In certain populations, the protective role of antibodies has been demonstrated. For example, higher titers of an antibody reactive to the LPS of a virulent strain of *A. actinomycetemcomitans* (serotype B) was shown to be protective for young individuals with generalized aggressive disease (15).

For most people suffering from periodontal disease, it is hypothesized that the innate and acquired immune responses are protective resulting either in minimal periodontal destruction or an arrested disease state. In individuals in whom either the innate or acquired response is altered, the result is likely to be aggressive/progressive destruction. An example of this is aggressive periodontitis where numerous studies have demonstrated abnormalities in neutrophil function. It is believed that it must be a "mild" alteration in function, because there may be no apparent infections elsewhere in the body (102).

THE HOST RESPONSE: A DOUBLE-EDGED SWORD

Although bacteria are capable of directly causing destruction of the periodontal tissues, most of the destruction that occurs is a result of an indirect process whereby host cells are activated producing tissue-degradative substances. Consequently, the host's protective nature may by countered by its destructive potential. Cytokines such as IL-1, IL-6, and IL-8 are likely to be important in the destructive process (5). IL-1 promotes bone resorption, stimulates release of the eicosanoid prostaglandin E_2 (PGE_2) by monocytes and fibroblasts, and stimulates the release of matrix metalloproteinases (MMPs) important in degradation of the extracellular matrix. IL-6 stimulates osteoclast formation and therefore may also play a role in bone resorption. IL-8, a chemoattractant for neutrophils, selectively stimulates MMP activity from these cells. Each of these cytokines is found in elevated levels in inflamed gingival tissues. Other tissue-destructive host-derived factors include tumor necrosis factor alpha and PGE_2, both of which stimulate MMP production and induce bone resorption. The individual or combined actions of these inflammatory molecules can result in significant tissue destruction.

NONBACTERIAL RISK FACTORS IN PERIODONTAL DISEASE

Bacterial plaque is the primary etiologic factor associated with periodontitis, yet there are several other variables that may place an individual at risk for developing disease (3, 99, 100, 101). Two of these variables are clearly defined risk factors: tobacco smoking and diabetes. A direct relationship exists between periodontal disease and the prevalence of smoking, and the prevalence and severity of periodontitis is significantly higher in patients with type I and type II diabetes. Several other less clearly defined factors should be included as part of a risk assessment for each patient. These include genetic factors, age, gender, socioeconomic status, stress, human immunodeficiency virus infection/acquired immunodeficiency syndrome, osteoporosis, infrequent dental visits, previous history of periodontal disease, and bleeding on probing.

Until recently, aggressive periodontal diseases were unique in their risk associated with genetic predisposition. A unique genetic marker for chronic periodontitis recently linked this form of periodontal disease to an inherited allele responsible for IL-1β overproduction (71). More studies are currently underway to define the role of this gene in other forms of periodontal disease and understand the significance it may have in performing and prescribing periodontal treatment. Meanwhile, twin studies demonstrate that chronic periodontitis has a 50% heritable component (94). These studies clearly demonstrate the multifactorial nature of periodontal diseases and the need for further research to better identify individuals at risk and for prescription of earlier and more definitive treatment.

PERIODONTAL THERAPY

The treatment of periodontal disease has primarily relied on mechanical therapy: root debridement performed either with or without surgical access to reduce the overall plaque mass. While specific microbial species are believed to play a role in the disease process, periodontal therapy today remains targeted toward removal of the plaque mass as opposed to elimination of specific pathogens. Benefits of mechanical debridement include: removal of calculus and endotoxin, disruption of the plaque biofilm complex, induction of potentially protective antibody responses to certain pathogens (31), and increased numbers of beneficial bacteria, such as streptococci (9). In addition, in the process of mechanical root debridement, specific subgingival pathogenic species are inadvertently removed or reduced to levels which result in improved clinical health and/or stabilization in periodontal maintenance patients (81, 103, 123).

Scaling and root planing (debridement) have routinely been shown to be effective in treatment of chronic periodontitis without the concomitant use of systemic or local antimicrobials (96). When performed as a part of routine periodontal maintenance, periodontal pathogens are suppressed to a level where an equilibrium is established between the host and the pathogen, which does not result in progressive loss of attachment in most patients (86, 112). Of equal importance is the necessity for good plaque control performed by the patient. Studies have shown that in shallow to moderately deep pockets, good oral hygiene can change the subgingival flora to one more compatible with periodontal health (138).

With the continued evolution of the specific plaque hypothesis, there is increased interest in chemical antimicrobials, which have the ability to suppress and/or eradicate the pathogenic players. In addition, periodontal pathogens, such as *A. actinomycetemcomitans* and *P. gingivalis,* that invade epithelium may not be as susceptible to standard mechanical debridement and require supplemental antibiotics and/or surgery for eradication (109, 129). Both systemic antimicrobials and locally delivered antimicrobial agents administered directly into periodontal pockets have been used in treatment of periodontal diseases.

Systemic antibiotics have been effective and are specifically recommended in the treatment of aggressive forms of periodontal disease (72, 136). In addition, they are effective in conjunction with scaling and root planing in deep periodontal pockets that are nonresponsive (46, 82, 137). Advantages of using systemic antibiotics in treatment of periodontal diseases include treatment of multiple sites and potential microbial reservoirs (tongue, tonsils, and buccal mucosa); treatment of organisms at the base of the pocket and in the tissue because of systemic absorption and delivery into oral tissues, gingival crevicular fluid, and saliva (137); availability of a variety of drugs and specific combinations from which to choose; and lower cost than locally delivered antimicrobials. Disadvantages of systemic antimicrobials include bacterial resistance, side effects (including superinfections and gastrointestinal irritation), compliance, and the fact that periodontal destruction is often localized to a few teeth.

Local delivery alleviates many concerns associated with systemic antibiotics and offers the ability to reach bacteria at the base of a pocket and retain activity for periods sufficient to have bactericidal or bacteristatic effects on offending pathogens. Considering that the gingival crevicular fluid is capable of being replaced 40 times in 1 h (45), the drug should ideally be substantive (retained on root surfaces) or be delivered in a slow- or controlled-release formulation. Local delivery results in a substantially higher drug concentration in the pocket than the equivalent systemic agent.

Local delivery of any antimicrobial is not, however, a substitute for systemic antibiotics when indicated in specific periodontal diseases. Antibiotic selection when choosing local delivery is empirical; therefore, in cases where one needs to know the specific bacteria and antimicrobial susceptibility (i.e., aggressive or nonresponsive disease), microbiologic testing and antibiotic susceptibility are recommended.

Periodontitis is a mixed infection. Today, drugs are available that target groups of microorganisms. However, broad-spectrum antibiotics are still widely used and have the disadvantage of killing beneficial bacteria as well. Judicious use of all antibiotics must be adhered to in light of this and increasing concerns of bacterial resistance. Finally, antimicrobials should not be used as a replacement for good mechanical therapy, but rather should be used in conjunction with mechanical therapy to optimize the therapeutic effectiveness of each. Although antimicrobials reduce the subgingival flora, their effectiveness against plaque as a part of a biofilm is not known. Bacterial life in a biofilm environment can be very different from the planktonic state. The architecture of the biofilm and its matrix may inhibit penetration of antimicrobials, the biofilm may contain inactivating substances, and phenotypic changes in biofilm bacteria, such as slower growth, may increase their resistance to antimicrobial agents. All of these factors may have an impact on the effectiveness of antimicrobial therapy. Therefore, as stated above, mechanical debridement remains an important component of periodontal therapy with antimicrobial therapy serving as an adjunct to this therapy.

Recently, new treatment strategies have been aimed at modulation of the host immunoinflammatory response. Therapeutic strategies now being used in clinical practice include administration of low-dose doxycycline, which inhibits matrix metalloproteinases, i.e., collagenase (16, 44). Other agents, which block specific cytokines or inhibit PGE_2, have also

shown therapeutic potential and continue to be evaluated (70).

Finally, because of the complex microbial picture in the pathogenesis of periodontal diseases, the development of a vaccine for treatment of periodontal disease will not occur readily. Unlike other infections whereby treatment correlates with elimination of the offending pathogen, the successful treatment of this polymicrobial infection occurs not by elimination of pathogens but by an alteration where a level of symbioses or homeostasis can occur between the offending bacteria and the defensive host.

SUMMARY

Periodontal diseases result from a polymicrobial infection of the subgingival crevice. Several primary players in the disease process have been identified and their virulence factors well-characterized. However, a vast number of pathogens potentially exist that have not been identified or characterized. The importance of the biofilm in plaque colonization and bacterial interactions and the impact these interactions have on expression or inhibition of specific virulence factors is not fully understood. What is realized, however, is that given the right combination of bacteria, indigenous colonizers may become opportunistic pathogens.

Currently, our therapy remains primarily directed toward controlling the bacterial etiology at the site of infection. Future treatment considerations should include reservoirs for the infection (i.e., buccal mucosa and tongue) and acquisition of the pathogens from family members (52, 135, 141). (Vertical and/or horizontal transmission has been shown both for *A. actinomycetemcomitans* and *P. gingivalis* [1, 2, 8, 133].) In addition, future research and treatment efforts will certainly continue in modulation of the host response and genetic heritability of periodontal diseases.

In the 19th and early 20th centuries, periodontal disease was believed to be a focus of oral sepsis serving as a seed of infection for inflammatory systemic diseases (59). The focal infection theory resulted in unnecessary and unsupported tooth extractions. In recent years, the connection of periodontal diseases with systemic diseases has been revisited and studies suggest that periodontal diseases may be a risk factor in preterm low birth weight deliveries, cardiovascular disease, diabetes, respiratory diseases, and other diseases (4). To support this, periodontal bacteria have been cultured from other target organs and prosthetic joints (49, 140). While the data are not entirely clear that periodontal diseases play a strong role in the development of other diseases, the systemic communications of this polymicrobial infection need to be further explored.

REFERENCES

1. **Alaluusua, S., M. Saarela, H. Jousimies-Somer, and S. Asikainen.** 1993. Ribotyping shows intrafamilial similarity in *Actinobacillus actinomycetemcomitans* isolates. *Oral Microbiol. Immunol.* **8:**225–229.

2. **Alaluusua, S., S. Asikainen, and C. H. Lai.** 1991. Intrafamilial transmission of *Actinobacillus actinomycetemcomitans. J. Periodontol.* **62:**207–210.

3. **American Academy of Periodontology.** 1996. Position paper. Epidemiology of periodontal diseases. *J. Periodontol.* **67:**935–945.

4. **American Academy of Periodontology.** 1998. Position paper. Periodontal disease as a potential risk factor for systemic diseases. *J. Periodontol.* **69:**841–850.

5. **American Academy of Periodontology.** 1999. Informational paper. The pathogenesis of periodontal diseases. *J. Periodontol.* **70:**457–470.

6. **Armitage, G. C.** 1999. Development of classification system for periodontal diseases and conditions. *Ann. Periodontol.* **4:**1–6.

7. **Asikainen, S., and C. Chen.** 1999. Oral ecology and person-to-person transmission of *Actinobacillus actinomycetemcomitans* and *Porphyromonas gingivalis. Periodontol. 2000* **20:**65–81.

8. **Asikainen, S., C. Chen, and J. Slots.** 1996. Likelihood of transmitting *Actinobacillus actinomycetemcomitans* and *Porphyromonas gingivalis* in families with periodontitis. *Oral Microbiol. Immunol.* **11:**387–394.

9. **Axelsson, P., and J. Lindhe.** 1981. The significance of maintenance care in the treatment of periodontal disease. *J. Clin. Periodontol.* **8:**281–294.

10. **Baehni, P., C. C. Tsai, W. P. McArthur, B. F. Hammond, and N. S. Taichman.** 1979. Interaction of inflammatory cells and oral microorganisms. VII. Detection of leukotoxic activity of a plaque-derived gram-negative microorganisms. *Infect. Immun.* **24:**233–243.

11. **Baer, P. N.** 1971. The case for periodontosis as a clinical entity. *J. Periodontol.* **42:**516–520.

12. **Beaty, T. H., J. A. Boughman, P. Yang, J. A. Astemborski, and J. B. Suzuki.** 1987. Genetic analysis of juvenile periodontitis in families ascertained through an affected proband. *Am. J. Hum. Genet.* **40:**443–452.

13. **Boughman, J. A., S. L. Halloran, D. Roulston, S. Schwartz, J. B. Suzuki, L. R. Weitkamp, R. E. Wenk, R. Wooten, and M. M. Cohen.** 1986. An autosomal-dominant form of juvenile periodontitis: its localization to chromosome 4 and linkage to dentinogenesis imperfecta and Gc. *J. Craniofac. Genet. Dev. Biol.* **6:**341–350.

14. **Bueno, L. C., M. P. Mayer, and J. M. DiRienzo.** 1998. Relationship between conversion of localized juvenile periodontitis-susceptible children from health to disease and *Actinobacillus actinomycetemcomitans* leukotoxin promoter structure. *J. Periodontol.* **69:**998–1007.

15. **Califano, J. V., J. C. Gunsolley, K. Nakashima, H. A. Schenkein, M. E. Wilson, and J. G. Tew.** 1996. Influence of anti-*Actinobacillus actinomycetemcomitans* Y4 (serotype b) lipopolysaccharide on severity of generalized early-onset periodontitis. *Infect. Immun.* **64:**3908–3910.

16. **Caton, J. G.** 1999. Evaluation of Periostat for patient management. *Compend. Cont. Educ. Dent.* **20:**451–456, 458–460, 462.

17. **Chan, E. C. S., and R. McLaughlin.** 2000. Taxonomy and virulence of oral spirochetes. *Oral Microbiol. Immunol.* **15:**1–9.

18. **Chen, P. B., L. B. Davern, J. Katz, J. H. Eldridge, and S. M. Michalek.** 1996. Host responses induced by co-infection with *Porphyromonas gingivalis* and *Actinobacillus actinomycetemcomitans* in a murine model. *Oral Microbiol. Immunol.* **11:**274–281.

19. **Clark, W. B., J. E. Beem, W. E. Nesbitt, J. O. Cisar, C. C. Tseng, and M. J. Levine.** 1989. Pellicle receptors for *Actinomyces viscosus* type I fimbriae in vitro. *Infect. Immun.* **57:**3003–3008.

20. **Conrads, G., A. Herrler, I. Moonen, F. Lampert, and N. Schnitzler.** 1999. Flow cytometry to monitor phagocytosis and oxidative burst of anaerobic periodontopathogenic bacteria by human polymorphonuclear leukocytes. *J. Periodontal Res.* **34:**136–144.

21. **Contreras, A., and J. Slots.** 2000 Herpesviruses in human periodontal disease. *J. Periodontal Res.* **35:**3–16.

22. **Cunningham, M. D., C. Seachord, K. Ratcliffe, B. Bainbridge, A. Aruffo, and R. P. Darveau.** 1996. *Helicobacter pylori* and *Porphyromonas gingivalis* lipopolysaccharides are poorly transferred to recombinant soluble CD14. *Infect. Immun.* **64:**3601–3608.

23. **Darenfed, J., D. Grenier, and D. Mayrand.** 1999. Acquisition of plasmin activity by *Fusobacterium nucleatum* subsp. *nucleatum* and potential contribution to tissue destruction during periodontitis. *Infect. Immun.* **67:**6439–6444.

24. **Darveau, R. P., A. Tanner, and R. C. Page.** 1997. The microbial challenge in periodontitis. *Periodontol. 2000* **14:**12–32.

25. **Darveau, R. P., C. M. Belton, R. A. Reife, and R. J. Lamont.** 1998. Local chemokine paralysis, a novel pathogenic mechanism for *Porphyromonas gingivalis*. *Infect. Immun.* **66:**1660–1665.

26. **Darveau, R. P., M. D. Cunningham, T. Bailey, C. Seachord, K. Ratcliffe, B. Bainbridge, M. Dietsch, R. C. Page, and A. Aruffo.** 1995. Ability of bacteria associated with chronic inflammatory disease to stimulate E-selectin expression and promote neutrophil adhesion. *Infect. Immun.* **63:**1311–1317.

27. **Dennison, D. K., and T. E. Van Dyke.** 1997. The acute inflammatory response and the role of phagocytic cells in periodontal health an disease. *Periodontol. 2000* **14:**54–78.

28. **Deshpande, R. M., M. B. Kahn, and C. A. Genco.** 1998. Invasion of aortic and heart endothelial cells by *Porphyromonas gingivalis*. *Infect. Immun.* **66:**5337–5343.

29. **Dorn, B. R., K. L. Leung, and A. Progulske-Fox.** 1998. Invasion of human oral epithelial cells by *Prevotella intermedia*. *Infect. Immun.* **66:**6054–6057.

30. **Ebersole, J. L., and M. A. Taubman.** 1994. The protective nature of host responses in periodontal diseases. *Periodontol. 2000* **5:**112–141.

31. **Ebersole, J. L., M. A. Taubman, D. J. Smith, and A. D. Haffajee.** 1985. Effect of subgingival scaling on systemic antibody responses to oral microorganisms. *Infect. Immun.* **48:**534–539.

32. **Ebisu, S., H. Nakae, H. Fukuhara, and H. Okada.** 1992. The mechanisms of *Eikenella corrodens* aggregation by salivary glycoprotein and the effect of the glycoprotein on oral bacterial aggregation. *J. Periodontal Res.* **27:**615–622.

33. **Ellen, R., M. Song, and C. McCullock.** 1994. Degradation of endogenous plasma membrane fibronectin concomitant with *Treponema denticola* 35405 adhesion to gingival fibroblasts. *Infect. Immun.* **62:**3033–3037.

34. **Fives-Taylor, P. M., D. H. Neyer, K. P. Mintz, and C. Brissette.** 1999. Virulence factors of *Actinobacillus actinomycetemcomitans*. *Periodontol. 2000* **20:**136–167.

35. **Fives-Taylor, P., D. Meyer, and K. Mintz.** 1993. Characteristics of *Actinobacillus actinomycetemcomitans* invasion of and adhesion to cultured epithelial cells. *Adv. Dent. Res.* **9:**55–62.

36. **Frandsen, E. V. G., J. Reinholdt, and M. Kilian.** 1987. Enzymatic and antigenic characterization of immunoglobulin A1 proteases from *Bacteroides* and *Capnocytophaga* spp. *Infect. Immun.* **55:**631–638.

37. **Ganeshkumar, N., M. Song, and B. C. McBride.** 1988. Cloning of a *Streptococcus sanguis* adhesin which mediates binding to saliva-coated hydroxyapatite. *Infect. Immun.* **56:**1150–1157.

38. **Ganz, T., and R. I. Lehrer.** 1995. Defensins. *Pharmacol. Ther.* **66:**191–205.

39. **Genco, R. J.** 1996. Current view of risk factors for periodontal diseases. *J. Periodontol.* **67**(Suppl.):1041–1049.

40. **Genco, R., D. Kornman, R. Williams, S. Offenbacher, J. Zambon, I. Ishikawa, M. Listgarten, B. Michalowicz, R. Page, H. Schenkein, J. Slots, S. Socransky, and T. Van Dyke.** 1996. Consensus report: periodontal diseases; pathogenesis and microbial factors. *Ann. Periodontol.* **1:**926–932.

41. **Gibbons, R. J., and J. van Houte.** 1980. Bacterial adherence and the formation of dental plaques, p. 63–104. *In* E. H. Beachey (ed.), *Bacterial Adherence.* Chapman & Hall, London, United Kingdom.

42. **Gibbons, R. J., D. I. Hay, and D. H. Schlesinger.** 1991. Delineation of a segment of adsorbed salivary acidic proline-rich proteins which promotes adhesion of *Streptococcus gordonii* to apatitic surfaces. *Infect. Immun.* **59:**2948–2954.

43. **Giuliana, G., P. Ammatuna, G. Pizzo, F. Capone, and M. D'Angelo.** 1997. Occurrence of invading bacteria in radicular dentin of periodontally diseased teeth: microbiological findings. *J. Clin. Periodontol.* **24:**478–485.

44. **Golub, L. M., H. M. Lee, M. E. Ryan, W. V. Giannobile, J. Payne, and T. Sorsa.** 1998. Tetracyclines inhibit connective tissue breakdown by multiple non-antimicrobial mechanisms. *Adv. Dent. Res.* **12:**12–26.

45. **Goodson, J. M.** 1989. Pharmacokinetic principles controlling efficacy of oral therapy. *J. Dent. Res.* **68:**1625–1632.

46. **Gordon, J. M., C. B. Walker, I. Lamster, T. West, S. Socransky, M. Seiger, and R. Fasciano.** 1985. Efficacy of clindamycin hydrochloride in refractory periodontitis. 12 month results. *J. Periodontol.* **56**(Suppl):75–80.

47. **Grenier, D.** 1991. Characteristics of hemolytic and hemagglutinating activities of *Treponema denticola*. *Oral Microbiol. Immunol.* **6:**246–249.

48. **Grenier, D., D. Mayrand, and B. McBride.** 1989. Further studies on the degradation of immunoglobulins by black-pigmented *Bacteroides*. *Oral Microbiol. Immunol.* **4:**12–18.

49. **Gristina, A. G.** 1987. Biomaterial-centered infection: microbial adhesion versus tissue integration. *Science* **237**:1588–1595.

50. **Grossi, S. G., J. J. Zambon, A. W. Ho, G. Koch, R. G. Dunford, E. E. Machtei, O. M. Norderyd, and R. J. Genco.** 1994. Assessment of risk for periodontal disease. I. Risk indicators for attachment loss. *J. Periodontol.* **65**:260–267.

51. **Grossi, S. G., R. J. Genco, E. E. Machtei, A. W. Ho, G. Koch, R. Dunford, J. J. Zambon, and E. Hausmann.** 1995. Assessment of risk for periodontal disease. II. Risk indicators for alveolar bone loss. *J. Periodontol.* **66**:23–29.

52. **Gunsolley, J. C., R. R. Ranney, J. J. Zambon, J. A. Burmeister, and H. A. Scheinkein.** 1990. *Actinobacillus actinomycetemcomitans* in families afflicted with periodontitis. *J. Periodontol.* **61**:643–648.

53. **Guthmiller, J. M., E. T. Lally, and J. Korostoff.** 2001. Beyond the specific plaque hypothesis: are highly leukotoxic strains of *Actinobacillus actinomycetemcomitans* a paradigm for periodontal pathogenesis? *Crit. Rev. Oral Biol. Med.* **12**:116–124.

54. **Haffajee, A. D., and S. S. Socransky.** 1994. Microbial etiological agents of destructive periodontal diseases. *Periodontol. 2000* **5**:78–111.

55. **Han, T. W., W. Shi, G. T.-J. Huang, S. Kinder Haake, N.-H. Park, H. Kuramitsu, and R. J. Genco.** 2000. Interactions between periodontal bacteria and human oral epithelial cells: *Fusobacterium nucleatum* adheres to and invades epithelial cells. *Infect. Immun.* **68**:3140–3146.

56. **Hart, T. C., M. L. Marazita, H. A. Schenkein, and S. R. Diehl.** 1992. Re-interpretation of the evidence for X-linked dominant inheritance of juvenile periodontitis. *J. Periodontol.* **63**:169–173.

57. **Haubek, D., K. Poulsen, J. Westergaard, G. Dahlen, and M. Kilian.** 1996. Highly toxic clone of *Actinobacillus actinomycetemcomitans* in geographically widespread cases of juvenile periodontitis in adolescents of African origin. *J. Clin. Microbiol.* **34**:1576–1578.

58. **Holt, S. C., L. Kesavalu, S. Walker, and C. A. Genco.** 1999. Virulence factors of *Porphyromonas gingivalis*. *Periodontol. 2000* **20**:168–238.

59. **Hughes, R. A.** 1994. Focal infection revisited. *Br. J. Rheumatol.* **33**:370–377.

60. **Iino, Y., and R. Hopps.** 1984. The bone-resorbing activities in tissue culture of lipopolysaccharides from the bacteria *Actinobacillus actinomycetemcomitans*, *Bacteroides gingivalis*, and *Capnocytophaga ochracea*, isolated from human mouths. *Arch. Oral Biol.* **29**:59–63.

61. **Ishihara, K., and K. Okuda.** 1999. Molecular pathogenesis of the cell surface proteins and lipids from *Treponema denticola*. *FEMS Microbiol. Lett.* **181**:199–204.

62. **Jansen, H. J., and J. S. van der Hoeven.** 1997. Protein degradation by *Prevotella intermedia* and *Actinomyces meyeri* supports the growth of non-protein-cleaving oral bacteria in serum. *J. Clin. Periodontol.* **24**:346–353.

63. **Johansson, A., L. Hanstrom, and S. Kalfas.** 2000. Inhibition of *Actinobacillus actinomycetemcomitans* leukotoxicity by bacteria from the subgingival flora. *Oral Microbiol. Immunol.* **15**:218–225.

64. **Jorgenson, R. J., L. S. Levin, S. T. Hutcherson, and C. F. Salinas.** 1975. Periodontosis in sibs. *Oral Surg.* **39**:396–402.

65. **Kagan, B. L., M. E. Selsted, T. Ganz, and R. I. Lehrer.** 1990. Antimicrobial defensin peptides form voltage-dependent ion-permeable channels in planar lipid bilayer membranes. *Proc. Natl. Acad. Sci. USA* **87**:210–214.

66. **Kilian, M.** 1981. Degradation of immunoglobulin A1, A2 and G by suspected principal periodontopathogens. *Infect. Immun.* **34**:757–765.

67. **Kilian, M., B. Thomsen, T. E. Petersen, and H. Bleeg.** 1983. Occurrence and nature of bacterial IgA proteases. *Ann. N. Y. Acad. Sci.* **409**:612–624.

68. **Kolenbrander, P. E.** 2000. Oral microbial communities: biofilms, interactions and genetic systems. *Annu. Rev. Microbiol.* **54**:413–437.

69. **Kolodrubetz, D., T. Dailey, J. Ebersole, and E. Kraig.** 1989. Cloning and expression of the leukotoxin gene from *Actinobacillus actinomycetemcomitans*. *Infect. Immun.* **57**:1465–1469.

70. **Kornman, K.** 1999. Host modulation as a therapeutic strategy in the treatment of periodontal disease. *Clin. Infect. Dis.* **28**:520–526.

71. **Kornman, K. S., A. Crane, H. Y. Wang, F. S. di Giovine, M. G. Newman, F. W. Pirk, T. G. Wilson, Jr., F. L. Higginbottom, and G. W. Duff.** 1997. The interleukin-1 genotype as a severity factor in adult periodontal disease. *J. Clin. Periodontol.* **24**:72–77.

72. **Kornman, K. S., M. G. Newman, D. J. Moore, and R. E. Singer.** 1994. The influence of supragingival plaque control on clinical and microbial outcomes following the use of antibiotics for the treatment of periodontitis. *J. Periodontol.* **65**:848–854.

73. **Kraig, E., T. Dailey, and D. Kolodrubetz.** 1990. Nucleotide sequence of the leukotoxin gene from *Actinobacillus actinomycetemcomitans*: homology to the alpha-hemolysin/leukotoxin gene family. *Infect. Immun.* **58**:920–929.

74. **Kremer, B. H. A., A. J. Herscheid, W. Papaioannou, M. Quirynen, and T. J. M. van Steenbergen.** 1999. Adherence of *Peptostreptococ-*

cus micros morphotypes to epithelial cells *in vitro*. *Oral Microbiol. Immunol.* **14**:49–55.

75. **Krisanaprakornkit, S., A. Weinberg, C. N. Perez, and B. A. Dale.** 1998. Expression of the peptide antibiotic human β-defensin 1 in cultured gingival epithelial cells and gingival tissue. *Infect. Immun.* **66**:4222–4228.

76. **Lally, E. T., E. E. Golub, I. R. Kieba, N. S. Taichman, J. Rosenbloom, J. C. Rosenbloom, C. W. Gibson, and D. R. Demuth.** 1989. Analysis of the *Actinobacillus actinomycetemcomitans* leukotoxin gene. Delineation of unique features and comparison to homologous toxins. *J. Biol. Chem.* **264**:15451–15456.

77. **Lally, E. T., I. R. Kieba, D. R. Demuth, J. Rosenbloom, E. E. Golub, N. S. Taichman, and C. W. Gibson.** 1989. Identification and expression of the *Actinobacillus actinomycetemcomitans* leukotoxin gene. *Biochem. Biophys. Res. Commun.* **159**:256–262.

78. **Lamkin, M. S., and F. G. Oppenheim.** 1993. Structural features of salivary function. *Crit. Rev. Oral Biol. Med.* **4**:251–259.

79. **Lamont, R. J., A. Chan, C. M. Belton, K. T. Izutsu, D. Vasel, and A. Weinberg.** 1995. *Porphyromonas gingivalis* invasion of gingival epithelial cells. *Infect. Immun.* **63**:3878–3885.

80. **Lamont, R. J., and H. F. Jenkinson.** 2000. Subgingival colonization by *Porphyromonas gingivalis*. *Oral Microbiol. Immunol.* **15**:341–349.

81. **Listgarten, M. A., P. Sullivan, C. George, L. Nitkin, E. S. Rosenberg, N. W. Chilton, and A. A. Kramer.** 1989. Comparative longitudinal study of 2 methods of scheduling maintenance visits: 4-year data. *J. Clin. Periodontol.* **16**:105–115.

82. **Loesche, W. J., J. Giordano, S. Soehren, R. Hutchinson, C. F. Rau, L. Walsh, and M. A. Schork.** 1996. Nonsurgical treatment of patients with periodontal disease. *Oral Surg. Oral Med. Oral Pathol.* **81**:533–543.

83. **Loesche, W. J.** 1976. Chemotherapy of dental plaque infections. *Oral Sci. Rev.* **9**:65.

84. **Madianos, P. N., P. N. Papapanou, and J. Sandros.** 1997. *Porphyromonas gingivalis* infection of oral epithelium inhibits neutrophil transepithelial migration. *Infect. Immun.* **65**:3983–3990.

85. **Madianos, P. N., P. N. Papapanou, U. Nannmark, G. Dahlén, and J. Sandros.** 1996. *Porphyromonas gingivalis* FDC381 multiplies and persists within human oral epithelial cells in vitro. *Infect. Immun.* **64**:660–664.

86. **Magnusson, I., J. Lindhe, T. Yoneyama, and B. Liljenberg.** 1984. Recolonization of a subgingival microbiota following scaling in deep pockets. *J. Clin. Periodontol.* **11**:193–207.

87. **Mathews, M., H. P. Jia, J. M. Guthmiller, G. Losh, S. Graham, G. K. Johnson, B. F. Tack, and P. B. McCray, Jr.** 1999. Production of β-defensin antimicrobial peptides by the oral mucosa and salivary glands. *Infect. Immun.* **67**:2740–2745.

88. **Mayer, M. P. A., L. C. Bueno, E. J. Hansen, and J. M. DiRienzo.** 1999. Identification of a cytolethal distending toxin gene locus and features of a virulence-associated region in *Actinobacillus actinomycetemcomitans*. *Infect. Immun.* **67**:1227–1237.

89. **Melnick, M., E. D. Shields, and D. Bixler.** 1976. Periodontosis: a phenotypic and genetic analysis. *Oral Surg.* **42**:32–41.

90. **Meyer, D. H., and P. M. Fives-Taylor.** 1997. The role of *Actinobacillus actinomycetemcomitans* in the pathogenesis of periodontal disease. *Trends Microbiol.* **5**:224–228.

91. **Meyer, D. H., J. E. Lippmann, and P. M. Fives-Taylor.** 1996. Invasion of epithelial cells by *Actinobacillus actinomycetemcomitans*: a dynamic, multistep process. *Infect. Immun.* **64**:2988–2997.

92. **Meyer, D. H., K. P. Mintz, and P. M. Fives-Taylor.** 1997. Models of invasion of enteric and periodontal pathogens into epithelial cells: a comparative analysis. *Crit. Rev. Oral Biol. Med.* **8**:389–409.

93. **Meyer, D. H., P. K. Sreenivasan, and P. M. Fives-Taylor.** 1991. Evidence for invasion of a human oral cell line by *Actinobacillus actinomycetemcomitans*. *Infect. Immun.* **59**:2719–2726.

94. **Michalowicz B. S., S. R. Diehl, J. C. Gunsolley, B. S. Sparks, C. N. Brooks, T. E. Koertge, J. V. Califano, J. A. Burmeister, and H. A. Scheinken.** 2000. Evidence of a substantial genetic basis for risk of adult periodontitis. *J. Periodontol.* **71**:1699–1707.

95. **Moore, W. E. C., and L. V. H. Moore.** 1994. The bacteria of periodontal disease. *Periodontol. 2000* **5**:66–77.

96. **Mousques, T., M. A. Listgarten, and R. W. Phillips.** 1980. Effect of scaling and root planing on the composition of human subgingival microflora. *J. Periodontal Res.* **15**:144–151.

97. **Offenbacher, S.** 1996. Periodontal diseases: pathogenesis. *Ann. Periodontol.* **1**:821–878.

98. **O'Toole, G., H. B. Kaplan, and R. Kolter.** 2000. Biofilm formation as microbial development. *Annu. Rev. Microbiol.* **54**:49–79.

99. **Page, R. C., and J. D. Beck.** Risk assessment for periodontal diseases. 1997. *Int. Dent. J.* **47**:61–87.

100. **Papapanou, P. N.** 1998. Risk assessments in the diagnosis and treatment of periodontal diseases. *J. Dent. Educ.* **62**:822–839.

101. **Pihlstrom, B. L.** 2001. Periodontal risk assessment, diagnosis and treatment planning. *Periodontol. 2000* **25**:37–58.

102. **Potempa, J., A. Banbula, and J. Travis.** 2000. Role of bacterial proteinases in matrix destruction and modulation of host responses. *Periodontol. 2000* **24**:153–192.

103. **Rams, T. E., M. A. Listgarten, and J. Slots.** 1996. Utility of 5 major putative periodontal pathogens and selected clinical parameters to predict periodontal breakdown in patients on maintenance care. *J. Clin. Periodontol.* **23**:346–354.

104. **Ranney, R. R., B. F. Debski, and J. G. Tew.** 1981. Pathogenesis of gingivitis and periodontal disease in children and young adults. *Pediatr. Dent.* **3**:89–100.

105. **Robertson, P. B., M. Lantz, P. T. Marucha, K. S. Kornman, C. L. Trummel, and S. C. Holt.** 1982. Collagenolytic activity associated with *Bacteriodes* species and *Actinobacillus actinomycetemcomitans. J. Periodontal Res.* **17**:275–283.

106. **Ruben, M. P.** 1979. Periodontosis—an analysis and clarification of its status as a disease entity. *J. Periodontol.* **50**:311–315.

107. **Saarela, M., J. E. Lippmann, D. H. Meyer, and P. M. Fives-Taylor.** 1999. *Actinobacillus actinomycetemcomitans apaH* is implicated in invasion of epithelial cells. *J. Dent. Res.* **78**(Special Issue):259.

108. **Sandros, J., P. N. Madianos, and P. N. Papapanou.** 1996. Cellular events concurrent with *Porphyromonas gingivalis* invasion of oral epithelium *in vitro. Eur. J. Oral Sci.* **104**:363–371.

109. **Sandros, J., P. Papapanou, and G. Dahlen.** 1993. *Porphyromonas gingivalis* invades oral epithelial cells *in vitro. J. Periodontal Res.* **28**:219–226.

110. **Saxén, L.** 1980. Heredity of juvenile periodontitis. *J. Clin. Periodontol.* **7**:276–288.

111. **Saxén, L., and H. R. Nevanlinna.** 1984. Autosomal recessive inheritance of juvenile periodontitis: a test of a hypothesis. *Clin. Genet.* **25**:332–335.

112. **Sbordone, L., L. Ramaglia, E. Gulletta, and V. Iacono.** 1990. Recolonization of the subgingival microflora after scaling and root planing in human periodontitis. *J. Periodontol.* **61**:579–584.

113. **Schenkels, L. C., E. C. Veerman, and A. V. Nieuw Amerongen.** 1995. Biochemical composition of human saliva in relation to other mucosal fluids. *Crit. Rev. Oral Biol. Med.* **6**:161–175.

114. **Schonwetter, B. S., E. D. Stolzenberg, and M. A. Zasloff.** 1995. Epithelial antibiotics induced at sites of inflammation. *Science* **267**:1645–1648.

115. **Shenker, B. J., L. A. Vitale, and D. A. Welham.** 1990. Immune suppression induced by *Actinobacillus actinomycetemcomitans:* effects on immunoglobulin production by human B cells. *Infect. Immun.* **58**:3856–3862.

116. **Shenker, B. J., M. E. Kushner, and C. C. Tsai.** 1982. Inhibition of fibroblast proliferation by *Actinobacillus actinomycetemcomitans. Infect. Immun.* **38**:986–992.

117. **Shenker, B. J., T. McKay, S. Datar, M. Miller, R. Chowhan, and D. Demuth.** 1999. *Actinobacillus actinomycetemcomitans* immunosuppressive protein is a member of the family of cytolethal distending toxins capable of causing a G2 arrest in human T cells. *J. Immunol.* **162**:4773–4780.

118. **Shenker, B. J., W. P. McArthur, and C. C. Tsai.** 1982. Immune suppression induced by *Actinobacillus actinomycetemcomitans.* I. Effects on human peripheral blood lymphocyte responses to mitogens and antigens. *J. Immunol.* **128**:148–154.

119. **Slots, J.** 1979. Subgingival microflora and periodontal disease. *J. Clin. Periodontol.* **6**:351–382.

120. **Slots, J.** 1986. Bacterial specificity in adult periodontitis. A summary of recent work. *J. Clin. Periodontol.* **13**:912–917.

121. **Slots, J.** 1999. *Actinobacillus actinomycetemcomitans* and *Porphyromonas gingivalis* in periodontal disease: introduction. *Periodontol. 2000* **20**:7–13.

122. **Slots, J., and C. Chen.** 1999. The oral microflora and human periodontal disease, p. 101–127. *In* G. W. Tannock (ed.), *Medical Importance of the Normal Microflora.* Kluwer Academic Publishers, London, United Kingdom.

123. **Slots, J., L. J. Emrich, R. J. Genco, and B. G. Rosling.** 1985. Relationship between some subgingival bacteria and periodontal pocket depth and gain or loss of periodontal attachment after treatment of adult periodontitis. *J. Clin. Periodontol.* **12**:540–552.

124. **Slots, J., and M. A. Listgarten.** 1988. *Bacteroides gingivalis, Bacteroides intermedius* and *Actinobacillus actinomycetemcomitans* in human periodontal diseases. *J. Clin. Periodontol.* **15**:85–93.

125. **Socransky, S. S.** 1977. Microbiology of periodontal disease: present status and future considerations. *J. Periodontol.* **48**:497–504.

126. **Socransky, S. S.** 1979. Criteria for the infectious agents in dental caries and periodontal disease. *J. Clin. Periodontol.* **6**(Extra Issue):16–19.

127. **Socransky, S. S., and A. D. Haffajee**, 1992. The bacterial etiology of destructive periodontal disease: current concepts. *J. Periodontol.* **63:**322–331.

128. **Socransky, S. S., A. D. Haffajee, M. A. Cugini, C. Smith, and R. L. Kent, Jr.** 1998. Microbial complexes in subgingival plaque. *J. Clin. Periodontol.* **25:**134–144.

129. **Sreenivasan, P. K., D. H. Meyer, and P. M. Fives-Taylor.** 1993. Requirements for invasion of epithelial cells by *Actinobacillus actinomycetemcomitans*. *Infect. Immun.* **61:**1239–1245.

130. **Sugai, M., T. Kawamoto, S. Y. Peres, Y. Ueno, H. Komatsuzawa, T. Fujiwara, H. Kurihara, H. Suginaka, and E. Oswald.** 1998. The cell cycle-specific growth-inhibitory factor produced by *Actinobacillus actinomycetemcomitans* is a cytolethal distending toxin. *Infect. Immun.* **66:**5008–5019.

131. **Sundqvist, G., D. Figdor, L. Hänström, S. Sörlin, and G. Sandström.** 1991. Phagocytosis and virulence of different stains of *Porphyromonas gingivalis*. *Scand. J. Dent. Res.* **99:**117–129.

132. **Theilade, E.** 1986. The non-specific theory in microbial etiology of inflammatory periodontal diseases. *J. Clin. Periodontol.* **13:**905–911.

133. **Tinoco, E., M. Sivakumar, and H. Preus.** 1998. The distribution and transmission of *Actinobacillus actinomycetemcomitans* in families with localized juvenile periodontitis. *J. Clin. Periodontol.* **25:**99–105.

134. **Tsai, C. C., W. P. McArthur, P. C. Baehni, B. F. Hammond, and N. S. Taichman.** 1979. Extraction and partial characterization of a leukotoxin from a plaque-derived gram-negative microorganism. *Infect. Immun.* **25:**427–439.

135. **Tuite-McDonnell, M., A. L. Griffen, M. L. Moeschberger, R. E. Dalton, P. A. Fuerst, and E. J. Leys.** 1997. Concordance of *Porphyromonas gingivalis* colonization in families. *J. Clin. Microbiol.* **35:**455–461.

136. **Van Winkelhoff, A. J., C. J. Tijhof, and J. de Graaff.** 1992. Microbiological and clinical results of metronidazole plus amoxicillin therapy in *Actinobacillus actinomycetemcomitans*-associated periodontitis. *J. Periodontol.* **63:**52–57.

137. **Van Winkelhoff, A. J., T. E. Rams, and J. Slots.** 1996. Systemic antibiotic therapy in periodontics. *Periodontol. 2000* **10:**45–78.

138. **Westfelt, E.** 1996. Rationale of mechanical plaque control. *J. Clin. Periodontol.* **23:**263–267.

139. **Wilson, M., and B. Henderson.** 1995. Virulence factors of *Actinobacillus actinomycetemcomitans* relevant to the pathogenesis of inflammatory periodontal diseases. *FEMS Microbiol. Rev.* **17:**365–379.

140. **Yuan A., P. C. Yang, L. Lee, D. B. Chang, S. H. Kuo, and K. T. Luh.** 1992. *Actinobacillus actinomycetemcomtians* with chest wall involvement and rib destruction. *Chest* **101:**1450–1452.

141. **Zambon, J. J., L. A. Christersson, and J. Slots.** 1983. *Actinobacillus actinomycetemcomitans* in human periodontal disease. Prevalence in patient groups and distribution of biotypes and serotypes within families. *J. Periodontol.* **54:**707–711.

142. **Zambon, J. J., V. I. Haraszthy, G. Hariharan, E. T. Lally, and D. R. Demuth.** 1996. The microbiology of early-onset periodontitis: association of highly toxic *Actinobacillus actinomycetemcomitans* strains with localized juvenile periodontitis. *J. Periodontol.* **67:**282–290.

ABSCESSES

Itzhak Brook

9

Abscesses that develop as a result of introduction of the normal endogenous flora into a normally sterile body site are often polymicrobial in nature. These flora can gain access to the sterile site by direct extension or secondary to laceration or perforation. Because of the uniqueness of the normal endogenous flora at the various body sites, the microbiology of such abscesses is generally predictable. This chapter describes the specific microbiology of polymicrobial abscesses that occur at various body sites. It also reviews the data that demonstrate the synergy between the aerobic and anaerobic components of these abscesses, and highlights the role of the bacterial capsule as a virulence factor that enhances the formation of an abscess.

THE ROLE OF NORMAL FLORA IN POLYMICROBIAL ABSCESSES

In most mucus membranes, anaerobes outnumber aerobic and facultative bacteria in ratios ranging from 10:1 to 10,000:1, with anaerobic gram-negative bacilli (AGNB) microorganisms predominating (12, 44). Species of the *Bacteroides fragilis* group that colonize the gastrointestinal tract are usually isolated in intra-abdominal and rectal abscesses; pigmented *Prevotella, Porphyromonas,* and *Fusobacterium* spp. that colonize the oral cavity are present mainly in oral cavity abscesses, and *Prevotella bivia* and *Prevotella disiens* that predominate in the cervical canal are most often recovered in pelvic abscesses. The predominant aerobes and facultative organisms in abdominal and rectal abscesses are *Enterobacteriaceae* and staphylococci, and *Neisseria gonorrhoeae* are common in pelvic abscesses (Fig. 1; Table 1).

The bacterial flora of the gastrointestinal tract (GIT) is very dynamic, and changes in the flora influence the type and severity of postperforation infection. The stomach and upper bowel flora contain 10^4 organisms or fewer/g, the lower ileum contains up to 10^8 organisms/g, and the colon contains up to 10^{11} organisms/g, most of which are anaerobes (46). The low number of organisms in the stomach is believed to be caused by the detrimental effect of the low pH of the stomach on the organisms ingested from the oropharynx. The contents of the gut slowly become alkaline at the lower intestine. This change, the effect of bile, and the decrease in oxygen tension in the lower intestine allow for selection of bile-resistant organisms and increase in the number of strict anaerobes. Numerous organisms in the upper GIT can, however, be found in patients

Itzhak Brook, Department of Pediatrics, Georgetown University School of Medicine, Washington, DC 20007.

Polymicrobial Diseases, Edited by Kim A. Brogden and Janet M. Guthmiller,
© 2002 ASM Press, Washington, D.C.

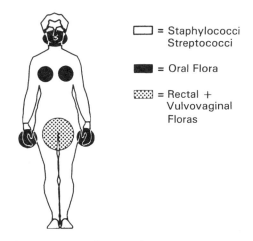

= Staphylococci
Streptococci

= Oral Flora

= Rectal +
Vulvovaginal
Floras

FIGURE 1 Distribution of organisms in abscesses, wounds, burns, and decubitus ulcers.

with decreased stomach acidity or with a shorter GIT or anastomosis.

The variations in the number of bacteria in the GIT account for the differences that are observed in cultures of the peritoneal cavity after perforations. Three different isolates per specimen and about 10^7 organisms/g were recovered from perforation of the small intestine, while 26 different bacterial isolates and 10^{12} organisms/g were isolated from specimens of colonic perforation (71). This high load of microorganisms is believed to account for the

higher frequency (50%) of the infections that follow colonic injury, compared with that after chest injuries (18%), found by Dellinger et al. (43). The higher number of organisms in the distal part of the colon also explains why infection developed in 45% of patients with descending-colon injuries, compared with about 13% in the other sites of the colon.

THE MICROBIOLOGY OF ABSCESSES OF ENDOGENOUS ORIGIN

Gram-positive anaerobic cocci are normal skin inhabitants and part of the normal fecal flora (44). These cocci are also isolated from intra-abdominal abscesses (6, 19–21, 23–25). They were isolated as frequently as AGNB from abscesses of the perineal region, and they were also frequently isolated from nonperineal cutaneous abscesses.

Organisms belonging to the *B. fragilis* group, which predominate in the feces, were cultured most frequently from abscesses of the perirectal area (46). *Prevotella melaninogenica,* which occurs in stool and in the oral cavity (44), also was recovered from this site and from the head.

The microbiology of intra-abdominal abscesses that develop following perforation of viscera is made of similar patterns of organisms

TABLE 1 Microbiologic characteristics of 676 cutaneous abscesses

Abscess location	No. of specimens	No. of specimens with indicated type of bacteria			No. of bacterial isolates/specimen		
		Aerobic only	Anaerobic only	Both	Aerobic	Anaerobic	Total
Head	158	45	51	62	0.8	1.4	2.2
Neck	43	20	14	9	1.0	1.7	2.7
Breast	40	7	18	15	0.7	1.4	2.1
Trunk	123	53	41	29	1.1	1.3	2.4
Arm	13	3	4	6	1.1	1.7	2.8
Hand	21	13	4	4	1.3	0.7	2.0
Leg	12	8	3	1	1.1	0.9	2.0
Inguinal	32	7	15	10	0.7	1.8	2.5
Buttock	35	8	15	12	0.7	1.4	2.1
Perirectal	136	9	55	72	0.9	2.2	3.1
Extragenital	63	4	23	36	0.9	1.9	2.8
Total	676	177	243	256			
Mean					0.9	1.6	2.5

TABLE 2 Predominant isolates in abscesses at various body sites

Infection site	Anaerobic bacteria	Facultative and miscellaneous bacteria
Skin and subcutaneous wounds and abscesses	*B. fragilis* group (rectal), *Prevotella* and *Porphyromonas* spp. (oral)	*S. aureus, S. pyogenes, E. coli* (rectal), *Enterobacteriaceae*
Head and neck	*Prevotella* and *Porphyromonas* spp., *Fusobacterium* spp., peptostreptococci	*S. pyogenes, S. aureus*
Abdomen	*B. fragilis* group, peptostreptococci, *Clostridium* spp.	*E. coli, Enterobacteriaceae*
Pelvis	*P. bivia, P. disiens, B. fragilis* group	*N. gonorrhoeae,* streptococci, *Chlamydia trachomatis, Enterobacteriaceae*

and is made up of the gastrointestinal flora at the level of the perforation (Table 2). The predominant anaerobic bacteria are the *B. fragilis* group, *Peptostreptococcus* spp., and *Clostridium* spp., while the most commonly isolated aerobic and facultative bacteria are *Enterobacteriaceae* and group D enterococci. These organisms were recovered from a variety of intra-abdominal (6), retroperitoneal (20), visceral (44, 46) [e.g., pancreatic (21), hepatic, and splenic (23)], and perirectal abscesses (25) [after diverticulitis rupture (19) and subphrenic (24)]. Similarity also exists in the microbiology of pelvic, vulvovaginal (27), and prostatic (5) abscesses that originate from the rectal and cervical flora (44, 46). The predominant anaerobic bacteria are *P. bivia, P. disiens,* and peptostreptococci, while the common aerobic and facultative bacteria include *Enterobacteriaceae, N. gonorrhoeae,* and group B streptococci (Table 2).

The microbiology of dental, orofacial, and neck abscesses is mainly made of oral flora organisms (Table 3) (9). These include peritonsillar (29), retropharyngeal (10), parotic (28), and cervical (22) lymph glands. The main anaerobes are pigmented *Prevotella, Porphyromonas, Fusobacterium,* and *Peptostreptococcus* spp. The most commonly isolated aerobes and facultative bacteria are *Streptococcus pyogenes* and *Staphylococcus aureus.*

The microbiology of skin and soft tissue abscesses is also related to their location (Fig. 1) (9, 17, 18, 26, 55). *S. pyogenes* and *S. aureus* that colonize the skin over the entire body can be recovered at all locations. The location of

the abscess is of paramount importance in the emergence of the other organism(s) that may also be involved in the infection. Under appropriate conditions of lowered tissue resistance, almost any of the common bacteria can initiate an infectious process. Cultures from lesions frequently contain several bacterial species; as might be expected, the organisms found most frequently are the "normal flora" of these regions (Table 1).

Aspirates from abscesses of the perineal and oral regions tend to yield organisms found in stool or mouth flora (17, 18, 55). Conversely, pus obtained from abscesses in areas remote from the rectum or mouth contain primarily constituents of the microflora indigenous to the skin such as *S. pyogenes* and *S. aureus.* Multiple anaerobic organisms usually are recovered from the perineal region, whereas only about one aerobe per abscess is present at other sites (18) (Table 1). Anaerobes also are more often recovered alone, without aerobes, from the perineal area. Mixed aerobic and anaerobic infections are more prevalent in the perirectal, head, finger, and nail bed areas. The similarities in the rates of isolation of mixed aerobic and anaerobic flora and the high rate of recovery of anaerobes in these areas are of particular interest. These similarities and the high rate of recovery can be caused by the introduction of mouth flora, which is predominantly anaerobic, onto the fingers by sucking or nail biting, which are common activities among children. This is parallel to the acquisition of infection following human bites and clenched fist in-

TABLE 3 Predominant isolates from abscesses

Parameter	Abdominal								Urogenital				Head and neck				
	Abdomen	Retroperitoneal	Diverticulitis	Perirectal	Liver	Spleen	Pancreatic	Subphrenic	Burtholm's cyst	Prostate	Testicular	Scrotal	Periapical	Cervical lymphadenitis	Parotic	Peritonsillar	Retropharyngeal
Reference	6	20	19	25	23	23	21	24	6	6	6	6	26	22	28	29	10
No. of patients	83	161	22	144	48	29	46	52	26	3	6	15	32	40	23	34	14
No. of aerobic bacteria																	
S. pyogenes		1		9	3	1		4				1		4	1	10	3
Enterococcus spp.		19	3	9	8	3	11	9				5					
S. aureus		11	1	34	4	4	6	5	2	1	1	5	1	8	8	6	5
M. catarrhalis	1															5	2
Haemophilus spp.													2			7	4
E. coli	57	60	15	19	11	5	18	28	6	2	1			1	2		
K. pneumoniae	8	20	3	3	5	3	12	3	2					1	1		
P. aeruginosa	4	9	1	4	2	1	5	3				2		1			
Enterobacter spp.	1	8	1	1			4	4	1								
Proteus spp.	2	8	1	12	2	3	3	4	3	1		1					
S. marcescens		6		2	3		3	3									
N. gonorrhoeae		4			1	1			4								
Other *Enterobacteriaceae*		20	2	16			6	2	3	2							
Subtotal	107	204	35	131	43	23	77	83	24	6	3	15	23	18	16	49	26

Anaerobic bacteria																	
Peptostreptococcus spp.	24	95	6	72	18	11	26	33	12	1	3	7	18	5	5	16	18
Veillonella spp.	2	10	1	6	3	1	6	6	2			1	2	1	1	5	3
Eubacterium spp.	2	6	1	11			1	4				1	2			1	4
P. acnes		13		2	3	3	4	4					1	4	4	3	1
C. perfringens	6	10	2	4	5	2	4	6	1								
Clostridium spp.	13	13	3	11	5	1	3	7				2					2
Fusobacterium spp.	4	14	1	21	10	3	5	5	2				9		3	11	14
B. fragilis	47	34	14	58	7	2	6	11	3	1	1	1	1	1	1	1	
B. fragilis group[a]	11	32	7	27	6	3	11	14	2	1	2		1		1		
P. melaninogenica	5	5	2	18	1	1	2	2	2		1	2	3	3	1	7	10
P. intermedia		7		12	2	2	3	3	1			1	2	2	3	3	4
P. asaccharolytica	4	3	1	20					3		1	2	1	2		5	4
P. oralis		2		2					1			1	4			1	3
P. disiens		1		6	1		1	1									
P. bivia		2		14					4		3						
Bacteroides spp.	3	12	1	19			4	7	6	1		6	4	2	1	4	11
P. gingivalis													7				
Subtotal	128	268	37	325	73	33	81	111	43	4	8	28	55	24	20	58	78
Total	235	472	72	256	116	56	158	194	67	10	11	33	78	42	36	107	104

[a] Other than B. fragilis.

juries in which anaerobic mouth flora was the source of most bacterial isolates (68).

The polymicrobial nature of abdominal, pelvic, and skin and soft tissue (proximal to the oral or rectal areas) abscesses is apparent in most patients, where the number of isolates in an infectious site varies between 2 and 6 (12, 44) (Tables 1 and 3). The average number of isolates is 3.6 in skin and soft tissue infections (2.6 anaerobes and 1.0 aerobe) per specimen (17, 18, 55), 5 in intra-abdominal infection (3.0 anaerobes and 2.0 aerobes) per specimen (6, 19–21, 23–25), and 4 in pelvic infections (2.8 anaerobes and 1.2 aerobes) per specimen (5, 27, 69). Polymicrobic infections are more pathogenic for experimental animals than those involving single organisms (1). The number of isolates in these polymicrobial abscesses varies from 2 to 6 (Tables 1 and 3), and generally is higher when reported in studies in which stricter methods for collection, transportation, and cultivation of anaerobic organisms are used (2, 10, 29, 68).

VIRULENCE OF ANAEROBIC BACTERIA

Although more than 400 bacterial species colonize in the colon, and more than 200 reside in oral cavities, the average number of bacterial species in infections associated with colonic perforation is five (44). The dominant anaerobic bacteria in this type of disease include the *B. fragilis* group, *Prevotella* and *Porphyromonas* spp. (previously called the *Bacteroides melaninogenicus* group), *Fusobacterium nucleatum, Clostridium perfringens,* and *Peptostreptococcus* spp. Thus, from the multiple anaerobic bacteria that make up the normal flora, only a few are common in the septic process; it is likely that their virulence is an important factor in their selection. The ability to produce a capsule (encapsulation) has been observed in all these anaerobic bacteria and may serve as an important virulence factor (48). Of all the anaerobes, *B. fragilis* group isolates are the most frequently encountered organisms in intra-abdominal abscesses or anaerobic bacteremia. Members of the *B. fragilis* group have several virulence factors and resist β-lactam antibiotics through production of the

enzyme β-lactamase (12, 44), possession of a capsule that inhibits phagocytosis (70), and the production of other enzymes and metabolic by-products. Succinic acid is an important metabolic by-product that can reduce polymorphonuclear migration (66). In addition to a capsule, anaerobic bacteria possess other important virulence factors. These include the production of superoxide dismutase and catalase, immunoglobulin proteases, coagulation-promoting and -spreading factors (such as hyaluronidase, collagenase, and fibrinolysin), and adherence factors (44, 48). Other factors that enhance the virulence of anaerobes include mucosal damage, oxidation-reduction potential drop, and the presence of hemoglobin or blood in an infected site.

ENCAPSULATION OF ANAEROBIC BACTERIA IN MIXED INFECTION AND ABSCESSES

Encapsulation of anaerobic bacteria defined by production of extracellular polysaccharide, termed glycocalyx (42), has been recognized as an important virulence factor. Several studies demonstrated the pathogenicity of encapsulated anaerobes and their ability to induce abscesses in experimental animals even when inoculated alone. Onderdonk et al. (60) correlated the formation of intra-abdominal abscesses in mice and rats by *B. fragilis* strains with the presence of capsule. Encapsulated *B. fragilis* strains or purified capsular polysaccharide alone induced abscesses, whereas nonencapsulated strains seldom caused abscesses unless they were combined with an aerobic organism. Simon et al. (67) showed that encapsulated *Bacteroides* strains resisted neutrophil-mediated killing, compared with nonencapsulated strains. Encapsulated *B. fragilis* strains adhered better to rat mesothelium than did nonencapsulated strains (62).

The susceptibility of pathogenic bacteria to phagocytosis and killing by polymorphonuclear leukocytes and macrophages is of major importance in determining the outcome of the host-pathogen interaction. Bjornson et al. (3) demonstrated phagocytosis and killing of *B. fragilis* by human leukocytes in vitro. Phagocytosis of *B. fragilis* in the presence of serum oc-curred in aerobic and anaerobic conditions. Ingham et al. (49) investigated the effect of *Bacteroides* spp. on the phagocytic killing of fac-ultative species. Killing of *B. fragilis* and *Proteus mirabilis* in mixtures in vitro was impaired when the concentration of *B. fragilis* was greater than 1×10^7 CFU/ml in the phago-cytic system. Tofte et al. (70) and Jones and Gemmell (50) reported that both phagocytic uptake and killing of facultative species were impaired at high concentrations of encapsu-lated *Bacteroides*. This inhibitory effect of *Bac-teroides* could be related to the effect of capsule on phagocytosis.

The presence of capsule in *B. fragilis* was shown to provide the organism with growth advantage in vivo over nonencapsulated iso-lates (65). Furthermore, encapsulated strains survived better in vitro than nonencapsulated variants when they were grown in an aerobic environment (65), and suppression of bacterial growth by the antimicrobial clindamycin was reduced in an encapsulated strain, as compared with a nonencapsulated one (30). Another re-cently described mechanism of protection in-dependent of encapsulation is the inhibition of polymorphonuclear migration due to the pro-duction of succinic acid by nonencapsulated *Bacteroides* spp. (66).

The importance of the capsular polysaccha-ride of *B. fragilis* as an immunogen was demon-strated when antibodies against it protected an-imals from early bacteriemia (52). However, prevention of the formation of intra-abdomi-nal abscess by this organism was found to be mediated by T cells (61).

The presence of a polysaccharide capsule, as defined by the electron microscopic visualiza-tion of a Ruthenium red-stained structure ex-ternal to the cell wall, has been documented for all members of the *B. fragilis* group (4, 41), and pigmented *Prevotella* and *Porphyromonas* (31), *Fusobacterium* spp. (37), and anaerobic cocci (40). However, because Ruthenium red stains some acidic polysaccharides as well as some lipopolysaccharides, some investigators consider immunochemical methods to be

more reliable for defining a true polysaccharide capsule (51).

The capsule of *B. fragilis* was studied more than any other anaerobic bacterium and was found to consist of two chemically distinct polysaccharides (A and B). Polysaccharide A is neutral at pH 7.3, but negatively charged at pH 8.6, and it contains predominantly galactose. Polysaccharide B is negatively charged at both pH 7.3 and 8.6 and contains fructose, galac-tose, quinovosamine, galacturonic acid, and galactosamine. These polysaccharides can give a complex multiprecipitin profile when react-ing with homologous antiserum in an immu-noelectrophoretic assay. The dual polysaccha-ride motif is a common feature of *B. fragilis* strains (63) that may result in different affinities for capsular detection stains such as Ruthe-nium red. This could also explain the diversity seen in electron microscopy analysis of *B. frag-ilis* cells (15, 64).

ENCAPSULATED ANAEROBIC BACTERIA IN CLINICAL INFECTIONS AND ABSCESSES

Aspirates obtained from infections next to mu-cous membrane surfaces generally contain a complex bacterial population consisting of sev-eral species (12, 44). Although anaerobes are components of mixed infections, their role and relative importance in the disease process are not always considered.

In an attempt to define the important pathogens among the isolates recovered from clinical specimens, we studied the virulence and importance of encapsulated bacterial iso-lates recovered from 13 clinical abscesses (35). This was done by injecting each of the 35 iso-lates (30 anaerobes and 5 aerobes) subcuta-neously (s.c.) into mice alone or in all possible combinations with the other isolates recovered from the same abscess. We then observed their ability to induce and/or survive in a subcuta-neous abscess. Sixteen of the isolates were en-capsulated; 15 of them were able to cause ab-scesses by themselves and were recovered from the abscesses even when inoculated alone. The other organisms, which were not encapsulated, were not able to induce abscesses when inoculated alone. However, some were able to survive when injected with encapsulated strains. Therefore, the possession of a capsule by an organism was associated with increased virulence, compared with the same organism's nonencapsulated counterparts, and might have allowed some of the other accompanying organisms to survive. We found this phenomenon to occur in *Bacteroides* spp., *Prevotella* spp., anaerobic gram-positive cocci, *Clostridium* spp., and *Escherichia coli*. Detection of a capsule in a clinical isolate may therefore suggest a pathogenic role of the organism in the infection.

Three studies support the importance of encapsulated anaerobic organisms in respiratory infections (13, 32, 34). The presence of encapsulated and abscess-forming organisms that belong to the pigmented *Prevotella* and *Porphyromonas* spp. in 25 children with acute tonsillitis and 23 children without tonsillar inflammation (control) was investigated (32). Encapsulated pigmented *Prevotella* and *Porphyromonas* were found in 23 of 25 children with acute tonsillitis, compared with 5 of 23 controls ($P < 0.001$). Subcutaneous inoculation into mice of the *Prevotella* and *Porphyromonas* strains that had been isolated from patients with tonsillitis produced abscesses in 17 of 25 instances, compared with 9 of 23 controls ($P < 0.05$). These findings suggest a possible pathogenic role for pigmented *Prevotella* and *Porphyromonas* spp. in acute tonsillar infection, and also suggest the importance of encapsulation in the pathogenesis of the infection.

In another study (13), the presence of encapsulated AGNB (pigmented *Prevotella* and *Porphyromonas* spp. and *Bacteroides* spp.) and anaerobic gram-positive cocci was investigated in 182 patients with chronic orofacial infections and in the pharynx of 26 individuals without inflammation. Forty-nine of the patients had chronic otitis media, 45 had cervical lymphadenitis, 37 had chronic sinusitis, 24 had chronic mastoiditis, 10 had peritonsillar abscesses, and 12 had periodontal abscesses. Of the 216 isolates of pigmented *Prevotella* and *Porphyromonas*, *B. fragilis* group, and anaerobic

cocci, 170 (79%) were found to be encapsulated in patients with chronic infections, compared with only 34 of 96 (35%) controls ($P < 0.001$).

The presence of encapsulated and piliated AGNB (mostly *B. fragilis* group and pigmented *Prevotella* and *Porphyromonas*) was investigated in isolates from blood, abscesses, and normal flora (34). Of the strains of AGNB isolated, 45 of 54 (83%) recovered from blood and 31 of 40 (78%) found in abscesses were encapsulated. In contrast, only 7 of 71 (10%) similar strains isolated from the feces or pharynx of healthy persons were encapsulated ($P < 0.001$). Pili were observed in 3 of 54 (6%) of strains isolated from blood, 30 of 40 (75%) of those recovered from abscesses ($P < 0.001$), and 49 of 71 (69%) of those found in normal flora ($P < 0.001$) (Fig. 2; shows only *B. fragilis* group). The predominance of encapsulated forms in all strains of AGNB in blood and in abscesses suggests an increased virulence of encapsulated forms compared with nonencapsulated isolates. In contrast, the presence of pili in AGNB recovered mostly from abscesses and normal flora suggests that this structure may play a role in the ability of these organisms to adhere to mucous membranes and may interfere with their ability to spread systematically. These findings illustrate the morphological differences that may be observed in AGNB from various anatomical sites.

The predominance of encapsulated *Bacteroides*, *Prevotella*, and *Porphyromonas* spp. recovered from blood and abscesses compared with their rate of encapsulation in the normal flora of the pharynx and feces suggests an in-

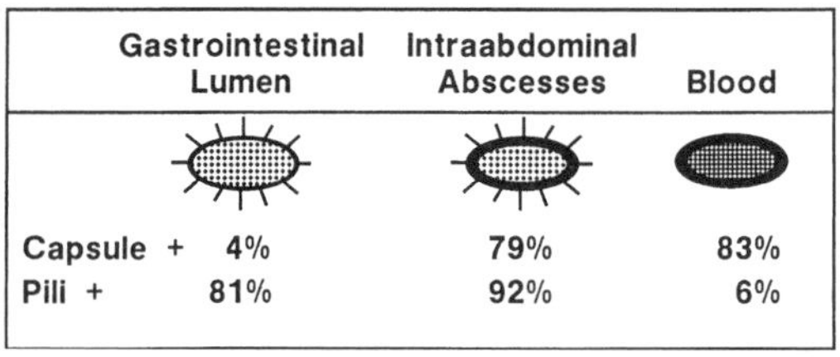

	Gastrointestinal Lumen	Intraabdominal Abscesses	Blood
Capsule +	4%	79%	83%
Pili +	81%	92%	6%

FIGURE 2 Dynamics of pili and capsule of *B. fragilis* group.

creased virulence of these strains as compared to nonencapsulated strains. In contrast to the emergence of encapsulated *Bacteroides* spp. in blood and abscesses, the presence of pili was less frequent in such strains recovered from blood. The rate of piliated strains was high among those recovered from abscesses.

Since most *Bacteroides, Prevotella,* and *Porphyromonas* spp. recovered from infected sites probably originate from the predominantly nonencapsulated endogenous flora of mucous membranes, they may express their capsules only during the inflammatory process. The frequent recovery of encapsulated AGNB in such conditions illustrates their increased virulence as compared with their nonencapsulated counterparts.

Complete eradication of experimental *Bacteroides* infection by means of metronidazole was not achieved when these organisms were encapsulated (11). Once the organisms become encapsulated, eradication of *Bacteroides* infection becomes difficult. Treatment of infections involving nonencapsulated *Bacteroides* spp., however, was more efficacious. Early treatment of anaerobic infections may therefore prevent the emergence of encapsulated AGNB, and subsequent bacteremia.

The recovery of a larger number of encapsulated anaerobic organisms from orofacial infections, abscesses, and blood of patients provides support for the potential pathogenic role of encapsulated organisms. Early and vigorous antimicrobial therapy, directed at both aerobic and anaerobic bacteria present in these mixed infections, may abort the infection before the emergence of encapsulated strains that contribute to the chronicity of the infection.

CAPSULE FORMATION IN EXPERIMENTAL ABSCESSES

The ability of the aerobic component in mixed infections to enhance the appearance of encapsulated anaerobic bacteria in these infections was studied in a s.c. abscess model in mice. The anaerobic bacteria with which they were inoculated were those commonly recovered in mixed infections.

Pigmented *Prevotella* and *Porphyromonas* spp. (31), *P. bivia* (14), *B. fragilis* group (16), and anaerobic and facultative gram-positive cocci (AFGPC) (40) did not induce abscess when isolates that contained only a few encapsulated organisms (<1%) were inoculated. However, when these relatively nonencapsulated isolates were inoculated, mixed with abscess-forming viable or nonviable bacteria ("helpers"), the *Bacteroides, Prevotella, Porphyromonas,* and AFGPC survived in the abscess and became heavily encapsulated (>50% of organisms had a capsule). Thereafter, these heavily encapsulated anaerobic isolates were able to induce abscesses when injected alone (Fig. 3). Of interest is the observed appearance of pili along with encapsulation in the *B. fragilis* group after coinoculation with *Klebsiella pneumoniae* (16).

Most of the helper strains were encapsulated; however, several of the strains were not encapsulated, but they were able to induce abscesses when inoculated alone. The helper organisms used in conjunction with pigmented *Prevotella* and *Porphyromonas* spp. and AFGPC were *S. aureus, S. pyogenes, Haemophilus influenzae, Pseudomonas aeruginosa, E. coli, K. pneumoniae,* and *Bacteroides* spp. (31, 40). For the *B. fragilis* group, these organisms were *E. coli, K. pneumoniae, S. aureus, S. pyogenes,* and *Enterococcus* spp. (16). *N. gonorrhoeae* was chosen as a helper for *B. fragilis,* and *Prevotella* and *Porphyromonas* spp. (14). Of interest is the observed inability of *N. gonorrhoeae* strains to survive in intra–abdominal abscesses and also their disappearance from s.c. abscesses within 5 days of inoculation with *Bacteroides* spp. and *P. bivia* (14).

The virulence of *Fusobacterium* spp. was also associated with the presence of a capsule. Only encapsulated strains of *F. nucleatum, Fusobacterium necrophorum,* and *Fusobacterium varium* were able to induce abscesses when inoculated alone (37). However, after passage in animals of nonencapsulated strains, none of these organisms acquired a capsule.

The presence of a thick granular cell wall (300 to 360 Å) before animal passage was associated with virulence of *Clostridium* spp. (38). Such structure was observed before inocula-

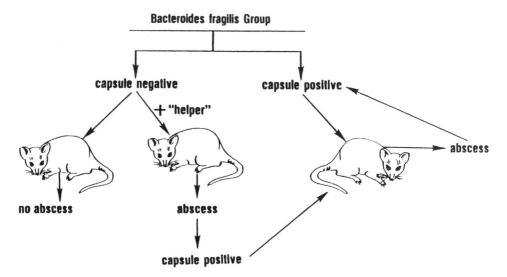

FIGURE 3 Encapsulation cycle of *B. fragilis* group after passage in mice. Helper is viable bacteria or formolized bacteria or capsular material.

tion into animals, only in *C. perfringens* and *Clostridium butyricum,* the only organisms capable of inducing an s.c. abscess when inoculated alone. This structure was observed in other *Clostridium* spp. only after their coinoculation with encapsulated *Bacteroides* spp. or *K. pneumoniae.* However, other undetermined factors may also contribute to the induction of an abscess, because most isolates of *Clostridium difficile* were not able to produce an abscess even though they possessed a thick wall.

The selection of encapsulated *Bacteroides* spp. and AFGPC with the assistance of other encapsulated or nonencapsulated but abscess-forming aerobic or anaerobic organisms may explain the conversion into pathogens of non-pathogenic organisms that are part of the normal host flora or are concomitant pathogens. Although such a phenomenon was not observed in *Fusobacterium* spp., the presence of a capsule in these organisms was a prerequisite for induction of s.c. abscesses. Some *Clostridium* spp. also manifested cell wall changes after animal passage that could be associated with increased virulence. Although the exact nature and chemical composition of the capsule or external cell wall may be different in each of the anaerobic species studied, the changes that were observed tended to follow similar patterns.

SIGNIFICANCE OF ANAEROBIC BACTERIA IN ABSCESSES MIXED WITH OTHER FLORA

Although anaerobic bacteria often are recovered mixed with other aerobic and facultative flora, their exact role in these infections and their relative contribution to the pathogenic process are unknown. The relative importance of the organisms present in an abscess caused by two bacteria (an aerobe and an anaerobe) and the effect of encapsulation on that relationship were determined by comparing the abscess sizes in (i) mice treated with antibiotics directed against one or both organisms and (ii) nontreated animals (36–39).

As judged by selective antimicrobial therapy, the possession of a capsule in most mixed infections involving AGNB generally made these organisms more important than their aerobic counterparts. In almost all instances, the aerobic counterparts in the infection were more important than nonencapsulated AGNB (39). Encapsulated members of the pigmented

Prevotella and *Porphyromonas* spp. were almost always more important in mixed infections than their aerobic counterparts (*S. pyogenes*, *Streptococcus pneumoniae*, *K. pneumoniae*, *H. influenzae*, and *S. aureus*). Encapsulated *B. fragilis* group organisms were more important than or as important as *E. coli* and enterococci, and less important than *S. aureus*, *S. pyogenes*, and *K. pneumoniae*.

In contrast to *Bacteroides* spp., encapsulated AFGPC were more often found to be less important than their aerobic counterparts (36). *Clostridium* and *Fusobacterium* spp. were less or equally important to enteric gram-negative rods (37, 38). Although *Fusobacterium*, AFGPC, and *Clostridium* spp. were generally equal to or less important than their aerobic counterpart, variations in the relationship existed. However, as determined by the abscess size, most of the anaerobic organisms enhanced mixed infection.

SYNERGY BETWEEN ANAEROBIC AND AEROBIC OR FACULTATIVE ANAEROBIC BACTERIA IN ABSCESSES

Several studies documented the synergistic effect of mixtures of aerobic and anaerobic bacteria in experimental infections. Altermeier (1) demonstrated the pathogenicity of bacteria isolates recovered from peritoneal cultures after appendiceal rupture. Pure cultures of individual isolates were relatively innocuous when implanted s.c. in animals, but combinations of facultative and anaerobic strains showed increased virulence. Similar observations were

reported by Meleney et al. (56) and Hite et al. (47).

We have evaluated the synergistic potentials between aerobic and anaerobic bacteria usually recovered in mixed infections (33). Each bacterium was inoculated s.c. into mice alone or mixed with another organism, and synergistic effects were determined by observing abscess formation and animal mortality. The tested bacteria included encapsulated *Bacteroides* spp., *Prevotella* spp., *Porphyromonas* spp., *Fusobacterium* spp., *Clostridium* spp., and anaerobic cocci. Facultative and anaerobic bacteria included *S. aureus*, *P. aeruginosa*, *E. coli*, *K. pneumoniae*, and *P. mirabilis*. In many combinations, the anaerobes significantly enhanced the virulence of each of the five aerobes (Tables 4 and 5). The most virulent combinations were between *P. aeruginosa* or *S. aureus* and anaerobic cocci or AGNB.

Enhancement of the growth of each bacterial component in mixed infection was evaluated by studying the relative growth of each bacterial component. This was done by comparing (i) the growth of each organism in an abscess when present with another organism with (ii) the growth of those bacteria when inoculated alone (7, 8, 38, 40).

S. pyogenes, *E. coli*, *S. aureus*, *K. pneumoniae*, and *P. aeruginosa* were enhanced by *B. fragilis*, *P. melaninogenica* (7, 8), *Peptostreptococcus* spp. (7), *Fusobacterium* spp. (37), and *Clostridium* spp. (38) except *C. difficile*. Although mutual enhancement of growth of both aerobic and anaerobic bacteria was noticed, the number of

TABLE 4 Synergy between anaerobic and aerobic and facultative bacteria

Aerobic facultative bacteria	Synergy[a] with anaerobic bacteria		
	Peptostreptococcus spp.	*B. fragilis*	*P. asaccharolytica*
P. aeruginosa	Yes	Yes	Yes
E. coli	No	Yes	Yes
K. pneumoniae	No	Yes	Yes
P. mirabilis	No	Yes	Yes
S. aureus	Yes	Yes	Yes

[a] Synergy was determined by demonstrating reduction of lethal dose in mice inoculated s.c.

TABLE 5 Synergy between anaerobic bacteria

Species	Synergy[a] with:				
	Peptostreptococcus spp.	*F. varium*	*F. nucleatum*	*C. perfringens*	*C. butyricum*
B. fragilis	Yes	Yes	Yes	Yes	No
P. asaccharolytica	Yes	Yes	Yes	No	No
F. varium	Yes			Yes	No
F. nucleatum	Yes			Yes	Yes
C. perfringens	No	Yes	Yes		
C. butyricum	No	No	Yes		

[a] Synergy was determined by demonstrating reduction in the number of bacteria needed to induce s.c. abscess in mice by s.c. inoculation of bacteria.

aerobic and facultative bacteria was increased many times more than their anaerobic counterparts. Encapsulated *Bacteroides* spp. were able to enhance the growth of aerobic and facultative anaerobic bacteria more than nonencapsulated organisms (Table 6) (7, 11). Exceptions to the mutual enhancement were noticed in combinations of organisms that generally are not recovered together in mixed infections, such as enterococci and *P. melaninogenica*. The observations above suggest that the aerobic and facultative bacteria benefit even more than do the anaerobes from their symbiosis.

The mutual enhancement between aerobic and facultative organisms and *B. fragilis* group was apparent in numerous combinations (8). An increase in the number of aerobic and facultative bacteria when combined with three members of the *B. fragilis* group was illustrated in almost all instances except for the one between *H. influenzae* and *B. fragilis* group (Fig. 4 and 5; Table 7). However, this is not surprising since this combination is rarely seen in clinical infections.

MECHANISMS OF SYNERGY

Several hypotheses have been proposed to explain microbial synergy in mixed infection (55). When this phenomenon occurs in mixtures of aerobic and anaerobic flora, it may be due to protection from phagocytosis and intracellular killing (49), production of essential growth factors (53), and lowering of oxidation-reduction potentials in host tissues (53). Obligate anaerobes can interfere with the phagocytosis and killing of aerobic bacteria (49). The ability of human polymorphonuclear leukocytes to phagocytose and kill *P. mirabilis* was impaired in vitro when the human serum used to opsonize the target bacterium was pretreated with live or dead organisms of various AGNB (50). *Porphyromonas gingivalis* cells or supernatant culture fluid was shown to possess the greatest inhibitory effect among the *Bacteroides* spp. (59). Supernatants of cultures of *B. fragilis* group, pigmented *Prevotella* and *Porphyromonas*, and *P. gingivalis* were capable of inhibiting the chemotaxis of leukocytes to the chemotactic factors of *P. mirabilis* (58).

Bacteria may also provide nutrients for each other. *Klebsiella* produces succinate, which supports *Porphyromonas asaccharolytica* (54), and oral diphtheroids produced vitamin K_1, which is a growth factor for *P. melaninogenica* (45).

Another possible mechanism that explains the synergistic effect of aerobic-anaerobic combinations is the lowering of local oxygen

TABLE 6 Average numbers of encapsulated and nonencapsulated *Bacteroides* spp. in mixed abscesses with *E. coli*

Species	No. of CFU/abscess (mean ± SD)	
	Encapsulated	Nonencapsulated
B. fragilis	10.9 ± 1.1	6.8 ± 0.9
B. thetaiotaomicron	11.3 ± 1.3	7.6 ± 0.7
B. vulgatus	10.2 ± 0.8	7.3 ± 0.9

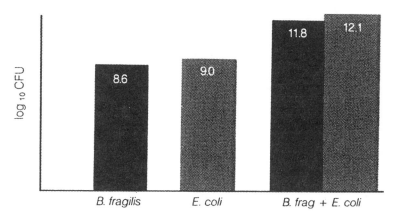

FIGURE 4   Number of *B. fragilis* and *E. coli* ($\log_{10}$ CFU) in s.c. abscesses induced by single and combined bacteria in mice. A mutual significant enhancement of growth of both *E. coli* and *B. fragilis* (*B. frag*) was noted in mixed infection compared with the number of these isolates when each was inoculated alone ($P > 0.05$). Similar mutual increases were also noticed in combinations of *B. ovatus* and *B. vulgatus* with *E. coli* (8).

concentrations and the oxidation-reduction potential by the aerobic bacteria. The resultant physical conditions are appropriate for replication and invasion by the anaerobic component of the infection. Such environmental factors are known to be critical for anaerobic growth in vitro and may apply with equal relevance to in vivo experimental animal studies. Mergenhagen et al. noted that the infecting dose of anaerobic cocci was significantly lowered

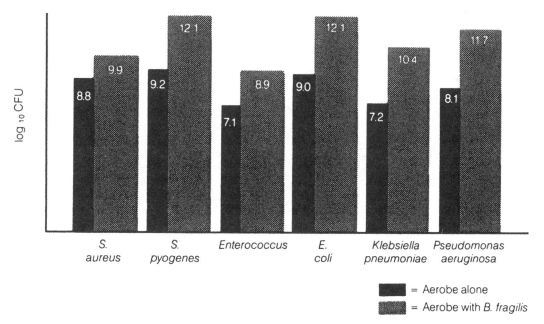

FIGURE 5   Change in number of aerobes when mixed in an abscess with *B. fragilis*. The increase in number of aerobic or facultative bacteria is illustrated by this bar graph (8).

TABLE 7 Average numbers of facultative and aerobic bacteria in subcutaneous abscesses induced by each organism alone combined with *B. fragilis* group

Organism	Avg no. of CFU/abscess[a]			
	Alone	With *B. fragilis*	With *B. vulgatus*	With *B. ovatus*
S. aureus	8.8	11.9★	12.2★	8.0
Group A streptococci	9.2	12.1★	12.7★	12.9★
Group D streptococci	7.1	8.9★	9.7★	9.5★
E. coli	9.0	12.1★	11.9★	11.8★
K. pneumoniae	7.2	10.4★	10.6★	9.9★
P. aeruginosa	8.1	11.7★	9.9★	10.0★
H. influenzae	6.3	6.9	5.4	6.7

[a]★, $P < 0.05$, between single and mixed infections.

when the inoculum was supplemented with chemical reducing agents (57). A similar effect may be produced by facultative bacteria, which may provide the proper conditions for establishing an anaerobic infection at a previously well-oxygenated site.

Demonstration of the synergistic potentials of anaerobic bacteria (such as the *B. fragilis* group, *Porphyromonas* and *Prevotella* spp., *Fusobacterium* spp., *Clostridium* spp., and anaerobic cocci) mixed with various aerobic and anaerobic bacteria further indicates their pathogenic role. Further studies are needed to investigate the exact mechanisms by which such synergy occurs, and the mode by which capsular material enhances it.

REFERENCES

1. **Altermeier, W. A.** 1942. The pathogenicity of the bacteria of appendicitis. *Surgery* **11:**374–378.
2. **Bennion, R. S., E. J. Baron, J. E. Thompson, Jr., J. Downes, P. Summanen, D. A. Talan, and S. M. Finegold.** 1990. The bacteriology of gangrenous and perforated appendicitis-revisited. *Ann. Surg.* **211:**165–171.
3. **Bjornson, A. B., W. A. Altemeier, and H. S. Bjornson.** 1976. Comparison of the in vitro bactericidal activity of human serum and leukocytes against *Bacteroides fragilis* and *Fusoacterium mortiferum* in aerobic and anaerobic environments. *Infect. Immun.* **14:**843–847.
4. **Bjornson, A. B., H. S. Bjornson, M. Ashraf, and T. J. Lang.** 1983. Quantitative variability in requirements for opsonization of strains within the *Bacteroides fragilis* group. *J. Infect. Dis.* **148:**667–675.
5. **Brook, I.** 1989. Anaerobic bacteria in suppurative genitourinary infections. *J. Urol.* **141:**889–893.
6. **Brook, I.** 1989. A 12 year study of aerobic and anaerobic bacteria in intra-abdominal and post surgical abdominal wound infections. *Surg. Gynecol. Obstet.* **169:**387–392.
7. **Brook, I.** 1988. Enhancement of growth of aerobic, anaerobic, and facultative bacteria in mixed infections with anaerobic and facultative gram-positive cocci. *J. Surg. Res.* **45:**222–227.
8. **Brook, I.** 1985. Enhancement of growth of aerobic and facultative bacteria in mixed infections with *Bacteroides* sp. *Infect. Immun.* **50:**929–931.
9. **Brook, I.** 1987. Microbiology of abscesses of the head and neck in children. *Ann. Otol. Rhinol. Laryngol.* **96:**429–433.
10. **Brook, I.** 1987. Microbiology of retropharyngeal abscesses in children. *Am. J. Dis. Child.* **141:**202–204.
11. **Brook, I.** 1988. Pathogenicity of encapsulated and non-encapsulated members of *Bacteroides fragilis* and *melaninogenicus* groups in mixed infection with *Escherichia coli* and *Streptococcus pyogenes*. *J. Med. Microbiol.* **27:**191–198.
12. **Brook, I.** 2002. *Pediatric Anaerobic Infection: Diagnosis and Management.* Marcel Dekker, New York, N.Y.
13. **Brook, I.** 1986. Recovery of encapsulated anaerobic bacteria from orofacial abscesses. *J. Med. Microbiol.* **22:**171–176.
14. **Brook, I.** 1986. The effect of encapsulation on the pathogenicity of mixed infection of *Neisseria gonorrhoea* and *Bacteroides* spp. *Am. J. Obstet. Gynecol.* **155:**421–428.

15. **Brook, I.** 1994. The role of encapsulated anaerobic bacteria in synergistic infections. *FEMS Microbiol. Rev.* **13:**65–74.

16. **Brook, I., J. C. Coolbaugh, and R. I. Walker.** 1984. Pathogenicity of piliated and encapsulated *Bacteroides fragilis. Eur. J. Clin. Microbiol.* **3:**207–209.

17. **Brook, I., and S. M. Finegold.** 1981. Aerobic and anaerobic bacteriology of cutaneous abscesses in children. *Pediatrics* **67:**891–895.

18. **Brook, I., and E. H. Frazier.** 1990. Aerobic and anaerobic bacteriology of wounds and cutaneous abscesses. *Arch. Surg.* **125:**1445–1551.

19. **Brook, I., and E. H. Frazier.** 2000. Aerobic and anaerobic microbiology in intra-abdominal infections associated with diverticulitis. *J. Med. Microbiol.* **49:**827–830.

20. **Brook, I., and E. H. Frazier.** 1998. Aerobic and anaerobic microbiology of retroperitoneal abscesses. *Clin. Infect. Dis.* **26:**938–941.

21. **Brook, I., and E. G. Frazier.** 1996. Microbiological analysis of pancreatic abscess. *Clin. Infect. Dis.* **22:**384–385.

22. **Brook, I., and E. H. Frazier.** 1998. Microbiology of cervical lymphadenitis in adults. *Acta Otolaryngol.* **118:**443–446.

23. **Brook, I., and E. H. Frazier.** 1998. Microbiology of liver and spleen abscesses. *J. Med. Microbiol.* **47:**1075–1080.

24. **Brook, I., and E. H. Frazier.** 1999. Microbiology of subphrenic abscesses: a 14-year experience. *Am. Surg.* **65:**1049–1053.

25. **Brook, I., and E. H. Frazier.** 1997. The aerobic and anaerobic bacteriology of perirectal abscesses. *J. Clin. Microbiol.* **35:**2974–2976.

26. **Brook, I., E. H. Frazier, and M. E. Gher.** 1991. Aerobic and anaerobic microbiology of periapical abscess. *Oral Microbiol. Immunol.* **6:**123–125.

27. **Brook, I., E. H. Frazier, and R. L. Thomas.** 1991. Aerobic and anaerobic microbiologic factors and recovery of beta-lactamase-producing bacteria from obstetric and gynecologic infection. *Surg. Gynecol. Obstet.* **172:**138–144.

28. **Brook, I., E. H. Frazier, and D. H. Thompson.** 1991. Aerobic and anaerobic microbiology of acute suppurative parotitis. *Laryngoscope* **101:**170–172.

29. **Brook, I., E. H. Frazier, and D. H. Thompson.** 1991. Aerobic and anaerobic microbiology of peritonsillar abscess. *Laryngoscope* **101:**289–292.

30. **Brook, I., and J. D. Gillmore.** 1994. Increased resistance of encapsulated *Bacteroides fragilis* to clindamycin. *Chemotherapy* **40:**16–20.

31. **Brook, I., J. D. Gillmore, J. C. Coolbaugh, and R. I. Walker.** 1983. Pathogenicity of encapsulated *Bacteroides melaninogenicus* group, *Bac-teroides oralis,* and *Bacteroides ruminicola* in abscesses in mice. *J. Infect.* **7:**281–286.

32. **Brook, I., and A. E. Gober.** 1983. *Bacteroides melaninogenicus,* its recovery from tonsils of children with acute tonsillitis. *Arch. Otolaryngol.* **109:**818–820.

33. **Brook, I., V. Hunter, and R. I. Walker.** 1984. Synergistic effects of anaerobic cocci, *Bacteroides, Clostridia, Fusobacteria,* and aerobic bacteria on mouse mortality and induction of subcutaneous abscess. *J. Infect. Dis.* **149:**924–928.

34. **Brook, I., L. A. Myhal, and C. H. Dorsey.** 1992. Encapsulation and pilus formation of *Bacteroides spp.* in formal flora abscesses and blood. *J. Infect.* **25:**251–257.

35. **Brook, I., and R. I. Walker.** 1983. Infectivity of organisms recovered from polymicrobial abscesses. *Infect. Immun.* **42:**986–989.

36. **Brook, I., and R. I. Walker.** 1984. Pathogenicity of anaerobic gram-positive cocci. *Infect. Immun.* **45:**320–324.

37. **Brook, I., and R. I. Walker.** 1986. Pathogenicity of *Fusobacterium* species. *J. Med. Microb.* **21:**93–100.

38. **Brook, I., and R. I. Walker.** 1986. Pathogenicity of some *Clostridium* species with other bacteria in mixed infection. *J. Infect.* **13:**245–253.

39. **Brook, I., and R. I. Walker.** 1984. Significance of encapsulated *Bacteroides melaninogenicus* and *Bacteroides fragilis* groups in mixed infections. *Infect. Immun.* **44:**12–15.

40. **Brook, I., and R. I. Walker.** 1985. The role of encapsulation in the pathogenicity of anaerobic gram-positive cocci. *Can. J. Microbiol.* **31:**176–180.

41. **Burt, S., S. Meldrum, D. R. Woods, and D. T. Jones.** 1978. Colonial variation capsule formation and bacteriophage resistance in *Bacteroides thetaiotaomicron. Appl. Environ. Microbiol.* **35:**439–443.

42. **Costerton, J. W., R. T. Irvin, and K. J. Cheng.** 1981. The role of bacterial surface structures in pathogenesis. *Crit. Rev. Microbiol.* **8:**303–338.

43. **Dellinger, E. P., M. R. Oreskovich, M. J. Wertz, V. Hamasaki, and E. S. Lennard.** 1984. Risk of infection following laparotomy for penetrating abdominal injury. *Arch. Surg.* **119:**20–27.

44. **Finegold, S. M.** 1977. *Anaerobic Bacteria in Human Disease.* Academic Press, Inc., New York, N.Y.

45. **Gibbons, R. J., and J. B. MacDonald.** 1960. Hemin and vitamin K compounds as required factors for the cultivation of certain strains of *Bacteroides melaninogenicus. J. Bacteriol.* **80:**164–170.

46. **Gorbach, S. L.** 1971. Intestinal microflora. *Gastroenterology* **50:**1110–1116.

47. **Hite, K. E., M. Locke, and H. C. Hesseltine.** 1949. Synergism in experimental infections with nonsporulating anaerobic bacteria. *Infect. Dis.* **84:**1–9.

48. **Hofstad, T.** 1992. Virulence factors in anaerobic bacteria. *Eur. J. Clin. Microbiol. Infect. Dis.* **11:** 1044–1048.

49. **Ingham, H. R., P. R. Sisson, D. Tharagonnet, J. B. Seldon, and A. A. Codd.** 1977. Inhibition of phagocytosis in vitro by obligate anaerobes. *Lancet* **ii:**1252–1254.

50. **Jones, G. R., and C. G. Gemmell.** 1982. Impairment by *Bacteroides* species of opsonization and phagocytosis of enterobacteria. *J. Med. Microbiol.* **15:**351–361.

51. **Kasper, D. L.** 1991. Immunochemical characterization of two surface polysaccharides of *Bacteroides fragilis*. *Infect. Immun.* **59:**2075–2082.

52. **Kasper, D. L., and A. B. Onderdonk.** 1982. Infection with *Bacteroides fragilis* pathogenesis and immunoprophylaxis in an animal model. *Scand. J. Infect. Dis.* **31**(Suppl.):28–33.

53. **Lev, M. K., K. C. Kridell, and A. F. Milford.** 1971. Succinate as a growth factor for *Bacteroides melaninogenicus*. *J. Bacteriol.* **108:**175–178.

54. **Mayrand, D., and B. G. McBride.** 1980. Ecological relationships of bacteria involved in a simple mixed anaerobic infection. *Infect. Immun.* **27:**44–50.

55. **Meislin, H. W., S. A. Lerner, M. H. Graves, M. D. McGehee, F. E. Kocka, J. A. Morello, and P. Rosen.** 1977. Cutaneous abscesses. Anaerobic and aerobic bacteriology and outpatient management. *Ann. Intern. Med.* **87:**145–149.

56. **Meleny, F., S. Olpp, H. D. Harvey, and H. Jern.** 1932. Peritonitis. Synergism of bacteria commonly found in peritoneal exudates. *Arch. Surg.* **25:**709–721.

57. **Mergenhagen, S. E., J. C. Thonard, and H. W. Scherp.** 1958. Studies on synergistic infections. Experimental infections with anaerobic streptococci. *J. Infect. Dis.* **103:**33–44.

58. **Namavar, F. A., M. J. J. Verweij, M. Bal, T. J. M. van Steenbergen, J. de Graaf, and D. M. MacLaren.** 1983. Effect of anaerobic bacteria on killing of *Proteus mirabilis* by human polymorphonuclear leukocytes. *Infect. Immun.* **40:**930–935.

59. **Namavar, F., A. M. J. J. Verweij-van Vught, W. A. C. Vel, M. Bal, and D. M. MacLaren.** 1984. Polymorphonuclear leukocyte chemotaxis by mixed anaerobic and aerobic bacteria. *J. Med. Microbiol.* **18:**167–172.

60. **Onderdonk, A. B., D. L. Kasper, D. L. Cisneros, and J. G. Bartlett.** 1977. The capsular polysaccharide of *Bacteroides fragilis* as a virulence factor: comparison of the pathogenic potential of encapsulated strains. *J. Infect. Dis.* **136:**82–89.

61. **Onderdonk, A. B., R. R. Markham, D. F. Zalenzik, R. L. Cineros, and D. L. Kasper.** 1982. Evidence for T cell-dependent immunity to *Bacteroides fragilis* in an intra-abdominal abscess model. *J. Clin. Invest.* **69:**9–16.

62. **Onderdonk, A. B., N. E. Moon, D. L. Kasper, and J. G. Bartlett.** 1978. Adherence of *Bacteroides fragilis* in vivo. *Infect. Immun.* **19:** 1083–1087.

63. **Pantosti, A., A. O. Tzianabos, B. G. Reinap, A. B. Onderdonk, and D. L. Kasper.** 1993. *Bacteroides fragilis* strains express multiple capsular polysaccharides. *J. Clin. Microbiol.* **31:**1850–1855.

64. **Patrick, S., J. H. Reid, and A. Coffey.** 1986. Capsulation of in vitro and in vivo frown *Bacteroides* species. *J. Gen. Microbiol.* **132:**1099–1109.

65. **Patrick, S., J. H. Reid, and M. H. Larkin.** 1984. The growth and survival of capsulate and non-capsulate *Bacteroides fragilis* in vivo and in vitro. *J. Med. Microbiol.* **17:**237–246.

66. **Rotstein, D., T. L. Pruett, V. D. Fiegel, R. D. Nelson, and R. L. Simmons.** 1985. Succinic acid, a metabolic byproduct of *Bacteroides* species, inhibits polymorphonuclear leukocytes function. *Infect. Immun.* **48:**402.

67. **Simon, G. L., M. S. Kelmpner, D. L. Kasper, and S. L. Gorbach.** 1982. Alteration in opsonophagocytic killing by neutrophils of *Bacteroides fragilis* associated with animal and laboratory passage: effect of capsular polysaccharide. *J. Infect. Dis.* **145:**72–79.

68. **Talan, D. A., D. M. Citron, F. M. Abrahamian, G. J. Moran, and E. J. Goldstein.** 1999. Bacteriologic analysis of infected dog and cat bites. Emergency Medicine Infection Study Group. *N. Engl. J. Med.* **340:**85–92.

69. **Thadepalli, H., S. L. Gorbach, and L. Keith.** 1973. Anaerobic infections of the female genital tract: bacteriology and therapeutic implementation. *Am. J. Obstet. Gynecol.* **117:**1034–1039.

70. **Tofte, R. W., P. U. Peterson, and D. Schmeling.** 1980. Opsonization of four *Bacteroides* species: role of the classical complement pathway and immunoglobulin. *Infect. Immun.* **27:**784–792.

71. **Weinstein, W. M., A. B. Onderdonk, J. G. Bartlett, T. J. Louie, and S. L. Gorbach.** 1975. Antimicrobial therapy of experimental intraabdominal sepsis. *J. Infect. Dis.* **132:**282–286.

ATROPHIC RHINITIS

Tibor Magyar and Alistair J. Lax

10

Atrophic rhinitis is a contagious respiratory disease of pigs that is highly prevalent throughout the world where modern pig husbandry is practiced. The clinical manifestation of this complex disease displays a wide scale of symptoms. These include partial or complete atrophy of one or both turbinate bones in the nose, twisting or shortening of the nose, nasal discharges, sneezing, nasal hemorrhage, and retarded growth rate.

Atrophic rhinitis was first described more than 170 years ago in Germany by Franque (54), who called this pathological condition "Schnüffelkrankheit" (sniffing disease). Since then numerous papers have been published on the etiology, pathogenesis, and control of the disease, yet these topics are still the subject of debate and controversy.

Some of the early attempts to explain etiology invoked heredity and nutritional factors (20, 47, 54, 93, 193). Later these were dropped as primary causes (129, 212), and the infectious nature of the disease came to the fore. Several agents were suspected to be etiological agents in the early studies. These in-cluded bacteria (*Pseudomonas, Actinomyces, Sphaerophorus, Corynebacterium,* or *Mycoplasma*), a virus (cytomegalovirus), and trichomonads (210, 213). However, only certain defined strains of *Bordetella bronchiseptica* and *Pasteurella multocida* proved to be able to constantly reproduce marked turbinate atrophy, the most characteristic lesion of atrophic rhinitis. This effect of *B. bronchiseptica* was first suggested by Switzer (210) and Cross and Claflin (39), and that of *P. multocida* by Gwatkin et al. (71) and Braend and Flatla (15), although it was some years before the link was proved.

After the first isolation of *B. bronchiseptica* from pigs, Switzer (210) demonstrated its unaided ability to induce significant turbinate atrophy. Later, several researchers reached a similar conclusion (16, 39, 104, 175, 196) resulting in the concept that *B. bronchiseptica* was the primary cause of atrophic rhinitis. At the same time, uncertainties that were supported by the following observations emerged.

1. In commercial pig herds the prevalence of infection with *B. bronchiseptica* greatly exceeded that of clinical atrophic rhinitis; the organism could be isolated from herds either with or without the clinical disease (61, 218).

Tibor Magyar, Veterinary Medical Research Institute, Hungarian Academy of Sciences, H-1143 Budapest, Hungary. *Alistair J. Lax,* Oral Microbiology, Guy's King's and St. Thomas' Dental Institute, King's College London, London SE1 9RT, United Kingdom.

We dedicate this chapter to the late Richard B. Rimler, who made many contributions to the study of atrophic rhinitis.

Polymicrobial Diseases, Edited by Kim A. Brogden and Janet M. Guthmiller,
© 2002 ASM Press, Washington, D.C.

One explanation for this observation could have been variations in virulence of the various strains of *B. bronchiseptica*. This was reported for isolates in the United States (176; B. J. Skelly, M. Pruss, R. Pellegrino, D. Andersen, and G. Abruzzo, *Proc. 6th Int. Pig Vet. Soc. Congr.*, p. 210, 1980), Canada (142), and the United Kingdom (30). However, Rutter et al. (184) found that *B. bronchiseptica* strains isolated in the United Kingdom from herds with or without progressive disease all caused turbinate lesions of similar severity.

2. Despite the ability of *B. bronchiseptica* to produce considerable turbinate atrophy in experimental infections, the lesions did not progress beyond the mild-to-moderate category (161). Even the most virulent of 10 United Kingdom isolates did not cause progressive turbinate atrophy or significant snout deformation in experimental infections (184).

3. Lesions induced by *B. bronchiseptica* infection appeared to regenerate over time (179, 217). This ability seemed to correlate with the age of the pigs at the time of experimental infection. In pigs infected at the age of 4 weeks, regeneration of the turbinates was noted 6 to 8 weeks after infection. When pigs were infected at 3 days of age, this process took 5 months (175).

Thus, the findings above strongly suggested that infection with *B. bronchiseptica* alone could not explain the disease, in particular, the severe lesions found in outbreaks of atrophic rhinitis.

The role of *P. multocida* was clarified after it was discovered that only a subset of *P. multocida* strains produced a heat-labile toxin (PMT) (96; M. F. de Jong, H. L. Oei, and G. J. Tetenburg, *Proc. 6th Int. Pig Vet. Soc. Congr.*, p. 211, 1980), and that only PMT-producing strains were able to cause irreversible turbinate atrophy in pigs (160, 161, 183). The etiological significance of toxin-producing *P. multocida* was confirmed by inoculation of pigs with cell extracts of toxin-producing *P. multocida* alone, either intranasally (96) or intraperitoneally (182), either of which reproduced the characteristic lesions of severe turbinate atrophy. The

role of PMT was confirmed when purified protein toxin was shown to induce the characteristic lesions after intranasal (44) or intraperitoneal (25) inoculation of gnotobiotic pigs. The ability of recombinant PMT to reproduce the signs of severe atrophic rhinitis was the final proof of the key role of PMT in the induced pathology (116).

These research findings strongly suggested that the severity and persistence of the changes that the two bacteria produced were different. *B. bronchiseptica* induced mild-to-moderate lesions that could regenerate by the time pigs reached slaughter weight, whereas toxigenic strains of *P. multocida* produced severe and irreversible turbinate atrophy. On these grounds, it was suggested that nonprogressive and progressive forms of atrophic rhinitis could be distinguished according to the principal etiological agents found (43).

The etiology of the disease is further complicated, however, by the poor capacity of *P. multocida* to colonize the intact nasal mucosa by itself. Rutter and Rojas (183) noticed only mild turbinate lesions in pigs infected with toxigenic *P. multocida* alone. This observation was confirmed by others (55, 100, 154). A productive *P. multocida* infection needs predisposing factors among which *B. bronchiseptica* preinfection is the most commonly recognized one. This interaction between the two pathogens classifies atrophic rhinitis as a member of the family of polymicrobial infections, and the disease will be reviewed with special attention to this aspect.

THE DISEASE

Clinical Signs

The clinical signs associated with atrophic rhinitis include sneezing; serous to mucopurulent nasal discharges; epistaxis; shortening and twisting of the snout; dark, crescent-shaped tear staining below the medial canthus of the eye; and reduced growth rates (181). Clinical signs usually become apparent from about 4 to 12 weeks of age onward (42). In severe outbreaks of the disease, all the signs above are seen in some pigs and some of the changes are present in others. However, most of these changes may be attributable to other factors as well, and the main pathognomonic sign is facial distortion because of disturbances in normal nasal bone development. The most common is brachygnathia superior, in which the upper jaw is shortened in relation to the lower, as a result of growth depression of the ossa nasales and maxillares. The skin and subcutis over the dorsum of the shortened snout are thrown into folds. When the disturbance of bone growth affects one side of the face more than the other, lateral deviation of the snout occurs. This facial deformity results from an underlying turbinate atrophy. With lateral deviation the atrophy is more pronounced on the side of the deviation. The prevalence of facial distortion varies among outbreaks, and visible turbinate atrophy is not accompanied with marked facial distortion in all pigs. Once turbinate atrophy has progressed into snout deformation, it does not resolve and the disease is chronic without causing serious mortality.

Pathological Changes

The dominant pathological lesion of atrophic rhinitis is an atrophy of the nasal turbinate bones as assessed by transverse section of the nasal cavity at the level of the first/second upper premolar teeth where the dorsal and ventral conchae are maximally developed in the normal pig (Fig. 1). The changes in the snout usually appear between 6 and 12 weeks of age of the pigs (181). In mild to moderate cases the ventral scrolls of the turbinates are the most commonly affected area; they vary from slightly shrunken to complete atrophy. In more severe cases, atrophy of the dorsal scrolls of the ventral turbinate and the dorsal and ethmoidal turbinates occurs. In the most severe form, all turbinate structures are completely absent. Lateral deviation of the nasal septum also is often observed. The very evident clinical signs of nasal atrophy have focused attention on this area. However, it is possible that pathology is also induced in other parts of the body, but has not been observed because it has not been looked for. For example, lesions have

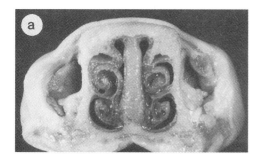

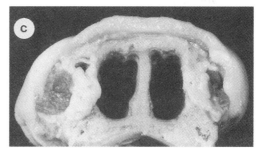

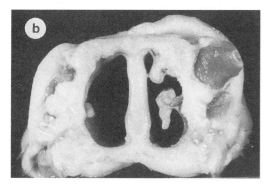

FIGURE 1 Cross-sections of snouts of 6-week-old pigs. (a) Uninfected pig showing normal anatomy of nasal structures. (b) Pig after infection with *B. bronchiseptica* and toxigenic *P. multocida*. The left dorsal turbinate is absent, and only a band of connective tissue remains from the left ventral turbinate. The right dorsal turbinate is slightly shrunken, and both scrolls of the right ventral turbinate show moderate atrophy. (c) Pig after infection with *B. bronchiseptica* and toxigenic *P. multocida*. There is complete absence of all turbinate structures accompanied with slight lateral deviation of the nasal septum.

been found in bladder epithelium during experimental infections (95).

Histopathology

Histopathological changes include hyperplasia and metaplasia of the nasal epithelium with the development of a stratified cuboidal type of cell, and marked thickening of the arterial walls in the lamina propria, with a dense infiltration of the submucosa with polymorphonuclear and mononuclear inflammatory cells. In severe cases, epithelial cells are disarranged and thrown into papillae or ridges and in some areas squamous cell metaplasia can be seen together with the loss of cilia from epithelial cells. Resorption of the osseous trabeculae of the turbinate bones also occurs, with replacement by a shrunken mass of fibrous tissue. Lesions in parenchymatous organs may also be present in cases of severe infection with toxigenic *P. multocida* (41, 180).

Parenteral injections with *P. multocida* toxin induced liver cirrhosis, renal failure, marked decrease of peripheral blood lymphocytes, and growth retardation (28; H. N. Becker, P. Reed, J. C. Woodard, and E. C. White, *Proc. 9th Int. Pig Vet. Soc. Congr.*, p. 249, 1986; P. R. Williams, R. M. Hall, and R. B. Rimler, *Proc. 9th Int. Pig Vet. Soc. Congr.*, p. 234, 1986). In addition, injection of PMT leads to gross proliferative changes that are discussed later.

Economic Importance

Atrophic rhinitis is thought to reduce growth rates, which makes it an economically important disease for pig producers (161). However, its economical importance has been variously estimated depending on whether a correlation was found between the presence of atrophic rhinitis and a reduction in growth rate (6, 102, 207, 208). Nevertheless, it is very likely that in moderate to severe outbreaks atrophic rhinitis can be of considerable economic importance (147, 163). An earlier proposal that severe turbinate atrophy predisposes pigs to pneumonia has not been confirmed (207, 208).

The picture is also not clear experimentally. Combined *B. bronchiseptica*-toxigenic *P. multocida* infection has frequently been found to reduce weight gain (51, 161, 162). Pedersen and Barfod (161, 162) reported that *B. bronchiseptica* infection, alone or in combination with nontoxigenic *P. multocida*, did not reduce weight gain, and concluded that toxigenic *P. multocida* was responsible for the impaired growth rate of the pigs. This view was supported by van Diemen et al. (220), who observed that lower weight gain in acetic acid-treated, *P. multocida*-infected pigs depended on the severity of the nasal lesions. Contrary to these findings, others have found reduced weight gain only in piglets infected with *B. bronchiseptica*, either alone or in combination with *P. multocida*, but not in the acetic acid-*P. multocida* challenge model (T. Magyar, V. L. King, and F. Kovács, submitted for publication).

Reduced growth rates may have several causes. Injection of toxin from *P. multocida* results in lower weight gains and may reflect a systemic effect of locally produced toxin. Alternatively, pigs with nasal damage may have a reduced food intake that could contribute to lower weight gains. Since PMT is known to affect several signal transduction pathways (see below), it is highly likely that it could have wide-ranging effects.

Treatment

Outbreaks of atrophic rhinitis can be treated by a combination of approaches. The overall goals of treatment are to reduce the prevalence of the etiological agents in young pigs by vaccination of the sow, medication of feed, and antibiotic treatment of piglets, and to manipulate housing and management circumstances to improve the overall environment for the pigs, which will reduce susceptibility to disease.

Antibiotic treatment can be given promptly to counteract an acute appearance of clinical atrophic rhinitis in a population and/or as a preventive measure when the risk of an outbreak is high. The sulfonamides were the first drugs applied successfully for the treatment of atrophic rhinitis (211), and are still widely used, either alone or in combination with other antibiotics, or potentiated with trimethoprim. In later surveys, most isolates of *B. bronchiseptica* of porcine origin proved to be sensitive to the tetracyclines

(166, 197). These drugs, especially their long-acting formulations, control bordetellosis in young pigs when administered via the parenteral route. The fluoroquinolones have also been recommended for porcine *B. bronchiseptica* (77). Most strains of *P. multocida* are sensitive to penicillin, tetracyclines, and chloramphenicol (197). Other antibiotics to which *P. multocida* may be sensitive, and that are frequently used against pasteurellosis, include penicillin-streptomycin, tylosin, lincomycin-spectinomycin, ampicillin, amoxicillin, spiramycin, quinolone derivatives, cephalosporins, and tiamulin. Their application for atrophic rhinitis, however, must be carefully balanced against the narrower antibiotic sensitivity pattern of *B. bronchiseptica*.

A general therapeutic strategy is to medicate the feed of the sow during the final month of gestation to reduce the infectious pressure transmitted to her offspring. In addition, suckling piglets can be medicated by carefully selected injections of antibiotics in therapeutic dosages four to eight times during the first 3 to 4 weeks of life. An interesting approach of specific treatment is the use of intranasal spraying of oxytetracycline in piglets (41).

It is generally accepted that atrophic rhinitis is associated with high population density in pig herds, poor hygiene, and poor management. Therefore, attention to these factors could help more specific measures in reducing of the prevalence of clinical disease and the damage caused by it.

Vaccination

Vaccination is widely used to try to reduce the prevalence of atrophic rhinitis in herds affected by the disease. Vaccination policy has evolved to reflect the prevailing opinion on the etiology of the disease. During the long period when *B. bronchiseptica* was regarded as the primary cause of progressive atrophic rhinitis, monovalent *B. bronchiseptica* vaccines were widely used. This type of vaccine was popular worldwide especially during the late 1970s and the 1980s. Although a reduction in the prevalence of clinical atrophic rhinitis was reported in several herds where the disease was endemic, considerable variations were reported (60). In the light of current knowledge, an effective *B. bronchiseptica* vaccine might be expected to reduce the severity of turbinate atrophy by (i) hindering colonization and subsequent turbinate damage caused by this pathogen and (ii) making circumstances less favorable for *P. multocida* colonization and so indirectly reducing the amount of *P. multocida* toxin present in the nasal cavity. On the other hand, it gives no protection against the activity of toxigenic *P. multocida*. Protection would be even less if other factors were responsible for enhancing toxigenic *P. multocida*. Thus, with the general acceptance of the polymicrobial nature of the disease, a modern vaccine is expected to provide protection against the harmful effect of both microorganisms. Most recently marketed atrophic rhinitis vaccines contain antigens from both *B. bronchiseptica* and *P. multocida*. Despite the detailed knowledge about the virulence determinants of *B. bronchiseptica*, this microbe is usually represented as a whole-cell bacterin. On the other hand, clarification of the crucial role of *P. multocida* toxin in the pathogenesis of progressive turbinate atrophy has resulted in the addition of purified, inactivated *P. multocida* toxin to the *B. bronchiseptica* component, either alone or in combination with whole-cell bacterins of toxigenic *P. multocida* strains of various serotypes.

Because of the view that *P. multocida* toxin might be the principal cause of atrophic rhinitis, monovalent PMT vaccines also appeared on the market. However, a monovalent *P. multocida* toxoid vaccine was less effective than a bivalent *B. bronchiseptica*-*P. multocida* vaccine when a severe *B. bronchiseptica*-*P. multocida* combined challenge was used (T. Magyar, F. Kovács, and K. K. Vestergaard-Nielsen, *Proc. 16th Int. Pig Vet. Soc. Congr.*, p. 479, 2000). This confirms the importance of *B. bronchiseptica* in atrophic rhinitis.

Some countries recommend immunization of sows complemented with vaccination of pigs. The immunization is intended to protect the piglets by the passive transfer of maternal antibodies. Sows are immunized twice during the first pregnancy, while a single vaccination is given before every subsequent farrowing. Vaccination of the pigs undoubtedly produces seroconversion, but its value is questionable because the infection exerts its main effects in younger animals. According to some reports, vaccination produced no differences in the prevalence or intensity of *B. bronchiseptica* infection, in the severity of clinical disease and turbinate atrophy in natural outbreaks (59), or in experimental infections (199). Some vaccine producers recommend the vaccination of piglets at 1 to 3 days of age, but no additional benefit was observed in a field study compared with immunization of sows alone (F. Kovács and T. Magyar, *Proc. 14th Int. Pig Vet. Soc. Congr.*, p. 254, 1996).

Prevention

Current vaccines only prevent the clinical manifestation of atrophic rhinitis; they do not exclude the causal agents from the herd. *B. bronchiseptica* is widely prevalent in the pig population. In addition, it is known to survive in natural waters (168), so its total eradication is not likely to be possible. Toxigenic *P. multocida* is less widely distributed in the pig population, and it may be possible to eliminate it from infected breeding farms after intensive vaccination for a period of more than 5 years (42). However, currently the only way to keep a herd free from the condition is the adoption of specific pathogen-free (SPF) conditions or a medicated and segregated early-weaning system (4), and the strict maintenance of an effective microbiological barrier based on a careful monitoring of the herds.

VIRULENCE DETERMINANTS EXPRESSED BY *B. BRONCHISEPTICA*

Bacterial species of the genus *Bordetella* are respiratory pathogens. *B. bronchiseptica* is widely distributed in nature. Besides turbinate atrophy and bronchopneumonia in swine, it causes respiratory disorders in a variety of other mammals, including dogs and rabbits (66), and an increasing number of cases in humans have also been reported (234). *B. pertussis* is the etiologic

agent of whooping cough, a respiratory disorder in humans, and is a close relative of *B. bronchiseptica*. The two bacteria have even been classified as a subspecies based on 23S RNA sequence comparison (150). Bordetellas express a variety of virulence factors (adhesins and toxins) that affect their interaction with the eukaryotic host and potentially with other bacteria. Intensive research has been conducted on the virulence determinants of *B. pertussis* and less on the other species. However, *B. bronchiseptica* shares most of its potential virulence factors with *B. pertussis* with the exception of pertussis toxin that is not expressed by *B. bronchiseptica*, so that research on *B. pertussis* has greatly helped us to understand *B. bronchiseptica*. For that reason some of what is described in this section refers to the properties of *B. pertussis*, but where possible we will describe the specific *B. bronchiseptica* virulence determinants.

Adhesion

Firm attachment to the target cell, a feature common to mucosal pathogens (8), is an essential prerequisite of colonization to avoid clearance by the flushing action of the cilia (mucociliary escalator). *B. bronchiseptica*, unlike *P. multocida*, seems to show a high affinity for attaching to the ciliated epithelial cells of the upper respiratory tract (29, 100, 133, 154, 235). Many *B. bronchiseptica* products, including fimbriae (pili), filamentous hemagglutinin (FHA), and pertactin, have been implicated as mediators of adhesion, although clarification of their exact role in colonization awaits further research.

FIMBRIAE

Yokomizo and Shimizu (235) first demonstrated that virulent porcine strains of *B. bronchiseptica* attached in vitro to the cilia of isolated nasal epithelial cells from pigs, whereas avirulent variants exhibited only weak adherence. With use of electron microscopy, hair-like fimbriae were shown to mediate the connection between the bacteria and the host tissue. Three different fimbrial subunit proteins were isolated from *B. bronchiseptica* (118), and postulated to have a role in the determination of host species specificity (21). More recently, *B. bronchiseptica* has been shown to express at least four fimbrial serotypes: Fim2, Fim3, FimX, and FimA, which are encoded by the *fim2, fim3, fimX,* and *fimA* genes, respectively (13, 187). Although these genes are unlinked on the chromosome, their protein products are assembled and secreted by a single apparatus encoded by the *fimBCD* locus (138). Mattoo et al. (138) constructed a Fim⁻ *B. bronchiseptica* mutant to assess the role of fimbriae in pathogenesis in vivo, and found that fimbriae increased the ability of *B. bronchiseptica* to establish tracheal colonization in rats. The number of bacteria recovered from the nasal cavity did not differ significantly between the mutant and the wild-type strain, indicating that site specificity may exist among the various adhesins and that fimbriae might not be involved in nasal colonization.

FILAMENTOUS HEMAGGLUTININ

Because of the frequent correlation between hemagglutinating activity and fimbriation of bacterial pathogens, hemagglutination assays have often been applied for the examination of bacterial adherence (158). Semjén and Magyar (194) showed that virulent isolates of *B. bronchiseptica* agglutinated red blood cells from several species including calf erythrocytes (calf-positive strains). Avirulent subcultures had lost their ability to agglutinate calf red blood cells but retained the rest of the original hemagglutination pattern (calf-negative strains). Calf-positive strains showed a considerable adherence to isolated swine nasal epithelial cells, while the calf-negative strains exhibited poor adherence. Thus, a bovine hemagglutinin of *B. bronchiseptica* may act as an adhesin. Ishikawa and Isayama (97) suggested that its receptor on mammalian cells was *N*-acetylneuraminic acid. With use of a sialic acid-specific lectin, a surface protein was purified that inhibited hemagglutinating activity for bovine erythrocytes (185). The purified protein had a molecular mass of approximately 200 kDa and appeared to be identical with *B. pertussis* FHA. This hemagglutinin inhibited the adherence of *B. bronchiseptica* to a rat cell line and acted as an adhesin.

FHA is regarded as the dominant attachment factor of *B. pertussis,* and is a primary component in acellular pertussis vaccines. Its biogenesis involves processing of a large precursor with a molecular mass of 367 kDa, which is modified at its N terminus (99) and cleaved at its C terminus (173) to form the mature 220-kDa FHA protein. FHA is produced and secreted at high levels by *B. pertussis* and at significantly lower levels by *B. bronchiseptica* strains (121), although a significant amount of FHA remains associated with the cell surface in *B. bronchiseptica* (173). FHA possesses at least three distinct attachment activities (128). One stimulates adherence to macrophages and possibly other leukocytes via CR3 integrins, another has a carbohydrate-binding site which mediates attachment to ciliated respiratory epithelial cells, and a third one displays a lectin-like activity for heparin, which can mediate adherence to nonciliated epithelial cells. The heparin-binding site is also required for FHA-mediated hemagglutination (141). Purified extracellular FHA binds both bacterial and host cell surfaces in vitro, suggesting that it may function as a bridge between the bacterium and the host (219). Moreover, it has been suggested that FHA is able to increase the adherence of other pathogens to the host (219). Such "piracy" of adhesins may enable bordetellas to interact with other respiratory pathogens and contribute to superinfection in mucosal diseases.

Comparison of a FHA⁻ knockout mutant with its parent strain in a rat respiratory model demonstrated that FHA is required for tracheal colonization (37). However, an ectopic FHA mutant strain that expressed only FHA, but not the other potential adhesins, failed to colonize, indicating that other factors are also required for tracheal colonization. Furthermore, the FHA⁻ mutant was still able to establish in the nasal cavity, suggesting again that a difference existed between nasal cavity and tracheal colonizations. This raises the possibility that *B. bronchiseptica* uses different adhesins for colonization at different anatomic sites.

PERTACTIN

P.68 pertactin is an outer membrane protein in *B. bronchiseptica,* so named because of its apparent molecular mass (144). The corresponding molecule produced by *B. pertussis* is P.69 pertactin (17, 27). Although P.69 pertactin has been demonstrated to be an agglutinogen (17), promoting adherence of *B. pertussis* to certain eukaryotic cells, probably via an Arg-Gly-Asp (RGD) motif (119, 120), the role of P.68 pertactin in adhesion of *B. bronchiseptica* to eukaryotic cells remains to be elucidated. *B. bronchiseptica,* formerly considered as an exclusively extracellular pathogen, can invade and persist intracellularly in a variety of eukaryotic cells, including phagocytes (7, 19, 52, 186, 190). Forde et al. (53) suggested that pertactin may have a role in promoting stable adhesion of *B. bronchiseptica* to macrophages.

The role of *B. bronchiseptica* pertactin in immunoprotection is more defined. Active or passive immunization of mice or piglets with pertactin preparations induces protective immunity against *B. bronchiseptica* infection (110, 144). A polymorphism in two repeated regions (designated regions 1 and 2) of the immunodominant epitopes of pertactin is believed to aid the bacterium in escaping from the immune responses of the host by displaying novel antigenic epitopes (14, 171).

The results summarized here suggest but do not prove the role of the various putative adhesins of *B. bronchiseptica* in the adhesion to the swine nasal epithelial cell, because most of the studies have tested nonporcine *B. bronchiseptica* isolates and have not been performed in pigs or on cells of porcine origin. Evidence that species and tissue specificity are likely to be important for *B. bronchiseptica* to infect and cause disease in pigs is increasing (30, 58, 152). Thus further studies are needed to confirm the role of various putative *Bordetella* adhesins in the pathogenesis of atrophic rhinitis.

Toxins

Bordetellas make several novel toxins. These include the tracheal cytotoxin and three protein toxins: adenylate cyclase toxin, dermonecrotic toxin (DNT), and, in the case of *B. pertussis,* pertussis toxin (PT).

ADENYLATE CYCLASE

The adenylate cyclase was discovered almost by chance in a *B. pertussis* vaccine preparation (232). Its appearance in the culture medium of growing bacteria marked it out from other bacterial adenylate cyclases and suggested that it could be a virulence determinant (83). Subsequent work showed that a substantial amount of the adenylate cyclase activity was located extracytoplasmically in the bacteria (85). A further, initially surprising finding was that the *Bordetella* adenylate cyclase was stimulated by the eukaryotic calcium-binding protein calmodulin (CaM) (233). The enzyme was also found in *B. bronchiseptica* (48), and later it was shown to be calmodulin dependent (114).

Transposon inactivation of the adenylate cyclase gene showed that it was essential for virulence in the mouse model (228), where it appeared to play a key role in colonization (67, 107). The adenylate cyclase can enter some cell types to raise cyclic AMP levels, which was might lead to "phagocyte impotence" as suggested (31). The invasive adenylate cyclase was shown to be a large molecule (78), although various other values for its molecular mass were published. This confusion was resolved when the *cya* gene was cloned, sequenced (62), and subsequently analyzed (63). The N terminus of the protein was enzymatically active and bound CaM. (This was the part found in the smaller adenylate cyclases that had been isolated.) The C-terminal part had striking homology to *Escherichia coli* hemolysin, a member of the RTX family of bacterial protein toxins. RTX toxins are pore-forming toxins that characteristically have flanking genes involved in the modification of the hemolytic protein and its transport from the bacteria. Homologous accessory genes were found in *Bordetella*

(63, 72). The domain of the adenylate cyclase that is homologous to RTX toxins provides the *Bordetella* hemolytic activity, but its main purpose appears to be to effect entry of the adenylate cyclase into host cells. The gene from *B. bronchiseptica* shows 98% identity to the *B. pertussis* gene (9).

The *Bordetella* adenylate cyclase is very active (233), and this probably explains its activation by CaM, which is a eukaryotic protein not found in bordetellas (233). The presence of such an active adenylate cyclase inside bordetellas might be detrimental to the regulation of gene function, although there appears to be no literature on *Bordetella* cyclic AMP-regulated genes, or might deplete ATP and be highly energy inefficient. The reliance on CaM ensures

that the enzyme is only active where needed, within a eukaryotic cell. This calmodulin sensitivity is similar to the other known toxic adenylate cyclase, that of *Bacillus anthracis* (124). Cyclic AMP is an important signaling molecule in eukaryotes (146, 214) which is produced in response to extracellular signals arriving at the cell membrane. These stimulate receptors coupled to the heterotrimeric G proteins G_i and G_s, which regulate the activity of membrane-bound adenylate cyclase. Cyclic AMP acts by binding to regulatory subunits of protein kinase A to stimulate release of the active enzyme, which has multiple effects within the cell (Fig. 2).

The *Bordetella* adenylate cyclase has caused macrophage apoptosis both in vitro (105) and

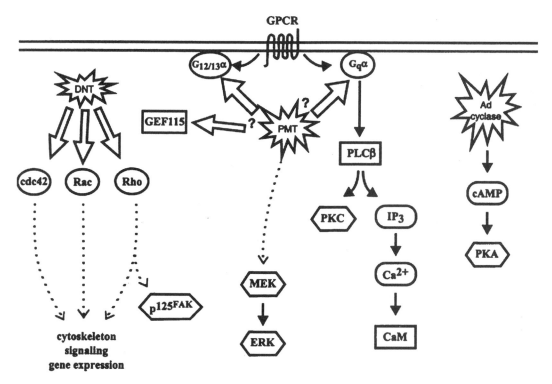

FIGURE 2 Diagram of some of the signal transduction pathways affected by the dermonecrotic (DNT) and adenylate cyclase (Ad cyclase) toxins from *B. bronchiseptica* and by the *P. multocida* toxin (PMT). Targets modified by the toxins are shown by open arrows. Direct interaction between molecules is shown by solid arrows, and interactions where the intervening components are either not shown or not known are indicated by dotted arrows. Abbreviations: GPCR, G-protein-coupled receptor; $G_q\alpha$ and $G_{12/13}\alpha$, the alpha subunits of the respective heterotrimeric G proteins; PKA, protein kinase A; cAMP, cyclic AMP; MEK, MAP kinase/extracellular signal-regulated kinase kinase; ERK, extracellular signal-regulated kinase.

in vivo (68), and also affects monocytes by modulating the tumor necrosis factor α and superoxide response (157). The toxin blocks phagocytosis by neutrophils (225). Very recently, the adenylate cyclase induced apoptosis in dendritic cells (B. P. Mahon, personal communication). In addition it has been shown that the adenylate cyclase affects platelet function by inhibiting their ability to aggregate, and this has had a direct effect on bleeding time in vivo (98). Similar experiments have been conducted with the B. bronchiseptica adenylate cyclase (80). Mutants with a nonpolar deletion in cyaA were as efficient as wild-type bacteria in killing macrophages, and this was attributed to the existence of type III delivered virulence factors. When this system was also mutated, the B. bronchiseptica adenylate cyclase was found to have a significant effect on killing. There was a minimal effect on bacterial colonization, but a significant effect on neutrophil infiltration and pathological damage.

Antibodies to the adenylate cyclase are protective, and it has been suggested that adenylate cyclase could be a valuable vaccine component (69, 84).

DERMONECROTIC TOXIN

DNT, or heat-labile toxin, was the first virulence factor to be identified in Bordetella (12). Its dermonecrotic nature was determined following subcutaneous injection (127). However, B. pertussis strains with a mutated DNT had 50% lethal doses (LD$_{50}$s) for mice that were identical to those of wild-type strains (226), suggesting that DNT is not essential for virulence. Similar observations were made with a naturally acquired DNT-negative B. bronchiseptica strain of porcine origin in both intravenously (131) and intracerebrally (123) inoculated mice. Nevertheless, DNT is found in all the Bordetella species where it is highly conserved (222), and it is regulated along with most of the other virulence genes by the bvg system (156, 227). Recently, there has been renewed interest in the toxin, as its mechanism of action has been identified. In addition, it has been clear for some time that

DNT from B. bronchiseptica has a role to play in atrophic rhinitis, as discussed later in this section.

DNT is a large intracellularly acting toxin that is taken up by target cells in a pH-dependent process (112). DNT acts on proteins of the Rho family (88, 92). These are small GTP-binding proteins that serve as molecular switches that interact with effector proteins when bound to GTP, but which contain an intrinsic GTPase and are inactive after hydrolysis of the GTP to GDP (174). They regulate many aspects of cellular function, including cytoskeletal organization and signaling pathways linked to gene expression and cell cycle progression. DNT appears to modify all members of the Rho family: Rho that is involved in stress fiber formation, Rac that regulates the appearance of membrane ruffling, and cdc42 that controls filopodia formation. DNT catalyzes either the deamidation (88) or transglutamination (137, 191) of glutamine 63 to inhibit the GTPase activity of the G protein. This results in its permanent activation, leading to the tyrosine phosphorylation and activation of the focal adhesion kinase (112), another key regulator of the cytoskeleton and intracellular signaling pathways. The equivalent modification induced by the E. coli cytotoxic necrotizing factor also leads via Rho to activation of the regulator of prostaglandin synthesis, COX-2 (216), and activation of the JNK via Rac or cdc42 (125), and it is likely that these effects will also occur with DNT. Since the Rho proteins have various effectors it is likely that cellular intoxication by DNT will lead to several sequelae (Fig. 2).

Cells treated with DNT display several morphological effects. Distinct membrane ruffling is observed, and the appearance of actin stress fibers and focal adhesions (92), linked to phosphorylation of the focal adhesion kinase (112). Quiescent resting cells are stimulated to enter the cell cycle and undergo DNA synthesis, but cytokinesis is blocked (89). All such effects can be attributed to activation of Rho proteins, since no evidence of activation of other signaling pathways exists (112).

Purification of DNT has proved to be difficult (238), and the field has been advanced most rapidly by the application of molecular biology. The gene sequence for DNT was first identified in *B. pertussis* (222), although expression of a recombinant DNT was first produced from *B. bronchiseptica* (170). The two proteins are practically identical. The start of the DNT sequence does not have a signal sequence, and there are no known accessory proteins that might aid secretion. Although it is possible that a novel mechanism for secretion exists, all available evidence suggests that DNT is only released on bacterial cell lysis (38, 153), and that DNT is released by dying bacterial cells to aid the remaining bacteria in an infection.

Intracellularly acting toxins often have two or three separate domains that mediate binding to the target cell, translocation of the enzymatically active part of the toxin across the membrane, and a catalytic domain (145). The only sequence homology to other proteins is in the C-terminal region of DNT to a similar region of cytotoxic necrotizing factor (222). This region is the catalytic site of both toxins, while the N-terminal regions of the proteins encode cell-binding and uptake functions (103, 122).

The role of DNT in bordetellosis remains elusive, in part, because its presence does not affect the LD_{50} of bordetellas for mice (226). However, the mouse is an unsatisfactory model for whooping cough (106, 159). In addition, DNT is produced by all *Bordetella* species and its expression is regulated like other virulence determinants (227). It also has a potent and specific activity. It is likely that DNT plays a subtle role, perhaps affecting bacterial clearance or immunity both to *Bordetella* and other pathogens. The ability of DNT to suppress immune function might be expected for a toxin that interferes with the normal functions of Rho proteins. Such effects would facilitate the secondary infection that is usually found in *Bordetella* disease. In addition DNT has a direct effect on bone formation as is discussed later. Thus, most observers now believe

that DNT has an important but undefined role in pathogenesis.

The importance of DNT in the pathogenesis of turbinate atrophy in pigs is more clearly established. This property of DNT was first suspected when Hanada et al. (76) showed that repeated intranasal inoculation of piglets with cell-free sonicated extracts from virulent *B. bronchiseptica* that contained high levels of DNT could produce nasal lesions similar to those seen in naturally occurring atrophic rhinitis. This view was supported by the comparison of a naturally acquired DNT− strain of porcine origin to a DNT+ strain also of porcine origin (131, 132). The mutant showed a similar production of adenylate cyclase-hemolysin and at least one adhesin (132). It exerted identical virulence in mice and colonized the nasal cavity of gnotobiotic pigs in a number comparable with the DNT+ strain, but only pigs infected with the latter strain developed turbinate atrophy. The slight possibility that other unknown differences between the strains could have been responsible for turbinate atrophy has been addressed by the use of genetically constructed isogenic DNT− strains. The parent and the mutant strains of *B. bronchiseptica* each possessed similar virulence for mice (134), but turbinate atrophy was only observed in pigs infected with the DNT+ strain, and not in those infected with the DNT− strain (S. L. Brockmeier, K. B. Register, T. Magyar, A. J. Lax, G. D. Pullinger, and R. A. Kunkle, submitted for publication). These data strongly suggest that DNT is required for the induction of turbinate atrophy in pigs that is linked to *B. bronchiseptica* infection.

TRACHEAL CYTOTOXIN

The production of tracheal cytotoxin is a common characteristic of *Bordetella* species (32, 64). Tracheal cytotoxin is a disaccharide-tetrapeptide derivative of the peptidoglycan layer of the cell wall that both structurally and functionally falls into the muramyl peptide family. Unlike most other gram-negative bacteria, *B. pertussis* releases a large amount of this glycopeptide into the culture supernatant, usually during log-phase growth (32). Exposure to purified tracheal cytotoxin specifically damages ciliated epithelial cells, causing ciliostasis and extrusion of these cells (33, 64, 65). It has been demonstrated in hamster trachea epithelial cells that the lactyl tetrapeptide portion of the molecule is responsible for its full toxic activity (130). Tracheal cytotoxin also has a toxic effect on other cells, impairing neutrophil function at low concentrations with toxicity found in larger quantities (40). The toxicity conferred by tracheal cytotoxin is caused by the induction of interleukin-1 in host cells (82), which activates host cell nitric oxide synthase leading to high levels of nitric oxide (NO) radicals (81). NO destroys iron-dependent enzymes, eventually inhibiting mitochondrial function and DNA synthesis in nearby host cells (82). The role of *B. bronchiseptica* tracheal cytotoxin has not been examined in detail. Dugal et al. (45) reported that a heat-stable substance of low molecular weight produced by *B. bronchiseptica,* possibly the tracheal cytotoxin, could induce ciliostasis of the tracheal epithelium with a concomitant accumulation of mucus.

Virulence Proteins Delivered by a Type III Secretion System

Type III secretion systems have been found in several gram-negative bacterial species, including bordetellas. This enables transfer of a set of bacterial proteins across the bacterial and the eukaryotic cell membranes, and thus facilitates the delivery of virulence factors directly into target cells. These systems consist of a secretion apparatus and an array of proteins released by this apparatus (34, 230). Yuk et al. (236) reported the presence of a cluster of type III secretion genes (*bscIJKLNO*), and demonstrated that the *bvg* locus regulated expression of *bscN* that is presumed to be involved in providing energy for type III secretion. Mutation of *bscN* led to several phenotypic alterations, including decreased cytotoxicity toward cultured cell lines, implicating *Bordetella* type III secretion in pathogenicity. *bscN*-mediated secretion is required for persistent colonization of the tra-

chea in a rat infection model. Further observations suggested that type III-secreted products of *B. bronchiseptica* interact with components of both innate and adaptive immune systems of the host (237). The mutants elicited higher titers of anti-*Bordetella* antibodies upon infection compared with wild-type bacteria. Type III secretion mutants also showed increased lethality in immunodeficient mice. Furthermore, *B. bronchiseptica* induced apoptosis in macrophages in vitro and inflammatory cells in vivo, and type III secretion was required for this process. At the same time, Winstanley et al. (231), examining *B. bronchiseptica* isolates from dogs and cats, found no correlation between the presence of type III secretion genes and the severity of respiratory disease and concluded that different clinical manifestations may be due to variations in gene expression or host factors, rather than the absence or presence of type III secretion genes.

The Regulation of *Bordetella* Virulence Determinants

Early experimentation with bordetellas showed that the main virulence characteristics were regulated in two ways: first, by an apparently irreversible phase shift in which virulence was rapidly lost upon repeated subculture (126), and second, by antigenic modulation whereby these characteristics could be reversibly controlled. The switch between the antigenic modes could be triggered by the addition of different salts or by cultivation at lower temperatures (113), or by nicotinic acid (192). *B. bronchiseptica* has a similar mechanism (155). The two switches are linked, with the loss of virulence on subculture resulting from in vitro selection of an infrequent mutation (114). This mutation occurs in a global regulator locus (*bvgAS*) that responds to environmental conditions (143, 206). The BvgAS regulatory system has been comprehensively reviewed (11, 36, 189, 198). A region of six cytosine bases at the promoter is clearly vulnerable to replication error, and insertional frameshift mutations have been identified in this locus (206), which would give the opportunity for reversion to the virulent phase. The *bvgAS* genes constitute a His-Asp phosphorelay relay system that regulates a wide variety of virulence determinants. Transcription of the *bvgAS* genes is controlled by four promoters, three of which are *bvg*-regulated. BvgS is a membrane-located histidine kinase. It is not known what signals BvgS responds to in vivo, although temperature is one possibility. BvgA is aspartic acid phosphorylated by BvgS and is a transcriptional activator that binds to the promoter elements of the regulated genes (177). It is interesting that the FHA gene is activated several hours prior to activation of toxin genes due to the differing affinities of phosphorylated BvgA for the respective promoter elements (188), implying that adhesion takes place before aggressins are expressed.

The BvgAS system regulates all elements of adhesion (FHA, pertactin, and fimbriae) and the dermonecrotic and adenylate cyclase toxins as well as the type III secretion system (Fig. 3); tracheal cytotoxin is not regulated by Bvg. In addition, several genes are repressed in the Bvg+ mode, the so-called *vrg* or *bvg*-repressed genes (109). These include motility (3) and the urease gene in *B. bronchiseptica* (140). The in vivo role of the *vrg* genes is unclear, as indeed is the role of *bvg* modulation. The various possibilities are discussed in some depth by Bock and Gross (11), who point out that *B. bronchiseptica* and *B. pertussis* express quite different *vrg* genes, and also that these genes, and *bvg*-mediated modulation, may either have a role

in environmental growth or in some as-yet not-understood aspect of pathogenesis. *B. bronchiseptica,* among the *Bordetella* species, is able to survive and even grow, among nutrient-poor circumstances, and at a temperature as low as 10°C (167, 168). Cotter and Miller (35) demonstrated that the Bvg− phase is advantageous for persistence under nutrient-limiting conditions compared with the Bvg+ phase. Furthermore, modulated *B. bronchiseptica* showed enhanced adhesion to ciliated porcine nasal epithelial cells in vitro (172) and gave increased colonization of the rat nasal cavity (18). *B. bronchiseptica* may have an environmental phase where the *bvg*-regulated virulence factors are redundant and not produced. At the same time, the increased adhesive ability coupled to reduced expression of virulence at reduced temperature might be beneficial for establishment in a host species and evasion of host defenses. In particular, this could lead to the establishment of a chronic infection. However, identification and characterization of the presumed adhesin and a better understanding of the potential role of modulated or phase-locked strains in vivo would be required to prove this hypothesis.

VIRULENCE DETERMINANTS EXPRESSED BY *P. MULTOCIDA*

P. multocida was one of the first bacteria to be linked to disease and then tamed by a vaccine, in Louis Pasteur's seminal work in 1881. Since

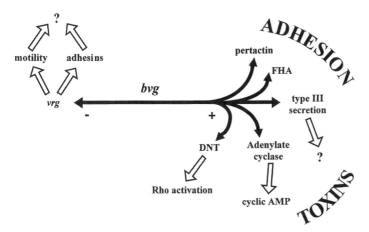

FIGURE 3 Diagram of some of the potential virulence determinants regulated by the *bvg* genes in *Bordetella* species. Abbreviations: *bvg, Bordetella* virulence gene; *vrg, vir (bvg)*-repressed gene; FHA, filamentous hemagglutinin.

then surprisingly little has been learned about its virulence. *P. multocida* causes two serious animal diseases in the developing world: fowl cholera and hemorrhagic septicemia in cattle. In the West, it is a major determinant of atrophic rhinitis in pigs and is the most common cause of infection in wounds inflicted by dogs and cats. Resurgent interest in this bacterium has led to new developments which should greatly aid further analysis of virulence, namely the publication of the complete genome sequence of an avian strain of *P. multocida* (139) and the application of signature-tagged mutagenesis to identify in vivo expressed genes that are likely to be important in pathogenesis (56). Nevertheless, the best understood virulence determinant in *P. multocida* is still the dermonecrotic toxin. This virulence factor is only found in a limited set of strains, mainly of porcine origin. Since this is of crucial importance in the disease of atrophic rhinitis, we discuss it in some detail.

The Effects of *P. multocida* Toxin

The discovery of PMT is linked to atrophic rhinitis research. The early suggestion of a role for *P. multocida* (71) was confused by the difficulty in correlating *P. multocida* presence with disease in the field, and resolved by the discovery that only some strains produced a toxin. Intraperitoneal injection of crude or partially purified extracts from toxigenic *P. multocida,* or purified recombinant PMT, also induced hyperplastic changes in the liver and urinary tract (25, 116, 182). This led to work using cultured fibroblast cells that defined its function in cells. The way that PMT acts on cells has been reviewed recently (115).

PMT has a novel mode of action and acts as a very effective mitogen, or growth promoter. PMT stimulates quiescent nongrowing Swiss 3T3 cells to undergo DNA synthesis and subsequent mitosis at low picomolar concentrations (178). It can also induce anchorage-independent growth in Rat-1 cells (86). PMT is extremely potent; it induces DNA synthesis equivalent to stimulation by 10% serum and is active at a far lower concentration than known growth factors such as platelet-derived growth factor, or neuropeptides such as bombesin. Like other toxins, PMT affects the regulation of intracellular signaling pathways. However, it targets a different set of signaling pathways from any other toxin.

PMT stimulates signaling cascades linked to phospholipase C (PLC). PMT action activates PLC to generate cellular diacylglycerol and inositol 1,4,5-trisphosphate (IP_3). The former leads to the membrane recruitment and activation of protein kinase C (PKC), which in turn leads to phosphorylation of the MARCKS/80K protein and other targets (203). IP_3 binds to receptors on calcium stores to induce the release of calcium (204). The released calcium binds to and activates effector proteins, most notably CaM. There is considerable evidence that PMT activates the PLCβ isoform of PLC via activation of the heterotrimeric G protein G_q, which is usually activated by membrane-spanning receptors. Murphy and Rozengurt (151) first suggested that PMT and bombesin might share a common mechanism. Direct evidence for G-protein activation was provided by using nucleotide analogues (151), and injection of cells with antibodies against G_q or G_q antisense cDNA that specifically blocked a PMT response (229). Similarly, antibodies against PLCβ1 blocked PMT action. Recently, Zywietz et al. (239) have added PMT to cell lines deficient in the α subunits of either G_q or G_{11} (two closely related members of the G_q family), or both, and shown that G_q but not G_{11} is involved in PMT-mediated stimulation of inositols. PMT action does not affect cyclic AMP concentration (178) suggesting that neither the G_s nor the G_i protein is targeted. PMT indirectly activates the mitogen-activated protein (MAP) kinases ERK1 and ERK2 (112). Activation is G_q dependent but PKC independent in HEK 293 cells (195).

PMT also stimulates signaling pathways linked to the cytoskeleton (111). The toxin induces actin stress fiber formation and assembly of focal contacts, leading to tyrosine phosphorylation of the focal adhesion kinase p125[FAK]. These changes are brought about by a signal transduction pathway that involves the Rho family of small GTPases (111), and which still functions in G_q-deficient cells (239). Rho is known to transmit signals through several effector kinases. The Rho kinase (ROK) is involved in p125^{FAK} activation (215). The details of the pathway linking ROK to actin stress fiber formation are known (202). In endothelial cells PMT induces an increase in cellular permeability and cytoskeletal rearrangements via the Rho/ROK pathway (49), which may explain some of the induced pathology. PMT action leads to phosphorylation of p125^{FAK} at the autophosphorylation site, Tyr^{397}, a high-affinity binding site for the Src kinase, resulting in association of p125^{FAK} with Src and its subsequent prolonged activation (215). These two tyrosine kinases each phosphorylate multiple substrates and promote proliferation (10, 223). A summary of the signaling pathways stimulated by PMT is shown in Fig. 2.

PMT is an intracellularly acting toxin (178) that undergoes a significant structural transition at about pH6 (200, 201). Such a transition might be functionally important for membrane translocation, as in other intracellularly acting toxins. PMT is thought to bind to ganglioside receptors on the cell surface, and may enter cells via non–clathrin-coated pits (165), but little is known about its uptake or possible processing. Toxin binding and cell entry are unlikely in themselves to lead to any cellular effects, since a PMT molecule with a cysteine-to-serine substitution at position 1165 near the C terminus showed no loss of structural integrity (224) and could bind to and enter cells (M. R. Baldwin and A. J. Lax, unpublished data), but was totally inactive including toxicity in animals (224). PMT is a large (146-kDa) protein (117, 164), and analysis of its protein sequence has provided valuable clues about function. A hydrophobic region near its N terminus is predicted to be helical (169). These properties are typical of a transmembrane region, and this region shows significant homology to the transmembrane region of the cytotoxic necrotizing factor (122). Recently, introduction of expressed C-terminal fragments into cells has been shown to induce DNA synthesis (22, 169). Addition of a large excess of N-terminal fragments blocked the activity of added wild-type toxin, indicating that the cell-binding domain is in this region (169).

The molecular target for PMT is not currently known, although the heterotrimeric G-protein G_q is one possible target. There is clear evidence that it is activated (151, 229, 239), and the observation that G_q but not the closely related G_{11} is involved in the PMT response (239) implies that activation involves an event that is specific for G_q. Since Rho protein activation by PMT is independent of PKC or Ca and does not require functional G_q (111, 239), G_q cannot be the sole target for PMT. Rho can be activated by several routes, and more than one may be involved. The heterotrimeric G-protein family G_{12}, which comprises G_{12} and G_{13}, signals to Rho via activation of a guanine nucleotide exchange factor, GEF115, to promote GTP binding to Rho and its subsequent activation (135). Alternatively, phosphoinositol 3-kinase interacts with G-proteins and can also activate Rho (23). Prolonged activation of such targets could explain all the observed effects (see also Fig. 2). The chemical modification induced by PMT has not been identified.

Regulation of PMT Expression

It was initially thought that a region upstream of the PMT gene was involved in negative regulation of its expression (164), but this turned out not to be the case (94). Further analysis of likely modulators of expression in vitro failed to identify any evidence of regulation (94), although it is entirely possible that regulation might occur in vivo.

ATROPHIC RHINITIS AND BONE METABOLISM

Bone is a complex tissue that is subject to constant remodeling throughout life. The two major cell types that comprise bone are osteoblasts, which form bone, and multinucleated osteoclasts, which are responsible for bone resorption. These cells are derived from different lineages: osteoblasts from mesenchymal stem cells, and osteoclasts from the monocyte/macrophage lineage (209). Various markers can be used to identify these cells and assess the stage of differentiation. Bone formation and resorption are known to be tightly coupled, and it appears that most systemic signals that regulate this process (e.g., hormones, growth factors, and cytokines) target osteoblasts, which in turn release signaling molecules that regulate control osteoclast differentiation and activity (209).

Bacterial Toxins and Bone Remodeling

It is clear that DNT from *B. bronchiseptica* and PMT from *P. multocida* have effects on bone metabolism. These have been investigated at various levels: (i) in the whole animal, primarily in the pig, but also some work in the mouse model; (ii) in bone explants; and (iii) in isolated cells. What happens in the experimental animal is most relevant to disease in the field, but it is impossible to analyze the molecular and cellular interactions in any detail. On the other hand, although working with isolated cells permits such analysis, it is not always possible to reproduce the in vivo situation. While early work used live bacterial infection, more recent work utilized bacterial extracts or purified toxins. There has been a much more thorough investigation of the effects of PMT than of DNT, partly because PMT is perceived as the main pathogenic factor in atrophic rhinitis and partly because it is more accessible experimentally.

B. BRONCHISEPTICA DNT AND BONE RESORPTION

The pig infection experiments with DNT-negative strains of *B. bronchiseptica* described above showed that DNT could cause bone resorption (132, 134). Injection of rats with a sublethal dose of purified DNT led to necrosis of periosteal cells and osteoblasts in calvaria and a severe reduction in bone matrix synthesis (91). DNT treatment of an osteoblast-like cell line inhibited the increase in the osteoblast marker alkaline phosphatase, suggesting that it blocked differentiation (90). It has not been established which of the Rho family proteins were responsible for these effects. It is also not known whether DNT acts directly on osteoclasts.

P. MULTOCIDA PMT AND BONE RESORPTION

In experimental animals injection of PMT at a low concentration, below the lethal level of about 1 μg kg of body weight^{-1}, leads to bone loss (116). It can also lead to proliferation in bladder and ureter epithelium (116, 182), as can experimental infection (95), but it is not known if such effects are found in naturally occurring atrophic rhinitis. Intraperitoneal injection of PMT leads to substantial liver and kidney damage, but it is unclear whether this is related to its mitogenic properties. The C1165S nonmitogenic mutant is completely nontoxic when injected at more than 1,000 times a lethal dose (224), supporting the notion that PMT has only one activity. Studies using in vitro organ culture models found that PMT induced bone resorption (50, 108, 205), but it was not clear whether PMT induced bone loss in pigs via the osteoblast and/or osteoclast.

PMT is a potent mitogen for primary osteoblasts (148; D. Harmey, A. J. Lax, and A. E. Grigoriadis, unpublished observation). PMT treatment leads to reduced alkaline phosphatase activity in osteoblast-like cells (148, 205) and also in primary osteoblasts (148). PMT also inhibits the ability of preosteoblasts to form mineralized nodules (70). It induces cytoskeletal rearrangements in these cells, thus highlighting the potential role of Rho family proteins in osteoblast differentiation and bone formation. We have recently analyzed this process in more detail and shown that PMT inhibits the differentiation of primary mouse osteoblast progenitor cells to fully differentiated bone nodules in vitro with a defined time window where cells are particularly sensitive to PMT (Harmey et al., unpublished). In addition, we have shown that PMT inhibits the expression of the osteoblast-specific marker genes alkaline phosphatase, Cbfa-1, and osteocalcin.

The effect on osteoclasts is less clear. Although it is generally accepted that osteoclast activity changes following PMT treatment, it is not clear whether this a direct effect of PMT on osteoclasts or via signals released by stimulated osteoblasts. There are data to support the latter view (149), though it is possible that both mechanisms are involved. Furthermore some studies have indicated that PMT leads to an increase in osteoclast activity (70, 101, 108, 136), whereas at least one other study suggests that PMT inhibits osteoclast function (1).

Thus, clearly there is much still to be done to unravel the mechanism of PMT-induced bone loss, not only in terms of defining the target cell involved, but also in identifying the molecular mechanisms involved in the osteoblast/osteoclast intercellular signaling.

THE INTERACTION BETWEEN B. BRONCHISEPTICA AND P. MULTOCIDA

There are three crucial stages in the pathogenesis of most infectious diseases: the pathogens must overcome the specific and nonspecific defense mechanisms of the host; they have to establish and multiply in or on the target tissue; and finally they should produce toxic or other harmful factors which are responsible, directly or indirectly, for the clinical signs of disease. As shown in this section, *B. bronchiseptica* and *P. multocida,* the two etiological agents of atrophic rhinitis, may share the tasks of fulfilling these stages.

Harris and Switzer (79) first reported that a type-D isolate of *P. multocida* failed to colonize the nasal cavity of pigs, but established and persisted if the animals had been previously infected with *B. bronchiseptica.* Since then it has been clearly established that toxigenic *P. multocida* needs some predisposing factor to colonize the nasal cavity in sufficient numbers to cause irreversible atrophy of the turbinate bones (161, 183). Gnotobiotic pigs infected with toxigenic *P. multocida* alone were colonized poorly, and only slight turbinate damage

was seen at slaughter, whereas in mixed infections with *B. bronchiseptica* and toxigenic *P. multocida* colonization by large numbers of *P. multocida* occurred and severe disease was produced (183). Other predisposing agents have also been discovered. Intranasal pretreatment with dilute acetic acid was found to successfully enhance colonization by toxigenic *P. multocida* in experimentally infected pigs (160). Histological changes were not detected in the nasal cavity 6 days after acetic acid treatment, and it was reported that acetic acid caused only transient modification of the nasal respiratory epithelium resulting in stagnation of the nasal mucus, which was presumed to make the nasal environment favorable to colonization by *P. multocida* (57). Aerial pollutants (e.g., dust and gaseous ammonia) can also contribute to the severity of lesions associated with atrophic rhinitis by facilitating colonization of the pig's upper respiratory tract by *P. multocida* (73–75). On the other hand, others did not find significant differences in the extent or frequency of conchal atrophy between ammonia-exposed pigs and controls, or in the frequency of isolation of toxigenic *P. multocida* from conchae and tonsils (5). In conclusion, *B. bronchiseptica,* which is highly prevalent in the pig population, still seems to be the most important predisposing factor, although other factors like chemical irritants and dust may also exacerbate the disease.

The ability of *B. bronchiseptica* to encourage *P. multocida* establishment and growth could result from a direct effect on colonization, by promoting direct bacterium-bacterium interaction to aid attachment, or by the induction of host damage that could lead to either enhanced binding or improved nutrient acquisition. Alternatively *B. bronchiseptica* infection could impair host response mechanisms, leading to better *P. multocida* colonization. There is currently insufficient information available to establish how many of these putative mechanisms operate, but there is evidence that several are involved.

Although the exact role for the array of putative adhesins expressed by *B. bronchiseptica* has not yet been clarified, it is clearly established that *B. bronchiseptica* has an outstanding capacity to attach firmly to nasal epithelial cells (235) and generate profound ultrastructural changes in the nasal mucosa (46). Tracheal rings either infected with *B. bronchiseptica* or treated with a cell-free *B. bronchiseptica* supernatant were reported to enhance *P. multocida* adherence, with the suggestion that tracheal cytotoxin was the important factor (45). Similarly, filtered supernatants of *B. bronchiseptica* sonicates enhanced *P. multocida* colonization in vivo (2). A further possible attachment mechanism is the so-called piracy of adhesins where pretreatment of ciliated cells or pathogenic bacteria with FHA can promote adherence to cilia in vitro and in vivo (219). Since *P. multocida* attaches poorly to nasal epithelial cells, utilization of extracellular FHA produced by *B. bronchiseptica* could contribute to its establishment in the nasal cavity, although this hypothesis needs further investigation. In summary, these observations suggest that *B. bronchiseptica* directly enhances *P. multocida* attachment.

The role of the *B. bronchiseptica* DNT in *P. multocida* colonization has been analyzed in some detail. Nasal colonization of pigs by *P. multocida* was substantially increased (by a factor of $>10^4$ CFU) by prior treatment with *B. bronchiseptica* (183) and resulted in an infection that persisted. A naturally occurring porcine isolate of *B. bronchiseptica* which did not produce DNT was compared with a wild-type strain for its ability to colonize and also to aid *P. multocida* colonization (26, 132). Later experiments used isogenic *dnt* mutant strains of *B. bronchiseptica* strains (134; Brockmeier et al., submitted). In all infection experiments using DNT-negative strains *P. multocida* colonized to lower levels (between 10- and 100-fold less) and declined after several days. An avirulent (Bvg−) variant of *B. bronchiseptica* was poorer at promoting *P. multocida* colonization than the *dnt* mutant strains (132). These results strongly suggest that DNT is the key factor that creates conditions in the nasal cavity most favorable for persistent colonization by large numbers of toxigenic *P. multocida*. Furthermore, these findings indicate

that other virulence determinants produced by virulent strains of *B. bronchiseptica* may assist the growth of *P. multocida* in the nasal cavity but to a lesser extent than DNT.

It has not been shown whether DNT enhances *P. multocida* colonization by causing local tissue damage or by affecting immune function, though both mechanisms are likely to play a role. Lesions in the nasal cavity induced by monoinfection of pigs with DNT producing *B. bronchiseptica*, namely, severe hyperplasia and dysplasia of the epithelium, squamous cell metaplasia, loss of cilia from epithelial cells, marked fibrosis of the lamina propria, and a mild to moderate resorption of bone, are not seen in infections with the DNT-negative strain (132). It is unknown which, if any, of these histopathological changes might promote colonization by toxigenic *P. multocida*. In addition the specific cellular effect of DNT on Rho function has been shown to paralyze immune cells (87, 159; Mahon, personal communication) and this is likely to be important in the disease. The *Bordetella* factors responsible for the enhancement of *P. multocida* growth in the absence of DNT have not been investigated. However one distinct possibility is that released adenylate cyclase could enhance *P. multocida* colonization given its well characterized effect on immune function. Tracheal cytotoxin and type III secretion products might also assist in the establishment of *P. multocida* through impairing ciliary activity and the immune reaction of the host, respectively.

The enhancement of colonization occurs in both directions, since it is also clear that *P. multocida* colonization can boost colonization by *B. bronchiseptica* (180). It is known that PMT treatment can decrease the antibody response to bystander antigens (221). Indeed it appears that the combined action of *B. bronchiseptica* DNT and PMT creates conditions favorable to the growth of both bacteria, which are not reproduced by the action of either toxin alone. Three key observations support this hypothesis. First, in *P. multocida* infected pigs the wild-type strain of *B. bronchiseptica* colonized in greater numbers than the DNT-negative strain, although they colonized in similar numbers when given as single infections (132). Furthermore, there was no difference in colonization by the DNT-negative strain of *B. bronchiseptica* in single infections or in combined infections with toxigenic *P. multocida*. This suggests that the enhanced colonization of *B. bronchiseptica* in pigs infected with *P. multocida* depended on the presence of the *B. bronchiseptica* DNT. Second, infection with toxigenic but not with nontoxigenic *P. multocida* enhanced the growth of *B. bronchiseptica* (180). Conversely, colonization by a nontoxigenic strain of *P. multocida* was increased only marginally in *B. bronchiseptica* infected pigs, whereas the growth of a toxigenic strain of *P. multocida* was greatly enhanced (183). This suggests that it is PMT which increased the growth of *B. bronchiseptica* and that the enhanced growth of *P. multocida* in *B. bronchiseptica*-infected pigs depends on the presence of PMT. Finally, in pigs pretreated intranasally with dilute acetic acid, toxigenic *P. multocida* colonized briefly in numbers as great as those seen in combined infections with *B. bronchiseptica* before declining abruptly, although the importance of PMT in promoting *P. multocida* colonization was emphasized by the observation that colonization was less if PMT was blocked by antibody (24). The damage in the turbinates of such pigs was as great as in combined infections, yet clearly the induced pathology did not permit continued colonization by *P. multocida* in large numbers. In summary, damage from PMT does not by itself support the growth of large numbers of *P. multocida* but does enhance colonization by *B. bronchiseptica* so long as DNT is also present. Conversely, colonization by *P. multocida* is increased in *B. bronchiseptica* infected pigs as long as the strain of *P. multocida* is toxigenic.

Finally, do the two bacteria synergize to produce turbinate damage and the other pathology that is seen in this disease? The degree of turbinate bone loss in mixed infection experiments seemed to correlate with the numbers of *P. multocida* present and by inference with the likely quantity of PMT released (26), and it is known that PMT alone can reproduce the severe loss of turbinate bone that characterizes the disease (44, 96, 116, 182). It remains unclear whether *Bordetella* DNT synergizes with PMT to lead to greater bone destruction, or other pathological changes. While DNT directly targets and activates proteins of the Rho family by chemical modification, PMT is likely to activate Rho more indirectly, and thus perhaps more transiently. In addition PMT affects other cell-signaling pathways. The analysis of potential synergistic reactions could best be tackled in vitro using purified toxins, and this has yet to be performed.

CONCLUSION

The question remains: what is atrophic rhinitis? The generally accepted most important signs of the disease are severe and persistent turbinate atrophy, snout deformation, and, perhaps more controversially, reduced growth rate. At the present stage of our knowledge, PMT seems to play a dominant role in developing these characteristic lesions, and so toxigenic *P. multocida* is considered to be the primary etiological agent of atrophic rhinitis. On the other hand, a substantial body of evidence shows that *P. multocida* is unable to fulfill its role without predisposing circumstances, a set of imprecisely determined changes to the nasal mucosa that creates a niche suitable for the establishment of this pathogen. From this point of view, atrophic rhinitis could be defined as a multifactorial disease because several factors seem able to assist colonization of the host by sufficient numbers of *P. multocida*. It could even be classed as an opportunistic pathogen. However, the specific synergistic interactions between *B. bronchiseptica* and *P. multocida* support the notion that it is a genuine polymicrobial disease, which in addition may serve as a useful model system for more complex mixed infections. Nevertheless, even for this relatively simple polymicrobial disease, further research is clearly necessary to achieve a deeper understanding of the molecular interactions involved, which, in turn, may lead to novel therapeutic approaches.

REFERENCES

1. **Ackermann, M. R., D. A. Adams, L. L. Gerken, M. J. Beckman, and R. B. Rimler.** 1993. Purified *Pasteurella multocida* protein toxin reduces acid phosphatase-positive osteoclasts in the ventral nasal concha of gnotobiotic pigs. *Calcif. Tissue Int.* **52**:455–459.

2. **Ackermann, M. R., R. B. Rimler, and J. R. Thurston.** 1991. Experimental model of atrophic rhinitis in gnotobiotic pigs. *Infect. Immun.* **59**:3626–3629.

3. **Akerley, B. J., D. M. Monack, S. Falkow, and J. F. Miller.** 1992. The *bvgAS* locus negatively controls motility and synthesis of flagella in *Bordetella bronchiseptica. J. Bacteriol.* **174**:980–990.

4. **Alexander, T. J. L., K. Thornton, G. Boon, R. J. Lysons, and A. F. Gush.** 1980. Medicated early weaning to obtain pigs free from pathogens endemic in the herd of origin. *Vet. Rec.* **106**:114–119.

5. **Andreasen, M., P. Baekbo, and J. P. Nielsen.** 2000. Lack of effect of aerial ammonia on atrophic rhinitis and pneumonia induced by *Mycoplasma hyopneumoniae* and toxigenic *Pasteurella multocida. J. Vet. Med. Ser. B* **47**:161–171.

6. **Bäckström, L., D. C. Hoefling, A. C. Morkoc, and R. P. Cowart.** 1985. Effect of atrophic rhinitis on growth rate in Illinois swine herds. *J. Am. Vet. Med. Assoc.* **187**:712–715.

7. **Banemann, A., and R. Gross.** 1997. Phase variation affects long-term survival of *Bordetella bronchiseptica* in professional phagocytes. *Infect. Immun.* **65**:3469–3473.

8. **Beachey, E. H.** 1981. Bacterial adherence: adhesin-receptor interactions mediating the attachment of bacteria to mucosal surfaces. *J. Infect. Dis.* **143**:325–345.

9. **Betsou, F., O. Sismeiro, A. Danchin, and N. Guiso.** 1995. Cloning and sequence of the *Bordetella bronchiseptica* adenylate cyclase-hemolysin-encoding gene. *Gene* **162**:165–166.

10. **Bjorge, J. D., A. Jakymiw, and D. J. Fujita.** 2000. Selected glimpses into the activation and function of Src kinase. *Oncogene* **19**:5620–5635.

11. **Bock, A., and R. Gross.** 2001. The BvgAS two-component system of *Bordetella* spp.: a versatile modulator of virulence gene expression. *Int. J. Med. Microbiol.* **291**:119–130.

12. **Bordet, J., and O. Gengou.** 1909. Le microbe de la coqueluche. *Ann. Inst. Pasteur* **20**:731–741.

13. **Boschwitz, J. S., H. G. J. van der Heide, F. R. Mooi, and D. A. Relman.** 1997. *Bordetella bronchiseptica* expresses the fimbrial structural subunit gene *fimA. J. Bacteriol.* **179**:7882–7885.

14. **Boursaux-Eude, C., and N. Guiso.** 2000. Polymorphism of repeated regions of pertactin in *Bordetella pertussis, Bordetella parapertussis* and *Bordetella bronchiseptica. Infect. Immun.* **68**:4815–4817.

15. **Braend, M., and J. L. Flatla.** 1954. Rhinitis infectiosa atroficans hos gris. *Nord. Vetmed.* **6**: 81–122.

16. **Brassine, M., A. Dewaele, and M. Gouffaux.** 1976. Intranasal infection with *Bordetella bronchiseptica* in gnotobiotic piglets. *Res. Vet. Sci.* **20**:162–166.

17. **Brennan, M. J., Z. M. Li, J. L. Cowell, M. E. Bisher, A. C. Steven, P. Novotny, and C. R. Manclark.** 1988. Identification of a 69-kilodalton nonfimbrial protein as an agglutinogen of *Bordetella pertussis. Infect. Immun.* **56**:3189–3195.

18. **Brockmeier, S. L.** 1999. Early colonization of the rat upper respiratory tract by temperature modulated *Bordetella bronchiseptica. FEMS Microbiol. Lett.* **174**:225–229.

19. **Brockmeier, S. L., and K. B. Register.** 2000. Effect of temperature modulation and *bvg* mutation of *Bordetella bronchiseptica* on adhesion, intracellular survival and cytotoxicity for swine alveolar macrophages. *Vet. Microbiol.* **73**:1–12.

20. **Brown, W. R., L. Krook, and W. G. Pond.** 1966. Atrophic rhinitis in swine. Etiology, pathogenesis and prophylaxis. *Cornell Vet.* **56**(Suppl. 1):1–108.

21. **Burns, E. H., Jr., J. M. Norman, M. D. Hatcher, and D. A. Bemis.** 1993. Fimbriae and determination of host species specificity of *Bordetella bronchiseptica. J. Clin. Microbiol.* **31**: 1838–1844.

22. **Busch, C., J. Orth, N. Djouder, and K. Aktories.** 2001. Biological activity of a C-terminal fragment of *Pasteurella multocida* toxin. *Infect. Immun.* **69**:3628–3634.

23. **Cantrell, D. A.** 2001. Phosphoinositide 3-kinase signalling pathways. *J. Cell Sci.* **114**:1439–1445.

24. **Chanter, N., and J. M. Rutter.** 1990. Colonisation by *Pasteurella multocida* in atrophic rhinitis of pigs and immunity to the osteolytic toxin. *Vet. Microbiol.* **25**:253–265.

25. **Chanter, N., J. M. Rutter, and A. MacKenzie.** 1986. Partial purification of an osteolytic toxin from *Pasteurella multocida. J. Gen. Microbiol.* **132**:1089–1097.

26. **Chanter, N., T. Magyar, and J. M. Rutter.** 1989. Interactions between *Bordetella bronchiseptica* and toxigenic *Pasteurella multocida* in atrophic rhinitis of pigs. *Res. Vet. Sci.* **47**:48–53.

27. **Charles, I. G., G. Dougan, D. Pickard, S. Chatfield, M. Smith, P. Novotny, P. Morrissey, and N. F. Fairweather.** 1989. Molecular cloning and characterization of protective outer membrane protein P.69 from *Bordetella pertussis. Proc. Natl. Acad. Sci. USA* **86**:3554–3558.

28. **Cheville, N. F., R. B. Rimler, and J. Thurston.** 1988. A toxin from *Pasteurella multocida* type D causes acute hepatic necrosis in pigs. *Vet. Pathol.* **25**:518–520.

29. Chung, W. B., M. T. Collins, and L. R. Bäckström. 1990. Adherence of *Bordetella bronchiseptica* and *Pasteurella multocida* to swine nasal ciliated epithelial cells in vitro. *APMIS* **98**:453–461.

30. Collings, L. A., and J. M. Rutter. 1985. Virulence of *Bordetella bronchiseptica* in the porcine respiratory tract. *J. Med. Microbiol.* **19**:247.

31. Confer, D. L., and J. W. Eaton. 1982. Phagocyte impotence caused by an invasive bacterial adenylate cyclase. *Science* **217**:948–950.

32. Cookson, B. T., and W. E. Goldman. 1987. Tracheal cytotoxin: a conserved virulence determinant of all *Bordetella* species. *J. Cell. Biochem.* **11B**(Suppl.):124.

33. Cookson, B. T., H.-L. Cho, L. A. Herwaldt, and W. E. Goldman. 1989. Biological activities and chemical composition of purified tracheal cytotoxin of *Bordetella pertussis*. *Infect. Immun.* **57**:2223–2229.

34. Cornelis, G. R., and F. Van Gijsegem. 2000. Assembly and function of type III secretory systems. *Annu. Rev. Microbiol.* **54**:735–774.

35. Cotter, P. A., and J. F. Miller. 1994. BvgAS-mediated signal transduction: analysis of phase-locked regulatory mutants of *Bordetella bronchiseptica* in a rabbit model. *Infect. Immun.* **62**:3381–3390.

36. Cotter, P. A., and J. F. Miller. 2000. Genetic analysis of the *Bordetella* infectious cycle. *Immunopharmacology* **48**:253–255.

37. Cotter, P. A., M. H. Yuk, S. Mattoo, B. J. Akerley, J. S. Boschwitz, D. A. Relman, and J. F. Miller. 1998. Filamentous hemagglutinin of *Bordetella bronchiseptica* is required for efficient establishment of tracheal colonization. *Infect. Immun.* **66**:5921–5929.

38. Cowell, J. L., E. L. Hewlett, and D. R. Manclark. 1979. Intracellular localization of the dermonecrotic toxin of *Bordetella pertussis*. *Infect. Immun.* **25**:896–901.

39. Cross, R. F., and R. M. Claflin. 1962. *Bordetella bronchiseptica* induced porcine atrophic rhinitis. *J. Am. Vet. Med. Assoc.* **141**:1467–1468.

40. Cundell, D. R., K. Kanthakumar, G. W. Taylor, W. E. Goldman, T. Flak, P. J. Cole, and R. Wilson. 1994. Effect of tracheal cytotoxin from *Bordetella pertussis* on human neutrophil function in vitro. *Infect. Immun.* **62**:639–643.

41. de Jong, M. F. 1983. Atrophic rhinitis caused by intranasal or intramuscular administration of broth-culture and broth-culture filtrates containing AR toxin of *Pasteurella multocida*, p. 136–146. *In* K. B. Pedersen and J. C. Nielsen (ed.), *Atrophic Rhinitis in Pigs*. Report EUR 8643 EN. Commission of the European Communities, Luxembourg, Luxembourg.

42. de Jong, M. F. 1999. Progressive and nonprogressive atrophic rhinitis, p. 355–384. *In* B. E. Straw, S. D'Allaire, W. L. Mengeling, and D. J. Taylor (ed.), *Diseases of Swine*, 8th ed. Iowa State University Press, Ames.

43. de Jong, M. F., and J. P. Nielsen. 1990. Definition of progressive atrophic rhinitis. *Vet. Rec.* **27**:93.

44. Dominick, M. A., and R. B. Rimler. 1986. Turbinate atrophy in gnotobiotic pigs intranasally inoculated with protein toxin isolated from type D *Pasteurella multocida*. *Am. J. Vet. Res.* **47**:1532–1536.

45. Dugal, F., M. Belanger, and M. Jacques. 1992. Enhanced adherence of *Pasteurella multocida* to porcine tracheal rings preinfected with *Bordetella bronchiseptica*. *Can. J. Vet. Res.* **56**:260–264.

46. Duncan, J. R., R. K. Ross, W. P. Switzer, and R. K. Ramsey. 1966. Pathology of experimental *Bordetella bronchiseptica* infection in swine: atrophic rhinitis. *Am. J. Vet. Res.* **27**:457–466.

47. Éliás, B., and D. Hámori. 1975. Adatok a sertés torzító orrgyulladásának kóroktanához. V. A genetikai tényezők szerepe. *Magy. Állatorv. Lapja* **30**:535–539.

48. Endoh, M., T. Takezawa, and Y. Nakase. 1980. Adenylate cyclase activity of *Bordetella* organisms. *Microbiol. Immunol.* **24**:95–104.

49. Essler, M., K. Hermann, M. Amano, K. Kaibuchi, J. Heesemann, P. C. Weber, and M. Aelfelbacher. 1998. *Pasteurella multocida* toxin increases endothelial permeability via Rho kinase and myosin light chain phosphatase. *J. Immunol.* **161**:5640–5646.

50. Felix, R., H. Fleisch, and P. L. Frandsen. 1992. Effect of *Pasteurella multocida* toxin on bone resorption in vitro. *Infect. Immun.* **60**:4984–4988.

51. Foged, N. T., J. P. Nielsen, and S. E. Jorsal. 1989. Protection against progressive atrophic rhinitis by vaccination with *Pasteurella multocida* toxin purified by monoclonal antibodies. *Vet. Rec.* **125**:7–11.

52. Forde, C. B., R. Parton, and J. G. Coote. 1998. Bioluminescence as a reporter of intracellular survival of *Bordetella bronchiseptica* in murine phagocytes. *Infect. Immun.* **66**:3198–3207.

53. Forde, C. B., X. Shi, J. Li, and M. Roberts. 1999. *Bordetella bronchiseptica*-mediated cytotoxicity to macrophages is dependent on *bvg*-regulated factors, including pertactin. *Infect. Immun.* **67**:5972–5978.

54. Franque, L. W. 1830. Was ist die Schnüffelkrankheit der Schweine? *Dtsch. Z. Gesamte Tierheilkd.* **1**:75–77.

55. Frymus, T., M. M. Wittenbrink, and K. Petzold. 1986. Failure to demonstrate adherence of *Pasteurella multocida* involved in atrophic rhinitis to swine nasal epithelial cells. *J. Vet. Med. Ser. B* **33**:140–144.

56. **Fuller, T. E., M. J. Kennedy, and D. E. Lowery.** 2000. Identification of *Pasteurella multocida* virulence genes in a septicemic mouse model using signature-tagged mutagenesis. *Microb. Pathog.* **29:** 25–38.

57. **Gagné, S., and B. Martineau-Doizé.** 1993. Nasal epithelial changes induced in piglets by acetic acid and by *B. bronchiseptica. J. Comp. Pathol.* **109:**71–81.

58. **Giardina, P. C., L. A. Foster, J. M. Musser, B. J. Akerley, J. F. Miller, and D. W. Dyer.** 1995. *bvg* repression of alcaligin synthesis in *Bordetella bronchiseptica* is associated with phylogenetic lineage. *J. Bacteriol.* **177:**6058–6063.

59. **Giles, C. J.** 1981. *Atrophic Rhinitis of Pigs: Studies on the Naturally-Occurring and Experimental Disease in England, with Particular Reference to* Bordetella bronchiseptica *Infection.* Ph.D. thesis. University of London, London, United Kingdom.

60. **Giles, C. J., and I. M. Smith.** 1983. Vaccination of pigs with *Bordetella bronchiseptica. Vet. Bull.* **53:**327–338.

61. **Giles, C. J., I. M. Smith, A. J. Baskerville, and E. Brothwell.** 1980. Clinical, bacteriological and epidemiological observation on infectious atrophic rhinitis of pigs in Southern England. *Vet. Rec.* **106:**25–28.

62. **Glaser, P., D. Ladant, O. Sezer, F. Pichot, A. Ullmann, and A. Danchin.** 1988a. The calmodulin-sensitive adenylate cyclase of *Bordetella pertussis:* cloning and expression in *Escherichia coli. Mol. Microbiol.* **2:**19–30.

63. **Glaser, P., H. Sakamoto, J. Bellalou, A. Ullmann, and A. Danchin.** 1988b. Secretion of cyclolysin, the calmodulin-sensitive adenylate cyclase-haemolysin bifunctional protein of *Bordetella pertussis. EMBO J.* **7:**3997–4004.

64. **Goldman, W. E., and B. T. Cookson.** 1988. Structure and functions of the *Bordetella* tracheal cytotoxin. *Tokai J. Exp. Clin. Med.* **13**(Suppl.): 187–191.

65. **Goldman, W. E., D. G. Klapper, and J. B. Baseman.** 1982. Detection, isolation, and analysis of a released *Bordetella pertussis* product toxic to cultured tracheal cells. *Infect. Immun.* **36:**782–794.

66. **Goodnow, R. A.** 1980. Biology of *Bordetella bronchiseptica. Microbiol. Rev.* **44:**722–738.

67. **Goodwin, M. S. M., and A. A. Weiss.** 1990. Adenylate cyclase is critical for colonization and pertussis toxin is critical for lethal infection by *Bordetella pertussis* in infant mice. *Infect. Immun.* **58:**3445–3447.

68. **Gueirard, P., A. Druilhe, M. Pretolani, and N. Guiso.** 1998. Role of adenylate cyclase-hemolysin in alveolar macrophage apoptosis during *Bordetella pertussis* infection in vivo. *Infect. Immun.* **66:**1718–1725.

69. **Guiso, N., M. Szatanik, and M. Rocancourt.** 1989. Protective activity of *Bordetella* adenylate cyclase-hemolysin against bacterial colonization. *Microb. Pathog.* **11:**423–431.

70. **Gwaltney, S. M., R. J. S. Galvin, K. B. Register, R. B. Rimler, and M. R. Ackermann.** 1997. Effects of *Pasteurella multocida* toxin on porcine bone marrow cell differentiation into osteoclasts and osteoblasts. *Vet. Pathol.* **34:**421–430.

71. **Gwatkin, R., L. Ozenis, and J. L. Byrne.** 1953. Rhinitis of swine. VII. Production of lesions in pigs and rabbits with a pure culture of *Pasteurella multocida. Can. J. Comp. Med. Vet. Sci.* **17:**215–217.

72. **Hackett, M., L. Guo, J. Shabanowitz, D. F. Hunt, and E. L. Hewett.** 1994. Internal lysine palmitoylation in adenylate cyclase toxin from *Bordetella pertussis. Science* **266:**433–435.

73. **Hamilton, T. D. C., J. M. Roe, and A. J. F. Webster.** 1996. Synergistic role of gaseous ammonia in etiology of *Pasteurella multocida*-induced atrophic rhinitis in swine. *J. Clin. Microbiol.* **34:** 2185–2190.

74. **Hamilton, T. D. C., J. M. Roe, C. M. Hayes, and A. J. F. Webster.** 1998. Effects of ammonia inhalation and acetic acid pretreatment on colonization kinetics of toxigenic *Pasteurella multocida* within upper respiratory tracts of swine. *J. Clin. Microbiol.* **36:**1260–1265.

75. **Hamilton, T. D. C., J. M. Roe, C. M. Hayes, P. Jones, G. R. Pearson, and A. J. F. Webster.** 1999. Contributory and exacerbating roles of gaseous ammonia and organic dust in the etiology of atrophic rhinitis. *Clin. Diagn. Lab. Immunol.* **6:**199–203.

76. **Hanada, M., K. Shimoda, S. Tomita, Y. Nakase, and Y. Nishiyama.** 1979. Production of lesions similar to naturally occurring swine atrophic rhinitis by cell-free sonicated extract of *Bordetella bronchiseptica. Jpn. J. Vet. Sci.* **41:**1–8.

77. **Hannan, P. C., P. J. O'Hanlon, and N. H. Rogers.** 1989. In vitro evaluation of various quinolone antibacterial agents against veterinary mycoplasmas and porcine respiratory bacterial pathogens. *Res. Vet. Sci.* **46:**202–211.

78. **Hanski, E., and Z. Farfel.** 1985. *Bordetella pertussis* invasive adenylate cyclase. *J. Biol. Chem.* **260:**5526–5532.

79. **Harris, D. L., and W. P. Switzer.** 1968. Turbinate atrophy in young pigs exposed to *Bordetella bronchiseptica, Pasteurella multocida* and combined inoculum. *Am. J. Vet. Res.* **29:**777–785.

80. **Harvill, E. T., P. A. Cotter, M. H. Yuk, and J. F. Miller.** 1999. Probing the function of *Bordetella bronchiseptica* adenylate cyclase toxin by manipulating host immunity. *Infect. Immun.* **67:** 1493–1500.

81. **Heiss, L. N., J. J. Lancaster, J. A. Corbett, and W. E. Goldman.** 1994. Epithelial autotoxicity of nitric oxide: role in the respiratory cytopathology of pertussis. *Proc. Natl. Acad. Sci. USA* **91:**267–270.

82. **Heiss, L. N., S. A. Moser, E. R. Unanue, and W. E. Goldman.** 1993. Interleukin-1 is linked to the respiratory epithelial cytopathology of pertussis. *Infect. Immun.* **61:**3123–3128.

83. **Hewlett, E., and J. Wolff.** 1976. Soluble adenylate cyclase from the culture medium of *Bordetella pertussis:* purification and characterization. *J. Bacteriol.* **127:**890–898.

84. **Hewlett, E. L., C. R. Manclark, and J. Wolff.** 1977. Adenylate cyclase in *Bordetella pertussis* vaccines. *J. Infect. Dis.* **136:**5216–5219.

85. **Hewlett, E. L., M. A. Urban, C. R. Manclark, and J. Wolff.** 1976. Extracytoplasmic adenylate cyclase of *Bordetella pertussis. Proc. Natl. Acad. Sci. USA* **73:**1926–1930.

86. **Higgins, T. E., A. C. Murphy, J. M. Staddon, A. J. Lax, and E. Rozengurt.** 1992. *Pasteurella multocida* toxin is a potent inducer of anchorage-independent cell growth. *Proc. Natl. Acad. Sci. USA* **89:**4240–4244.

87. **Horiguchi, Y., H. Matsuda, H. Koyama, T. Nakai, and K. Kume.** 1992. *Bordetella bronchiseptica* dermonecrotizing toxin suppressed in vivo antibody responses in mice. *FEMS Microbiol. Lett.* **90:**229–234.

88. **Horiguchi, Y., N. Inoue, M. Masuda, T. Kashimoto, J. Katahira, N. Sugimoto, and M. Matsuda.** 1997. *Bordetella bronchiseptica* dermonecrotizing toxin induces reorganization of actin stress fibers through deamidation of Gln-63 of the GTP-binding protein Rho. *Proc. Natl. Acad. Sci. USA* **94:**11623–11626.

89. **Horiguchi, Y., N. Sugimoto, and M. Matsuda.** 1993. Stimulation of DNA synthesis in osteoblast-like MC3T3-E1 cells by *Bordetella bronchiseptica* dermonecrotic toxin. *Infect. Immun.* **61:**3611–3615.

90. **Horiguchi, Y., T. Nakai, and K. Kume.** 1991. Effects of *Bordetella bronchiseptica* dermonecrotic toxin on the structure and function of osteoblastic clone MC3T3-E1 cells. *Infect. Immun.* **59:**1112–1116.

91. **Horiguchi, Y., T. Okada, N. Sugimoto, Y. Morikawa, J. Katahira, and M. Matsuda.** 1995. Effects of *Bordetella bronchiseptica* dermonecrotizing toxin on bone formation in calvaria of neonatal rats. *FEMS Immunol. Med. Microbiol.* **12:**29–32.

92. **Horiguchi, Y., T. Senda, N. Sugimoto, J. Katahira, and M. Matsuda.** 1995. *Bordetella bronchiseptica* dermonecrotizing toxin stimulates assembly of actin stress fibers and focal adhesions by modifying the small GTP-binding protein rho. *J. Cell. Sci.* **108:**3243–3251.

93. **Horváth, Z., L. Papp, and B. Éliás.** 1972. Studies of Ca and P metabolism in atrophic rhinitis of swine. II. Bone Ca and P contents of healthy and pigs affected with atrophic rhinitis. *Acta Vet. Hung.* **22:**45–51.

94. **Hoskins, I. C., and A. J. Lax.** 1996. Constitutive expression of *Pasteurella multocida* toxin. *FEMS Microbiol. Lett.* **141:**189–193.

95. **Hoskins, I. C., L. H. Thomas, and A. J. Lax.** 1997. Nasal infection with *Pasteurella multocida* causes proliferation of bladder epithelium in gnotobiotic pigs. *Vet. Rec.* **140:**22.

96. **Il'ina, Z. M., and I. Zasukhin.** 1975. Role of *Pasteurella* toxins in the pathogenesis of infectious atrophic rhinitis. *Sb. Nauchn. Rab. Sib. Zon Nauch. Vet. Inst. Omsk* **25:**76–86.

97. **Ishikawa, H., and Y. Isayama.** 1987. Evidence for sialyl glycoconjugates as receptors for *B. bronchiseptica* on swine nasal mucosa. *Infect. Immun.* **55:**1607–1609.

98. **Iwaki, M., K. Kamachi, N. Heveker, and T. Konda.** 1999. Suppression of platelet aggregation by *Bordetella pertussis* adenylate cyclase toxin. *Infect. Immun.* **67:**2763–2768.

99. **Jacob-Dubuisson, F., C. Buisine, N. Mielcarek, E. Clement, F. D. Menozzi, and C. Locht.** 1996. Amino-terminal maturation of the *Bordetella* pertussis filamentous haemagglutinin. *Mol. Microbiol.* **19:**65–78.

100. **Jacques, M., N. Parent, and B. Foiry.** 1988. Adherence of *Bordetella bronchiseptica* and *Pasteurella multocida* to porcine nasal epithelial cells. *Can. J. Vet. Res.* **52:**283–285.

101. **Jutras, I., and B. Martineau-Doizé.** 1996. Stimulation of osteoclast-like cell formation by *Pasteurella multocida* toxin from hemopoietic progenitor cells in mouse bone marrow cultures. *Can. J. Vet. Res.* **60:**34–39.

102. **Kabay, M. J., A. R. Mercy, J. M. Lloyd, and G. M. Robertson.** 1992. Vaccine efficacy for reducing turbinate atrophy and improving growth rate in piggeries with endemic atrophic rhinitis. *Aust. Vet. J.* **69:**101–103.

103. **Kashimoto, T., J. Katahira, W. R. Cornejo, M. Masuda, A. Fukuoh, T. Matsuzawa, T. Ohnishi, and Y. Horiguchi.** 1999. Identification of functional domains of *Bordetella* dermonecrotizing toxin. *Infect. Immun.* **67:**3727–3732.

104. **Kemeny, L. J.** 1972. Experimental atrophic rhinitis produced by *Bordetella bronchiseptica* culture in young pigs. *Cornell Vet.* **62:**477–485.

105. **Khelef, N., A. Zychlinsky, and N. Guiso.** 1993. *Bordetella pertussis* induces apoptosis in macrophages: role of adenylate cyclase-hemolysin. *Infect. Immun.* **61:**4064–4071.

106. **Khelef, N., C.-M. Bachelet, B. B. Vargaftig, and N. Guiso.** 1994. Characterization of murine lung inflammation after infection with parental *Bordetella pertussis* and mutants deficient in adhesins or toxins. *Infect. Immun.* **62:**2893–2900.

107. **Khelef, N., H. Sakamoto, and N. Guiso.** 1992. Both adenylate cyclase and hemolytic activities are required by *Bordetella pertussis* to initiate infection. *Microb. Pathog.* **12:**227–235.

108. **Kimman, T. G., C. W. G. M. Löwik, L. J. A. van de Wee-Pals, C. W. Thesingh, P. Defize, E. M. Kamp, and O. L. M. Bijvoet.** 1987. Stimulation of bone resorption by inflamed nasal mucosa, dermonecrotic toxin-containing conditioned medium from *Pasteurella multocida,* and purified dermonecrotic toxin from *P. multocida. Infect. Immun.* **55:**2110–2116.

109. **Knapp, S., and J. J. Mekalanos.** 1988. Two *trans*-acting regulatory genes (vir and mod) control antigenic modulation in *Bordetella pertussis. J. Bacteriol.* **170:**5059–5066.

110. **Kobisch, M., and P. Novotny.** 1990. Identification of a 68-kilodalton outer membrane protein as the major protective antigen of *Bordetella bronchiseptica* by using specific-pathogen-free piglets. *Infect. Immun.* **58:**352–357.

111. **Lacerda, H. M., A. J. Lax, and E. Rozengurt.** 1996. *Pasteurella multocida* toxin, a potent intracellularly acting mitogen, induces p125^FAK and paxillin tyrosine phosphorylation, actin stress fiber formation, and focal contact assembly in Swiss 3T3 cells. *J. Biol. Chem.* **271:**439–445.

112. **Lacerda, H. M., G. D. Pullinger, A. J. Lax, and E. Rozengurt.** 1997. Cytotoxic necrotizing factor 1 from *Escherichia coli* and dermonecrotic toxin from *Bordetella bronchiseptica* induce p21^rho-dependent tyrosine phosphorylation of focal adhesion kinase and paxillin in Swiss 3T3 cells. *J. Biol. Chem.* **272:**9587–9596.

113. **Lacey, B. W.** 1960. Antigenic modulation of *Bordetella pertussis. J. Hyg. Camb.* **58:**57–93.

114. **Lax, A. J.** 1985. Is phase variation in *Bordetella* caused by mutation and selection? *J. Gen. Microbiol.* **131:**913–917.

115. **Lax, A. J., and A. E. Grigoriadis.** 2001. *Pasteurella multocida* toxin: the mitogenic toxin that stimulates signalling cascades to regulate growth and differentiation. *Int. J. Med. Microbiol.* **291:**261–268.

116. **Lax, A. J., and N. Chanter.** 1990. Cloning of the toxin gene from *Pasteurella multocida* and its role in atrophic rhinitis. *J. Gen. Microbiol.* **136:**81–87.

117. **Lax, A. J., N. Chanter, G. D. Pullinger, T. Higgins, J. M. Staddon, and E. Rozengurt.** 1990. Sequence analysis of the potent mitogenic toxin of *Pasteurella multocida. FEBS Lett.* **277:**59–64.

118. **Lee, S. W., A. Way, and E. G. Osen.** 1986. Purification and subunit heterogeneity of pili of *Bordetella bronchiseptica. Infect. Immun.* **51:**586–593.

119. **Leininger, E., C. A. Ewanowich, A. Bhargava, M. S. Peppler, J. G. Kenimer, and M. J. Brennan.** 1992. Comparative roles of the Arg-Gly-Asp sequence present in the *Bordetella pertussis* adhesins pertactin and filamentous hemagglutinin. *Infect. Immun.* **60:**2380–2385.

120. **Leininger, E., M. Roberts, J. G. Kenimer, I. G. Charles, N. Fairweather, P. Novotny, and M. J. Brennan.** 1991. Pertactin, an arg-gly-asp containing *Bordetella pertussis* surface protein that promotes adherence of mammalian cells. *Proc. Natl. Acad. Sci. USA* **88:**345–349.

121. **Leininger, E., P. G. Probst, M. J. Brennan, and J. G. Kenimer.** 1993. Inhibition of *Bordetella pertussis* filamentous hemagglutinin-mediated cell adherence with monoclonal antibodies. *FEMS Microbiol. Lett.* **80:**31–38.

122. **Lemichez, E., G. Flatau, M. Bruzzone, P. Boquet, and M. Gauthier.** 1997. Molecular localization of the *Escherichia coli* cytotoxic necrotizing factor CNF1 cell-binding and catalytic domains. *Mol. Microbiol.* **24:**1061–1070.

123. **Lendvai, N., T. Magyar, and G. Semjén.** 1992. Cross-protection studies on *Bordetella bronchiseptica* in mice using an intracerebral challenge model. *Vet. Microbiol.* **31:**191–196.

124. **Leppla, S. H.** 1982. Anthrax toxin edema factor: a bacterial adenylate cyclase that increases cyclic AMP concentrations in eukaryotic cells. *Proc. Natl. Acad. Sci. USA* **79:**3162–3166.

125. **Lerm, M., J. Selzer, A. Hoffmeyer, U. R. Rapp, K. Aktories, and G. Schmidt.** 1999. Deamidation of Cdc42 and Rac by *Escherichia coli* cytotoxic necrotizing factor 1: activation of c-jun N-terminal kinase in HeLa cells. *Infect. Immun.* **67:**496–503.

126. **Leslie, P. H., and A. D. Gardner.** 1931. The phases of *Haemophilus pertussis. J. Hyg. Camb.* **31:**531–545.

127. **Livey, I., and A. C. Wardlaw.** 1984. Production and properties of *Bordetella pertussis* heat labile toxin. *J. Med. Microbiol.* **17:**91–103.

128. **Locht, C., P. Bertin, F. D. Menozzi, and G. Renauld.** 1993. The filamentous haemagglutinin, a multifaceted adhesion produced by virulent *Bordetella* spp. *Mol. Microbiol.* **4:**653–660.

129. **Logomarsino, J. V., W. G. Pond, B. E. Sheffy, and L. Krook.** 1974. Turbinate morphology in pigs inoculated with *Bordetella bronchiseptica* and fed high or low calcium diets. *Cornell Vet.* **64:**573–583.

130. **Luker, K. E., A. N. Tyler, G. R. Marshall, and W. E. Goldman.** 1995. Tracheal cytotoxin structural requirements for respiratory epithelial damage in pertussis. *Mol. Microbiol.* **16:**733–743.

131. **Magyar, T.** 1990. Virulence and lienotoxicity of *Bordetella bronchiseptica* in mice. *Vet. Microbiol.* **25:**199–207.

132. **Magyar, T., N. Chanter, A. J. Lax, J. M. Rutter, and G. A. Hall.** 1988. The pathogenesis of turbinate atrophy in pigs caused by *Bordetella bronchiseptica. Vet. Microbiol.* **18:**135–146.

133. **Magyar, T., N. Lendvai, G. Semjén, and L. Réthy.** 1983. Investigation of the biological activities of *Bordetella bronchiseptica.* II. Adherence to the target cell. *Ann. Immunol. Hung.* **23:**361–366.

134. **Magyar, T., R. Glávits, G. D. Pullinger, and A. J. Lax.** 2000. The pathological effect of the *bordetella* dermonecrotic toxin in mice. *Acta Vet. Hung.* **48:**397–406.

135. **Mao, J., H. Yuan, W. Xie, and D. Wu.** 1998. Guanine nucleotide exchange factor GEF115 specifically mediates activation of Rho and serum response factor by the G protein α subunit Gα13. *Proc. Natl. Acad. Sci. USA* **95:** 12973–12976.

136. **Martineau-Doizé, B., I. Caya, S. Gagné, I. Jutras, and G. Dumas.** 1993. Effects of *Pasteurella multocida* toxin on the osteoclast population of the rat. *Comp. Pathol.* **108:**81–91.

137. **Masuda, M., L. Betancourt, T. Matsuzawa, T. Kashimoto, T. Takao, Y. Shimonishi, and Y. Horiguchi.** 2000. Activation of Rho through a cross-link with polyamines catalyzed by *Bordetella* dermonecrotizing toxin. *EMBO J.* **19:**521–530.

138. **Mattoo, S., J. F. Miller, and P. A. Cotter.** 2000. Role of *Bordetella bronchiseptica* fimbriae in tracheal colonization and development of a humoral immune response. *Infect. Immun.* **68:**2024–2033.

139. **May, B. J., Q. Zhang, L. L. Li, M. L. Paustian, T. S. Whittam, and V. Kapur.** 2001. Complete genomic sequence of *Pasteurella multocida,* Pm70. *Proc. Natl. Acad. Sci. USA* **98:**3460–3465.

140. **McMillan, D. J., M. Shojaei, G. S. Chhatwal, C. A. Guzmán, and M. J. Walker.** 1996. Molecular analysis of the *bvg*-repressed urease of *Bordetella bronchiseptica. Microb. Pathog.* **21:**379–394.

141. **Menozzi, F. D., R. Mutombo, G. Renauld, C. Gantiez, J. H. Hannah, E. Leininger, M. J. Brennan, and C. Locht.** 1994. Heparin-inhabitable lectin activity of the filamentous hemagglutinin adhesin of *Bordetella pertussis. Infect. Immun.* **62:**769–778.

142. **Miniats, O. P., and J. A. Johnson.** 1980. Experimental atrophic rhinitis in gnotobiotic pigs. *Can. J. Comp. Med.* **44:**358–365.

143. **Monack, D. M., B. Aricò, R. Rappuoli, and S. Falkow.** 1989. Phase variants of *Bordetella bronchiseptica* arise by spontaneous deletions in the *vir* locus. *Mol. Microbiol.* **3:**1719–1728.

144. **Montaraz, J. A., P. Novotny, and J. Ivanyi.** 1985. Identification of a 68-kilodalton protective protein antigen from *Bordetella bronchiseptica. Infect. Immun.* **47:**744–751.

145. **Montecucco, C., E. Papini, and G. Schiavo.** 1994. Bacterial protein toxins penetrate cells via a four-step mechanism. *FEBS Lett.* **346:**92–98.

146. **Montminy, M.** 1997. Transcriptional regulation by cyclic AMP. *Annu. Rev. Biochem.* **66:** 807–822.

147. **Muirhead, M. R.** 1979. Respiratory diseases of pigs. *Br. Vet. J.* **135:**497–508.

148. **Mullan, P. B., and A. J. Lax.** 1996. *Pasteurella multocida* toxin is a mitogen for bone cells in primary culture. *Infect. Immun.* **64:**959–965.

149. **Mullan, P. B., and A. J. Lax.** 1998. *Pasteurella multocida* toxin stimulates bone resorption by osteoclasts via interaction with osteoblasts. *Calcif. Tissue Int.* **63:**340–345.

150. **Muller, M., and A. Hildebrandt.** 1993. Nucleotide sequence of the 285 RNA genes from *Bordetella pertussis, B. parapertussis, B. bronchiseptica* and *B. avium,* and their implications for phylogenic analysis. *Nucleic Acids Res.* **21:**3320.

151. **Murphy, A. C., and E. Rozengurt.** 1992. *Pasteurella multocida* toxin selectively facilitates phosphatidylinositol 4,5-bisphosphate hydrolysis by bombesin, vasopressin, and endothelin. *J. Biol. Chem.* **267:**25296–25303.

152. **Musser, J. M., D. A. Bemis, H. Ishikawa, and R. K. Selander.** 1987. Clonal diversity and host distribution in *Bordetella bronchiseptica. J. Bacteriol.* **169:**2793–2803.

153. **Nakai, T., A. Sawata, and K. Kume.** 1985. Intracellular locations of dermonecotic toxins in *Pasteurella multocida* and *Bordetella bronchiseptica. Am. J. Vet. Res.* **46:**870–874.

154. **Nakai, T., K. Kume, H. Yoshikawa, T. Oyamada, and T. Yoshikawa.** 1988. Adherence of *Pasteurella multocida* or *Bordetella bronchiseptica* to the swine nasal epithelial cell in vitro. *Infect. Immun.* **56:**234–240.

155. **Nakase, Y.** 1957. Studies on Hemophilus bronchisepticus II: phase variation of H. bronchisepticus. *Kitasato Arch. Exp. Med.* **30:**73–78.

156. **Nakase, Y.** 1957. Studies on Hemophilus bronchisepticus III: differences of biological properties between phase I and phase III of H. bronchisepticus. *Kitasato Arch. Exp. Med.* **30:**79–84.

157. **Njamkepo, E., F. Pinot, D. François, N. Guiso, B. S. Polla, and M. Bachelet.** 2000. Adaptive responses of human monocytes infected by *Bordetella pertussis:* the role of adenylate cyclase hemolysin. *J. Cell. Physiol.* **183:**91–99.

158. **Ofek, I., and E. H. Beachey.** 1980. Bacterial adherence, p. 3–29. *In* E. H. Beachey (ed.), *Receptors and Recognition,* series B6. Chapman and Hall, London, United Kingdom.

159. **Parton, R., E. Hall, and A. C. Wardlaw.** 1994. Responses to *Bordetella pertussis* mutant strains and to vaccination in the coughing rat model of pertussis. *J. Med. Microbiol.* **40:**307–312.

160. **Pedersen, K. B., and F. Elling.** 1984. The pathogenesis of atrophic rhinitis in pigs induced by toxigenic *Pasteurella multocida. J. Comp. Pathol.* **94:**203–214.

161. **Pedersen, K. B., and K. Barfod.** 1981. The aetiological significance of *Bordetella bronchiseptica* and *Pasteurella multocida* in atrophic rhinitis of swine. *Nord. Vetmed.* **33:**513–522.

162. **Pedersen, K. B., and K. Barfod.** 1982. Effect on the incidence of atrophic rhinitis of vaccination of sows with vaccine *Pasteurella multocida* toxin. *Nord. Vetmed.* **34:**293–302.

163. **Penny, R. H. C., and J. C. Penny.** 1976. Priorities for pig research. *Vet. Rec.* **99:**451–453.

164. **Petersen, S. K.** 1990. The complete nucleotide sequence of the *Pasteurella multocida* toxin gene and evidence for a transcriptional repressor, TxaR. *Mol. Microbiol.* **4:**821–830.

165. **Pettit, R. K., M. R. Ackermann, and R. B. Rimler.** 1993. Receptor-mediated binding of *Pasteurella multocida* dermonecrotic toxin to canine osteosarcoma and monkey kidney (vero) cells. *Lab. Investig.* **69:**94–100.

166. **Pijpers, A., B. van Klingeren, E. J. Schoevers, J. H. M. Verheijden, and A. S. J. P. A. M. Van Miert.** 1989. In vitro activity of five tetracyclines and some other antimicrobial agents against four porcine respiratory tract pathogens. *J. Vet. Pharmacol. Ther.* **12:**267–276.

167. **Porter, J. F., and A. C. Wardlaw.** 1993. Long-term survival of *Bordetella bronchiseptica* in lakewater and in buffered saline without added nutrients. *FEMS Microbiol. Lett.* **110:**33–36.

168. **Porter, J. F., R. Parton, and A. C. Wardlaw.** 1991. Growth and survival of *Bordetella bronchiseptica* in natural waters and in buffered saline without added nutrients. *Appl. Environ. Microbiol.* **57:**1202–1206.

169. **Pullinger, G. D., R. Sowdhamini, and A. J. Lax.** 2001. Localization of functional domains of the mitogenic toxin of *Pasteurella multocida. Infect. Immun.* **69:**7839–7850.

170. **Pullinger, G. D., T. E. Adams, P. B. Mullan, T. I. Garrod, and A. J. Lax.** 1996. Cloning, expression, and molecular characterization of the dermonecrotic toxin gene of *Bordetella* spp. *Infect. Immun.* **64:**4163–4171.

171. **Register, K. B.** 2001. Novel genetic and phenotypic heterogeneity in *Bordetella bronchiseptica* pertactin. *Infect. Immun.* **69:**1917–1921.

172. **Register, K. B., and M. R. Ackermann.** 1997. A highly adherent phenotype associated with virulent Bvg$^+$-phase swine isolates of *Bordetella bronchiseptica* grown under modulating conditions. *Infect. Immun.* **65:**5295–5300.

173. **Renauld-Mongenie, G., J. Cornette, N. Mielcarek, F. D. Menozzi, and C. Locht.** 1996. Distinct roles of the N-terminal and C-terminal precursor domains in the biogenesis of the *Bordetella pertussis* filamentous hemagglutinin. *J. Bacteriol.* **178:**1053–1060.

174. **Ridley, A. J.** 1996. Rho: theme and variations. *Curr. Biol.* **6:**1256–1264.

175. **Ross, R. F., J. R. Duncan, and W. P. Switzer.** 1963. Turbinate atrophy in swine produced by pure cultures of *Bordetella bronchiseptica. Vet. Med.* **58:**566–570.

176. **Ross, R. F., W. P. Switzer, and J. P. Duncan.** 1967. Comparison of pathogenicity of various isolates of *Bordetella bronchiseptica* in young pigs. *Can. J. Comp. Med.* **31:**53–57.

177. **Roy, C. R., J. F. Miller, and S. Falkow.** 1989. The *bvgA* gene of *Bordetella pertussis* encodes a transcriptional activator required for coordinate regulation of several virulence genes. *J. Bacteriol.* **171:**6338–6344.

178. **Rozengurt, E., T. Higgins, N. Chanter, A. J. Lax, and J. M. Staddon.** 1990. *Pasteurella multocida* toxin: potent mitogen for cultured fibroblasts. *Proc. Natl. Acad. Sci. USA* **87:**123–127.

179. **Rutter, J. M.** 1981. Quantitative observations on *Bordetella bronchiseptica* infection in atrophic rhinitis of pigs. *Vet. Rec.* **108:**451–454.

180. **Rutter, J. M.** 1983. Virulence of *Pasteurella multocida* in atrophic rhinitis of gnotobiotic pigs infected with *Bordetella bronchiseptica. Res. Vet. Sci.* **34:**287.

181. **Rutter, J. M.** 1985. Atrophic rhinitis in swine. *Adv. Vet. Sci. Comp. Med.* **29:**239–279.

182. **Rutter, J. M., and A. Mackenzie.** 1984. Pathogenesis of atrophic rhinitis in pigs: a new perspective. *Vet. Rec.* **114:**89–90.

183. **Rutter, J. M., and X. Rojas.** 1982. Atrophic rhinitis in gnotobiotic piglets: differences in the pathogenicity of *Pasteurella multocida* in combined infections with *Bordetella bronchiseptica. Vet. Rec.* **110:**531–535.

184. **Rutter, J. M., L. M. Francis, and B. F. Sansom.** 1982. Virulence of *Bordetella bronchiseptica* from pigs with or without atrophic rhinitis. *J. Med. Microbiol.* **15:**105–116.

185. **Sakurai, Y., H. Suzuki, and E. Terada.** 1993. Purification and characterisation of haemagglutinin from *Bordetella bronchiseptica*. *J. Med. Microbiol.* **39:**388–392.

186. **Savelkoul, P. H., B. Kremer, J. G. Kusters, B. A. van der Zeijst, and W. Gaastra.** 1993. Invasion of HeLa cells by *Bordetella bronchiseptica*. *Microb. Pathog.* **14:**161–168.

187. **Savelkoul, P. H. M., D. P. G. de Kerf, R. J. Willems, F. R. Mooi, B. A. M. van der Zeijst, and W. Gaastra.** 1996. Characterization of the *fim2* and *fim3* fimbrial subunit genes of *Bordetella bronchiseptica*: roles of Fim2 and Fim3 fimbriae and flagella in adhesion. *Infect. Immun.* **64:**5098–5105.

188. **Scarlato, V., B. Arico, A. Prugnola, and R. Rappuoli.** 1991. Sequential activation and environmental regulation of virulence genes in *Bordetella pertussis*. *EMBO J.* **10:**3971–3975.

189. **Scarlato, V., B. Arico, M. Domenighini, and R. Rappuoli.** 1993. Environmental regulation of virulence factors in *Bordetella* species. *Bioessays* **15:**99–104.

190. **Schipper, H., G. F. Krohne, and R. Gross.** 1994. Epithelial cell invasion and survival of *Bordetella bronchiseptica*. *Infect. Immun.* **62:**3008–3011.

191. **Schmidt, G., U.-M. Goehring, J. Schirmer, M. Lerm, and K. Aktories.** 1999. Identification of the C-terminal part of *Bordetella* dermonecrotic toxin as a transglutaminase for Rho GTPases. *J. Biol. Chem.* **274:**31875–31881.

192. **Schneider, D. R., and C. D. Parker.** 1983. Effect of pyridines on phenotypic properties of *Bordetella pertussis*. *Infect. Immun.* **38:**548–553.

193. **Seifert, H.** 1971. Genetic aspects of atrophic rhinitis in the pig. *Monatsh. Vetmed.* **26:**770–772.

194. **Semjén, G., and T. Magyar.** 1985. A bovine haemagglutinin of *Bordetella bronchiseptica* responsible for adherence. *Acta Vet. Hung.* **33:**129–136.

195. **Seo, B., E. W. Choy, S. Maudsley, W. E. Miller, B. A. Wilson, and L. M. Luttrell.** 2000. *Pasteurella multocida* toxin stimulates mitogen-activated protein kinase via $G_{q/11}$-dependent transactivation of the epidermal growth factor receptor. *J. Biol. Chem.* **275:**2239–2245.

196. **Shimizu, T., M. Nakagawa, S. Shibata, and K. Suzuki.** 1971. Atrophic rhinitis produced by intranasal inoculation of *Bordetella bronchiseptica* in hysterectomy produced colostrum-deprived pigs. *Cornell Vet.* **61:**696–705.

197. **Sisak, F., M. Gois, and F. Kuksa.** 1978. The sensitivity of the strains of *Bordetella bronchiseptica, Pasteurella multocida* and *Mycoplasma hyorhinis,* isolated from pigs, to antibiotics and chemotherapeutics. *Vet. Med.* (Prague) **23:**531.

198. **Smith, A. M., C. A. Guzman, and M. J. Walker.** 2001. The virulence factors of *Bordetella pertussis*: a matter of control. *FEMS Microbiol. Rev.* **25:**309–333.

199. **Smith, I. M., C. J. Giles, and A. J. Baskerville.** 1982. The immunisation of pigs against experimental infection with *Bordetella bronchiseptica*. *Vet. Rec.* **110:**488–494.

200. **Smyth, M. G., I. G. Sumner, and A. J. Lax.** 1999. Reduced pH causes structural changes in the potent mitogenic toxin of *Pasteurella multocida*. *FEMS Microbiol. Lett.* **180:**15–20.

201. **Smyth, M. G., R. W. Pickersgill, and A. J. Lax.** 1995. The potent mitogen *Pasteurella multocida* toxin is highly resistant to proteolysis but becomes susceptible at lysosomal pH. *FEBS Lett.* **360:**62–66.

202. **Somlyo, A. P., and A. V. Somlyo.** 2000. Signal transduction by G-proteins, Rho-kinase and protein phosphatase to smooth muscle and non-muscle myosin II. *J. Physiol.* **522:**177–185.

203. **Staddon, J. M., N. Chanter, A. J. Lax, T. E. Higgins, and E. Rozengurt.** 1990. *Pasteurella multocida* toxin, a potent mitogen, stimulates protein kinase C-dependent and -independent protein phosphorylation in Swiss 3T3 cells. *J. Biol. Chem.* **265:**11841–11848.

204. **Staddon, J. M., C. J. Barker, A. C. Murphy, N. Chanter, A. J. Lax, R. H. Michell, and E. Rozengurt.** 1991. *Pasteurella multocida* toxin, a potent mitogen, increases inositol 1,4,5-trisphosphate and mobilizes Ca^{2+} in Swiss 3T3 cells. *J. Biol. Chem.* **266:**4840–4847.

205. **Sterner-Kock, A., B. Lanske, S. Überschär, and M. J. Atkinson.** 1995. Effects of the *Pasteurella multocida* toxin on osteoblastic cells in vitro. *Vet. Pathol.* **32:**274–279.

206. **Stibitz, S., W. Aaronson, D. Monack, and S. Falkow.** 1989. Phase variation in *Bordetella pertussis* by frameshift mutation in a gene for a novel two-component system. *Nature* **338:**266–269.

207. **Straw, B. E., A. D. Leman, and R. A. Robinson.** 1984. Pneumonia and atrophic rhinitis in pigs from a test station: a follow-up study. *J. Am. Vet. Med. Assoc.* **185:**1544–1546.

208. **Straw, B. E., E. J. Burgi, and H. D. Hilley.** 1983. Pneumonia and atrophic rhinitis in pigs from a test station. *J. Am. Vet. Med. Assoc.* **182:**607–611.

209. **Suda, T., N. Takahashi, N. Udagawa, E. Jimi, M. T. Gillespie, and T. J. Martin.**

1999. Modulation of osteoclast differentiation and function by the new members of the tumor necrosis factor receptor and ligand families. *Endocr. Rev.* **20**:345–357.

210. **Switzer, W. P.** 1956. Infectious atrophic rhinitis: concept that several agents may cause turbinate atrophy. *Am. J. Vet. Res.* **17**:478–484.

211. **Switzer, W. P.** 1963. Elimination of *Bordetella bronchiseptica* from the nasal cavity of swine by sulphonamide therapy. *Vet. Med.* **58**:571–574.

212. **Switzer, W. P.** 1981. Bordetellosis, p. 497–507. *In* A. D. Leman, R. D. Glock, W. L. Mengeling, R. H. C. Penny, E. Scholl, and B. Straw (ed.), *Diseases of Swine,* 5th ed. Iowa State University Press, Ames.

213. **Switzer, W. P., and D. O. Farrington.** 1975. Infectious atrophic rhinitis, p. 687–711. *In* H. W. Dunne and A. D. Leman (ed.), *Diseases of Swine,* 4th ed. Iowa State University Press, Ames.

214. **Taylor, S. S., J. A. Buechler, and W. Yonemoto.** 1990. cAMP-dependent protein kinase: framework for a diverse family of regulatory enzymes. *Annu. Rev. Biochem.* **59**:971–1005.

215. **Thomas, W., G. D. Pullinger, A. J. Lax and E. Rozengurt.** 2001. *Escherichia coli* cytotoxic necrotizing factor and *Pasteurella multocida* toxin induce FAK autophosphorylation and src association. *Infect. Immun.* **69**:5931–5935.

216. **Thomas, W., Z. K. Ascott, D. Harmey, L. W. Slice, E. Rozengurt, and A. J. Lax.** 2001. Cytotoxic necrotizing factor from *Escherichia coli* induces RhoA-dependent expression of the cyclooxygenase-2 gene. *Infect. Immun.* **69**:6839–6845.

217. **Tornoe, N., and N. C. Nielsen.** 1976. Inoculation experiments with *Bordetella bronchiseptica* strains in SPF pigs. *Nord. Vetmed.* **28**:233–242.

218. **Tornoe, N., N. C. Nielsen, and J. Svendsen.** 1976. *Bordetella bronchiseptica* isolations from the nasal cavity of pigs in relation to atrophic rhinitis. *Nord. Vetmed.* **28**:1.

219. **Tuomanen, E.** 1986. Piracy of adhesins: attachment of superinfecting pathogens to respiratory cilia by secreted adhesins of *Bordetella pertussis. Infect. Immun.* **54**:905–908.

220. **van Diemen, P. M., M. F. de Jong, G. de Vries Reilingh, and J. W. van der Hel P, Schrama.** 1994. Intranasal administration of *Pasteurella multocida* toxin in a challenge-exposure model used to induce subclinical signs of atrophic rhinitis in pigs. *Am. J. Vet. Res.* **55**:49–54.

221. **van Diemen, P. M., G. de Vries Reilingh, and H. K. Parmentier.** 1996. Effect of *Pasteurella multocida* toxin on in vivo immune responses in piglets. *Vet. Q.* **18**:141–146.

222. **Walker, K. E., and A. A. Weiss.** 1994. Characterization of the dermonecrotic toxin in members of the genus *Bordetella. Infect. Immun.* **62**:3817–3828.

223. **Wang, D., J. R. Grammer, C. S. Cobbs, J. E. Stewart, Z. Liu, R. Rhoden, T. P. Hecker, Q. Ding, and C. L. Gladson.** 2000. p125 focal adhesion kinase promotes malignant astrocytoma cell proliferation in vivo. *J. Cell Sci.* **113**:4221–4230.

224. **Ward, P. N., A. J. Miles, I. G. Sumner, L. H. Thomas, and A. J. Lax.** 1998. Activity of the mitogenic *Pasteurella multocida* toxin requires an essential C-terminal residue. *Infect. Immun.* **66**:5636–5642.

225. **Weingart, C. L., and A. A. Weiss.** 2000. *Bordetella pertussis* virulence factors affect phagocytosis by human neutrophils. *Infect. Immun.* **68**:1735–1739.

226. **Weiss, A. A., and M. S. M. Goodwin.** 1989. *Bordetella pertussis* mutants in the infant mouse model. *Infect. Immun.* **57**:3757–3764.

227. **Weiss, A. A., and S. Falkow.** 1984. Genetic analysis of phase change in *Bordetella pertussis. Infect. Immun.* **43**:263–269.

228. **Weiss, A. A., E. L. Hewlett, G. A. Myers, and S. Falkow.** 1984. Pertussis toxin and extracytoplasmic adenylate cyclase as virulence factors of *Bordetella pertussis. J. Infect. Dis.* **150**:219–221.

229. **Wilson, B. A., X. Zhu, M. Ho, and L. Lu.** 1997. *Pasteurella multocida* toxin activates the inositol triphosphate signaling pathway in *Xenopus* oocytes via $G_q\alpha$-coupled phospholipase C-$\beta1$. *J. Biol. Chem.* **272**:1268–1275.

230. **Winstanley, C., and C. A. Hart.** 2001. Type III secretion systems and pathogenicity islands. *J. Med. Microbiol.* **50**:116–126.

231. **Winstanley, C., B. A. Hales, L. M. Sibanda, S. Dawson, R. M. Gaskell, and C. A. Hart.** 2000. Detection of type III secretion system genes in animal isolates of *Bordetella bronchiseptica. Vet. Microbiol.* **72**:329–337.

232. **Wolff, J., and G. H. Cook.** 1973. Activity of thyroid membrane adenylate cyclase. *J. Biol. Chem.* **248**:350–355.

233. **Wolff, J., G. H. Cook, A. R. Goldhammer, and S. A. Berkowitz.** 1980. Calmodulin activates prokaryotic adenylate cyclase. *Proc. Natl. Acad. Sci. USA* **77**:3841–3844.

234. **Woolfrey, B. F., and J. A. Moody.** 1991. Human infections associated with *Bordetella bronchiseptica. Clin. Microbiol. Rev.* **4**:243–255.

235. **Yokomizo, Y., and T. Shimizu.** 1979. Adherence of *Bordetella bronchiseptica* to swine nasal epithelial cells and its possible role in virulence. *Res. Vet. Sci.* **27**:15–21.

236. **Yuk, M. H., E. T. Harvill, and J. F. Miller.** 1998. The BvgAS virulence control system regulates type III secretion in *Bordetella bronchiseptica*. *Mol. Microbiol.* **28:**945–959.

237. **Yuk, M. H., E. T. Harvill, P. A. Cotter, and J. F. Miller.** 2000. Modulation of host immune responses, induction of apoptosis and inhibition of NF-kappaB activation by the *Bordetella* type III secretion system. *Mol. Microbiol.* **35:**991–1004.

238. **Zhang, Y. L., and R. D. Sekura.** 1991. Purification and characterization of the heat-labile toxin of *Bordetella pertussis*. *Infect. Immun.* **59:** 3754–3759.

239. **Zywietz, A., A. Gohla, M. Shmelz, G. Schultz, and S. Offermanns.** 2001. Pleiotropic effects of *Pasteurella multocida* toxin are mediated by G_q-dependent and -independent mechanisms. *J. Biol. Chem.* **276:**3840–3845.

POLYMICROBIAL DISEASES INVOLVING VIRUSES AND BACTERIA

IV

COOPERATION BETWEEN VIRAL AND BACTERIAL PATHOGENS IN CAUSING HUMAN RESPIRATORY DISEASE

Harry Smith and Clive Sweet

Viruses that most commonly attack the human respiratory tract are influenza virus, parainfluenza viruses, respiratory syncytial virus (RSV), adenoviruses, measles virus, rhinoviruses, and coronaviruses (64). The main bacterial pathogens found in this tract are *Streptococcus pneumoniae, Streptococcus pyogenes, Haemophilus influenzae, Staphylococcus aureus, Neisseria meningitidis, Mycobacterium tuberculosis, Bordetella pertussis,* and, in immunocompromised patients, *Pseudomonas aeruginosa* (37). This chapter describes how some of these viruses and bacteria can cooperate to cause respiratory diseases which are more severe than those caused by either pathogen alone. Clinical, pathological, and epidemiological observations on natural disease, which suggest that such cooperation occurs, are examined first. This is followed by experiments using either animal models or, occasionally, human infections which prove the case. Finally, possible mechanisms to explain the increased severity of disease arising from dual infections are explained.

Harry Smith, Medical School, University of Birmingham, Birmingham B15 2TT, United Kingdom. *Clive Sweet,* School of Biosciences, University of Birmingham, Birmingham B15 2TT, United Kingdom.

OBSERVATIONS ON NATURAL DISEASE

The best and most studied example of virus-bacterium cooperation in the respiratory tract involves influenza virus. Influenza in humans is predominantly an upper respiratory tract infection; it is not usually fatal, but sometimes the lungs become infected, and this may have lethal consequences (51, 64). Most deaths in influenza epidemics arise from secondary bacterial infections, which were a scourge to humankind before the advent of antibiotics and even now are troublesome (6, 15, 27, 51, 60, 90). The bacteria concerned are predominantly *S. pneumoniae, H. influenzae, S. aureus,* and *N. meningitidis* (6, 15, 27, 51, 60, 90, 100). Indeed, the incidences of influenza, pneumococcal infection, and meningococcal disease show a seasonal association: they all peak in the winter months (14, 52). During the 1918 to 1919 influenza pandemic, around 40 million people died. Some deaths appeared to be due to viral pneumonia, since they occurred rapidly after the onset of symptoms, often with acute pulmonary hemorrhage or edema. However, clinical and pathological evidence indicates that the majority of people succumbed to secondary bacterial pneumonia (100).

Polymicrobial Diseases, Edited by Kim A. Brogden and Janet M. Guthmiller,
© 2002 ASM Press, Washington, D.C.

In respiratory disease of children, cooperation of bacteria with RSV may occur more frequently than with influenza virus. For example, in a serological study of the etiology of community-acquired pneumonia in children, 39% of the children with viral infection had a concomitant bacterial infection, and the most frequent combination for those under the age of 5 years was RSV with *S. pneumoniae* (38). As with influenza, both RSV infection and pneumococcal disease peak in the winter months (52). RSV has been associated with other bacteria too, e.g., *B. pertussis* (2, 68) and *S. aureus* (12). Other respiratory viruses have been implicated in bacterial interactions but to a lesser degree. Human parainfluenza virus was found, together with *S. pneumoniae,* in an outbreak of pneumonia in a long-term care facility (26). Adenoviruses also may predispose patients to respiratory bacterial infections (21, 30), and associations between adenovirus and *B. pertussis* in severe respiratory disease of children have been noted (2, 93). Measles virus seems to exacerbate tuberculosis (24). Also, in 182 cases of measles-associated pneumonia of children, mixed infection was found in 53% of the patients, with *S. pneumoniae* being the most common finding in blood cultures (74). In contrast to most respiratory viruses, rhinoviruses and coronaviruses that cause the common cold appear to act alone. In 200 young adults with common colds, virus etiology was established for 138 cases (105 had rhinoviruses, and 17 had coronaviruses), but evidence of bacterial infection was found in only 7 of the patients (65).

In sudden infant death syndrome (SIDS), a common cause of postperinatal mortality (31, 69), there is often a history of upper respiratory tract infection and inflammatory changes are sometimes visible at postmortem (13, 104). Several respiratory viruses have been associated with SIDS; they include RSV, influenza virus, parainfluenza virus, adenovirus, and rhinovirus (91, 110). Also, changes in bacterial populations in the nasopharynx, particularly an increase in *S. aureus* and enterobacteria, have been associated with SIDS (9, 101).

These observations on naturally occurring human disease clearly show that viruses and bacteria are found together in severe respiratory disease. However, there is no specific evidence for cooperation between them except for in influenza, for which histopathology indicates that most deaths following viral infection are due to secondary bacterial infections.

PROOF THAT VIRUSES COOPERATE WITH BACTERIA IN PRODUCING DISEASE

In many experiments using animal models, bacterial infections have been superimposed at various times after inoculation of viruses. Enhancement of bacterial infection was demonstrated by comparisons of the bacterial contents of appropriate tissues with those of animals receiving bacteria alone. Exacerbation of disease was shown by more-severe lesions or higher death rates than for animals receiving either the bacteria or viruses alone. The classical investigation using an animal model was that of Shope in 1931 (94) using influenza virus and *H. influenzae* in pigs. However, mice have been the experimental animals used for most investigations. Examples are as follows. Influenza virus enhanced respiratory infections with pneumococci (36, 59, 97), staphylococci (43), *Listeria monocytogenes* (28), group B streptococci (49), and *Bacillus thuringiensis* (39). Sendai virus enhanced respiratory infections with *Mycoplasma pulmonis* (41). Reovirus enhanced staphylococcal infection (53), and cytomegalovirus enhanced *P. aeruginosa* infection (33). Observations for other animal models included increased infection with *H. influenzae* in RSV-infected cotton rats (71), the effect of influenza virus on colonization of the nasopharynx of chinchillas by different phenotypes of *S. pneumoniae* (102), and enhanced streptococcal infection following influenza virus infection of ferrets (10, 29). Neonatal ferrets infected with influenza virus provided an animal model for SIDS. An intranasally administered virulent strain (clone 7a) killed the neonates, and the pathology of some was akin to that seen in SIDS. In contrast to the virulent strain, killing of the neonates by a less virulent strain (PR8) could be prevented by antibiotic treatment, indicating that it was due to virus exacerbation of naturally acquired bacterial infection (42).

For obvious reasons, humans have not been deliberately infected with respiratory viruses followed by bacterial pathogens to study the progress of subsequent bacterial infection as described above for animal models. However, the effect of experimental influenza A virus infection of volunteers on selection of pathogens from the natural nasopharyngeal flora has been studied; *S. pneumoniae* was not isolated from any subject prior to virus challenge but was isolated in substantial numbers from 15% of the subjects on the sixth day following challenge (105). Also, cells and fluids have been harvested, either from patients with natural infections or volunteers experimentally infected with viruses, and interacted with pathogenic bacteria in vitro in biological tests related to infection. For example, *S. aureus, H. influenzae,* and *S. pneumoniae* showed enhanced adherence to pharyngeal cells obtained from volunteers infected with influenza virus compared with cells from uninfected controls (23). Other examples are given below.

MECHANISMS OF COOPERATION

To cause disease, microorganisms must infect mucous surfaces, penetrate into the tissues, grow in the tissue environment, inhibit host defense mechanisms, and cause damage to the host (96). Viruses can increase the ability of bacterial pathogens to achieve one or more of these steps. Also, there is one example of bacteria enhancing viral growth in host cells. The mechanisms are discussed in relation to infections of the respiratory tract.

Infection of the Mucous Surface

Bacterial infection of respiratory tract surfaces could occur more easily if mucociliary clearance was impaired by virus attack. In fact, bacterial pulmonary infection is common in primary ciliary dyskinesia (80). Viruses are thought to impair ciliary action. RSV infection caused a loss of cilia from human bronchial cells in vitro (103). Influenza virus infection caused damage to ciliated columnar epithelium and the bronchial epithelial lining (107). Nevertheless, the results of early work with animal models indicated that virus infection does not impair mucociliary clearance. In mice infected with influenza virus, ciliated epithelium was damaged but mucociliary clearance was unaffected (34). Similarly, in mice infected with Sendai virus, tracheobronchial clearance of inhaled radiotracer-labeled bacteria was not significantly altered (30).

Enhanced adherence to host cells by bacteria would also increase infection of the respiratory tract, and this does occur as a result of virus attack. This is proved by two types of experiments: adherence to cell lines infected with virus in vitro (Table 1) and adherence to cells

TABLE 1 Enhanced bacterial adherence to cell lines when infected with viruses in vitro

Virus	Cell line	Bacteria	Reference
Influenza A virus	MDCK	*S. aureus*	88
	HeLa	*S. aureus, S. pyogenes, S. pneumoniae*	92
	HEp-2	*S. pneumoniae, N. meningitidis*	20
RSV	HEp-2	*S. aureus*	84
		H. influenzae	79
		B. pertussis	83
	A549	*H. influenzae*	47
Adenovirus	A549	*S. pneumoniae*	32

TABLE 2 Enhanced bacterial adherence to tissues or cells of virus-infected animals or humans

Adherence observed	Virus	Animal or humans	Tissue or harvested cells	Bacterium	Reference
In vivo	Influenza A virus	Mouse	Tracheal	*S. pneumoniae*	73
	Influenza A virus	Mouse	Tracheal	Group B streptococci	48
	Influenza A virus	Mouse	Tracheal	*P. aeruginosa*	75
	Influenza A virus	Mouse	Nasopharynx	*S. pneumoniae,* *H. influenzae*	40
	Influenza A virus	Ferret	Nasopharynx	*S. aureus,* group B streptococci	85
	RSV	Cotton rat	Nasopharynx	*H. influenzae*	71
In vitro	Influenza A virus	Volunteers	Pharyngeal	*S. aureus, S. pneumoniae,* *H. influenzae*	23
	Nonspecific	Patients	Pharyngeal	*S. aureus*	23
	Influenza A virus	Chinchilla	Tracheal	*H. influenzae*	4

of virus-infected animals or people examined either in vivo or in vitro (Table 2). Now there is much interest in the molecular bases for the enhanced adherence.

Virus-induced change in host cell membranes is the most likely cause of increased bacterial adherence. For example, viral glycoproteins expressed on host cell membranes could act as receptors for bacteria. In the case of influenza virus, both its hemagglutinin (HA) and neuraminidase are inserted into host cell membranes (64). An early study (88) indicated that influenza virus HA on infected MDCK cells was a receptor for group B streptococci because the adherence was blocked by antibodies to the HA. Also, the adherence could be blocked by treatment with neuraminidase (17), which suggests that adherence was mediated through sialic acid on the HA oligosaccharide. In a more recent study, alteration in the glycoconjugate structure of murine nasopharyngeal mucosae brought about by influenza virus infection was detected by changes in lectin binding patterns (40).

Neither antibody nor neuraminidase treatment inhibited increased staphylococcal adherence to influenza virus-infected MDCK cells, so other receptor mechanisms must also be involved. Two studies suggest that these mechanisms are complex. The bacterial adhesins mediating the binding of staphylococci to virus-infected cells are more heat labile than those involved in staphylococcal binding to

uninfected cells, and two staphylococcal proteins, clumping factor and protein A, act as adhesins for normal but not virus-infected cells (18, 87). The natures of the cell receptors are unknown. One possible mechanism for staphylococcal adherence to virus-infected cells in vivo was suggested by an earlier study (3). Protein A on the surface of staphylococci is known to interact with antibody (37). In vivo, infected cells may be coated with viral antibody, thus providing a receptor for staphylococcal protein A. Indeed, adherence of protein A-containing staphylococci, but not that of strains lacking protein A, was enhanced by treating influenza virus-infected cells with antibody (3). This mechanism could operate for other viruses.

Glycoproteins F and G of RSV are inserted into the membrane of infected HEp-2 cells, and glycoprotein G is involved in the increased binding of *N. meningitidis* to these cells (77). Also in HEp-2 cells, RSV infection up-regulated normal host cell receptors such as CD14, CD15, and CD18, and CD14 and CD15 were associated with the increased adherence of a nonpiliated strain of *N. meningitidis* (78).

Extracellular matrices can provide a vehicle for cross-linking bacteria with virus-induced alterations of host cell membranes. For example, the adhesion of group A streptococci to influenza A virus-infected cells is enhanced by addition of fibrinogen (86). Oligosaccharides on neuraminidase, HA, or both, expressed on virus-infected cell surfaces, may be responsible for binding the fibrinogen because addition of tunicamycin, an inhibitor of glycosylation of viral proteins, decreased the fibrinogen-mediated adherence (86).

Penetration into the Tissues

The denudation of epithelial cells that results from infection with influenza virus must aid penetration into the tissues. Thus, staphylococci appear to attack only those parts of the respiratory tract damaged by viral attack (67). Epithelial damage by other viruses could have similar effects.

Growth in the Tissue Environment

An early study indicated that fluid exuded onto mucous surfaces as the result of virus attack could increase bacterial growth. In mice, infection with influenza virus alone induced lung edema, and virus-free edema fluid from such mice enhanced the ability of pneumococci to produce pneumonia in other mice not previously infected with influenza virus (35). The factors involved are unknown.

Inhibition of Host Defense Mechanisms

There are three types of defense against bacterial attack that could be inhibited by virus infection: nonspecific humoral factors, such as complement-mediated killing by normal serum; nonspecific phagocytosis by neutrophils and macrophages at the beginning of infection; and the later specific-antibody- and cell-mediated response (96). With regard to humoral factors, some viruses, notably, herpesviruses, poxviruses, and human immunodeficiency virus type 1, are able to interfere with complement, either by incorporation of cellular complement regulatory protein CD55 into the virion envelope or cell membrane (95) or by expression of viral molecules that mimic functions of complement regulatory protein (7). Also, the viruses can bind to the third component of complement, C3, directly or block C5 and properdin binding to C3 (62). However,

we are not aware of reports showing that respiratory viruses are able to interfere with the complement system or that these viruses interfere with the action of host humoral factors on bacteria. Viral immunosuppression is dealt with in chapter 19; hence, interference with the nonspecific action of phagocytes is the subject of this section.

Numerous experiments with respiratory viruses show that the capacity of neutrophils and macrophages to deal with bacterial infection is substantially reduced by virus attack. Only a few examples are cited here. Human neutrophils, after interaction with influenza virus in vitro, showed decreased chemotaxis and phagocytic activity in interactions with staphylococci (58). In vivo, rat neutrophil exudation and mobility were depressed by influenza virus infection (82). Macrophage chemotaxis towards bacteria was inhibited by influenza virus infection in vitro (55, 72). Also, experiments with a monocytic cell line (THP-1) showed that RSV depressed tumor necrosis factor alpha production and bactericidal activity against *H. influenzae* and *S. pneumoniae* (76). In vivo, influenza virus infection of mice inhibited accumulation of macrophages at inflammatory sites (54) and impaired their capacity to remove staphylococci from the lungs (43). Both ingestion and killing of bacteria by alveolar macrophages are inhibited (109). Inhaled staphylococci were ingested equally by alveolar macrophages of normal mice and those infected with Sendai virus, but the bacteria were killed in the former cells and grew in the latter (30).

With regard to the mechanism of reduction in bactericidal power of neutrophils and macrophages, influenza virus infection impairs lysozyme production by both types of phagocytes (70, 108), while Sendai virus inhibits phagolysosome fusion in mouse alveolar macrophages (44). Superoxide generation is also inhibited in influenza virus-infected phagocytes (19). Interestingly, dual infection of neutrophils with influenza A virus and *S. pneumoniae* caused significantly more H_2O_2 production than either pathogen alone, but the increased respiratory burst contributed to diminished neutrophil survival (22). Finally, neutrophil and macrophage apoptosis is accelerated by influenza virus infection (16, 25, 61), and this would decrease the overall antibacterial activity.

Cause Damage to the Host

Bacteria can damage the host by producing toxins and/or inducing cytokines and inflammation (96). There is research regarding SIDS which indicates that viral infection can exacerbate the effect of toxins and the induction of inflammatory cytokines in the respiratory tract.

We noted above that in SIDS there is an increase of *S. aureus* and enterobacteria in the nasal flora, and it has been suggested that bacterial toxins may contribute to SIDS (66). Staphylococcal enterotoxins and the toxic shock syndrome toxin have been identified in the tissues from over half of SIDS cases from five countries (8). The possibility that virus infection can enhance the lethal effects of bacterial toxins was examined by using the neonatal ferret model for SIDS (45). Staphylococcal α and γ toxins, endotoxin, and diphtheria toxins were lethal for 5-day-old ferrets. Their toxicities were enhanced in 1-day-old animals infected with influenza virus PR8, from 3-fold with staphylococcal γ toxin to 14-fold for staphylococcal α toxin, 84-fold for endotoxin, and 219-fold for diphtheria toxin. No increased viral replication occurred in any tissue; thus, the effects of the toxins were exacerbated by the infection, not vice versa. Neonates died suddenly without clinical symptoms, similarly to human babies dying from SIDS. Pathological examination showed inflammation in the upper respiratory tract, lung edema and collapse, and early bronchopneumonia in the animals treated with toxin and influenza virus but not in those treated with toxin or virus alone. Thus, bacterial toxins could play a role in SIDS, this being more likely with a concomitant influenza virus infection.

The increased toxicity of staphylococcal α toxin and diphtheria toxin may follow from the enhancement of membrane leakage in virus-infected cells. This was detected by the release of α-amino[^{14}C]isobutyric acid from ferret Mpf cells (46). The release, induced by staphylococcal α toxin and diphtheria toxin, was enhanced significantly when the cells had been previously infected with influenza virus PR8, although infection with virus alone did not increase the release of radiolabel compared with that of untreated cells. The mechanism of enhancement of release is unclear, but it occurs 0.5 to 2 h after inoculation and viral membrane-endosome fusion is essential. As stated above, the increase in lethality in the ferret neonatal model is accompanied by inflammation in the upper respiratory tract and lung edema. The reason for these effects may be that the enhanced cellular permeability leads to the release of histamine and other inflammatory mediators such as interleukin 1, tumor necrosis factor, and platelet-activating factor.

Endotoxin has no effect on the membrane permeability of ferret Mpf cells either alone or after influenza virus PR8 infection (46), so changes in membrane permeability probably play no part in the viral enhancement of its toxicity for neonates. However, cytokine release from human peripheral blood leukocytes was increased by infection with influenza virus (63). This release could be the reason for the upper respiratory tract inflammation seen in SIDS and in the neonatal ferret model.

Cleavage of Influenza A Virus HA by Bacterial Proteases

Cell entry of influenza A virus by receptor-mediated endocytosis requires cleavage of its HA (81). During viral entry, the HA undergoes a conformational change in the acidic environment of the endosome (11). Proteolytic cleavage of precursor HA into HA1 and HA2 exposes the amino-terminal fusion peptide of HA2, resulting in fusion of the viral envelope within the endosomal membrane. Cleavage of HA is important in viral pathogenicity and tissue tropism because it is necessary for spread of infection throughout the host (81). The HAs of mammalian and nonpathogenic avian influenza virus strains are usually cleaved by the proteases in only a few cell types, thus causing only local respiratory infection. On the other hand, the HAs of some avian influenza strains of the H5 and H7 subtypes are cleaved by proteases in a broad range of cells and consequently cause systemic infection. The major structural property that determines the difference in protease sensitivity is the link between HA1 and HA2 in the uncleaved precursor. In HA showing restricted cleavage, the link usually consists of a single arginine residue, whereas highly cleavable HAs have multiple basic residues in this position, forming the consensus sequence R-X-K/R-R (56, 81).

Early studies showed that trypsin was required for cleavage of HA in vitro (57). The HAs of the pathogenic avian viruses are susceptible to host intracellular proteases such as furin; this is not so for the HAs of the mammalian viruses, which are cleaved predominantly by extracellular serine proteases (50, 81, 106). The specific proteases that confer cleavage activation of HA in respiratory infection of humans are not clear, although proteases have been found in nasal washings of children with upper respiratory tract infections (5). Host proteases such as thrombin and plasmin cleave the HAs of some but not all influenza viruses (89).

The proteases of respiratory tract bacteria could contribute to cleavage of influenza virus HA in vivo. This was first shown for the protease of *S. aureus* (98, 99) and then for those of other bacteria in the respiratory tract, e.g., *Streptomyces griseus* and *Aerococcus viridans* (57, 89). HA cleavage by *S. aureus* and *A. viridans* not only conferred virus infectivity and the ability to replicate in vitro but also augmented virus replication and pathogenicity in mice (89, 98, 99). Another possible method for bacteria to enhance influenza virus infection is by activation of host proteases which could cause cleavage of HA, e.g., staphylokinase, streptokinase, and a protease from *Serratia marcescens* which facilitates HA cleavage activation by generating plasmin from plasminogen (1, 89).

SUMMARY AND CONCLUSION

Clinical observations and epidemiology indicate that viruses and bacteria can cooperate to produce more severe respiratory disease in humans than occurs with either infection alone. Experimental studies of mixed infection in animal models and occasionally humans have confirmed this. The mechanisms involved have been probed, and it has been demonstrated that viruses can aid bacteria in all aspects of their pathogenesis, namely, infection and penetration of mucous surfaces, growth in the host environment, interference with host defense, and the causation of damage to the host. Conversely, bacterial proteases may help influenza virus to infect cells of the respiratory tract by cleaving the viral HA.

The important practical conclusion is that successful vaccination against respiratory virus diseases may contribute to protection against bacterial attack.

REFERENCES

1. **Akaike, T., A. Molla, M. Ando, S. Araki, and H. Maeda.** 1989. Molecular mechanism of complex infection by bacteria and virus analyzed by a model using serratial protease and influenza virus in mice. *J. Virol.* **63:**2252–2259.
2. **Aoyama, T., Y. Ide, J. Watanabe, Y. Takeuchi, and A. Imaizumi.** 1996. Respiratory failure caused by dual infection with *Bordetella pertussis* and respiratory syncytial virus. *Acta Paediatr. Jpn.* **38:**282–285.
3. **Austin, R. M., and C. A. Daniels.** 1978. The role of protein A in attachment of staphylococci to influenza-infected cells. *Lab. Investig.* **39:**128–132.
4. **Bakaletz, L. O., T. M. Hoeph, T. F. DeMaria, and D. J. Lim.** 1988. The effect of antecedent influenza A virus infection on the adherence of *Haemophilus influenzae* to chinchilla tracheal cells. *Am. J. Otolaryngol.* **9:**127–134.
5. **Barbey-Morel, C., T. Oeltmann, K. Edwards, and P. Wright.** 1987. Role of the respiratory tract proteases in infectivity of influenza A virus. *J. Infect. Dis.* **155:**667–672.
6. **Barker, W. H., and J. P. Mullooly.** 1982. Pneumonia and influenza deaths during epidemics: implications for prevention. *Arch. Intern. Med.* **142:**85–89.
7. **Barrett, J. W., J. X. Cao, S. Hota-Mitchell, and G. McFadden.** 2001. Immunomodulatory proteins of myxoma virus. *Semin. Immunol.* **13:**73–84.
8. **Blackwell, C. C., A. E. Gordon, V. S. James, D. A. C. MacKenzie, M. Mogensen-**

Buchannan, O. R. El Ahmer, O. M. Al Madani, K. Toro, Z. Cuskas, P. Sotonyi, D. M. Weir, and A. Busuttil. The role of bacterial toxins in sudden infant death syndrome (SIDS). *Int. J. Med. Microbiol.*, in press.

9. Blackwell, C. C., D. A. C. MacKenzie, V. S. James, R. A. Elton, A. A. Zorgani, D. M. Weir, and A. Busuttil. 1999. Toxigenic bacteria and sudden infant death syndrome (SIDS): nasopharyngeal flora during the first year of life. *FEMS Immunol. Med. Microbiol.* 25:51–58.

10. Brightman, I. J. 1935. Streptococcus infection occurring in ferrets inoculated with human influenza virus. *Yale J. Biol. Med.* 8:127–135.

11. Bullough, P. A., F. M. Hughson, J. J. Skehel, and D. C. Wiley. 1994. Structure of influenza haemagglutinin at the pH of membrane fusion. *Nature* 371:37–43.

12. Carfrae, D. C., E. J. Bell, and N. R. Grist. 1982. Fatal hemorrhagic pneumonia in an adult due to respiratory syncytial virus and *Staphylococcus aureus*. *J. Infect.* 4:79.

13. Carpenter, R. G., A. Gardener, E. Pursall, P. M. McWeeny, and S. Norn. 1979. Identification of some infants at risk of dying unexpectedly and justifying intensive study. *Lancet* ii:343–346.

14. Cartwright, K. A. V., D. M. Jones, A. J. Smith, J. M. Stuart, E. B. Kaesmarski, and S. R. Palmer. 1991. Influenza A and meningococcal disease. *Lancet* 338:554–557.

15. Cate, T. R. 1998. Impact of influenza and other community-acquired viruses. *Semin. Respir. Infect.* 13:17–23.

16. Colamussi, M. L., M. R. White, E. Crouch, and K. L. Hartshorn. 1999. Influenza virus A accelerates neutrophil apoptosis and markedly potentiates apoptotic effects of bacteria. *Blood* 93:2395–2403.

17. Davison, V. E., and B. A. Sanford. 1981. Adherence of *Staphylococcus aureus* to influenza A virus-infected Madin-Darby canine kidney cell cultures. *Infect. Immun.* 32:118–126.

18. Davison, V. E., and B. A. Sanford. 1982. Factors influencing adherence of *Staphylococcus aureus* to influenza A virus-infected cell cultures. *Infect. Immun.* 37:946–955.

19. Dyer, R. M., S. Majumdar, S. D. Douglas, and H. M. Korchak. 1994. Bovine parainfluenza-3 virus selectively depletes a calcium-dependent, phospholipid-dependent protein kinase C and inhibits superoxide anion generation in bovine alveolar macrophages. *J. Immunol.* 153:1171–1179.

20. El Ahmer, O. R., M. W. Raza, M. M. Ogilvie, D. M. Weir, and C. C. Blackwell. 1999. Binding of bacteria to HEp-2 cells infected with influenza A virus. *FEMS Immunol. Med. Microbiol.* 23:331–341.

21. El-Sheikh, S. M., S. M. El-Assouli, K. A. Mohammed, and M. Albar. 1998. Bacteria and viruses that cause respiratory tract infections during the pilgrimage (Haj) season in Makkah, Saudi Arabia. *Trop. Med. Int. Health* 3:205–209.

22. Englelich, G., M. White, and K. L. Hartshorn. 2001. Neutrophil survival is markedly reduced by incubation with influenza virus and *Streptococcus pneumoniae*: role of respiratory burst. *J. Leukoc. Biol.* 69:50–56.

23. Fainstein, F., D. M. Musher, and T. R. Cate. 1980. Bacterial adherence to pharyngeal cells during viral infections. *J. Infect. Dis.* 141:172–176.

24. Fenner, F., and D. O. White. 1976. *Medical Virology,* 2nd ed. Academic Press, London, United Kingdom.

25. Fesq, H., N. Bacher, M. Nain, and D. Gemsa. 1994. Programmed cell death (apoptosis) in human monocytes infected with influenza A virus. *Immunobiology* 190:175–182.

26. Fiore, A. E., C. Iverson, T. Messmer, D. Erdman, S. M. Lett, D. F. Talkington, L. J. Anderson, B. Fields, G. M. Carlone, R. F. Breiman, and M. S. Cetron. 1998. Outbreak of pneumonia in a long term care facility: antecedent human parainfluenza virus 1 infection may predispose to bacterial pneumonia. *J. Am. Geriatr. Soc.* 46:1112–1117.

27. Floret, D. 1997. Virus-bacteria co-infections. *Arch. Pediatr.* 4:1119–1124.

28. Gardner, I. D. 1980. Effect of influenza virus infection on susceptibility of bacteria in mice. *J. Infect. Dis.* 142:704–706.

29. Glover, R. E. 1941. Spread of infection from the respiratory tract of the ferret. II. Association of influenza A virus and streptococcus group C. *Br. J. Exp. Pathol.* 22:98–107.

30. Green, G. M., G. J. Jakab, R. B. Low, and G. S. Davis. 1977. Defense mechanisms of the respiratory membrane. *Am. Rev. Respir. Dis.* 115:479–514.

31. Guntheroth, W. G. 1989. *Crib Death: the Sudden Infant Death Syndrome.* Futura Publishing, New York, N.Y.

32. Hakansson, A., A. Kidd, G. Wadell, H. Sabharwal, and C. Svanborg. 1994. Adenovirus infection enhances in vitro adherence of *Streptococcus pneumoniae*. *Infect. Immun.* 62:2707–2714.

33. Hamilton, J. R., and J. C. Overall. 1978. Synergistic infection with murine cytomegalovirus and *Pseudomonas aeruginosa* in mice. *J. Infect. Dis.* 137:775–782.

34. Harford, C. G., and A. Hamlin. 1952. Effect of influenza virus on cilia and epithelial cells in the bronchi of mice. *J. Exp. Med.* 95:173–189.

35. **Harford, C. G., and M. Hara.** 1950. Pulmonary edema in influenza pneumonia of the mouse and the relation of fluid in the lung to the inception of pneumococcal pneumonia. *J. Exp. Med.* **91:**245–259.

36. **Harford, C. G., V. Leidler, and M. Hara.** 1949. Effect of the lesion due to influenza virus on the resistance of mice to inhaled pneumococci. *J. Exp. Med.* **89:**53–68.

37. **Hausler, W. J., and M. Sussman (ed.).** 1998. *Topley and Wilson's Microbiology and Microbial Infection,* 9th ed., vol. 3. *Bacterial Infections.* Arnold, London, United Kingdom.

38. **Heiskanen-Kosma, T., M. Korppi, C. Jokinen, S. Kurki, L. Heiskanen, H. Juvonen, S. Kallinen, M. Sten, A. Tarkiainen, P. R. Ronnberg, M. Kleemola, P. H. Makela, and M. Leinonen.** 1998. Etiology of childhood pneumonia: serologic results of a prospective, population based study. *Pediatr. Infect. Dis. J.* **17:**986–991.

39. **Hernandez, E., F. Ramisse, P. Gros, and J.-D. Cavallo.** 2000. Super-infection by *Bacillus thuringiensis* H34 or 3a3b can lead to death in mice infected with the influenza A virus. *FEMS Immunol. Med. Microbiol.* **29:**177–181.

40. **Hirano, T., Y. Kurono, I. Ichimiya, M. Suzuki, and G. Mogi.** 1999. Effects of influenza A virus on lectin-binding patterns in murine nasopharyngeal mucosa and on bacterial colonization. *Otolaryngol. Head Neck Surg.* **121:**616–621.

41. **Howard, C. J., E. J. Stott, and G. Taylor.** 1978. The effect of pneumonia induced in mice with *Mycoplasma pulmonis* on resistance to subsequent bacterial infection and the effect of respiratory infections with Sendai virus on resistance of mice to *Mycoplasma pulmonis. J. Gen. Microbiol.* **109:**79–87.

42. **Husseini, R. H., M. H. Collie, D. L. Rushton, C. Sweet, and H. Smith.** 1983. The role of naturally-acquired bacterial infection in influenza-related death in neonatal ferrets. *Br. J. Exp. Pathol.* **64:**559–569.

43. **Jakab, G. J., G. A. Warr, and M. E. Knight.** 1979. Pulmonary and systemic defences against challenge with *Staphylococcus aureus* in mice with pneumonia due to influenza A virus. *J. Infect. Dis.* **140:**105–108.

44. **Jakab, G. J., G. A. Warr, and P. L. Sonnes.** 1980. Alveolar macrophage ingestion and phagosome-lysosome fusion defect associated with virus pneumonia. *Infect. Immun.* **27:**960–968.

45. **Jakeman, K. J., D. I. Rushton, H. Smith, and C. Sweet.** 1991. Exacerbation of bacterial toxicity to infant ferrets by influenza virus: possible role in sudden infant death syndrome. *J. Infect. Dis.* **163:**35–40.

46. **Jakeman, K. J., H. Smith, and C. Sweet.** 1991. Influenza virus enhancement of membrane leakiness induced by staphylococcal α toxin, diphtheria toxin and streptolysin S. *J. Gen. Virol.* **72:**111–115.

47. **Jiang, Z., N. Nagata, E. Molina, L. O. Bakaletz, H. Hawkins, and J. A. Patel.** 1999. Fimbria-mediated enhanced attachment of nontypeable *Haemophilus influenzae* to respiratory syncytial virus-infected respiratory epithelial cells. *Infect. Immun.* **67:**187–192.

48. **Jones, W. T., and J. H. Menna.** 1982. Influenza type-A virus-mediated adherence of type 1A group-B streptococci to mouse tracheal tissue in vivo. *Infect. Immun.* **38:**791–794.

49. **Jones, W. T., J. H. Menna, and D. E. Wennerstrom.** 1983. Lethal synergism induced in mice by influenza type-A virus and type-1A group-B streptococci. *Infect. Immun.* **41:**618–623.

50. **Kawaoka, Y., and R. G. Webster.** 1988. Sequence requirements for cleavage activation of influenza virus hemagglutinin expressed in mammalian cells. *Proc. Natl. Acad. Sci. USA* **85:**324–328.

51. **Kilbourne, E. D.** 1987. *Influenza.* Plenum Publishing Corp., New York, N.Y.

52. **Kim, P. E., D. M. Musher, W. P. Glezen, M. C. Rodriguez-Barradas, W. K. Nahm, and C. E. Wright.** 1996. Association of invasive pneumococcal disease with season, atmospheric conditions, air pollution and isolation of respiratory viruses. *Clin. Infect. Dis.* **22:**100–106.

53. **Klein, J. O., G. M. Green, J. G. Tiles, E. H. Kass, and M. Finland.** 1969. Effect of intranasal virus infection on antibacterial activity of mouse lung. *J. Infect. Dis.* **119:**43–50.

54. **Kleinerman, E. S., C. A. Daniels, R. P. Pollsson, and R. Snyderman.** 1976. Effect of virus infection on the inflammatory response. Depression of macrophage accumulation in influenza infected mice. *Am. J. Pathol.* **85:**373–382.

55. **Kleinerman, E. S., R. Snyderman, and C. A. Daniels.** 1974. Depression of human monocyte chemotaxis by *Herpes simplex,* and influenza viruses. *J. Immunol.* **113:**1562–1567.

56. **Klenk, H. D., and R. Rott.** 1988. The molecular biology of influenza virus pathogenicity. *Adv. Virus Res.* **34:**247–281.

57. **Klenk, H. D., R. Rott, and M. Orlich.** 1977. Further studies on the activation of influenza virus by proteolytic cleavage of the haemagglutinin. *J. Gen. Virol.* **36:**151–161.

58. **Larson, H. E., R. P. Parry, C. Gilchrist, A. Luquetti, and D. A. J. Tyrrell.** 1977. Influenza viruses and staphylococci *in vitro:* some interactions with polymorphonuclear and epithelial cells. *Br. J. Exp. Pathol.* **58:**281–292.

59. **LeVine, A. M., V. Koeningsknecht, and J. M. Stark.** 2001. Decreased pulmonary clearance of *S. pneumoniae* following influenza A infection in mice. *J. Virol. Methods* **94:**173–186.

60. **Louria, D. B., H. L. Blumenfeld, J. T. Ellis, E. D. Kilbourne, and D. E. Rogers.** 1959. Studies on influenza in the pandemic of 1957–58. II. Pulmonary complications of influenza. *J. Clin. Investig.* **38:**213–265.

61. **Lowry, R. J., and D. S. Dimitrov.** 1995. Induction of apoptosis in J774.1 macrophages by influenza-virus. *Mol. Biol. Cell* **6:**2063–2071.

62. **Lubinski, J., L. Y. Wang, D. Mastellos, A. Sahu, J. D. Lambris, and H. M. Friedman.** 1999. In vivo role of complement-interacting domain of herpes simplex virus type 1 glycoprotein gC. *J. Exp. Med.* **190:**1637–1646.

63. **Lundemose, J. B., H. Smith, and C. Sweet.** 1993. Cytokine release from human peripheral blood leucocytes incubated with endotoxin with or without prior infection with influenza virus: relevance to the sudden infant death syndrome. *Int. J. Exp. Pathol.* **74:**291–297.

64. **Mahy, B. W. J., and L. Collier (ed.).** 1998. *Topley and Wilson's Microbiology and Microbial Infection,* 9th ed., vol. 1. *Virology.* Arnold, London, United Kingdom.

65. **Makela, M. J., T. Puhakka, O. Ruuskanen, M. Leinonen, P. Saikku, M. Kimpimaki, S. Blomqvist, T. Hyypia, and P. Arstila.** 1998. Viruses and bacteria in the etiology of the common cold. *J. Clin. Microbiol.* **36:**539–542.

66. **Morris, J. A., D. Haran, and A. Smith.** 1987. Hypothesis: common bacterial toxins are a possible cause of sudden infant death syndrome. *Med. Hypotheses* **22:**211–222.

67. **Mulder, J., and J. F. P. Hers.** 1972. *Influenza.* Wolters-Noordhoff, Groningen, The Netherlands.

68. **Nelson, W. L., R. S. Hopkins, M. H. Roe, and M. P. Glode.** 1986. Simultaneous infection with *Bordetella pertussis* and respiratory syncytial virus in hospitalized children. *Pediatr. Infect. Dis. J.* **5:**540–544.

69. **OPCS.** 1988. *Monitor on Sudden Infant Deaths 1985–1987.* Her Majesty's Stationery Office, London, United Kingdom.

70. **Pang, G., R. Clancy, M. Gong, M. Ortega, Z. G. Ren, and G. Reeves.** 2000. Influenza virus inhibits lysozyme secretion by sputum neutrophils in subjects with chronic bronchial sepsis. *Am. J. Respir. Crit. Care Med.* **161:**718–722.

71. **Patel, J., H. Faden, S. Sharma, and P. L. Ogra.** 1992. Effect of respiratory syncytial virus on adherence, colonization and immunity of nontypeable *Haemophilus influenzae*: implications for otitis media. *Int. J. Pediatr. Otorhinolaryngol.* **23:**15–23.

72. **Pike, M. C., C. A. Daniels, and R. Snyderman.** 1977. Influenza-induced depression of monocyte chemotaxis: reversal by levamisole. *Cell. Immunol.* **32:**234–238.

73. **Plotkowski, M.-C., E. Puchelle, G. Beck, J. Jacquot, and C. Hannoun.** 1986. Adherence of type 1 *Streptococcus pneumoniae* to tracheal epithelium of mice infected with influenza A/PR8 virus. *Am. Rev. Respir. Dis.* **134:**1040–1044.

74. **Quiambao, B. P., S. R. Gatchalian, P. Halonen, M. Lucero, L. Sombrero, F. J. Paladin, O. Meurman, J. Merin, and P. Ruutu.** 1998. Co-infection is common in measles-associated pneumonia. *Pediatr. Infect. Dis. J.* **17:**89–93.

75. **Ramphal, A., P. M. Small, J. W. Shands, W. Fischlschwiegen, and P. A. Small.** 1980. Adherence of *Pseudomonas aeruginosa* to tracheal cells injured by influenza infection or by endotracheal tubulation. *Infect. Immun.* **27:**614–619.

76. **Raza, M. W., C. C. Blackwell, R. A. Elton, and D. M. Weir.** 2000. Bactericidal activity of a monocytic cell line (THP-1) against common respiratory tract bacterial pathogens is depressed after infection with respiratory syncytial virus. *J. Med. Microbiol.* **49:**227–233.

77. **Raza, M. W., C. C. Blackwell, M. M. Ogilvie, A. T. Saadi, J. Stewart, R. A. Elton, and D. M. Weir.** 1994. Evidence for the role of glycoprotein-G of respiratory syncytial virus in binding of *Neisseria meningiditis* to HEp-2 cells. *FEMS Immunol. Med. Microbiol.* **10:**25–30.

78. **Raza, M. W., O. R. El Ahmer, M. M. Ogilvie, C. C. Blackwell, A. T. Saadi, R. A. Elton, and D. M. Weir.** 1999. Infection with respiratory syncytial virus enhances expression of native receptors for non-pilate *Neisseria meningiditis* on HEp-2 cells. *FEMS Immunol. Med. Microbiol.* **23:**115–124.

79. **Raza, M. W., M. M. Ogilvie, C. C. Blackwell, J. Stewart, R. A. Elton, and D. M. Weir.** 1993. Effect of respiratory syncytial virus infection on binding of *Neisseria meningitidis* and *Haemophilus influenzae* type b to a human epithelial cell line (Hep-2). *Epidemiol. Infect.* **119:**339–347.

80. **Reynolds, H. Y., and E. K. Root.** 1991. Bronchiectasis and broncholithiasis, p. 1069–1071. *In* J. D. Wilson, E. Braunwald, K. J. Isselbacher, R. G. Petersdorf, J. B. Martin, A. S. Fauci, and E. K. Root (ed.), *Harrison's Principles of Internal Medicine.* McGraw-Hill, New York, N.Y.

81. **Rott, R., H. D. Klenk, Y. Nagai, and M. Tashiro.** 1995. Influenza viruses, cell enzymes and pathogenicity. *Am. J. Respir. Crit. Care Med.* **152**(Suppl.)**:**S16–S19.

82. **Ruutu, P.** 1977. Depression of rat neutrophil exudation and motility by influenza virus. *Scand. J. Immunol.* **6:**1113–1120.

83. **Saadi, A. T., C. C. Blackwell, S. D. Essery, M. W. Raza, O. R. El-Almer, D. A. C. MacKenzie, V. S. James, D. M. Weir, M. M. Ogilvie, R. A. Elton, A. Busuttil, and J. W. Keeling.** 1996. Developmental and environmental factors that enhance binding of *Bordetella pertussis* to human epithelial cells in relation to sudden infant death syndrome (SIDS). *FEMS Immunol. Med. Microbiol.* **16:**51–59.

84. **Saadi, A. T., C. C. Blackwell, M. W. Raza, V. S. James, J. Stewart, R. A. Elton, and D. M. Weir.** 1993. Factors enhancing adherence of toxigenic staphylococci to epithelial cells and their possible role in sudden infant death syndrome. *Epidemiol. Infect.* **110:**507–517.

85. **Sanford, B. A., and M. A. Ramsay.** 1987. Bacterial adherence to the upper respiratory tract of ferrets infected with influenza A virus (42525). *Proc. Soc. Exp. Biol. Med.* **185:**120–128.

86. **Sanford, B. A., V. E. Davison, and M. A. Ramsay.** 1982. Fibrinogen-mediated adherence of group A streptococcus to influenza A virus-infected cell cultures. *Infect. Immun.* **38:**513–520.

87. **Sanford, B. A., V. E. Davison, and M. A. Ramsay.** 1986. *Staphylococcus aureus* adherence to influenza A virus-infected and control cell-cultures: evidence for multiple adhesins. *Proc. Soc. Exp. Biol. Med.* **181:**104–111.

88. **Sanford, B. A., A. Shelokov, and M. A. Ramsay.** 1978. Bacterial adherence to virus infected cells: a cell culture model of bacteria superinfection. *J. Infect. Dis.* **137:**176–181.

89. **Scheiblauer, H., M. Reinacher, M. Toshiro, and R. Rott.** 1992. Interaction between bacteria and influenza A virus in the development of influenza pneumonia. *J. Infect. Dis.* **166:**783–791.

90. **Schwarzmann, S. W., J. L. Adler, R. J. Sullivan, and W. M. Marine.** 1971. Bacterial pneumonia during the Hong Kong influenza epidemic of 1968–69. Experience in a city-county hospital. *Arch. Intern. Med.* **127:**1037–1041.

91. **Scot, D. J., P. S. Gardener, J. McQuillan, A. N. Stanton, and M. A. P. S. Downham.** 1978. Respiratory viruses and cot death. *Br. Med. J.* **2:**12–13.

92. **Selinger, D. S., W. P. Reed, and L. C. McLaren.** 1981. Model for studying bacterial adherence to epithelial cells infected with viruses. *Infect. Immun.* **32:**941–944.

93. **Severien, C., N. Teig, F. Riedel, J. Hohendahl, and C. Reiger.** 1995. Severe pneumonia and chronic lung disease in a young child with adenovirus and *Bordetella pertussis* infection. *Pediatr. Infect. Dis. J.* **14:**400–401.

94. **Shope, R. E.** 1931. Swine influenza. III. Filtration experiments and etiology. *J. Exp. Med.* **54:**373–385.

95. **Smith, G. L.** 1999. Vaccinia virus immune evasion. *Immunol. Lett.* **65:**55–62.

96. **Smith, H.** 1995. The revival of interest in mechanisms of bacterial pathogenicity. *Biol. Rev.* **70:**277–316.

97. **Takase, H., H. Nitanai, E. Yamamura, and T. Otani.** 1999. Facilitated expansion of pneumococcal colonization from the nose to the lower respiratory tract in mice preinfected with influenza virus. *Microbiol. Immunol.* **43:**905–907.

98. **Tashiro, M., P. Ciborowski, H. Klenk, G. Pulverer, and R. Rott.** 1987. Role of staphylococcus protease in the development of influenza pneumonia. *Nature* **325:**536–537.

99. **Tashiro, M., P. Ciborowski, M. Reinacher, G. Pulverer, H.-D. Klenk, and R. Rott.** 1987. Synergistic role of staphylococcal proteases in the induction of influenza virus pathogenicity. *Virology* **157:**421–430.

100. **Taubenberger, J. K., A. H. Reid, and T. G. Fanning.** 2000. The 1918 influenza virus: a killer comes into view. *Virology* **274:**241–245.

101. **Telford, D. R., J. A. Morris, P. Hughes, A. R. Conway, S. Lee, A. J. Barson, and D. B. Drucker.** 1989. The nasopharyngeal bacterial flora in the sudden infant death syndrome. *J. Infect.* **18:**125–130.

102. **Tong, H. H., J. N. Weiser, M. A. James, and T. F. DeMaria.** 2001. Effect of influenza A virus on nasopharyngeal colonization and otitis media induced by transparent or opaque phenotype variants of *Streptococcus pneumoniae* in the chinchilla model. *Infect. Immun.* **69:**602–606.

103. **Tristam, D., W. Hicks, and R. Hard.** 1998. Respiratory syncytial virus and human bronchial epithelium. *Arch. Otolaryngol. Head Neck Surg.* **124:**777–783.

104. **Valdes-Dapena, M. A.** 1967. Sudden and unexpected death in infancy: a review of the world literature 1954–1966. *Pediatrics* **39:**123–138.

105. **Wadowsky, R. M., S. M. Mietzner, D. P. Skoner, W. J. Doyle, and P. Fireman.** 1995. Effect of experimental influenza A virus infection on isolation of *Streptococcus pneumoniae* and other aerobic bacteria from the oropharynges of allergic and nonallergic adult subjects. *Infect. Immun.* **63:**1153–1157.

106. **Walker, J. A., S. S. Molloy, G. Thomas, T. Sakaguchi, T. Yoshida, T. M. Chambers, and Y. Kawaoka.** 1994. Sequence specificity of furin, a proprotein-processing endoprotease, for the hemagglutinin of a virulent avian influenza virus. *J. Virol.* **68:**1213–1218.

107. **Walsh, J., L. Dietlein, F. Low, G. Burch, and W. Mogabgab.** 1960. Bronchotracheal response in human influenza. *Arch. Intern. Med.* **108:**376–388.

108. **Warr, G. A., G. J. Jakab, T. W. Chan, and M. F. Tsan.** 1979. Effects of viral pneumonia on lung macrophage lysosomal enzymes. *Infect. Immun.* **24:**577–579.

109. **Warshauer, D., E. Goldstein, T. Akers, W. Lippert, and M. Kim.** 1977. Effect of influenza viral infection on the ingestion and killing of bacteria by alveolar macrophages. *Am. Rev. Respir. Dis.* **115:**269–277.

110. **Zink, P., J. Drescher, W. Verhagen, J. Flik, and H. Milbrandt.** 1987. Serological evidence of recent influenza virus A (H_3N_2) infections in forensic cases of the sudden infant death syndrome (SIDS). *Arch. Virol.* **93:**223–232.

RESPIRATORY VIRUSES AND BACTERIA IN CATTLE

Douglas C. Hodgins, Jennifer A. Conlon,
and Patricia E. Shewen

12

Bovine respiratory disease is the principal source of economic loss for the North American beef industry and a significant health problem in the dairy industry as well (151). The pathogenesis typically involves some combination of predisposing stress which compromises respiratory defense mechanisms and coincidental primary infection with one or more respiratory viruses. Viral infection and the host's response to it further compromise defense and facilitate colonization of deeper pulmonary tissues by bacteria normally carried in the nasopharynx, especially members of the family *Pasteurellaceae* (54). Often called pneumonic pasteurellosis, this disease syndrome has a multifactorial nature that is better captured in its designation as the bovine respiratory disease complex (BRD) (47). Catastrophic outbreaks or "wrecks" involving large numbers of animals typically follow a week to 10 days after shipment of calves to feedlots, hence the alternative name "shipping fever," but isolated cases in home-reared calves and dairy animals are also recognized. Clinical diagnosis, based on the presence of lethargy or depression, re-

duced feed intake, fever, increased respiratory rate, and dyspnea, with or without nasal discharge, is often made without attempt to identify the offending viruses or bacteria, leaving the diagnosis as undifferentiated bovine respiratory disease (UBRD). Treatment with broad-spectrum antibiotics may assist recovery in many animals, though feed conversion, weight gain, and the resulting economic return can be seriously compromised in those that recover. Prevention would be the preferred intervention, and many vaccines targeting the various bacteria and viruses implicated in BRD have been developed over the last 70 or more years. Those developed in the past decade or so have shown enhanced efficacy but at best protect only 75% of vaccinated animals and provide no protection in outbreaks where the causative organisms are not those most commonly targeted by vaccines. Thus, the search to identify pathogenic mechanisms and virulence factors for both viral and bacterial contributors to disease continues, and as a result the importance of certain defense mechanisms in protection of the respiratory tract is being investigated.

The viruses most frequently associated with BRD include infectious bovine rhinotracheitis virus, a type 1 bovine herpesvirus (BHV1), parainfluenza virus type 3 (PI3), bovine respi-

Douglas C. Hodgins and Patricia E. Shewen, Department of Pathobiology, Ontario Veterinary College, University of Guelph, Guelph, Ontario N1G 2W1, Canada. *Jennifer A. Conlon,* Biocor Animal Health, 2720 North 84th St., Omaha, NE 68134.

Polymicrobial Diseases, Edited by Kim A. Brogden and Janet M. Guthmiller,
© 2002 ASM Press, Washington, D.C.

ratory syncytial virus (BRSV), and bovine viral diarrhea virus (BVDV). Other viruses which may be involved and could be underestimated are bovine adenovirus and bovine coronavirus (BCV). In addition, there are several viruses which are occasionally implicated by serological evidence but for which no clear or consistent association has been made: bovine calicivirus, bovine parvovirus, BHV4, bovine reovirus, bovine enterovirus, bovine rhinovirus, and malignant catarrhal fever virus.

Secondary bacterial pneumonia is typically attributed to members of the family *Pasteurellaceae*, including *Mannheimia haemolytica* (formerly *Pasteurella haemolytica*), *Pasteurella multocida*, and *Haemophilus somnus*.

Other bacteria that have been isolated with some frequency are mycoplasmas, especially *Ureaplasma diversum, Mycoplasma dispar, Mycoplasma bovis*, and *Mycoplasma bovirhinis*.

Chlamydia spp. have been recovered from pneumonic lungs of cattle with BRD, coincidentally with *Pasteurellaceae* and mycoplasmas (108). Although chlamydiae alone do cause primary respiratory disease, their role in UBRD is uncertain and their coincidental isolation may be merely that.

Pasteurellaceae are commensal inhabitants of the upper respiratory tract in cattle, from which they are normally inhaled in small numbers and rapidly cleared by the mucociliary escalator of the trachea and large bronchi (53). This clearance may be impaired when the animals are stressed by changes in weather, change in feed or housing, or transport. Endogenous release of stress hormones has been shown to increase mucus production and decrease ciliary activity, impair recruitment of neutrophils into pulmonary tissue, and reduce the phagocytic activity of resident alveolar macrophages. In addition, the numbers of bacteria isolated from the nasopharynx and tonsillar regions increase during transport or similarly stressful changes in environment (53). While the mechanism for this enhanced bacterial colonization is not known, the result is an increase in the numbers of inhaled bacteria that is coincident with reduced nonspecific defenses. Furthermore, one direct result of the mixing of calves from different farms of origin, as occurs in assembly of the feedlot herd, is the transmission of respiratory viruses from apparently healthy carriers to their naive pen-mates. Many of those viruses, which are known to predispose animals for development of pneumonic pasteurellosis, have direct effects on bacterial clearance mechanisms in the lung, affecting especially the ability of virus-infected alveolar macrophages to take up and kill inhaled bacteria (71). In addition, the antigen-specific immune response to the virus results in killing of virus-infected epithelial cells and macrophages, further compromising clearance and rendering the host extremely vulnerable. The importance of the antiviral immune response in facilitating bacterial pneumonia is clearly demonstrated in experimental models of bovine pneumonia in which the interval between viral challenge and bacterial challenge is critical for production of disease and corresponds directly to the point when antiviral antibodies are first detected in serum (64). Pneumonia can be induced experimentally with bacteria alone but only by direct pulmonary inoculation (intrabronchial instillation or transthoracic injection) using larger numbers of bacteria than are needed for aerosol or intranasal challenge following viral prechallenge (87).

BOVINE RESPIRATORY VIRUSES

BHV1

BHV1 infection has been associated with a variety of clinical syndromes resulting from infection of the genital, respiratory, or digestive tract: abortion, encephalitis, mastitis, and tracheitis (130). Clinical manifestations reflect both the route of exposure and the virus subtype, as well as the naiveté of the animals. Fulminating disease of the upper respiratory tract, classical infectious bovine rhinotracheitis, is observed following infection with BHV1 subtypes 1 and 2a in unvaccinated animals or herds with no prior history of BHV1 infection (148). Endemic infection is more common in most regions of the world; typically, seropositive rates approach 40% of animals within herds (22). When BHV1 infection is endemic, or in herds where vaccination is practiced, clinical respiratory disease is mild or inapparent and most often observed in young animals (140). It is this form of disease which is associated with predisposition to pneumonic pasteurellosis or other bacterial pneumonias. Infection with BHV1 can occur simultaneously with other respiratory viruses, most commonly with BVDV and PI3.

At least some of the mechanisms by which BHV1 predisposes to bacterial pneumonia have been deduced from study of experimental infection. Intranasal aerosol exposure of neonatal or weanling calves to BHV1 resulted in mucosal lesions of the pharyngeal tonsil, characterized by an initial loss of microvilli and goblet cells which progressed to necrosis of the epithelium and adjacent lymphoid tissue and leukocyte exudation (117). Briggs and Frank (25) observed illness and increased nasal mucus 3 to 10 days after intranasal exposure of calves to BHV1. Various measures of serum leakage and cell death increased on day 3 and peaked 5 to 7 days postinfection, and increased elastase activity preceded colonization by *M. haemolytica*. These changes may facilitate bacterial colonization by cleavage of epithelial cell surface fibronectin and mucus and exposure of receptors. An earlier study demonstrated that intranasal vaccination with live infectious bovine rhinotracheitis virus vaccine appeared to enhance bacterial colonization of the upper respiratory tract as determined from nasal and tracheal swabs (152). Following endobronchial inoculation of BHV1, infection could be demonstrated in bronchial, bronchiolar, and alveolar epithelial cells and resulted in degeneration and focal necrosis of the epithelium in the lower respiratory tract. Both virus and viral antigen could be demonstrated in desquamated epithelial cells and alveolar macrophages recovered by bronchoalveolar lavage (88). Conlon and coworkers (40) demonstrated impairment of the relaxation response of tracheal and bronchial smooth muscle following aerosol challenge and suggested that

disruption of normal homeostatic bronchodilatory mechanisms may predispose infected animals to secondary bacterial infections due to excessive airway constriction and subsequent compromise of lung defenses. The composition of lung surfactant is also affected by infection with BHV1 or PI3, potentially altering its effects on inhaled bacteria (51).

Other innate defenses may be compromised by BHV1 infection. Warren et al. (145) observed reduced influx of neutrophils into the lungs of BHV1-infected calves in response to subsequent challenge with *M. haemolytica* and speculated that the virus infection altered the cytokine-mediated responsiveness of the lung endothelium. This agreed with an earlier study which demonstrated impaired direct migration, ingestion of bacteria, and nitroblue tetrazolium reduction by neutrophils following experimental (1 to 7 days) or natural (1 to 28 days) infection, while random migration, adherence, and aggregation were increased (45).

Alveolar macrophages are permissive to productive and nonproductive infection with BHV1. Bovine alveolar macrophages harvested 6 days after experimental infection with BHV1 or PI3 had reduced expression of Fc or C3b receptors and were significantly impaired in their ability to phagocytize opsonized bacteria (29). This impairment may be cytokine mediated. In vitro infection of alveolar macrophages with BHV1 had no significant effect on receptor-mediated phagocyte binding, but the addition of lavage fluids from calves infected by aerosol 6 days previously decreased both antibody Fc-mediated and complement C3b-mediated binding (30). In vitro infection of bovine alveolar macrophages with PI3, BVDV, or BHV1 also results in increased procoagulant activity, suggesting that initial viral infection may induce fibrin deposition in alveoli prior to establishment of a secondary bacterial infection (91).

BHV1 infection may affect antigen-specific as well as nonspecific defense mechanisms. Several researchers have demonstrated that the mitogenic response of peripheral blood mononuclear cells stimulated by concanavalin A is suppressed during BHV1 infection. This effect was associated with a deficit of responder T cells, specifically, a selective depletion of circulating CD8 cells coincident with increased T helper (CD4 cell) activity as indicated by elevated levels of interleukin 2 (IL-2) production 2 to 5 days postinfection (58). However, Carter and coworkers (35) found that proliferation in response to IL-2 by IL-2-dependent lymphocyte cultures was reduced, suggesting potential for failure in the induction phase of antigen-specific immunity despite increased T helper activity. In that study, inhibition of mitogenesis approached 100% even though less than 1 cell in 1,000 was productively infected with BHV1. In addition, lymphopenia is observed in vivo 2 to 8 days postinfection with BHV1. There is a significant decrease in the percentage of T cells and non-T, non-B cells but a significant increase in B cells and monocytes. These monocytes and B cells have increased expression of Fc receptor and an apparent decrease in major histocompatibility complex (MHC) class II expression, suggesting a bias against antigen presentation (58).

PI3

Bovine PI3 has been associated with both acute and chronic pneumonia in cattle. In one recent study of 120 calves transported to western feedlots in the United States, 104 (87.5%) were treated for UBRD and 16 (13.3%) died. PI3 was isolated from seven of nine lungs cultured, and 71 of 104 surviving calves (68.3%) seroconverted to PI3 (55). Infection with PI3 is often concurrent with BHV1 and/or BVDV infection. Ghram and coworkers (56) observed that calves infected with BHV1 and PI3 developed clinical signs including fever, cough, and nasal and ocular discharges. Animals infected with both viruses appeared more depressed and showed higher rectal temperatures, while those infected with PI3 alone had milder disease.

Infection with PI3 may predispose to bacterial pneumonia as a consequence of effects on phagocyte function (26). PI3 infection of alveolar macrophages both in vivo and in vitro has been associated with decreased ability to kill bacteria, including inhibition of phagosome-lysosome fusion, and enhanced production of the metabolites of arachidonic acid which may be inhibitory to other phagocyte functions (71). Dyer and coworkers (48) demonstrated that infection of bovine alveolar macrophages with PI3 inhibited oxygen-dependent bacterial killing by selective inhibition of calcium-independent phosphatidylserinediglyceride-dependent protein kinase C activity. Such inhibition of the oxygen-dependent bactericidal function of macrophages and disturbances in signal transduction would contribute to bacterial superinfection. Brown and Ananaba (29) found that alveolar macrophages harvested from lavage fluid 6 days after infection with PI3 had reduced expression of Fc or C3b receptors, which significantly impaired their ability to phagocytize opsonized bacteria. Subsequent studies confirmed these findings and showed that the addition of lavage fluids from infected calves decreased both Fc-mediated and C3b-mediated binding in macrophages harvested from uninfected animals, suggesting that a cytokine or other soluble factor mediated this inhibition (30).

PI3-infected macrophages or monocytes have been shown to depress mitogen-induced lymphocyte proliferation in vitro while simultaneously causing nonproductive or abortive infection in lymphocytes (15). While this effect on lymphocytes may reduce viral infectivity in vivo, it also has the potential to inhibit the protective immune response. The same researchers subsequently showed that PI3-infected alveolar macrophages inhibit the lymphocyte response to concanavalin A and IL-2 and speculated that this was due to infection of lymphocytes by cell-to-cell contact with infected macrophages (16). Other workers (141) suggest that PI3 adversely affects lymphocyte proliferation because it interferes with the accessory role of macrophages.

Despite the effects of PI3 on lymphocytes, infected animals do mount antigen-specific immune responses to the virus. Bovine peripheral blood lymphocytes were shown to have maximum cytotoxic activity against PI3-infected cells between 5 and 9 days postinfection (14). This corresponds temporally with the optimum time for bacterial secondary infection in experimental challenge models. Killing of PI3-infected cells in vitro has been observed with neutrophils, alveolar macrophages, and lymphocytes (23). When the target cells are virus-infected phagocytes or lymphocytes, host defenses against other organisms would be compromised. The same workers (23) found that addition of specific antibody increased killing by neutrophils, monocytes, and lymphocytes but inhibited killing by alveolar macrophages. Subsequent in vivo work confirmed that alveolar macrophages were capable of killing PI3-infected cells early in infection, but this capability declined after antibodies to PI3 were detectable, 5 days postinfection (2). Other researchers found that cultured alveolar macrophages release tumor necrosis factor alpha (TNF-α) when stimulated by exposure to PI3 in the presence of neutralizing antibodies (21). It is probable that the inhibitory effects of antiviral antibody on infected macrophages alter the ability of these cells to deal with other organisms.

PI3 infection has the potential to alter airway smooth muscle reactivity. Four days after experimental intratracheal inoculation of PI3 in guinea pigs, Folkerts and coworkers (52) observed a 45% increase in histamine-induced contraction of tracheal smooth muscle, and the number of inflammatory cells in the airways was 1.5 times higher than in controls. This tracheal hyperreactivity was also associated with an increase in inflammatory bronchoalveolar cells. Similarly, 6 days after aerosol infection of calves with PI3, there was increased histamine content in mast cells and enhanced ionophore-induced release (90). These reactions, typically associated with type 1 hypersensitivity responses, suggest inflammatory responses to PI3 infection which could ultimately have adverse effects on respiratory clearance and which might facilitate pulmonary colonization by bacteria.

BRSV

BRSV has been established as a common pathogen in respiratory disease (10, 13, 127, 128) and has been demonstrated to interact with bacterial pathogens in establishing pneumonia in cattle (101, 127). BRSV occurs within the cattle population around the world. Although difficult to isolate, the prevalence of the virus is inferred by the presence of BRSV-specific serum antibodies (7, 13). The most likely method of transmission of BRSV from animal to animal is by aerosol and through contaminated nasal secretions. Three to 5 days after infection, clinical disease occurs (20). Spread of the virus is rapid within a naive herd, and high morbidity rates (60 to 80%) have been reported by various researchers, including van der Poel et al. (139). Severe clinical disease has been related to age and is most commonly seen in calves less than 6 months old (99).

BRSV has been demonstrated to infect both ciliated and nonciliated epithelial cells in the respiratory tract, causing necrotizing bronchiolitis and interstitial pneumonia (31, 32, 36, 49). Infiltration of the lung by neutrophils and other inflammatory cells is presumed to be due to cytokine and chemokine release from virally infected cells (32).

Both Trigo et al. (138) and later Sharma and Woldehiwet (118) demonstrated that lambs which were experimentally infected with BRSV were more susceptible to infection with *M. haemolytica* than those not exposed to the virus. Although not conclusively proven, it is thought that BRSV alters the normal function of macrophages, neutrophils, and lymphocytes. In vitro challenge of peripheral blood mononuclear cells with BRSV decreases the proliferative response to phytohemagglutinin (86, 119).

Another closely related pneumovirus, human respiratory syncytial virus (HRSV), has been shown to infect immune cells, resulting in immunosuppression in the host (46). Recent studies with HRSV have demonstrated high-level expression of chemokines by virus-infected epithelial cells of the lower airway (156), suggesting a mechanism for recruitment of neutrophils, monocytes, eosinophils, NK cells, T lymphocytes, and dendritic cells into airways. Although necessary for defense against the infection, immunopathology associated with this inflammatory response no doubt contributes to respiratory pathology. Additionally, HRSV has been reported to stimulate production of inflammatory mediators, including gamma interferon (IFN-γ) and prostaglandins (98, 105). Keles and coworkers (66) demonstrated that both inactivated BRSV and live BRSV were capable of suppressing the lymphocyte proliferative response to phytohemagglutinin, probably through release of inhibitory substances from mononuclear cells. Other researchers were able to demonstrate that mononuclear cells exposed to HRSV released inhibitors to IL-1 (86, 111, 114) and IFN-α (105), resulting in decreased cellular function. Furthermore, alveolar macrophages which have been infected with BRSV produce a decreased level of nitric oxide (116), an important bacteriocidal compound produced in response to bacterial invasion. Still, others argue that the level of replication of BRSV in alveolar macrophages is low and the impact on alveolar macrophage function is questionable (12). There is some indication that not all strains of BRSV produce the same effect on pulmonary immune cell function (137).

BVDV

The role of BVDV in shipping fever pneumonia in feedlot cattle remains controversial in spite of decades of research (59, 100, 106). BVDV has been reported to be the virus most commonly isolated from pneumonic lungs of cattle (107). Serological evidence suggests that multiple infections with respiratory viruses are common in young calves suffering from respiratory disease and that BVDV is present in the majority of these multiple infections (55, 110). In experimental studies, inoculation of susceptible calves with BVDV alone typically leads to mild or moderately severe respiratory disease (19, 27, 104), but labored abdominal breathing with fevers over 41°C has been noted with a

Canadian type 2 noncytopathic strain (9). In some studies, infection with BVDV followed by inoculation, after several days, with *M. haemolytica* has resulted in severe pneumonic disease (102, 104). In short-term studies, Lopez and coworkers did not find an effect of BVDV infection on lung clearance of *M. haemolytica;* the authors, however, did not reject the possibility that other mechanisms besides impaired bacterial clearance could mediate pathogenic effects of BVDV (80, 81). Differences in pneumopathogenicity of BVDV strains have been documented (65, 102); both cytopathic and noncytopathic strains were represented among those classified as pneumopathogenic.

In epidemiological studies, rates of seroconversion to BVDV vary widely (59), as do the risks of developing pneumonia associated with this seroconversion. A number of feedlot studies, however, have found serological support for a role of BVDV in UBRD (82, 83, 89). Several studies have examined the clinical effects of concurrent infection with BRSV and BVDV (27, 50). Clinical signs of respiratory disease were more severe with mixed infection, and immune responses to BRSV were considered to be delayed by the presence of BVDV infection. Potgieter and coworkers investigated the effects of experimentally induced BVDV infection on respiratory infection with BHV1 (103). Inoculation of calves with BHV1 alone was associated with isolation of virus mainly from the upper respiratory tract, with lower titers of virus present in lung tissue. Inoculation with BVDV 7 days prior resulted in high titers of BHV1 being isolated from both upper and lower respiratory tracts and from liver, spleen, brain, and intestinal tract tissues, indicating impairment of host defenses. BVDV has also been reported to influence clearance of endogenous bacteria in the lungs, leading to bacteremia in BVDV-infected calves (109).

In vivo and in vitro studies have documented multiple effects of BVDV on the functional capabilities of the bovine immune system. Welsh and coworkers (147) have investigated effects on alveolar macrophages. Macrophages recovered from bronchoalveolar lavage fluids from calves experimentally infected with cytopathic BVDV had decreased expression of both Fc and complement receptors. Phagocytic and microbicidal activities were impaired, as well as the ability to exert a chemotactic effect on neutrophils. Effects on receptor expression and phagocytic ability could also be shown in alveolar macrophages from uninfected calves infected in vitro (79, 147). It is anticipated that these effects on alveolar macrophages would reduce the ability to clear *M. haemolytica* and other bacterial pathogens from the lung.

Olchowy and coworkers have investigated the effects of cytopathic and noncytopathic BVDV strains on the procoagulant activities of alveolar macrophages (91). Inoculation of cell cultures with BVDV increased procoagulant activity. At low doses of virus, the presence of lipopolysaccharide (LPS) stimulated a further increase. These findings suggest that in the bovine lung, infection with BVDV can lead to fibrin deposition in the alveoli, impeding clearance of bacteria and promoting colonization.

BVDV has been shown to increase production of prostaglandin E2 by monocytes in vitro (146) and is associated with decreased expression of MHC class II molecules on peripheral blood mononuclear cells in infected calves (9), effects anticipated to reduce or delay antigen-specific immune responses.

Bovine Adenovirus

Although adenovirus infections of cattle were documented before 1960 (68), their role in clinical diseases in cattle remains controversial. Ten serotypes of bovine adenovirus have been identified (155). The virus is encountered worldwide in cattle, with particular serotypes predominating from time to time in a particular geographic region (33). Although adenoviruses have been isolated from the respiratory tracts of pneumonic calves, isolation from clinically healthy cattle is more frequent (136). Some serologic studies have supported a role for bovine adenoviruses (11, 34, 76) in bovine respiratory disease, while evidence was lacking

in other studies (13, 128). Several serotypes of bovine adenovirus have been shown to induce disease in newborn colostrum-deprived calves (33, 75). In several studies, vaccination reduced the incidence of pneumonic disease in calves (33, 85).

Adenovirus infection is common in sheep, in which, in contrast to the situation in cattle, isolation of adenovirus from diseased animals is more common than from healthy animals (28). Six serotypes of ovine adenoviruses are recognized (155). Infection of colostrum-deprived lambs with serotype 6 ovine adenovirus leads to clinical respiratory disease, and infection with both adenovirus and *M. haemolytica* leads to more severe and more prolonged disease (42, 74).

Adair and coworkers have examined the effects of bovine adenovirus type 1 on bovine alveolar macrophages in vitro (3). A decrease in expression of Fc and complement receptors and a decrease in the ability to phagocytose and kill *Candida krusei* were noted. Effects of a type 2 strain of adenovirus were less dramatic. The effects of human adenovirus infection on adhesion of *Haemophilus influenzae* and *Streptococcus pneumoniae* to respiratory epithelial cells in vitro was investigated by Hakansson and coworkers (60). When serotypes of adenovirus associated with respiratory tract infections were used, binding by adherent strains of *S. pneumoniae* was increased. The authors suggested that expression of receptors used by *S. pneumoniae* was increased by adenovirus infection.

BCV

Interest in BCV as a respiratory pathogen contributing to BRD (pneumonic pasteurellosis) in feedlot calves is relatively recent. Work by Storz and coworkers (125) in the mid-1990s documented high rates of isolation of BCV from nasal swabs collected on arrival at feedlots from calves with respiratory disease. More recent studies have confirmed this observation (78, 124) and noted, in addition, that high titers of serum immunoglobulin G2 (IgG2) antibody to BCV were associated with protection against respiratory disease. A prospective study that included monitoring of nasal shedding of *M. haemolytica,* as well as BCV and five other respiratory viruses, also found that calves that remained clinically normal had high titers of serum antibody to BCV on feedlot arrival and did not subsequently shed BCV (123). BCV was isolated from lung tissue of 18 calves and *M. haemolytica* was isolated from lung tissue of 25 calves of a total of 26 calves dying with respiratory disease. Nasal shedding of BCV and serological evidence of viral infection in 12 lots of feedlot cattle in Ohio, Texas, and Nebraska were examined by Lathrop and coworkers (72, 73). Shedding of BCV varied from 0 to 36%, depending on the origin of the calves, year of study, and location of the feedlot. Over 60% of the calves seroconverted to BCV by 28 days after feedlot arrival. Calves shedding BCV and responding serologically had an estimated 1.6-times-increased risk of being treated for respiratory disease. Canadian studies examining calves in seven feedlots in Alberta and Ontario found that over 80% of calves have serum antibodies to BCV on feedlot arrival (84, 89). Rates of seroconversion to BCV in the first month in the feedlot varied from 50 to 100% in different groups. The very high incidence of BCV exposure in these studies made inferences about the causal role of BCV in respiratory disease difficult.

Laboratory studies have suggested several mechanisms whereby respiratory infection with BCV may decrease resistance to bacterial pathogens. Respiratory isolates of BCV with acetylesterase activity capable of releasing acetate from the normal glycocalyx lining of the bovine respiratory tract have been found. It is postulated that this modification of the glycocalyx enhances adhesion of *M. haemolytica* and *P. multocida* to host cells in the lower respiratory tract (77, 123, 126).

Oleszak and coworkers have investigated binding of the Fc portion of immunoglobulins by S peplomer proteins of various coronaviruses (92–96). The S proteins of mouse hepatitis virus, transmissible gastroenteritis virus, and BCV bind immunoglobulins of murine, swine, and bovine origins, respectively, but do not bind F(ab′)$_2$ fragments. This property could interfere with opsonization of both bacteria and viruses by preventing interaction of antibodies with Fc receptors on macrophages and neutrophils or by interfering with binding of complement component C1q with the Fc portion of bound antibodies, preventing initiation of the classical pathway of complement activation. Either scenario would decrease uptake and destruction of pathogens and permit their replication.

The M and E structural proteins of coronaviruses (including transmissible gastroenteritis virus and BCV) have been shown to be potent inducers of IFN-α synthesis by peripheral blood mononuclear cells (17, 18, 37). IFN-α is an early cytokine and has proinflammatory properties in common with TNF-α and IL-1. IFN-α has synergistic effects with TNF-α and IL-1, and each can induce expression of the other (142). TNF-α and IL-1 both induce infiltration of neutrophils into the lung and thus are of central importance in the pathogenesis of bacterial pneumonias. High-level expression of IFN-α theoretically could contribute to either protection or disease pathogenesis; work with porcine respiratory coronavirus in pigs suggests, however, that infection with respiratory coronavirus in combination with exposure to bacterial LPS leads to enhanced expression of both TNF-α and IL-1 and exacerbation of respiratory disease (143). Experimental evidence suggests that IFN-α induces expression of adhesion molecules by endothelial cells (142) and mediates infiltration of CD8 T lymphocytes into lung tissue (57, 58). The implications of these observations for polymicrobial infections involving BCV in cattle have not been explored experimentally.

BACTERIAL PNEUMONIA IN CATTLE

Pasteurellaceae

The severe pneumonic damage characterized by pulmonary invasion of *M. haemolytica* and other bacteria is associated with the production of virulence factors which facilitate colonization of the lower respiratory tract (39). Production of neuraminidase and neutral protease may enhance the bacterium's ability to adhere and colonize the respiratory epithelium (151). Lung injury characterized by vascular damage, excess fibrin effusion, and neutrophil infiltration results from the host's response to LPS produced by this gram-negative organism (1, 150, 151). The large influx of neutrophils into the lung is a hallmark of infection with *M. haemolytica* and has been associated with pathology, possibly as a result of neutrophil lysis by the leukotoxin (Lkt) of *M. haemolytica* (133, 154). Animals chemically depleted of neutrophils and then challenged with *M. haemolytica* were demonstrated to have reduced lesions (24).

The Lkt of *M. haemolytica,* a member of the RTX family of toxins, is a pore-forming, Ca^{2+}-dependent cytolysin with specificity for ruminant leukocytes and platelets (38, 120). Low concentrations of Lkt activate neutrophils and induce apoptosis of leukocytes (43, 122). This may be important in the progression of pneumonic pasteurellosis, since apoptosis would limit the initial inflammatory response, allowing the organism to colonize and replicate within the lung (131). Additionally, Lkt has been shown to suppress leukocyte respiratory burst, stimulate lysosomal degranulation, and inhibit phagocytosis and bacterial killing (44, 151). Any of these activities would enhance the organism's ability to establish within the lung.

Other pathogens often associated with bacterial pneumonia in cattle include *P. multocida* and *H. somnus* (87). Like *M. haemolytica,* both are normal inhabitants of the upper respiratory tract of cattle. *P. multocida* is considered to be less virulent than *M. haemolytica,* and in experimental challenge studies, more organisms are required to produce primary pneumonia (8). The organism may cause acute fibrinous bronchopneumonia or may be associated with chronic suppurative bronchopneumonia. Very little is known about the virulence factors of *P. multocida* that contribute to pulmonary pathogenicity. The capsular polysaccharide may allow the organism to evade phagocytosis and complement-mediated killing (44). Production of neuraminidase has been correlated with growth of *P. multocida* in vitro (149). Although not serologically related to the neuraminidase of *M. haemolytica,* this neuraminidase may also enhance colonization and adhesion in deeper pulmonary structures (87).

In general, pneumonia attributed to *H. somnus* is more subacute or chronic than that caused by infection with either *M. haemolytica* or *P. multocida* (101, 121). Lesions associated with *H. somnus* infection include necrotizing bronchiolitis and alveolitis. It is unclear if necrotizing airway lesions are due to colonization by this organism or a predisposing infection with respiratory viruses such as BRSV (32). One of the important virulence factors of *H. somnus* is thought to be its lipooligosaccharide (LOS), which functions similarly to the LPS of *M. haemolytica* and *P. multocida* (41). LOS of *H. somnus* is responsible for endothelial changes that can trigger thrombosis in alveolar vessels and cause subsequent lung damage (132). Additionally, *H. somnus* can trigger apoptosis of bovine neutrophils (153), probably a mechanism by which the organism evades killing by the host.

Mycoplasma and *Ureaplasma* Species
Mycoplasma mycoides subsp. *mycoides* (small colony type [SC]) (144), *M. bovis, M. dispar,* and *U. diversum* have been associated with respiratory tract disease in cattle (61, 112). *M. mycoides* subsp. *mycoides* SC causes contagious bovine pleuropneumonia, an enzootic disease in cattle in Africa, Asia, and parts of Europe with major economic impact (115). *M. bovis, M. dispar,* and *U. diversum* contribute to respiratory disease in housed calves and feedlot cattle. *M. bovirhinis* has been isolated from the lower respiratory tract of calves (4, 97), but evidence of a role in lung disease remains elusive. Epidemiological evidence points to a role of *M. bovis* and *M. dispar* in pneumonia of feedlot calves (83, 113). Isolation of multiple species of mycoplasmas from pneumonic lungs has been noted in some studies (69, 70, 134).

M. dispar has effects on tracheal epithelial cells that range from ciliostasis (63) to degenerative changes and death (5). Experimental infection of calves with *M. dispar* leads to decreased clearance of *Serratia marcescens* (5), suggesting that *M. dispar* infection facilitates infection by other bacterial species. *M. bovis* infection, in contrast, has less effect on the function of ciliated epithelium but invades deeper into lung parenchyma, incites a stronger cellular response, and induces more lung damage (63).

Mycoplasma species can alter phagocytic function. In the absence of opsonizing antibodies, capsular material of *M. dispar* not only inhibits uptake of itself, but also prevents activation of macrophages by other stimuli (6). In vitro, killing of *Escherichia coli* by bovine neutrophils is inhibited by mycoplasma products (62). *M. bovis* interacts with bovine neutrophils in vitro to impair the respiratory burst (135).

Some mycoplasma species exhibit mitogenic activity for B and T lymphocytes, and a peptide of *Mycoplasma arthritidis* has been shown to be a superantigen for T cells. Mitogenic stimulation of B and T cells induces proliferation of lymphocyte clones which are irrelevant for protection (against mycoplasmas and coinfecting organisms) but may contribute to autoimmune disease (112).

U. diversum has been shown to have protease activity against bovine IgA (67). Because this protease activity cleaves IgA regardless of the antibody specificity, it affects immunity to other pathogens at the same mucosal site and may augment other infectious processes.

SUMMARY

In conclusion, there is ample evidence to support the synergistic effect of combined viral and bacterial infections in bovine respiratory disease. The fact that predisposition can be attributed to more than one virus and the realization that no single bacterium is responsible for the resulting pneumonia support the notion that despite differences in the details of mechanisms that facilitate secondary infection, the overarching effect is impairment of host defense. This effect may be mediated by direct action of the organism, for example, destruc-

tion of the epithelial barrier through infection of epithelial cells, but indirect effects which alter the innate and/or specific immune response are key in these scenarios. Such effects include alterations in mucus secretion or the activity of cilia which affect the mucociliary escalator; impaired phagocytic uptake and/or killing by alveolar macrophages, a dysfunction which impedes clearance of inhaled organisms from the deeper reaches of the lung; alterations in neutrophil migration and activity which impair augmentation of clearance through inflammatory recruitment; inhibition of the responsiveness of lymphocytes to mitogens and antigens which limits antigen-specific responses to the organisms; and the apparently paradoxical effects of specific antibodies which can accentuate the defects of virus-infected phagocytes and which may lead to further loss of defense though complement-mediated killing of infected neutrophils, macrophages, monocytes, lymphocytes, or epithelial cells. Understanding the reactions which facilitate and result from mixed infections is critical for the development of effective measures for control and prevention of bovine respiratory disease.

REFERENCES

1. **Ackermann, M. R., and K. A. Brogden.** 2000. Response of the ruminant respiratory tract to *Mannheimia (Pasteurella) haemolytica*. *Microbes Infect./Inst. Pasteur* **2**:1079–1088.
2. **Adair, B. M., H. E. Bradford, M. S. McNulty, and J. C. Foster.** 1999. Cytotoxic interactions between bovine parainfluenza 3 virus and bovine alveolar macrophages. *Vet. Immunol. Immunopathol.* **67**:285–294.
3. **Adair, B. M., M. S. McNulty, and J. C. Foster.** 1992. Effects of two adenoviruses (type 1 and type 8) on functional properties of bovine alveolar macrophages in vitro. *Am. J. Vet. Res.* **53**: 1010–1014.
4. **Allen, J. W., L. Viel, K. G. Bateman, and S. Rosendal.** 1992. Changes in the bacterial flora of the upper and lower respiratory tracts and bronchoalveolar lavage differential cell counts in feedlot calves treated for respiratory diseases. *Can. J. Vet. Res.* **56**:177–183.
5. **Almeida, R. A., and R. F. Rosenbusch.** 1994. Impaired tracheobronchial clearance of

bacteria in calves infected with Mycoplasma dispar. *Zentbl. Vet. Med. B* **41**:473–482.

6. **Almeida, R. A., M. J. Wannemuehler, and R. F. Rosenbusch.** 1992. Interaction of *Mycoplasma dispar* with bovine alveolar macrophages. *Infect. Immun.* **60**:2914–2919.

7. **Ames, T. R.** 1993. The epidemiology of BRSV infection. *Vet. Med.* **88**:881–885.

8. **Ames, T. R., R. J. F. Markham, J. Opuda-Asibo, J. R. Leininger, and S. K. Maheswaran.** 1985. Pulmonary response to intratracheal challenge with *Pasteurella haemolytica* and *Pasteurella multocida. Can. J. Comp. Med.* **49**:395–400.

9. **Archambault, D., C. Beliveau, Y. Couture, and S. Carman.** 2000. Clinical response and immunomodulation following experimental challenge of calves with type 2 noncytopathogenic bovine viral diarrhea virus. *Vet. Res.* **31**:215–227.

10. **Baker, J. C.** 1993. The characteristics of respiratory syncytial viruses. *Vet. Med.* **88**:1190–1195.

11. **Baker, J. C., T. R. Ames, and R. E. Werdin.** 1986. Seroepizootiologic study of bovine respiratory syncytial virus in a beef herd. *Am. J. Vet. Res.* **47**:246–253.

12. **Baker, J. C., J. A. Ellis, and E. G. Clark.** 1997. Bovine respiratory syncytial virus. *Vet. Clin. N. Am. Food Anim. Pract.* **13**:425–454.

13. **Baker, J. C., R. E. Werdin, T. R. Ames, F. J. Markham, and V. L. Larson.** 1986. Study on the etiologic role of bovine respiratory syncytial virus in pneumonia of dairy calves. *J. Am. Vet. Med. Assoc.* **189**:66–70.

14. **Bamford, A. I., B. M. Adair, and J. C. Foster.** 1995. Primary cytotoxic response of bovine peripheral blood leukocytes. *Vet. Immunol. Immunopathol.* **45**:85–95.

15. **Basaraba, R. J., P. R. Brown, W. W. Laegreid, R. M. Silflow, J. F. Everman, and R. W. Leid.** 1993. Suppression of lymphocyte proliferation by parainfluenza virus type 3-infected bovine alveolar macrophages. *Immunology* **79**:179–188.

16. **Basaraba, R. J., W. W. Laegreid, P. R. Brown, R. M. Silflow, R. A. Brown, and R. W. Leid.** 1994. Cell-to-cell contact not soluble factors mediate suppression of lymphocyte proliferation by bovine parainfluenza virus type 3. *Viral Immunol.* **7**:121–132.

17. **Baudoux, P., L. Besnardeau, C. Carrat, P. Rottier, B. Charley, and H. Laude.** 1998. Interferon alpha inducing property of coronavirus particles and pseudoparticles. *Adv. Exp. Med. Biol.* **440**:377–386.

18. **Baudoux, P., C. Carrat, L. Besnardeau, B. Charley, and H. Laude.** 1998. Coronavirus pseudoparticles formed with recombinant M and

E proteins induce alpha interferon synthesis by leukocytes. *J. Virol.* **72**:8636–8643.

19. **Baule, C., G. Kulcsar, K. Belak, M. Albert, C. Mittelholzer, T. Soos, L. Kucsera, and S. Belak.** 2001. Pathogenesis of primary respiratory disease induced by isolates from a new genetic cluster of bovine viral diarrhea virus type I. *J. Clin. Microbiol.* **39**:146–153.

20. **Belknap, E. B.** 1993. Recognizing the clinical signs of BRSV infection. *Vet. Med.* **88**:886–887.

21. **Bienhoff, S. E., G. K. Allen, and J. N. Berg.** 1992. Release of tumor necrosis factor-alpha from bovine alveolar macrophages stimulated with bovine respiratory viruses and bacterial endotoxins. *Vet. Immunol. Immunopathol.* **30**:341–357.

22. **Boelaert, F., P. Biront, B. Soumare, M. Dispas, E. Vanopdenbosch, J. P. Vermeersch, A. Raskin, J. Dufey, D. Berkvens, and P. Kerkhofs.** 2000. Prevalence of bovine herpesvirus-1 in the Belgian cattle population. *Vet. Med.* **45**:285–295.

23. **Bradford, H. E., B. M. Adair, M. S. McNulty, and J. C. Foster.** 1992. Cytotoxicity of bovine leukocytes for parainfluenza type-3 virus infection. *Vet. Immunol. Immunopathol.* **31**:115–127.

24. **Breider, M. A., R. D. Walker, F. M. Hopkins, T. W. Schultz, and T. L. Bowersock.** 1988. Pulmonary lesions induced by *Pasteurella haemolytica* in neutrophil sufficient and neutrophil deficient calves. *Can. J. Vet. Res.* **52**:205–209.

25. **Briggs, R. E., and G. H. Frank.** 1992. Increased elastase activity in nasal mucus associated with nasal colonization by *Pasteurella haemolytica* in infectious bovine rhinotracheitis virus-infected calves. *Am. J. Vet. Res.* **53**:631–635.

26. **Briggs, R. E., M. Kehrli, and G. H. Frank.** 1988. Effect of infection with parainfluenza-3 virus and infectious rhinotracheitis virus on neutrophil functions in calves. *Am. J. Vet. Res.* **49**:682–686.

27. **Brodersen, B. W., and C. L. Kelling.** 1998. Effect of concurrent experimentally induced bovine respiratory syncytial virus and bovine viral diarrhea virus infection on respiratory tract and enteric diseases in calves. *Am. J. Vet. Res.* **59**:1423–1430.

28. **Brogden, K. A., H. D. Lehmkuhl, and R. C. Cutlip.** 1998. Pasteurella haemolytica complicated respiratory infections in sheep and goats. *Vet. Res.* **29**:233–254.

29. **Brown, T. T., and G. Ananaba.** 1988. Effect of respiratory infections caused by bovine herpes virus-1 and parainfluenza-3 virus on bovine alveolar macrophage function. *Am. J. Vet. Res.* **49**:1447–1451.

30. **Brown, T. T., and K. Shin.** 1990. Effect of bovine herpesvirus-1 or parainfluenza-3 virus on

immune receptor-mediated functions of bovine alveolar macrophages in the presence or absence of virus-specific serum or pulmonary lavage fluids collected after virus infection. *Am. J. Vet.* **51:** 1616–1622.

31. **Bryson, D. G.** 1993. Necropsy findings associated with BRSV pneumonia. *Vet. Med.* **88:**894–899.

32. **Bryson, D. G., H. J. Ball, M. McAliskey, W. McConnell, and S. J. McCullough.** 1990. Pathological, immunocytochemical and microbiological findings in calf pneumonias associated with *Haemophilus somnus* infection. *J. Comp. Pathol.* **103:**433–443.

33. **Burki, F.** 1990. Bovine adenoviruses, p. 161–169. *In* Z. Dinter and B. Morein (ed.), *Virus Infections of Ruminants.* Elsevier, Amsterdam, The Netherlands.

34. **Caldow, G. L., S. Edwards, A. R. Peters, P. Nixon, G. Ibata, and R. Sayers.** 1993. Associations between viral infections and respiratory disease in artificially reared calves. *Vet. Rec.* **133:**85–89.

35. **Carter, J. J., A. D. Weinberg, A. Pollard, R. Reeves, J. A. Magnuson, and N. S. Magnuson.** 1989. Inhibition of T-lymphocyte mitogenic responses and effects on cell functions by bovine herpesvirus 1. *J. Virol.* **63:**1525–1530.

36. **Castleman, W. L., S. K. Chandler, and D. O. Slauson.** 1985. Experimental bovine respiratory syncytial virus infection in conventional calves: ultrastructural respiratory lesions. *Am. J. Vet. Res.* **46:**554–560.

37. **Charley, B., and H. Laude.** 1988. Induction of alpha interferon by transmissible gastroenteritis coronavirus: role of transmembrane glycoprotein E1. *J. Virol.* **62:**8–11.

38. **Clinkenbeard, K. D., and M. L. Upton.** Lysis of bovine platelets by *Pasteurella haemolytica* leukotoxin. *Am. J. Vet. Res.* **52:**453–457.

39. **Confer, A. W., R. J. Panciera, K. D. Clinkenbeard, and D. A. Mosier.** 1990. Molecular aspects of virulence of *Pasteurella haemolytica. Can. J. Vet. Res.* **54:**S48–S52.

40. **Conlon, P. D., P. O. Ogunbiyi, R. J. Perron, and P. Eyre.** 1987. Effects of infectious bovine rhinotracheitis virus infections on bovine airway reactivity. *Can. J. Vet. Res.* **51:**345–349.

41. **Corbeil, L. B.** 1990. Molecular aspects of some virulence factors of *Haemophilus somnus:* bovine reproductive and respiratory disease. *Can. J. Vet. Res.* **54:**S57–S62.

42. **Cutlip, R. C., H. D. Lehmkuhl, K. A. Brogden, and N.-J. Hsu.** 1996. Lesions in lambs experimentally infected with ovine adenovirus serotype 6 and *Pasteurella haemolytica. J. Vet. Diagn. Investig.* **8:**296–303.

43. **Czuprynski, C. J., E. J. Noel, O. Oriz-Carranza, and S. Srikumaran.** 1991. Activation of bovine neutrophils by partially purified *Pasteurella haemolytica* leukotoxin. *Infect. Immun.* **59:**3126–3133.

44. **Czuprynski, C. J., and A. K. Sample.** 1990. Interaction of *Haemophilus-Actinobacillus-Pasteurella* bacteria with phagocytic cells. *Can. Vet. J.* **54:**S36–S40.

45. **Deptula, W.** 1991. Phagocytic activity of neutrophils (PMN cells) in cattle infected with IBR/IPV virus (bovine herpesvirus 1–BHV-1). *Pol. Arch. Weter.* **31:**153–165.

46. **Dormurat, F., N. J. Roberts, E. E. Walsh, and R. Dagan.** 1985. Respiratory syncytial virus infection of human mononuclear leukocytes *in vitro* and *in vivo. J. Infect. Dis.* **152:**895–902.

47. **Dyer, R. M.** 1982. The bovine respiratory disease complex: a complex interaction of host, environment and infectious factors. *Compend. Contin. Educ.* **4:**S296–S304.

48. **Dyer, R. M., S. Majumdar, S. D. Douglas, and H. M. Korchak.** 1994. Bovine parainfluenza-3 virus selectively depletes a calcium-independent, phospholipid-dependent kinase C and inhibits superoxide anion generation in alveolar macrophages. *J. Immunol.* **153:**1170–1171.

49. **Ellis, J. A., H. Philibert, K. West, E. Clark, K. Martin, and D. Haines.** 1996. Fatal pneumonia in adult dairy cattle associated with active infection with bovine respiratory syncytial virus. *Can. Vet. J.* **37:**103–105.

50. **Elvander, M., C. Baule, M. Persson, L. Egyed, A. Ballagi-Pordany, S. Belak, and S. Alenius.** 1998. An experimental study of a concurrent primary infection with bovine respiratory syncytial virus (BRSV) and bovine viral diarrhoea virus (BVDV) in calves. *Acta Vet. Scand.* **39:** 251–264.

51. **Engen, R. L., and T. T. Brown.** 1991. Changes in phospholipid of alveolar lining material in calves after aerosol exposure to bovine herpesvirus-1 or parainfluenza-3. *Am. J. Vet. Res.* **52:**675–677.

52. **Folkerts, G., M. Janssen, and F. P. Nijkamp.** 1990. Parainfluenza-3 induced hyperreactivity of the guinea pig trachea coincides with an increased number of bronchoalveolar cells. *Br. J. Clin. Pharmacol.* **30:**159S–161S.

53. **Frank, G.** 1989. Pasteurellosis of cattle, p. 197–222. *In* C. Adlam and J. M. Rutter (ed.), *Pasteurella and Pasteurellosis.* Academic Press, London, United Kingdom.

54. **Frank, G. H., and R. E. Briggs.** 1992. Colonization of the tonsils of calves with *Pasteurella haemolytica. Am. J. Vet. Res.* **53:**481–484.

55. **Fulton, R. W., C. W. Purdy, A. W. Confer, J. T. Saliki, R. W. Loan, R. E. Briggs, and L. J. Burge.** 2000. Bovine viral diarrhea viral infections in feeder calves with respiratory disease: interactions with Pasteurella spp., parainfluenza-3

virus, and bovine respiratory syncytial virus. *Can. J. Vet. Res.* **64**:151–159.

56. **Ghram, A., P. G. Reddy, J. L. Morrill, F. Blecha, and H. C. Minocha.** 1989. Bovine herpesvirus-1 and parinfluenza-3 interactions: clinical and immunological response in calves. *Can. J. Vet. Res.* **53**:62–67.

57. **Griebel, P. J., H. Bielefeldt Ohmann, M. Campos, L. Qualtiere, W. C. Davis, M. J. Lawman, and L. A. Babiuk.** 1989. Bovine peripheral blood leukocyte population dynamics following treatment with recombinant bovine interferon-alpha I1. *J. Interferon Res.* **9**:245–257.

58. **Griebel, P. J., L. Qualtiere, W. C. Davis, A. Gee, H. Bielefeldt Ohmann, M. J. Lawman, and L. A. Babiuk.** 1987. T lymphocyte population dynamics and function following a primary bovine herpesvirus type-1 infection. *Viral Immunol.* **1**:287–304.

59. **Grooms, D. L.** 1998. Role of bovine viral diarrhea virus in the bovine respiratory disease complex. *Bovine Pract.* **32**:7–12.

60. **Hakansson, A., A. Kidd, G. Wadell, H. Sabharwal, and C. Svanborg.** 1994. Adenovirus infection enhances in vitro adherence of *Streptococcus pneumoniae. Infect. Immun.* **62**:2707–2714.

61. **Howard, C. J.** 1983. Mycoplasmas and bovine respiratory disease: studies related to pathogenicity and the immune response—a selective review. *Yale J. Biol. Med.* **56**:789–797.

62. **Howard, C. J., and G. Taylor.** 1983. Interaction of mycoplasmas and phagocytes. *Yale J. Biol. Med.* **56**:643–648.

63. **Howard, C. J., L. H. Thomas, and K. R. Parsons.** 1987. Comparative pathogenicity of Mycoplasma bovis and Mycoplasma dispar for the respiratory tract of calves. *Isr. J. Med. Sci.* **23**:621–624.

64. **Jakab, G. J., and E. C. Dick.** 1973. Synergistic effect in viral bacterial infection: combined infection of the murine respiratory tract with Sendai virus and *Pasteurella pneumotropica. Infect. Immun.* **8**:762–768.

65. **Jewett, C. J., C. L. Kelling, M. L. Frey, and A. R. Doster.** 1990. Comparative pathogenicity of selected bovine viral diarrhea virus isolates in gnotobiotic lambs. *Am. J. Vet. Res.* **51**:1640–1644.

66. **Keles, I., A. K. Sharma, Z. Woldehiwet, and R. D. Murray.** 1999. The effects of bovine respiratory syncytial virus on normal ovine lymphocyte responses to mitogens or antigens *in vitro. Comp. Immunol. Microbiol. Infect. Dis.* **22**:1–13.

67. **Kilian, M., and E. A. Freundt.** 1984. Exclusive occurrence of an extracellular protease capable of cleaving the hinge region of human immunoglobulin A1 in strains of Ureaplasma urealyticum. *Isr. J. Med. Sci.* **20**:938–941.

68. **Klein, M., E. Earley, and J. Zellat.** 1959. Isolation from cattle of a virus related to human adenovirus. *Proc. Soc. Exp. Biol. Med.* **102**:1–4.

69. **Knudtson, W. U., D. E. Reed, and G. Daniels.** 1986. Identification of Mycoplasmatales in pneumonic calf lungs. *Vet. Microbiol.* **11**:79–91.

70. **Kusiluka, L. J., B. Ojeniyi, and N. F. Friis.** 2000. Increasing prevalence of Mycoplasma bovis in Danish cattle. *Acta Vet. Scand.* **41**:139–146.

71. **Laegreid, W. W., H. D. Liggitt, R. M. Silflow, J. R. Evermann, S. M. Taylor, and R. W. Leid.** 1989. Reversal of virus-induced alveolar macrophage bactericidal dysfunction by cyclooxygenase inhibition in vitro. *J. Leukoc. Biol.* **45**:293–300.

72. **Lathrop, S. L., T. E. Wittum, K. V. Brock, S. C. Loerch, L. J. Perino, H. R. Bingham, F. T. McCollum, and L. J. Saif.** 2000. Association between infection of the respiratory tract attributable to bovine coronavirus and health and growth performance of cattle in feedlots. *Am. J. Vet. Res.* **61**:1062–1066.

73. **Lathrop, S. L., T. E. Wittum, S. C. Loerch, L. J. Perino, and L. J. Saif.** 2000. Antibody titers against bovine coronavirus and shedding of the virus via the respiratory tract in feedlot cattle. *Am. J. Vet. Res.* **61**:1057–1061.

74. **Lehmkuhl, H. D., J. A. Contreras, R. C. Cutlip, and K. A. Brogden.** 1989. Clinical and microbiologic findings in lambs inoculated with Pasteurella haemolytica after infection with ovine adenovirus type 6. *Am. J. Vet. Res.* **50**:671–675.

75. **Lehmkuhl, H. D., M. H. Smith, and R. E. Dierks.** 1975. A bovine adenovirus type 3: isolation, characterization, and experimental infection in calves. *Arch. Virol.* **48**:39–46.

76. **Lehmkuhl, H. D., M. H. Smith, and P. M. Gough.** 1979. Neutralizing antibody to bovine adenovirus serotype 3 in healthy cattle and cattle with respiratory tract disease. *Am. J. Vet. Res.* **40**:580–583.

77. **Lin, X. Q., V. N. Chouljenko, K. G. Kousoulas, and J. Storz.** 2000. Temperature-sensitive acetylesterase activity of haemagglutinin-esterase specified by respiratory bovine coronaviruses. *J. Med. Microbiol.* **49**:1119–1127.

78. **Lin, X. Q., K. L. O'Reilly, J. Storz, C. W. Purdy, and R. W. Loan.** 2000. Antibody responses to respiratory coronavirus infections of cattle during shipping fever pathogenesis. *Arch. Virol.* **145**:2335–2349.

79. **Liu, L., H. D. Lehmkuhl, and M. L. Kaeberle.** 1999. Synergistic effects of bovine respiratory syncytial virus and non-cytopathic bovine viral diarrhea virus infection on selected bovine alveolar macrophage functions. *Can. J. Vet. Res.* **63**:41–48.

80. **Lopez, A., M. G. Maxie, L. Ruhnke, M. Savan, and R. G. Thomson.** 1986. Cellular inflammatory response in the lungs of calves ex-

posed to bovine viral diarrhea virus, Mycoplasma bovis, and Pasteurella haemolytica. *Am. J. Vet. Res.* **47**:1283–1286.

81. **Lopez, A., M. G. Maxie, M. Savan, H. L. Ruhnke, R. G. Thomson, D. A. Barnum, and H. D. Geissinger.** 1982. The pulmonary clearance of Pasteurella haemolytica in calves infected with bovine virus diarrhea or Mycoplasma bovis. *Can. J. Comp. Med.* **46**:302–306.

82. **Martin, S. W., K. G. Bateman, P. E. Shewen, S. Rosendal, and J. E. Bohac.** 1989. The frequency, distribution and effects of antibodies, to seven putative respiratory pathogens, on respiratory disease and weight gain in feedlot calves in Ontario. *Can. J. Vet. Res.* **53**:355–362.

83. **Martin, S. W., K. G. Bateman, P. E. Shewen, S. Rosendal, J. G. Bohac, and M. Thorburn.** 1990. A group level analysis of the associations between antibodies to seven putative pathogens and respiratory disease and weight gain in Ontario feedlot calves. *Can. J. Vet. Res.* **54**:337–342.

84. **Martin, S. W., E. Nagy, P. E. Shewen, and R. J. Harland.** 1998. The association of titers to bovine coronavirus with treatment for bovine respiratory disease and weight gain in feedlot calves. *Can. J. Vet. Res.* **62**:257–261.

85. **Mattson, D. E., J. R. Wangelin, and R. L. Sweat.** 1987. Vaccination of dairy calves with bovine adenovirus type 3. *Cornell Vet.* **77**:351–361.

86. **McCarthy, D. O., F. M. Dormurat, J. E. Nichols, and N. J. Roberts.** 1989. Interleukin-1 inhibitor production by human mononuclear leukocytes and leukocyte subpopulations exposed to respiratory syncytial virus: analysis and comparison with response to influenza virus. *J. Leukoc. Biol.* **46**:189–198.

87. **Mosier, D.** 1997. Bacterial pneumonia. *Vet. Clin. N. Am. Food Anim. Pract.* **13**:483–494.

88. **Narita, M., K. Kimura, N. Tamimura, and T. Tsuboi.** 2000. Pneumonia induced by endobronchial inoculation of calves with bovine herpes virus-1. *J. Comp. Pathol.* **122**:185–192.

89. **O'Connor, A., S. W. Martin, E. Nagy, P. Menzies, and R. Harland.** 2001. The relationship between the occurrence of undifferentiated bovine respiratory disease and titer changes to bovine coronavirus and bovine viral diarrhea virus in 3 Ontario feedlots. *Can. J. Vet. Res.* **65**:137–142.

90. **Ogunbiyi, P. O., W. D. Black, and P. Eyre.** 1988. Parainfluenza-3 virus-induced enhancement of histamine release from calf lung mast cells—effect of levamisole. *J. Vet. Pharmacol. Ther.* **11**:338–344.

91. **Olchowy, T. W., D. O. Slauson, and P. N. Bochsler.** 1997. Induction of procoagulant activity in virus infected bovine alveolar macrophages and the effect of lipopolysaccharide. *Vet. Immunol. Immunopathol.* **58**:27–37.

92. **Oleszak, E. L.** 1994. Molecular mimicry between Fc receptors and viral antigens. *Arch. Immunol. Ther. Exp.* **42**:83–88.

93. **Oleszak, E. L., J. Kuzmak, B. Hogue, R. Parr, E. W. Collisson, L. S. Rodkey, and J. L. Leibowitz.** 1995. Molecular mimicry between Fc receptor and S peplomer protein of mouse hepatitis virus, bovine corona virus, and transmissible gastroenteritis virus. *Hybridoma* **14**:1–8.

94. **Oleszak, E. L., and J. L. Leibowitz.** 1990. Immunoglobulin Fc binding activity is associated with the mouse hepatitis virus E2 peplomer protein. *Virology* **176**:70–80.

95. **Oleszak, E. L., S. Perlman, and J. L. Leibowitz.** 1992. MHV S peplomer protein expressed by a recombinant vaccinia virus vector exhibits IgG Fc-receptor activity. *Virology* **186**:122–132.

96. **Oleszak, E. L., S. Perlman, R. Parr, E. W. Collisson, and J. L. Leibowitz.** 1993. Molecular mimicry between S peplomer proteins of coronaviruses (MHV, BCV, TGEV and IBV) and Fc receptor. *Adv. Exp. Med. Biol.* **342**:183–188.

97. **Otto, P., M. Elschner, P. Reinhold, H. Kohler, H. J. Streckert, S. Philippou, H. Werchau, and K. Morgenroth.** 1996. A model for respiratory syncytial virus (RSV) infection based on experiment aerosol exposure with bovine RSV in calves. *Comp. Immunol. Microbiol. Infect. Dis.* **19**:85–97.

98. **Panuska, J. R., N. M. Cirino, F. Midulla, J. E. Despot, E. R. McFadden, and Y. T. Huan.** 1990. Productive infection of isolated human alveolar macrophages by respiratory syncytial virus. *J. Clin. Invest.* **86**:113–119.

99. **Pirie, H. M., L. Petrie, E. M. Allen, and C. R. Pringle.** 1981. Acute fatal pneumonia in calves due to respiratory syncytial virus. *Vet. Rec.* **108**:411–416.

100. **Potgieter, L. N.** 1997. Bovine respiratory tract disease caused by bovine viral diarrhea virus. *Vet. Clin. N. Am. Food Anim. Pract.* **13**:471–481.

101. **Potgieter, L. N., R. G. Helman, W. Greene, M. A. Breider, E. T. Thurber, and R. H. Peetz.** 1988. Experimental bovine respiratory tract disease with *Haemophilus somnus*. *Vet. Pathol.* **25**:124–130.

102. **Potgieter, L. N., M. D. McCracken, F. M. Hopkins, and J. S. Guy.** 1985. Comparison of the pneumopathogenicity of two strains of bovine viral diarrhea virus. *Am. J. Vet. Res.* **46**:151–153.

103. **Potgieter, L. N., M. D. McCracken, F. M. Hopkins, and R. D. Walker.** 1984. Effect of bovine viral diarrhea virus infection on the distribution of infectious bovine rhinotracheitis virus in calves. *Am. J. Vet. Res.* **45:**687–690.

104. **Potgieter, L. N., M. D. McCracken, F. M. Hopkins, R. D. Walker, and J. S. Guy.** 1984. Experimental production of bovine respiratory tract disease with bovine viral diarrhea virus. *Am. J. Vet. Res.* **45:**1582–1585.

105. **Preston, F. M., P. L. Beier, and J. H. Pope.** 1995. Identification of the respiratory syncytial virus-induced immunosuppressive factor produced by human peripheral blood mononuclear cells *in vitro* as interferon alpha. *J. Infect. Dis.* **172:**919–926.

106. **Radostits, O. M., and H. G. Townsend.** 1989. The controversy surrounding the role of the bovine virus diarrhea virus (B.V.D.V.) in the pathogenesis of pneumonic pasteurellosis in cattle. *Bovine Proc.* **21:**111–114.

107. **Reggiardo, C.** 1979. Role of BVD virus in shipping fever of feedlot cattle. Case studies and diagnostic considerations. *Am. Assoc. Vet. Lab. Diagnosticians* **22:**315–320.

108. **Reggiardo, C., T. J. Fhurmann, G. L. Meerdink, and E. J. Bicknell.** 1989. Diagnostic features of chlamydia infection in dairy calves. *J. Vet. Diagn. Investig.* **1:**305–308.

109. **Reggiardo, C., and M. L. Kaeberle.** 1981. Detection of bacteremia in cattle inoculated with bovine viral diarrhea virus. *Am. J. Vet. Res.* **42:**218–221.

110. **Richer, L., P. Marois, and L. Lamontagne.** 1988. Association of bovine viral diarrhea virus with multiple viral infections in bovine respiratory disease outbreaks. *Can. Vet. J.* **29:**713–717.

111. **Roberts, N. J., A. H. Prill, and T. N. Mann.** 1986. Interleukin 1 and interleukin 1 inhibitor production by human macrophages exposed to influenza virus or respiratory syncytial virus: respiratory syncytial virus is a potent inducer of inhibitor activity. *J. Exp. Biol.* **163:**511–519.

112. **Rosendal, S.** 1993. Mycoplasma, p. 297–311. *In* C. L. Gyles and C. O. Thoen (ed.), *Pathogenesis of Bacterial Infections in Animals,* 2nd ed. Iowa State University Press, Ames.

113. **Rosendal, S., and S. W. Martin.** 1986. The association between serological evidence of mycoplasma infection and respiratory disease in feedlot calves. *Can. J. Vet. Res.* **50:**179–183.

114. **Salkind, A. R., and N. J. Roberts.** 1992. Recent observations regarding the pathogenesis of recurrent respiratory syncytial virus infections: implications for vaccine development. *Vaccine* **10:**519–523.

115. **Schneider, H. P., J. J. van der Lugt, and O. J. B. Hubschle.** 1994. Contagious bovine pleuropneumonia, p. 1485–1494. *In* J. A. W. Coetzer, G. R. Thomson, and R. C. Tustin (ed.), *Infectious Diseases of Livestock, with Special Reference to Southern Africa.* Oxford University Press, Cape Town, South Africa.

116. **Schrijver, R. S.** 1998. Immunobiology of bovine respiratory syncytial virus infections. *Tijdschr. Diergeneeskd.* **123:**658–662.

117. **Schuh, J. C., H. Bielefeldt Ohmann, L. A. Babiuk, and C. E. Doige.** 1992. Bovine herpesvirus-1-induced pharyngeal tonsil lesions in neonatal and weanling calves. *J. Comp. Pathol.* **106:**243–253.

118. **Sharma, R., and Z. Woldehiwet.** 1990. Increased susceptibility to *Pasteurella haemolytica* infection in lambs infected with bovine respiratory syncytial virus. *J. Comp. Pathol.* **103:**411–419.

119. **Sharma, R., and Z. Woldehiwet.** 1991. Depression of lymphocyte response to phytohaemagglutinin in lambs experimentally infected with bovine respiratory syncytial virus. *Res. Vet. Sci.* **50:**152–156.

120. **Shewen, P. W., and B. N. Wilkie.** 1982. Cytoxin of *Pasteurella haemolytica* acting on bovine leukocytes. *Infect. Immun.* **35:**91–94.

121. **Stephens, L. R.** 1990. Positive and negative aspects of host immune response to *Haemophilus, Actinobacillus* and *Pasteurella. Can. J. Vet. Res.* **54:**S41–S44.

122. **Stevens, P. K., and C. J. Czuprynski.** 1996. *Pasteurella haemolytica* leukotoxin induces bovine leukocytes to undergo morphologic changes consistent with apoptosis in vitro. *Infect. Immun.* **64:**2687–2694.

123. **Storz, J., X. Lin, C. W. Purdy, V. N. Chouljenko, K. G. Kousoulas, F. M. Enright, W. C. Gilmore, R. E. Briggs, and R. W. Loan.** 2000. Coronavirus and *Pasteurella* infections in bovine shipping fever pneumonia and Evans' criteria for causation. *J. Clin. Microbiol.* **38:**3291–3298.

124. **Storz, J., C. W. Purdy, X. Lin, M. Burrell, R. E. Truax, R. E. Briggs, G. H. Frank, and R. W. Loan.** 2000. Isolation of respiratory bovine coronavirus, other cytocidal viruses, and Pasteurella spp from cattle involved in two natural outbreaks of shipping fever. *J. Am. Vet. Med. Assoc.* **216:**1599–1604.

125. **Storz, J., L. Stine, A. Liem, and G. A. Anderson.** 1996. Coronavirus isolation from nasal swab samples in cattle with signs of respiratory tract disease after shipping. *J. Am. Vet. Med. Assoc.* **208:**1452–1455.

126. **Storz, J., X. M. Zhang, and R. Rott.** 1992. Comparison of hemagglutinating, receptor-de-

stroying, and acetylesterase activities of avirulent and virulent bovine coronavirus strains. *Arch. Virol.* **125:**193–204.

127. **Stott, E. J., and G. Taylor.** 1985. Respiratory syncytial virus: brief review. *Arch. Virol.* **84:** 1–52.

128. **Stott, E. J., L. H. Thomas, A. P. Collins, S. Crouch, J. Jebbett, G. S. Smith, P. D. Luther, and R. Caswell.** 1980. A survey of virus infections of the respiratory tract of cattle and their association with disease. *J. Hyg.* **85:** 257–270.

129. Reference deleted.

130. **Straub, O. C.** 1991. BHV1 infections: relevance and spread in Europe. *Comp. Immunol. Microbiol. Infect. Dis.* **14:**175–186.

131. **Sun, Y., K. D. Clinkenbeard, C. Clarke, L. Cudd, S. Highlander, and S. Mady Dabo.** 1999. *Pasteurella haemolytica* leukotoxin induced apoptosis of bovine lymphocytes involves DNA fragmentation. *Vet. Microbiol.* **65:**153–166.

132. **Sylte, M. J., L. B. Corbeil, T. J. Inzana, and C. J. Czuprynski.** 2001. *Haemophilus somnus* induces apoptosis in bovine endothelial cells in vitro. *Infect. Immun.* **69:**1650–1660.

133. **Tatum, F. M., R. E. Briggs, S. S. Sreevatsan, E. S. Zehr, S. L. Hsuan, L. O. Whiteley, T. R. Ames, and S. K. Maheswaran.** 1998. Construction of an isogenic leukotoxin deletion mutant of *Pasteurella haemolytica* serotype 1: characterization and virulence. *Microbiol. Pathog.* **24:**37–46.

134. **Tegtmeier, C., A. Uttenthal, N. F. Friis, N. E. Jensen, and H. E. Jensen.** 1999. Pathological and microbiological studies on pneumonic lungs from Danish calves. *Zentbl. Vet Med.* **46:**693–700.

135. **Thomas, C. B., P. Van Ess, L. J. Wolfgram, J. Riebe, P. Sharp, and R. D. Schultz.** 1991. Adherence to bovine neutrophils and suppression of neutrophil chemiluminescence by Mycoplasma bovis. *Vet. Immunol. Immunopathol.* **27:**365–381.

136. **Thomson, G. R.** 1994. Adenovirus infections, p. 901–908. *In* J. A. W. Coetzer, G. R. Thomson, and R. C. Tustin (ed.), *Infectious Diseases of Livestock, with Special Reference to Southern Africa.* Oxford University Press, Cape Town, South Africa.

137. **Trigo, E. G., H. D. Liggitt, J. F. Evermann, R. G. Breeze, I. Y. Huston, and R. Silflow.** 1985. Effect of in vitro inoculation of bovine respiratory syncytial virus on bovine pulmonary alveolar macrophage function. *Am. J. Vet. Res.* **46:**1098–1103.

138. **Trigo, F. G., R. G. Breeze, H. D. Liggitt, J. F. Evermann, and E. Trigo.** 1984. Interaction of bovine respiratory syncytial virus and

Pasteurella haemolytica in the ovine lung. *Am. J. Vet. Res.* **45:**1671–1678.

139. **Van der Poel, W. H., M. C. Mourits, M. Nielen, K. Frakena, J. T. Van Oirschot, and Y. H. Schukken.** 1995. Bovine respiratory syncytial virus reinfections and decreased milk yields in dairy cattle. *Vet. Q.* **17:** 77–81.

140. **Van Nieuwstadt, A. P., and J. Verhoeff.** 1983. Epidemiology of BHV-1 virus infections in dairy herds. *J. Hyg.* **91:**309–318.

141. **Van Reeth, K., and B. Adair.** 1997. Macrophages and respiratory viruses. *Pathol. Biol.* **45:**184–192.

142. **Van Reeth, K., and H. Nauwynck.** 2000. Proinflammatory cytokines and viral respiratory disease in pigs. *Vet. Res.* **31:**187–213.

143. **Van Reeth, K., H. Nauwynck, and M. Pensaert.** 2000. A potential role for tumour necrosis factor-alpha in synergy between porcine respiratory coronavirus and bacterial lipopolysaccharide in the induction of respiratory disease in pigs. *J. Med. Microbiol.* **49:**613–620.

144. **Walker, R. L.** 1999. Mollicutes, p. 165–172. *In* D. C. Hirsh and Y. C. Zee (ed.), *Veterinary Microbiology.* Blackwell Science, Malden, Mass.

145. **Warren, L. M., L. A. Babiuk, and M. Campos.** 1996. Effects of BHV-1 on PMN adhesion to bovine lung endothelia. *Vet. Immunol. Immunopathol.* **55:**73–82.

146. **Welsh, M. D., and B. M. Adair.** 1995. Prostaglandin E2 production by bovine virus diarrhoea virus infected cell culture and monocytes, p. 63–67. *In* M. Schwyzer, M. Akermann, G. Bertoni, R. Kocherhans, K. McCullough, M. Engels, R. Wittek, and R. Zanoni (ed.), *Immunobiology of Virus Infections. Proceedings of the 3rd Congress of the European Society for Veterinary Virology, Interlaken, Switzerland.* Fondation Marcel Merieux, Lyon, France.

147. **Welsh, M. D., B. M. Adair, and J. C. Foster.** 1995. Effect of BVD virus infection on alveolar macrophage functions. *Vet. Immunol. Immunopathol.* **46:**195–210.

148. **Wentink, G. H., J. T. van Oirschot, and J. Verhoeff.** 1993. Risk of infection with bovine herpes virus 1 (BHV1): a review. *Vet. Q.* **15:** 30–33.

149. **White, D. J., W. L. Jolley, C. W. Purdy, and D. C. Strauss.** 1995. Extracellular neuraminidase production by a *Pasteurella multocida* A:3 strain associated with bovine pneumonia. *Infect. Immun.* **63:**1703–1709.

150. **Whiteley, L. O., S. K. Maheswaran, D. J. Weiss, and T. R. Ames.** 1991. Alterations in pulmonary morphology and peripheral coagulation profiles caused by intratracheal inoculation of live and ultraviolet light-killed *Pasteurella*

haemolytica A1 in calves. *Vet. Pathol.* **28:**275–285.

151. **Whiteley, L. O., S. K. Maheswaran, D. J. Weiss, T. R. Ames, and M. S. Kannan.** 1992. *Pasteurella haemolytica* A1 and bovine respiratory disease. *J. Vet. Intern. Med.* **6:**11–22.

152. **Woldehiwet, A., B. Mamache, and T. G. Rowan.** 1990. The effects of age, environmental temperature and relative humidity on the bacterial flora of the upper respiratory tract in calves. *Br. Vet. J.* **146:**211–218.

153. **Yang, Y. F., M. J. Sylte, and C. J. Czuprynski.** 1998. Apoptosis: a possible tactic of *Haemophilus somnus* for evasion of killing by bovine neutrophils? *Microb. Pathog.* **24:**351–359.

154. **Yoo, H. S., B. S. Rajagopal, S. K. Maheswaran, and T. R. Ames.** 1995. Purified Pasteurella haemolytica leukotoxin induces expression of inflammatory cytokines from bovine alveolar macrophages. *Microb. Pathog.* **18:** 237–252.

155. **Zee, Y. C.** 1999. Adenoviridae, p. 346–349. *In* D. C. Hirsh and Y. C. Zee (ed.), *Veterinary Microbiology.* Blackwell Science, Malden, Mass.

156. **Zhang, Y., B. A. Luxon, A. Casola, R. P. Garofalo, M. Jamaluddin, and A. R. Brasier.** 2001. Expression of respiratory syncytial virus-induced chemokine gene networks in lower airway epithelial cells revealed by cDNA microarrays. *J. Virol.* **75:**9044–9058.

PORCINE RESPIRATORY
DISEASE COMPLEX

Susan L. Brockmeier, Patrick G. Halbur, and Eileen L. Thacker

13

Respiratory disease in pigs is arguably the most important health concern for swine producers today. In 1995, the National Animal Health Monitoring System reported respiratory disease as the leading cause of mortality in nursery and grower-finisher units (75). Data collected from 1990 to 1994 in high-health herds revealed a 58% prevalence of pneumonia at slaughter (preconference workshop on PigMON slaughter monitoring, 1990–1994, A. D. Leman Swine Conference, 1995). As with respiratory disease in humans and other species, respiratory disease in swine is often the result of a combination of primary and opportunistic infectious agents. In addition, adverse environmental and management conditions play an important role in the multifactorial nature of respiratory disease in pigs (Fig. 1).

Even though many potential bacterial pathogens colonize the nasal cavity or tonsils of pigs, normal respiratory defense mechanisms prevent damage or spread to the lung. Thus, it is common to categorize pathogens as either primary pathogens, capable of subverting these defense mechanisms and establishing infection on their own, or opportunistic pathogens, which take advantage of the virulence mechanisms of the primary pathogens to establish infections. Some of the bacterial agents may act as both primary and opportunistic invaders depending on the situation. Although primary respiratory infectious agents can cause serious disease on their own, more often uncomplicated infections with these agents are mild and transient. It is when these primary infections become complicated with opportunistic bacteria that more serious and chronic respiratory disease results and the most economic loss is incurred. Primary agents in pigs include viral agents like porcine reproductive and respiratory syndrome virus (PRRSV), swine influenza virus (SIV), pseudorabies virus (PRV), and possibly porcine respiratory coronavirus (PRCV) and porcine circovirus type 2 (PCV2) and bacterial agents like *Mycoplasma hyopneumoniae*, *Bordetella bronchiseptica*, and *Actinobacillus pleuropneumoniae*. The most common opportunistic agent is *Pasteurella multocida*, but other common opportunistic agents include *Haemophilus parasuis*, *Streptococcus suis*, *Actinobacillus suis*, and *Arcanobacterium pyogenes*. *Salmonella choleraesuis*, *A. suis*, and *A. pyogenes* can also cause primary respiratory disease probably through a blood-borne route.

Susan L. Brockmeier, Respiratory Diseases of Livestock Research Unit, National Animal Disease Center, USDA Agricultural Research Service, Ames, IA 50010. *Patrick G. Halbur*, Veterinary Diagnostic and Production Animal Medicine, College of Veterinary Medicine, Iowa State University, Ames, IA 50011. *Eileen L. Thacker*, Veterinary Medical Research Institute, Iowa State University, Ames, IA 50011.

Polymicrobial Diseases, Edited by Kim A. Brogden and Janet M. Guthmiller,
© 2002 ASM Press, Washington, D.C.

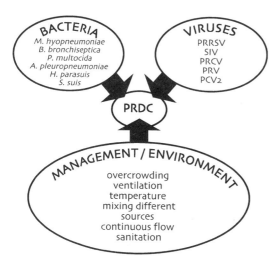

FIGURE 1 Interaction of viral, bacterial, and adverse management conditions which result in porcine respiratory disease complex (PRDC).

Noninfectious causes (management and environmental factors) are significant contributors to respiratory disease, either by increasing transmission and spread of the pathogens or by creating unfavorable conditions which result in increased stress for the animal or damage to the respiratory tract. During the past 30 years, swine production has intensified with larger herd sizes and confinement rearing perhaps contributing to an increase in respiratory disease. It is not unusual to have hundreds to a thousand or more pigs in an enclosed or semienclosed building, which emphasizes the importance of proper ventilation and waste removal for the respiratory health of pigs. Overcrowding and/or improper ventilation can lead to overheating or chilling, increased stress, and increased ammonia and dust levels which have a negative impact on the respiratory tract defenses. Management practices such as continuous pig flow, where young pigs are continuously being brought into the building as older pigs are removed for market, and mixing of pigs from multiple sources and age groups contribute to the spread of disease. Many respiratory pathogens are so ubiquitous that it is hard to

find a herd that is free from them; thus, it is not uncommon for herds to be circulating multiple pathogens at any given time.

To offset the obvious problem of keeping large numbers of pigs in a confined space, management practices have been developed to decrease infectious disease transmission and establish healthier herds. Although high-health management practices decrease the overall infection level of a herd, in large herds these practices may also result in a low level, or subpopulation, of infected pigs which can persist, spreading the agents to naive pigs when maternal immunity is waning later in the finishing stage. Even under the best circumstances disease can sometimes enter the herd through aerosol or vector transmission or through introduction of subclinically infected animals. This can cause severe outbreaks in animals raised without exposure to disease which are immunologically naive.

The term porcine respiratory disease complex (PRDC) was used to describe pneumonia of multiple etiology causing clinical disease and failure to gain weight later in the finishing process (15 to 20 weeks of age). The etiology of PRDC varies between and within production systems and over time within the same system. On most farms with PRDC, one or two viruses, *M. hyopneumoniae,* and several opportunistic bacteria work in combination to induce losses associated with respiratory disease. In addition to the pathogens long known to induce respiratory disease, several emerging and changing pathogens play an important role in the development of PRDC. The emergence of PRRSV in the latter part of the 1980s resulted in significant changes in the health status of the worldwide swine population. In addition to PRRSV, several other respiratory pathogens have emerged, including PCV2, PRCV, and new strains of SIV (H3N2). Since it was first described, the term PRDC has also been used to describe pneumonia of mixed etiology at other stages of production. In this chapter, we discuss PRDC in the broader sense of mixed respiratory infections that occur in swine of any age.

ETIOLOGICAL AGENTS

Table 1 summarizes field case data from the Iowa State University Veterinary Diagnostic Laboratory for 1993 to 2000. A clear trend towards increasing case numbers of pneumonia due to PRRSV, SIV, PCV2, *M. hyopneumoniae*, *P. multocida*, *S. suis*, *B. bronchiseptica*, and *A. suis* is demonstrated. The increased incidence of PRRSV, PCV2, and *A. suis*-induced pneumonia is most remarkable. The sixfold increase in SIV can in large part be explained by the introduction of subtype H3N2 into the United States in 1998. The number of cases of pneumonia due to PRV, *A. pleuropneumoniae*, and *S. choleraesuis* is steady or decreasing.

The following is not an exhaustive list of the respiratory pathogens found in swine, but a brief description of the most commonly isolated or studied pathogens for which interactions have been demonstrated. There are many reasons why potentially important pathogens may be overlooked. Diagnosticians may not be actively looking for bacteria or viruses not thought to be important, or even known to exist; or the initiating agent may no longer be present when overt disease with an opportunistic agent is noticed. Isolation or detection of agents may be difficult or, on the contrary, the agents may be so ubiquitous that their role is difficult to ascertain. For example, chlamydial infection is apparently so widespread in pigs that >90% seroconvert by 2 to 3 months

of age (A. A. Andersen, personal communication). Disease has been reproduced in gnotobiotic pigs inoculated with *Chlamydia*, but since it is isolated from diseased as well as normal pigs, its importance in causing clinical respiratory disease in the field has yet to be determined (85). Emerging pathogens such as PCV2 may be found to contribute significantly to respiratory disease in pigs. Recent evidence suggests that porcine parvovirus may be an important cofactor in disease caused by PCV2. No doubt there will be changes in the perceived importance of pathogens as well as continued emergence and reemergence of pathogens, as there have been in the past.

PRRSV

PRRSV is a widely disseminated pathogen of swine capable of causing both reproductive and respiratory disease. PRRS was first recognized as acute outbreaks of reproductive failure in the late 1980s. PRRSV is a member of the family *Arteriviridae*. It is important to remember that considerable genetic, antigenic, and virulence differences exist among PRRSV isolates. Depending on strain, dose, and immune status, some farms may be subclinically infected with PRRSV while others experience severe reproductive and/or respiratory disease. Neonatal and nursery pigs may experience high fevers, anorexia, dyspnea, tachypnea, conjunctivitis, and failure to thrive. Coughing is not a feature

TABLE 1 Pneumonia case diagnoses at Iowa State University Veterinary Diagnostic Laboratory from 1993 to 2000

Agent	No. of cases of pneumonia diagnosed								Trend
	1993	1994	1995	1996	1997	1998	1999	2000	
PRRSV	120	367	708	714	869	859	981	1,587	13×
P. multocida	360	376	563	638	653	715	815	971	3×
M. hyopneumoniae	218	357	417	624	731	894	867	823	4×
S. suis	200	188	297	348	351	474	714	639	3×
SIV	117	175	291	384	447	350	694	627	6×
PCV2	0	0	0	1	20	111	290	456	456×
A. pleuropneumoniae	262	235	220	298	271	230	178	224	Flat
B. bronchiseptica	77	76	100	99	130	150	161	206	3×
S. choleraesuis	302	274	292	259	197	205	310	177	1/2×
A. suis	9	10	16	23	32	28	44	141	14×

of uncomplicated PRRSV infection. Grow-finish pigs infected with PRRSV exhibit respiratory disease that varies from no detectable signs to fatal pneumonia depending on the strain of PRRSV and the types of coinfections.

Field and experimental data support a marked difference in pneumovirulence of PRRSV isolates within and between geographical areas across the world (46). Neonatal and nursery pigs may have mildly to severely and multifocally to diffusely affected, mottled-tan, rubbery lungs that fail to collapse. Experimentally induced lesions of pneumonia are evident by 3 days postinoculation (DPI) and are most severe at 7 to 10 DPI, and if uncomplicated, the lesions induced by most isolates resolve by 14 to 28 DPI. Enlarged tan lymph nodes develop after 10 DPI and are the most consistent PRRSV-induced gross lesions. Microscopic examination of lungs reveals interstitial pneumonia in young pigs characterized by alveolar septal infiltration with mononuclear cells, type 2 pneumocyte hypertrophy and hyperplasia, and alveolar exudate consisting of mixed mononuclear cells and necrotic debris. Lymphohistiocytic encephalitis, myocarditis, and rhinitis may be observed with some strains.

Following oronasal exposure, PRRSV replicates in macrophages and dendritic cells in tonsils, upper respiratory tract, and lungs resulting in viremia by 6 to 12 h postinfection. Further replication occurs in the lungs, lymph nodes, spleen, thymus, bone marrow, heart, and other tissues. Viremia may persist for several weeks despite the presence of circulating antibodies. In growing pigs, PRRSV is shed in saliva, respiratory tract secretions, oropharyngeal secretions, and urine. Isolation of PRRSV from oropharyngeal samples for up to 157 days after experimental intranasal inoculation of conventional pigs provides evidence of persistent infection of growing pigs (123). Sows infected at 85 to 90 days of gestation may give birth to persistently infected pigs in which viral RNA could be detected for 210 days or more (9). Preweaning mortality is high and respiratory disease is severe in these persistently infected pigs, and they may

be an important source of virus dissemination and persistence.

PRRSV infection results in destruction and decreased function of pulmonary alveolar macrophages and pulmonary intravascular macrophages, damage to the mucociliary apparatus, changes in T-cell subpopulations, and possibly decreased function of antigen-presenting cells such as dendritic cells and macrophages. Infection of macrophages by PRRSV has a profound impact on the respiratory immune system of the pig. Despite infection and lysis of macrophages, no evidence of reduced lymphocyte response to antigens has been reported, and enhanced antibody responses to experimentally administered antigens has been described (1, 70, 101). These findings are in direct conflict with field reports from producers and veterinarians in the field who report an increase in secondary infections associated with PRRSV disease outbreaks. These conflicting views suggest that PRRSV is immunomodulatory in nature instead of classically immunosuppressive.

PRRSV induces cell lysis of pulmonary alveolar macrophages and pulmonary intravascular macrophages which are the primary sites of replication of the virus in the lung (45, 104). Within 1 week of infection, a dramatic decrease in the number of pulmonary alveolar macrophages has been observed, with the function of remaining macrophages severely compromised (71). However, it has also been demonstrated that no more than 2% of pulmonary alveolar macrophages stained positively for PRRSV antigen during acute infection, suggesting that depletion of pulmonary alveolar macrophages would be difficult to explain by lysis of infected macrophages alone (32). In addition to lysis of cells, studies have demonstrated apoptosis of macrophages in PRRSV-infected lung tissues (95). PRRSV appears to induce apoptosis in bystander cells, thus damaging more macrophages than just those infected with the virus, which might explain the reduction in number of alveolar macrophages and circulating monocytes (95). PRRSV-induced damage to pulmonary intravascular macrophages and pulmonary alveolar macrophages is believed to result in increased susceptibility to bacterial pneumonia and septicemia (102–104).

There is clinical evidence that PRRSV is associated with outbreaks of other pathogens, and PRRSV is the most common virus isolated from cases of PRDC. Experimentally, studies found that PRRSV-infected pigs showed an increased septicemia and mortality when challenged with *S. suis* and increased pulmonary infections with *B. bronchiseptica* (11, 42, 47, 102). In contrast, experimental infection of PRRSV with other pathogens, including *P. multocida*, *M. hyopneumoniae*, and transmissible gastroenteritis virus (TGEV), failed to identify an increase in clinical disease associated with coinfections (12, 23, 28, 99, 121). Primary infection with both PRRSV and *B. bronchiseptica*, however, predisposed pigs to secondary pulmonary infection with *P. multocida* (12). In contrast to the expected exacerbation of mycoplasmal pneumonia by PRRSV and *M. hyopneumoniae*, it was found that *M. hyopneumoniae* increased the severity and duration of PRRSV-induced pneumonia independent of the timing of infection with either pathogen (99). There is also evidence of PRRSV interaction with other respiratory viruses such as PRCV and SIV in pigs, and alteration in the typical disease response to pathogens such as *H. parasuis* (97, 114, 118). Thus, the mechanisms that enable PRRSV infection to increase the incidence of secondary infections as observed in the field have been frustrating to demonstrate experimentally. These results demonstrate the truly complex nature of mixed respiratory disease in pigs. Even though PRRSV itself may not result in the dramatic increase in susceptibility to secondary infections that would be predicted by the field evidence, it may tip the balance in combination with other respiratory pathogens or adverse environmental conditions.

SIV

Swine influenza is caused by type A influenza viruses, which are members of the family *Orthomyxoviridae*. Subtype classification is by antigenic and genetic properties of surface proteins hemagglutinin (H) and neuraminidase (N). There are 15 hemagglutinins (H1 to H15) and 9 neuraminidases (N1 to N9). Subtype H1N1 is widespread in North America, Europe, and Asia. Before 1998, swine influenza in the United States was caused almost exclusively by subtype H1N1. Beginning in mid-1998, subtype H3N2 quickly became widespread in the United States. On the basis of cases submitted to Iowa State University in 1998 to 2000, more than 50% of the influenza cases were diagnosed as subtype H3N2 (90). An even more recent report from Indiana in 2000 has confirmed the presence of H1N2 in the United States (59).

Several recent examples of antigenic drift of SIV exist. Antigenic drift occurs within a subtype and involves a series of point mutations. Mutations that affect neutralizing epitopes may produce antigenic variants. Since 1988 in Canada, unique pneumonia outbreaks described as proliferative and necrotizing pneumonia have been associated with an antigenic variant of H1N1 SIV (72). Microscopic lesions of proliferative and necrotizing pneumonia are characterized by necrotizing bronchiolitis, marked type 2 pneumocyte proliferation, abundant alveolar exudate, and hyaline membranes along alveolar septa. Analysis of a Quebec strain associated with proliferative and necrotizing pneumonia revealed a variant of H1N1 with considerable genomic divergence (drift) from current North American isolates (84). In 1992 in the United States, A/Swine/Nebraska/1/92 H1N1 was isolated and found to be antigenically and genetically distinct from classical swine H1N1 (77).

Antigenic shifts are more dramatic changes in which an entirely new virus arises from reassortment of genes from two different viruses resulting in a completely new H or N component. In 1992 in England, H1N7 was identified in pigs and is thought to be the result of reassortment between human and equine isolates (16). An H1N2 virus was isolated from pigs experiencing respiratory disease in Scotland in

1994 and was determined to be a result of reassortment between human and swine viruses (17). Genetic reassortment between avian and swine influenza viruses has been reported in Italy (24). Genetic analysis indicates that the virus associated with recent swine flu outbreaks in the midwestern United States (IA H3N2) is a reassortment of human H3N2 and swine H1N1. It appears to be distinct from European and Asian H3N2 viruses from pigs.

Evidence suggests that there has been continuous circulation of a human H3N2 virus in pigs in Europe for quite some time (78). In January 1992, respiratory disease suddenly increased in the swine population of England. The isolate A/swine/England/195852/92 was typical of the isolates from this outbreak and was distinguishable from classical and European swine viruses in hemagglutination inhibition tests using monoclonal antibodies to the H1 hemagglutinin (20). Convalescent-phase sera from this outbreak tested negative in hemagglutination inhibition tests with the classical United Kingdom prototype H1N1 and H3N2 swine influenza viruses. The isolate was later confirmed to be an avian H1N1 isolate based on genetic and antigenic analysis (19). Experimental inoculation of pigs resulted in disease and lesions similar to classical SIV (18). Avian H1N1 viruses have also been isolated from pigs in China (44).

Severity of SIV disease varies with the age and immune status of the pig, the particular influenza isolate involved, and concurrent infections. Acute (epizootic) swine influenza is characterized by an acute onset of respiratory disease with high morbidity and low mortality. Dyspnea, labored abdominal respiration, paroxysmal barking cough, prostration, and fever are characteristic. Infection of naive pregnant sows or gilts may result in abortion storms that persist for 2 to 3 weeks. Sickness in adult animals and subsequent reproductive disease appears to be more common and severe in recent cases of H3N2 SIV outbreaks in the United States. Rapid recovery of individual animals usually occurs in 2 to 6 days if uncomplicated. Passive antibody for SIV is generally protective and wanes by 8 to 12 weeks of age. Loss of protective passively acquired antibody explains why SIV-induced disease is most common in 12- to 24-week-old pigs. If a naive sow herd is infected, influenza can be expected and is commonly observed in suckling and nursery pigs.

SIV induces multifocal to diffuse pneumonia with dark red-tan, mottled areas affecting 20 to 100% of the lung tissue. Lesions are often cranioventral in distribution. The lungs are often congested and airways contain blood-tinged foam. Enlarged and hyperemic mediastinal and tracheobronchial lymph nodes are common. Microscopic examination reveals bronchointerstitial pneumonia characterized by necrotizing bronchitis and bronchiolitis, alveolar septal infiltration with mixed inflammatory cells, type 2 pneumocyte hypertrophy and hyperplasia, and filling of airways and alveolar spaces with proteinaceous fluid and mixed inflammatory cells.

In contrast to PRRSV, the immune response to SIV infection is rapid and fairly effective. SIV is typically isolated only within the first 7 days after infection. The antibody response can occur as quickly as 3 days after inoculation (67). Isotype-specific antibodies have been found in nasal secretions 5 to 10 days after inoculation with an increase in immunoglobulin M antibodies correlating to viral clearance (51). Production of SIV-specific, antibody-producing cells has been found in both the upper and lower respiratory tract, and immunoglobulin A appears to be the predominant isotype (66). There is apparently minimal cross-immunity between the different subtypes of SIV, so pigs can contract each of the different subtypes, all of which can potentially induce respiratory disease.

SIV is most commonly spread from pig to pig via nasopharyngeal secretions. The virus attaches to the cilia, and viral replication begins in the epithelium of the upper respiratory tract. Infection spreads to bronchi and bronchioles resulting in loss of cilia, extrusion of mucus, exudation of neutrophils and macrophages, and necrosis and metaplasia of airway epithelium. Extension of virus infection to alveolar epithelium, endothelium, and alveolar macrophages results in flooding of alveoli with serofibrinous exudate.

Although SIV is frequently isolated from pigs with PRDC and seroconversion is common in grow-finish pigs, its role in the pathogenesis of PRDC is less clear. Pigs may be predisposed to bacterial pneumonia due to damage to the mucociliary apparatus and decreased macrophage function. SIV may precipitate a more severe disease in combination with other respiratory viruses as well. Coinfection with either PRRSV or *M. hyopneumoniae* increased the severity and duration of respiratory disease (100, 114). In contrast, there were fewer viruses isolated from pigs infected with both SIV and PRCV organisms (65, 118).

PRCV

PRCV, a member of the family *Coronaviridae,* is a variant of TGEV with altered tropism from the enteric tract to the respiratory tract. The main difference between TGEV and PRCV is a deletion in the S gene of PRCV (83). The significance of PRCV infection was recently reviewed (79) and is essentially threefold: (i) some strains may induce or contribute to respiratory disease, (ii) it is difficult to distinguish PRCV serologically from TGEV, and (iii) PRCV may provide some cross-protection against TGEV.

Herds may be seropositive to PRCV without evidence of respiratory disease. European and U.S. researchers have reported a range of clinical respiratory signs in experimentally inoculated pigs. The first isolates of PRCV were demonstrated to be nonpathogenic or mildly pathogenic, whereas more recent isolates appear to be moderately or highly pathogenic. Experimental inoculations may result in varying degrees of anorexia, lethargy, pyrexia, dyspnea, tachypnea, weight loss, or death. Field and experimental evidence supports a synergistic role of PRCV and other common swine viral respiratory pathogens.

Characteristic lesions vary from inapparent to severe, multifocal, tan-mottling, or consolidation of the lung. Microscopic examination reveals bronchointerstitial pneumonia characterized by necrosis, metaplasia, and proliferation of bronchiolar epithelium and increased neutrophils and macrophages in alveolar spaces.

In endemically infected herds, most pigs appear to become naturally infected at 5 to 8 weeks of age despite having some passive antibody protection at this time. PRCV replicates primarily in the epithelium of the upper respiratory tract and subsequently invades the bronchi and bronchiolar epithelium with extension to the peribronchiolar and alveolar regions. Decreased pulmonary alveolar macrophage function of PRCV-infected macrophages may also play a role in decreased defense. The role of this virus in complicated respiratory disease in swine is unclear, but it is not uncommon to isolate this virus in conjunction with PRRSV and/or SIV, and this may increase susceptibility to secondary bacterial infections.

PRV

PRV is supposed to be eradicated from the U.S. swine population in the near future. However, it continues to be a serious concern in much of the world. If present, PRV can be an important contributor to PRDC. PRV (also known as Aujeszky's disease virus) is an alphaherpesvirus which has a predilection for the respiratory and nervous system. Clinical signs depend on the strain of PRV, the challenge dose, and the age and immune status of the pig infected (63). In general, high-mortality central nervous system disease occurs in young pigs, while low-mortality respiratory signs occur in older pigs. Respiratory disease typically consists of a rhinitis with sneezing and nasal discharge which may progress to pneumonia with coughing and labored breathing. Systemic signs include fever, depression, and anorexia. In some cases, disease is subclinical with only decreased weight gain. Pseudorabies can also cause abortions in pregnant animals. The PRV-induced immune response is well characterized. Seroconversion occurs consistently between 7 and 10 days after infection, with serum-neutralizing antibodies appearing within 8 to 10 days. Although the immune response effectively controls the viremia, PRV becomes latent in the trigeminal ganglia and tonsil allowing possible recrudescence during times of stress (25).

Gross lesions in the respiratory tract include fibrinonecrotic rhinitis, tonsillitis, laryngitis which may extend to the trachea and lung resulting in pneumonia characterized by pulmonary edema, hemorrhage, and foci of necrosis; however, definitive gross lesions in growing pigs are often absent. Neonatal pigs may have miliary foci of necrosis in the spleen and liver. The most definitive PRV-induced microscopic lesion is severe lymphohistiocytic encephalitis with perivascular cuffing, gliosis, glial nodule formation, neuronophagia, and neuronal necrosis. This may be difficult to distinguish from severe PRRSV-induced lesions. Microscopic lesions in the lung are characterized by pulmonary congestion and hemorrhage and patchy to diffuse alveolar septal thickening and multifocal necrosis. Eosinophilic intranuclear inclusion bodies may be associated with foci of necrosis in the lung and liver.

PRV initially replicates in the epithelium of the nasopharynx and tonsil and subsequently spreads to regional lymph nodes and the nervous system after which there is a viremia and spread of the virus throughout tissues of body. Virus-induced damage to the mucosa of the upper respiratory tract results in damage to the mucociliary apparatus. PRV can also be isolated from alveolar macrophages of infected pigs. Together, this results in impaired defense mechanism of the respiratory tract (55). Experimentally, pseudorabies virus has exacerbated disease with several bacterial diseases such as *A. pleuropneumoniae, P. multocida, S. suis, M. hyopneumoniae,* PRRSV, and possibly *H. parasuis* (30, 41, 56, 74, 89, 94).

PCV

PCV is a very small, single-stranded, circular DNA virus in the family *Circoviridae*. PCV was originally detected as a noncytopathic contaminant of continuous PK/15 cells (106) and that isolate is now known as PCV1. Hines and Luk-ert (52) associated PCV infection with congenital tremors in 1994. The congenital tremor strain of PCV was thought to be PCV1; however, the presence of PCV2 nucleic acid was recently identified in central nervous system tissues from pigs exhibiting congenital tremors (98). Interest in PCV has greatly increased since it was associated with postweaning multisystemic wasting syndrome (PMWS) in Canada (36, 49). Since that time, several groups in North America and Europe have associated porcine circovirus with PMWS (62, 73, 93). Strains of PCV from cases of PMWS differ considerably from PK/15 strains based on sequence analysis (48, 68, 73) and are tentatively classified as PCV2.

The most common clinical signs of PMWS include progressive weight loss (wasting) and chronic pneumonia (tachypnea and dyspnea). Morbidity within a group is usually low (5 to 50%); however, mortality among affected pigs is often very high. Icterus, paleness, and diarrhea are less commonly reported. PCV2 has also been associated with gastric ulcers and with porcine dermatitis and nephropathy syndrome (87). Pigs in the late-nursery to mid-finishing phase (6 to 18 weeks) are most commonly affected. It can be very difficult clinically to distinguish PMWS from PRRSV and secondary infections. PRRSV and PCV are frequently detected together in cases of PMWS.

Characteristic gross lesions of PMWS include markedly enlarged tan lymph nodes, rubbery-tan lungs that fail to collapse, and less commonly enlarged "waxy" kidneys or mottled-tan livers. Diagnosis of PMWS is based on identification of unique microscopic lesions (86). Characteristic microscopic lesions include depletion of lymphoid follicles and granulomatous inflammation of the lymphoid tissues, liver, pancreas, and a variety of other tissues. Lung lesions are characterized by lymphohistiocytic interstitial pneumonia of variable severity. There are varying degrees of airway epithelial sloughing and fibroplasia in the lamina propria. Bronchiolitis and bronchitis obliterans fibrosa is common in severe cases.

Multinucleate syncytial cells may be present in alveolar spaces. Macrophages in B-cell-dependent areas of lymphoid tissues often contain clusters of variably sized basophilic intracytoplasmic "grape-like clusters" of inclusion bodies. The lymphoid depletion, granulomatous inflammation, and inclusion bodies are most easily identified in tonsils and Peyer's patches.

We are just beginning to understand the pathogenesis of porcine circoviruses. The PCV1 strain from persistently infected continuous PK/15 cells was found to be nonpathogenic in colostrum-deprived pigs (3). Ellis et al. demonstrated a high degree of correlation between the presence of PCV2 and lesions of PMWS in pigs from more than 70 herds in Canada (36). Evidence continues to point toward PCV2 as the primary cause or at least an integral component of PMWS. PCV2 apparently is essential but perhaps not sufficient by itself to induce PMWS (64). The importance of concurrent infection(s) with other pathogens such as porcine parvovirus (PPV), adenovirus, PRRSV, and other pathogens is under continued investigation.

M. hyopneumoniae

M. hyopneumoniae is the primary pathogen associated with enzootic pneumonia, which occurs when *M. hyopneumoniae* is combined with opportunistic bacteria such as *P. multocida*. *M. hyopneumoniae*, one of the smallest known bacteria, is a mucosal pathogen that colonizes the respiratory tract by attaching to the cilia of the epithelium by adhesin proteins. Adherence to the cilia by *M. hyopneumoniae* results in clumping and loss of cilia, and epithelial cell death, with a consequent reduced function of the mucociliary apparatus (31). The decrease in the mucociliary apparatus is thought to be a significant contributor to the increased incidence of secondary bacterial infections associated with *M. hyopneumoniae* infection. Mycoplasmal pneumonia is a high-morbidity, low-mortality disease characterized by a chronic nonproductive cough. Incubation takes 10 to 16 days, and it spreads slowly so evidence of disease in the herd is often unnoticed

until pigs are 3 to 6 months old. Gross lesions appear as purple to gray areas of consolidation of the lung with a cranial ventral distribution. Early microscopic lesions consist of accumulations of neutrophils in the lumina and around airways and in alveoli. As the disease progresses, there are perivascular, peribronchial, and peribronchiolar accumulations of lymphocytes.

The complex, chronic pathogenesis of respiratory disease mediated by *M. hyopneumoniae* appears to depend on evasion or alteration of the host immune response. Immunopathologic changes are a major component of mycoplasmal pneumonia, although little is known about the mechanisms or the underlying immune and inflammatory responses. The effect of *M. hyopneumoniae* on the immune system is conflicting. Pulmonary alveolar macrophages from pigs infected concurrently with *M. hyopneumoniae* and *A. pleuropneumoniae* exhibited decreased phagocytic capability (22). *M. hyopneumoniae* has a nonspecific stimulatory (mitogenic) effect on lymphocytes (69). In addition, inflammation, as demonstrated by the production of proinflammatory cytokines, seems to play an important role in the pneumonia induced by *M. hyopneumoniae* and its effect on other pathogens within the respiratory system of the pig (6, 7, 101). Although an inflammatory response is important in controlling respiratory pathogens, the tissue injury and disease subsequent to *M. hyopneumoniae* infection appears to be induced more by the host than by the microbe itself.

Disease due to *M. hyopneumoniae*, although chronic, tends to be mild if uncomplicated, and most cases of mycoplasmal pneumonia are mixed infections. *M. hyopneumoniae* along with PRRSV and *P. multocida* is the most common combination of pathogens in PRDC. *M. hyopneumoniae* has been shown experimentally to predispose to infection with *P. multocida* and *A. pleuropneumoniae* (5, 27, 124). Recent research demonstrated that *M. hyopneumoniae* enhances the severity and duration of PRRSV-induced pneumonia (99). Inflammation appears to be an important factor in the potentiation of PRRSV-induced pneumonia by *M. hyopneumoniae* as demonstrated by increased levels of proinflammatory cytokines by both pathogens (99, 105).

B. bronchiseptica

B. bronchiseptica is a gram-negative bacterium closely related to *Bordetella pertussis* but it does not produce the pertussis toxin. *B. bronchiseptica* causes rhinitis and mild to moderate turbinate atrophy and predisposes to infection with toxigenic strains of *P. multocida* which causes the progressive form of atrophic rhinitis. (The interaction between *B. bronchiseptica* and toxigenic *P. multocida* in atrophic rhinitis is the subject of chapter 10.) Lesions associated with the upper respiratory tract include mucosal inflammatory lesions with loss of cilia and atrophy of the turbinates (35). *B. bronchiseptica* also causes primary pneumonia in neonatal pigs and secondary pneumonia in older pigs. In primary *Bordetella* pneumonia, severity of pneumonic lesions peaks between 10 and 14 DPI when red, consolidated areas are noticeable in the lung (34). By 21 DPI these lesions become tan and contracted (34). Early histologic lesions of the lung are characterized by alveolar hemorrhage and neutrophilic infiltrates in alveoli and bronchioles. This is followed by epithelialization of alveoli and fibrosis.

Like *M. hyopneumoniae*, *B. bronchiseptica* is associated with ciliated cells of the upper and lower respiratory tract and has multifactorial virulence mechanisms. *B. bronchiseptica* produces virulence factors which are regulated by a two-component sensory transduction system encoded by the *bvg* locus (82). Some of the virulence factors that are positively regulated by *bvg* include purported adhesins such as filamentous hemagglutinin, pertactin and fimbriae, and dermonecrotic and adenylate cyclase-hemolysin toxins. The dermonecrotic toxin contributes to turbinate atrophy and pneumonia, while the adenylate cyclase-hemolysin is thought to be responsible for alveolar macrophage cytotoxicity (13, 14). Another virulence factor not regulated by the *bvg*

locus is the tracheal cytotoxin which is released from the bacterial peptidoglycan and is thought to be responsible for epithelial and cilial damage.

B. bronchiseptica has been shown to increase colonization and/or exacerbate disease with *P. multocida, S. suis,* and *H. parasuis* (12, 29, 119, 120; S. L. Brockmeier and M.V. Palmer, *Proc. 82nd Conf. Res. Work Anim. Dis.,* abstr. 180, 2001). Coinfection with PRRSV and *B. bronchiseptica* leads to increased severity of clinical disease and predisposes to pneumonic lesions with *B. bronchiseptica* (11). In addition, whereas PRRSV or *B. bronchiseptica* by itself does not increase susceptibility to *P. multocida* pneumonia, a combination of the two does (12).

P. multocida

P. multocida is a gram-negative bacterium which is a cause of atrophic rhinitis and pneumonia in pigs. There are five capsular serotypes of *P. multocida,* but only A and D are usually found in swine. Serotype A is most commonly isolated from lungs and serotype D from cases of atrophic rhinitis, but both types have been associated with both diseases (61, 80). The dermonecrotic toxin (*Pasteurella* toxin) is the primary virulence factor responsible for producing the turbinate atrophy seen in atrophic rhinitis. *B. bronchiseptica* predisposes to this condition (111). The role of the toxin in pneumonic lesions is less defined. Many isolates from pneumonic lesions are not toxigenic, but some studies have indicated that toxigenic strains may be more virulent (61). The capsule, especially for capsular type A, may be an important virulence factor in avoidance of phagocytosis (40). Experimentally, it is difficult to infect pigs with pure cultures of *P. multocida,* even though studies indicate it is commonly carried in the tonsil of pigs; thus, it is usually considered an opportunistic infection. However, there have been recent reports of an increasing number of cases of severe bronchopneumonia often with pleuritis associated with singular infection with *P. multocida* type A or type D; therefore, certain isolates may be more virulent and should perhaps be considered as primary pathogens (P. G. Halbur, unpublished data). Several viruses and bacteria have been shown to predispose to infection with this organism (5, 12, 26, 27, 41). Clinical signs and lesions are usually superimposed on that of a primary agent, usually involving chronic occasional cough, labored breathing, and failure to grow. Well-demarcated red to gray colored consolidation of the lung with a cranial-ventral distribution is common. There may be pleuritis, pleural adhesions, and/or abscesses as well. Microscopically lobular purulent bronchopneumonia is seen.

A. pleuropneumoniae

A. pleuropneumoniae is a gram-negative bacterium which is the most common cause of pleuropneumonia in pigs. There are 12 capsular serotypes of A. pleuropneumoniae. Serotypes 1, 5, and 7 are the most common in the United States, and types 1, 2, 5, and 7 are most common in Europe. Outbreaks of A. pleuropneumoniae are usually precipitated by stress, environmental changes, or viral or mycoplasmal infection. The disease may present clinically as a peracute form with sudden death; an acute form with clinical signs characterized by fever, lethargy, dyspnea, cyanosis, recumbency, and froth from the nose; or a subacute/chronic form which develops after disappearance of acute signs with intermittent cough, slow growth, and exercise intolerance. Depending on the stage of disease, pathologic lesions consist of fibrinohemorrhagic pleuropneumonia that is firm, dark-red, friable, necrotic, and often in dorsocaudal portions. The dark lesions form abscess-like nodules as the disease becomes more chronic and the fibrinous pleuritis progresses into fibrous adhesions. Microscopic examination reveals fibrinosuppurative and necrohemorrhagic pleuropneumonia.

A. pleuropneumoniae is spread by direct contact or aerosol over short distances. Survivors of acute infection frequently become chronic carriers, with the organisms persisting in necrotic lung tissues, tonsils, and occasionally the nasal cavity. A marked difference in viru-

lence exists between serotypes and strains within serotypes. A. pleuropneumoniae can colonize the tonsil and adhere to alveolar epithelium where production of three Apx toxins (ApxI, ApxII, and ApxIII) cause damage to endothelial and epithelial cells of the lung and alveolar macrophages (39). The damage to the lungs associated with A. pleuropneumoniae infection is caused by both the production of Apx toxins, lipopolysaccharides (LPS), and the production of proinflammatory cytokines (10, 38, 57, 76). LPS release results in profound endotoxemia with induction of coagulation and inflammatory pathways. The capsule may prevent digestion by phagocytes, and the bacteria are resistant to complement (88). Production of the cytokines interleukin-1β (IL-1β), IL-8, and tumor necrosis factor (TNF) may contribute to the development of lesions. Chronic forms of the disease may be exacerbated by other respiratory infections. Experimentally, coinfection with M. hyopneumoniae causes more severe disease than with either pathogen alone and the Apx toxins predisposed to pulmonary infection with P. multocida (26).

H. parasuis

H. parasuis is a gram-negative bacterium which causes polyserositis (Glasser's disease) and pneumonia in swine. In stressed young pigs, it causes a sporadic disease within a few days of inoculation which is characterized by systemic invasion and bacteremia and results in a polyserositis syndrome (serofibrinous to fibrinopurulent peritonitis, pleuritis, pericarditis, meningitis, and arthritis). Clinical signs include fever, anorexia, swollen joints with lameness, dyspnea, and central nervous system signs. Fifteen serovars of H. parasuis have been identified, but many isolates are nontypable. Serovars 4 and 5 are isolated most frequently in conjunction with clinical disease in the United States. Virulence may be associated with certain of these serovars; however, disease induced by different isolates of the same serovar can differ significantly. Experimental evidence indicates that H. parasuis may colonize the nasal cavity and trachea initially, resulting in loss of cilia and damage to ciliated epithelium, even though the organism does not appear to be closely associated with these cells (108, 109). Damage to the mucosal epithelial cells may facilitate invasion. Others have reported finding the bacteria in the tonsil rather than the nasal cavity. After initial colonization, invasion resulting in a bacteremia and subsequent systemic spread occurs, but the factors responsible for this are unknown. The incidence of isolation of this organism from cases of pneumonia has increased with the increased incidence of PRDC in healthy herds. Pneumonia is not a common sequela with experimental infections and may be due to interactions with other pathogens, as shown when there was accidental inoculation of *H. parasuis* with pseudorabies virus which resulted in pneumonia (74). Other interactions, such as with PRRSV, have been harder to demonstrate experimentally (91, 92, 96, 97). When isolated from the lung, pneumonic lesions are typical of bacterial pneumonia consisting of fibrinopurulent bronchopneumonia.

S. suis

S. suis is a gram-positive bacterium commonly carried in the tonsil and nasal cavity of pigs which causes sporadic systemic and respiratory disease. Transmission from dam to offspring occurs early; therefore, early weaning practices have been unable to break the transmission cycle. At least 35 capsular serotypes of *S. suis* exist. Capsular type 2 is the most common type isolated from diseased pigs. The earliest sign of disease is usually fever followed by bacteremia which can result in meningitis with central nervous system signs, arthritis with lameness, polyserositis, endocarditis, and pneumonia. *S. suis* invades tonsils and reaches the lymph nodes via lymphatics. Infected monocytes may distribute the organism throughout the body and to the brain. Virulence factors are not well characterized. Several potential virulence factors of *S. suis* have been identified such as fimbriae and hemagglutinins, which may act as adhesins, and the capsule, which may inhibit phagocytosis. Other potential virulence factors include muramidase-release protein, extracel-

lular factor, immunoglobulin G (IgG)-binding protein, albumin-binding protein, a hemolysin (suilysin), and purine immunosuppressive factor (15). However, none of these factors appear to completely correlate with ability to cause disease, and thus virulence is probably multifactorial. Lesions induced by *S. suis* include fibrinopurulent meningitis or polyserositis and suppurative bronchopneumonia. Once again, as with *H. parasuis,* while it is not uncommon to isolate *S. suis* from pneumonic lesions in the field, pneumonia is not typically produced with experimental infections; thus, mixed infections may play a role in inducing pulmonary lesions. PRV, PRRSV, and *B. bronchiseptica* have been shown to predispose pigs to disease with *S. suis* (43, 47, 56, 102, 119, 120).

Other Pathogens

Several other pathogens including porcine cytomegalovirus, paramyxovirus, encephalomyocarditis virus, hemagglutinating encephalomyocarditis virus, adenovirus, *S. choleraesuis, A. suis,* and *A. pyogenes* are less frequently involved in PRDC.

As seen from the discussions above, it is difficult to give an all-inclusive description of PRDC. As stated before, the term PRDC was initially used to describe a late-finishing respiratory disease where pigs failed to gain weight, but mixed respiratory infections in pigs can occur at any age and involve a myriad of both viral and bacterial pathogens. The clinical presentation can be very broad and include not only respiratory signs, but systemic signs of disease as well, depending on the organisms involved. Respiratory signs can vary and include sneezing if there is rhinitis, coughing of varying frequency and productiveness, and labored breathing. It is not uncommon for respiratory signs to be mild with the major signs of disease being poor growth, roughened hair coat, anorexia, decreased weight gain, and lethargy. Disseminated or systemic signs of disease can include central nervous system disturbances, swollen joints and lameness, reproductive failure, or even sudden death. Pathological findings can also be broad and overlapping in nature, so it can be difficult to discern from just clinical signs and pathology what pathogens are causing problems without additional diagnostics to identify the agents involved.

MECHANISMS OF DISEASE PATHOGENESIS

The specific pathogenesis mechanisms of PRDC are largely unknown. Primary bacterial and viral pathogens have virulence factors that allow them to overcome natural defenses in the respiratory tract and cause overt disease by themselves. Mechanisms by which primary agents alter the defense of the respiratory tract are not entirely understood, but include damage to the ciliated or pulmonary epithelium of the respiratory tract, altered function of pulmonary macrophages, production of adhesins that may be used by other bacteria to attach to respiratory epithelium, and immunomodulatory effects (Fig. 2). To complicate matters further, several pathogens may work together to break down different defenses leaving the respiratory tract susceptible to several less pathogenic organisms.

The multifactorial nature of respiratory disease in pigs has been implicated for some time on the basis of diagnostic and field examination, and one might think that experimentally reproducing lesions through coinfection experiments would be easily accomplished. However, this is not always the case, and it is often difficult to experimentally reproduce disease with dual infections. This may be because of the virulence of strains used, timing of coinfection, and difficulty in reproducing environmental or management stressors. In addition, differences in age, genetic makeup, immune status, and existing pathogen or flora status (conventionally reared versus gnotobiotic pigs) alters the susceptibility of pigs to disease. Thus, reproduction of experimental results between laboratories or even by the same laboratory has been difficult at times.

PRDC is observed in differing management and facility schemes, including but not limited to intensive production systems. Because PRDC is not caused by a single entity but rather is a multifactorial disease, the pathogens isolated from pigs vary between and within

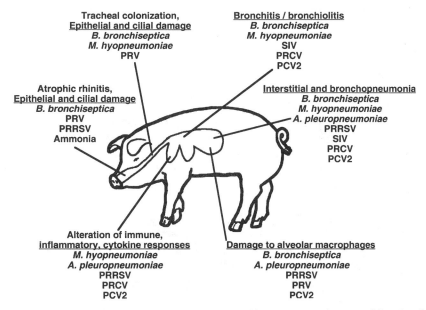

FIGURE 2 Areas and defense mechanisms which are affected by primary pathogens of the pig, allowing them and opportunistic pathogens to establish infection.

production units. As the number of pathogens in an animal increases, the interaction between individual organisms becomes more complex and the intricate patterns and roles of each become increasingly difficult to elucidate. Although the pathogenesis is known for most of these common respiratory pathogens, less is known about the host responses to these agents. The following section is a discussion of some of the successful models of mixed infection and theories as to the pathogenic mechanisms of interaction.

Polymicrobial Disease Involving Viruses and Bacteria

Epidemiological evidence that secondary bacterial infections often follow viral respiratory diseases is well documented. Although some of these superinfections have been replicated experimentally, specific mechanisms of interactions are poorly understood and often inferred based on pathogenesis of the viral infections. PRV, PRCV, SIV, and PRRSV are all common viral respiratory pathogens of pigs, and all have been variously implicated in increasing the incidence of bacterial respiratory disease in herds which circulate the viruses.

PRV

The fact that the United States as well as many other countries have ongoing eradication programs for PRV testifies to the importance of this pathogen for swine. Although its incidence has decreased in recent years due to eradication efforts, it is still is an important problem in many pig-producing areas of the world. The virus by itself can cause respiratory, neurologic, and reproductive disease. In older animals, where the disease tends to be mild or subclinical, secondary respiratory disease has been associated with circulation of this virus in the herd. This led to studies which demonstrated that PRV had a profound effect on the development of lesions with many bacterial pathogens of pigs such as *P. multocida, S. suis, A. pleuropneumoniae, H. parasuis,* and *M. hyopneumoniae* (41, 56, 74, 89, 94). In all cases lesions in coinfected pigs were more extensive and severe

than for pigs inoculated with the single agents alone. In some experiments PRV lowered the threshold for infection with the bacterial agent, an important point when one considers the field situation where infectious dose exposure is probably not as great as experimental exposure. In addition, PRV was able to exert effects when given before, concurrently with, or after infection with bacterial pathogens.

The mechanisms by which PRV predisposes to secondary bacterial infection are not definitively known but probably involve breakdown of general defenses rather than specific viral-bacterial interactions, since infection with this virus predisposes to so many bacterial species. PRV replicates in alveolar macrophages and monocytes and causes a lytic infection. Destruction of these important cells that are involved in both innate and active immunity may cause immunosuppression. Such functions as phagocytosis, killing of phagocytized bacteria, antibody-dependent and -independent cytotoxicity, alpha interferon (IFN-α) production, phagosome-lysosome fusion, and O_2 production after stimulation with opsonized zymosan have been shown to be reduced in PRV-infected macrophages (40, 53, 54). PRV causes necrotic rhinitis and has been shown to disrupt ciliary activity in the respiratory mucosa and thus mechanical damage may contribute to decreased clearance, increased adherence and increased nutrient supply (74).

PRCV

Although infection with PRCV is fairly common, and its interaction with other viruses has been examined, no studies have examined the impact of this infection on bacterial diseases. However, in a study examining the effects of coexposure to PRCV and LPS, exposure to virus or LPS alone was subclinical, but coexposure resulted in severe respiratory disease (116). Increases in TNF-α and IL-1 were induced with the combination of both PRCV and LPS and the increase in TNF-α, but not IL-1, correlated with clinical signs. Therefore, there is some indication that exposure to high endotoxin concentrations in swine buildings or coinfection with gram-negative bacteria could precipitate disease in PRCV-infected pigs.

SIV

SIV is one of the most common pathogens isolated from cases of PRDC. Infection with SIV causes an acute high-morbidity, low-mortality, respiratory disease in swine which, if uncomplicated, recedes quickly. Secondary bacterial infections can be the most important complicating factors in SIV outbreaks. Examining the effects of SIV on subsequent infection with bacteria has been somewhat limited given the difficulty in experimentally reproducing disease with SIV alone. Infection studies with SIV and *M. hyopneumoniae* found that, although pigs infected with both agents exhibited more severe respiratory clinical disease, the effects were more additive than synergistic with the pneumonia induced by each following a normal course over time (100). Since both *M. hyopneumoniae* and SIV disrupt the airway epithelium, the combination of the two may lead to an increase in opportunistic infections over what is seen with each agent alone. Although not demonstrated in pigs, a mixed infection with SIV and *A. pleuropneumoniae* in mice showed synergism with increased mortality after mixed infection. Cleavage of the hemagglutinin of influenza viruses by proteases is required for infectivity. Research has shown that some bacterial proteases can cleave the hemagglutinins of several influenza viruses and thus potentiate infection with the virus. However, no bacterial isolates from pigs have demonstrated cleavage activation of influenza virus hemagglutinin (21).

PRRSV

Since PRRSV emerged in the 1980s, an increase in concurrent respiratory disease has been noted on farms where pigs are also infected with PRRSV, and PRRSV is often isolated from cases of PRDC. This, in addition to the fact that experimental infection with PRRSV isolates often resulted in minimal respiratory disease by itself, led to the theory that

PRRSV might interact with other respiratory pathogens to produce clinical signs of disease. However, the relationship has been difficult to prove experimentally. In coinfection studies with PRRSV and other agents, there have been reports ranging from no interaction to increased incidence and severity of disease, sometimes with conflicting results between laboratories using the same infectious agents.

Initial studies with PRRSV and bacterial pathogens such as *A. pleuropneumoniae, H. parasuis, S. suis, S. choleraesuis, P. multocida,* and *M. hyopneumoniae* showed that the virus had minimal if any effect on the severity of these bacterial diseases (28, 81, 110). Since then, experimental evidence has shown that PRRSV may interact with some of these pathogens, although not always in a straightforward manner. For example, two additional studies have failed to demonstrate any interaction of PRRSV with *P. multocida,* even though these two pathogens are the most common isolates from cases of PRDC (12, 23, 28). However, prior infection with both *B. bronchiseptica* and PRRSV did predispose pigs to pulmonary infection with *P. multocida,* where neither alone could (12). The relationship among these pathogens was discovered after initial studies were conducted examining the effects of PRRSV on subsequent challenges of either *P. multocida* or *B. bronchiseptica.* As already pointed out no interaction between PRRSV and *P. multocida* could be detected. Challenge with *P. multocida* alone did not result in clinical signs of disease or detectible colonization. When *P. multocida* was given after infection with PRRSV, there was still no colonization with *P. multocida.* However, PRRSV did predispose pigs to pneumonia with *B. bronchiseptica* (11). Clinical signs, febrile response, and decreased weight gain were more severe in the coinoculated group than in the other groups infected with either agent alone. Pigs in the group that received only *B. bronchiseptica* lacked gross or microscopic lung lesions, and *B. bronchiseptica* was not cultured from lung tissue. In the group inoculated with *B. bronchiseptica* and PRRSV, 80% of the pigs had gross and microscopic lesions consistent with bacterial bronchopneumonia, and *B. bronchiseptica* was isolated from these lesions. Pigs inoculated with only PRRSV had lesions of interstitial pneumonia, and no bacteria were isolated from the lungs. Further investigation demonstrated that *B. bronchiseptica* predisposed to infection of the upper respiratory tract, but not the lung, with *P. multocida*. This led to the theory that the combination of PRRSV and *B. bronchiseptica* may leave pigs more susceptible to pulmonary infection with opportunistic bacteria. Challenge with *P. multocida* following coinfection with PRRSV and *B. bronchiseptica* resulted in increased colonization of the nasal cavity and tonsil with *P. multocida,* as well as isolation of all three agents from pneumonic lesions.

Studies examining the effects of PRRSV infection on subsequent infection with *H. parasuis* indicated that pigs infected with both PRRSV and *H. parasuis* actually had fewer clinical signs and lesions of polyserositis (1 of 10) than pigs infected with *H. parasuis* alone (7 of 10) (97). The coinfected group did have 3 of 10 pigs die suddenly of unknown causes, possibly septic shock. *H. parasuis* was cultured from multiple sites in both groups, and distribution of virus and bacteria as seen by immunohistochemistry was the same (92). At 7 days after PRRSV infection, alveolar macrophages collected from pigs had decreased uptake of opsonized *H. parasuis* and decreased superoxide anion production; at 9 days there was increased intracellular survival of *H. parasuis* and decreased superoxide anion production (96). These effects were not seen at earlier times. Although studies have shown that macrophages from PRRSV-infected pigs have decreased functions, others have shown an enhancement of humoral and cell-mediated functions. Thus, immunomodulation may be responsible for the differences in clinical presentation between the PRRSV and *H. parasuis* group and the *H. parasuis*-only group.

A study looking at the interaction of PRRSV and *S. choleraesuis* demonstrated that, although coinfection with both resulted in in-creased clinical signs, pigs which received dexamethasone in addition to the PRRSV and *S. choleraesuis* were most severely affected with increased mortality and with increased replication and shedding of both organisms (122). This study points out that PRRSV may work as a cofactor with stress from environmental factors to increase susceptibility to disease.

The combination of PRRSV and *M. hyopneumoniae* produces another unique interaction. Rather than PRRSV increasing disease caused by *M. hyopneumoniae,* infection with *M. hyopneumoniae* potentiated and prolonged PRRSV-induced pneumonia clinically, macroscopically, and microscopically (99). The levels of *M. hyopneumoniae* or PRRSV were not increased in tissues in dually infected pigs, which suggests the effect was not due to increased viral or bacterial replication. However, *M. hyopneumoniae* is known to have immunomodulatory effects, it is mitogenic for swine lymphocytes, and activation of the immune system and inflammatory response may enhance recruitment of macrophages to the lung, which results in persistent PRRSV replication contributing to the prolongation of viral pneumonia. Increased production of proinflammatory cytokines was detected in a coculture system of *M. hyopneumoniae*-infected tracheal ring explants and PRRSV-infected alveolar macrophages; thus, the combination of the two may be needed to induce the changes needed for prolongation of PRRSV-induced pneumonia seen in coinfection (105).

Finally, PRRSV has been shown to predispose to colonization and disease with *S. suis* (42, 102). In one of these studies, both a virulent and an attenuated vaccine strain of PRRSV predisposed to *S. suis* infection, but the virulent strain was more efficient than the vaccine strain in doing so. Pulmonary intravascular macrophages are prominent in pigs and are thought to be primarily responsible for clearance of blood-borne pathogens. Pulmonary intravascular macrophages are as permissive to PRRSV replication as alveolar macrophages, and viral antigen has been seen in both immunohistologically (104). Clearance of intravenous copper particles was used to examine the effects of low (vaccine strain)- and high-virulence PRRSV strains on pulmonary intravascular macrophage function. Copper concentrations in the lung of high-virulence PRRSV-infected pigs were significantly lower than in lungs of control and low-virulence pigs at 7, 10, and 14 DPI (103). These results support the hypothesis that PRRSV infection may make pigs more susceptible to bacterial septicemia. In vitro, PRRSV decreased the numbers of macrophages in culture and affected some functions of both intravascular and alveolar macrophages, such as superoxide anion production, although there was no evidence for decreased ability to phagocytize *Staphylococcus aureus* or kill the bacteria (103, 104). Thus, whether it is a decrease in numbers or function of macrophages, or both, which result in decreased clearance is unknown. Lesions of rhinitis, including alteration of the epithelial surface and loss of cilia, have been reported with PRRSV. Thus, mechanical damage of the respiratory tract as well as effects on alveolar macrophage clearance may leave the animal more susceptible to systemic invasion of bacteria, and damage to intravascular macrophages may exacerbate dissemination.

Polymicrobial Viral Disease

PRCV, SIV, AND PRRSV

Field studies have shown that multiple viral infections are common in pigs entering the finishing herd (117). Because of this, the laboratories of van Reeth, Nauwynck, and Pensaert have extensively examined mixed viral infections with PRCV, SIV (H1N1 strain), and PRRSV. Their studies have focused on the role the early-response proinflammatory cytokines IFN-α, TNF-α, and IL-1 have in pathogenesis and potential interactions. These cytokines are thought to play roles in respiratory disease through such local actions as neutrophil migration and activation, alteration of pulmonary function, antiviral effects, and systemic effects such as induction of fever, anorexia, and the acute-phase response. Infections with each of

these viruses were examined independently, and it was found that these viruses behave differently with regard to the early cytokine response elicited (112, 115). SIV infection in pigs resulted in clinical signs, lung epithelial desquamation, and neutrophil infiltration. Levels of TNF-α, IFN-α, and IL-1 were all elevated 18 to 24 h after inoculation with SIV, and increased levels of these cytokines correlated with increases in bronchoalveolar lavage cell numbers, neutrophil infiltration, as well as onset and degree of clinical signs. PRCV was subclinical but caused mild bronchointerstitial pneumonitis and neutrophil infiltration and resulted in an increase in IFN-α. PRRSV induced anorexia, lethargy, and marked infiltration with mononuclear cells in alveolar septa and bronchoalveolar fluids, and there was an increase in IL-1 from 3 to 10 DPI.

After determining the effects of each virus by itself, interaction between viruses was examined by using coinfection models in pigs. In a study examining the combined effects of PRCV and SIV in pigs, disease appeared more severe in coinfected animals than in pigs infected with SIV alone. Pigs infected with PRCV only were not included since PRCV results in subclinical disease. Although clinical signs appeared worse in the coinfected animals, prior infection with PRCV decreased replication and shedding of SIV and it was speculated that the high IFN-α levels induced by PRCV were responsible for inhibition of SIV replication (118).

With conventionally raised pigs, dual infections with PRRSV and PRCV or PRRSV and SIV were examined. Disease, including fever, decreased weight gain, and respiratory dyspnea, was more pronounced in dually infected animals (114). When these experiments were repeated with gnotobiotic pigs, the clinical outcome was different than with conventional pigs. In gnotobiotic pigs, clinical signs were milder, there was decreased morbidity, and the effect of the coinfection appeared additive of the two single infections rather than synergistic (113). In the gnotobiotic pigs coinfected with PRRSV and PRCV, TNF-α was undetectable and IL-1 and IFN-α were similar to what is seen with PRRSV and PRCV alone, respectively. Differences between the conventionally raised pigs and the gnotobiotic pigs may have played a role in the different clinical outcomes. The conventional pigs may have had other contributing pathogens that were not detected. Whether or not the effects seen were synergistic or additive, coinfection probably compromised a broader spectrum of defense mechanisms, leaving the pigs especially vulnerable to secondary bacterial infections.

PCV2 AND PPV

Several groups have attempted to experimentally reproduce characteristic PMWS lesions with filtered tissue homogenates or cell culture material. Ellis et al. reproduced most of the lesions typical of PMWS in gnotobiotic pigs inoculated with filtered cell culture material and filtered lymphoid tissues from pigs with naturally acquired PMWS (37). However, both PCV2 and PPV and antibodies to these viruses were detected in the experimentally inoculated pigs. Balasch et al. also reproduced some of the lesions consistent with PMWS in conventional pigs inoculated with tissue homogenates from pigs with PMWS (8). Allan et al. (2) and Kennedy et al. (60) subsequently inoculated colostrum-deprived pigs with PCV2 alone, PPV alone, or the combination of PCV2 and PPV and reproduced severe clinical disease, death, and lesions typical of PMWS in the pigs dually inoculated with PCV2 and PPV. Only mild lesions of PMWS were reproduced in pigs inoculated with PCV2 alone. Krakowka et al. further confirmed the synergistic relationship of PCV2 and PPV in gnotobiotic pigs by reproducing clinical disease and lesions typical of PMWS in coinfected pigs (64). Infection with a combination of PCV2 and PRRSV has been shown to potentiate replication and distribution of PCV2 and results in a more severe clinical outcome than with either virus by itself (4, 50). Mittal et al. demonstrated colocalization of porcine circovirus with porcine adenovirus in pigs with naturally occurring PMWS (S. K. Mittal, M.

Kiupel, G. W. Stevenson, L. Anothayanontha, J. Choi, and C. L. Kanitz, *Proc. World Assoc. Vet. Lab. Diagn.*, p. 62, 1999). Recent evidence suggests that activation of macrophages in lymphoid tissues may lead to potentiation of PCV2 replication and development of clinical disease and lesions typical of PMWS (4, 64).

Polymicrobial Bacterial Disease

As discussed previously, numerous bacteria are capable of causing respiratory disease in pigs. Some of these agents are considered primary pathogens because of their ability to readily establish infection and cause disease on their own. *M. hyopneumoniae*, *A. pleuropneumoniae*, and *B. bronchiseptica* fall into this category. Many of the secondary bacteria of pigs readily colonize the tonsil and nasal cavity of pigs without causing disease until some insult comes along which allows them to replicate to a greater extent and infect deeper tissues. Although uncomplicated infections with bacteria such as *H. parasuis* and *S. suis* are occasionally diagnosed, more often than not there is an underlying factor which contributes to the development of disease with these pathogens. With other bacteria like *P. multocida*, it is very difficult to reproduce disease without prior insult. Because of this relationship, research has focused on the ability of these primary pathogens, especially *M. hyopneumoniae* and *B. bronchiseptica*, to predispose to secondary bacteria.

M. HYOPNEUMONIAE,
A. PLEUROPNEUMONIAE, AND
P. MULTOCIDA

Diagnostic examinations of cases of enzootic pneumonia in pigs has long indicated a relationship between *M. hyopneumoniae* and *P. multocida*. Several experimental studies confirmed the fact that inoculation with *M. hyopneumoniae* alone caused only mild disease and lung lesions, while inoculation with *P. multocida* alone caused no disease and was rarely even recoverable. But if pigs were given both *M. hyopneumoniae* and *P. multocida*, pigs developed higher fever, a more severe cough, and more extensive lung lesions from which both organisms were isolated (5, 27). *M. hyopneumoniae* is thought to compromise defense mechanisms of the respiratory tract by damaging the epithelial surface and causing ciliostasis, thus increasing the ability of *P. multocida* to infect lower respiratory tissues. Compromising cilial function decreases clearance of microorganisms and mucus; some studies have shown that *P. multocida* adheres to the mucus of the respiratory tract. Most pneumonic isolates of *P. multocida* are type A and nontoxigenic, but type D and toxigenic *P. multocida* have been isolated from pneumonia as well (61, 80). Capsular type A has a large hyaluronic acid capsule which in vitro has been shown to interfere with phagocytosis by alveolar macrophages; however, the relevance of this is in question since other studies have found that little capsule is produced in vivo (40, 58). It is unknown whether the *Pasteurella* dermonecrotic toxin plays a role in the development of pneumonia as it does with atrophic rhinitis. The immune response induced by *M. hyopneumoniae* is believed to play a role in lesion development and may cause immunosuppression and increased susceptibility to secondary infection. In experiments with *P. multocida*, if pigs were vaccinated before challenge with *M. hyopneumoniae* or if the pigs were allowed to recover from *M. hyopneumoniae* challenge, they were not susceptible to subsequent *P. multocida* challenge (5).

In addition to predisposing to *P. multocida* infection, *M. hyopneumoniae* had a synergistic effect with *A. pleuropneumoniae,* and lesions in coinfected pigs were more severe than with either agent given alone or what would be additive of individual infections (124). Alveolar macrophages collected from pigs infected with either *M. hyopneumoniae* or *A. pleuropneumoniae* had increased phagocytosis, whereas alveolar macrophages collected from pigs coinfected with both *M. hyopneumoniae* and *A. pleuropneumoniae* had decreased phagocytic abilities (22). Combined challenges of pigs with *P. multocida* and the cytotoxins of *A. pleuropneumoniae* caused more severe lung lesions than did inoculation of either factor alone (26). The cytotoxins of *A. pleuropneumoniae* are cytotoxic for alveolar macrophages and epithelial and endothelial cells; thus, destruction of normal architecture, decreased clearance due to mechanical damage, and decreased phagocytosis all may contribute to secondary infection with *P. multocida.*

B. BRONCHISEPTICA

B. bronchiseptica is another primary pathogen of pigs which by itself may only cause mild disease, but its interaction with other bacteria, especially toxigenic *P. multocida,* has been well documented. Discussion of the interactions of *B. bronchiseptica* and toxigenic *P. multocida* in atrophic rhinitis of pigs is the subject of chapter 10. Experiments we have conducted to examine the interactions of *B. bronchiseptica* with *P. multocida* on pulmonary lesions showed that *B. bronchiseptica* predisposes the upper respiratory tract but not the lungs to colonization with nontoxigenic type A, *P. multocida,* the most common type isolated from pneumonic lesions of pigs (12). Prior inoculation with both *B. bronchiseptica* and PRRSV resulted in enhanced colonization of the nasal cavity and tonsils with *P. multocida* and in recovery of *P. multocida* from the lungs (12). This is an example where neither primary pathogen by itself resulted in predisposition to an opportunistic infection but the combination of primary pathogens did, which may more realistically mimic the complex infections seen in the field.

B. bronchiseptica has also been shown to predispose to disease with *S. suis.* Preinoculation of pigs with *B. bronchiseptica* before *S. suis* resulted in increased clinical signs and fever, increased isolation of *S. suis,* increased pneumonia and disseminated lesions due to *S. suis,* and increased mortality (119, 120). We are now examining whether *B. bronchiseptica* predisposes to colonization and disease with *H. parasuis* and have found that *B. bronchiseptica* increases colonization of the nasal cavity with *H. parasuis* (Brockmeier and Palmer, *82nd Conf. Res. Work Anim. Dis.*)

Possible mechanisms by which *B. bronchiseptica* predisposes to infection with other bacteria include use of adhesins secreted by *B. bronchiseptica,* toxin-induced turbinate atrophy, damage to ciliated epithelium, and other innate defense mechanisms. *B. pertussis,* a close relative of *B. bronchiseptica,* has been shown to enhance adhesion of secondary bacteria. *Streptococcus pneumoniae* and *Haemophilus influenzae* acquired the ability to adhere to cilia which were pretreated with filamentous hemagglutinin or pertussis toxin, two proteins which are secreted by *B. pertussis* and known to mediate adherence to the cilia of respiratory epithelium (107). *B. bronchiseptica* does not produce pertussis toxin but does produce filamentous hemagglutinin; thus, this could be a method by which *B. bronchiseptica* increases adhesion of other bacteria in pigs. Pretreatment with *B. bronchiseptica* has been shown to increase adhesion of *P. multocida* to tracheal explants, but the specific mechanism for this has not been explored (33).

As with *M. hyopneumoniae, B. bronchiseptica* is known to cause attenuation of the epithelium and loss of cilia, probably because of the tracheal cytotoxin which is produced by this bacterium. The dermonecrotic toxin of *B. bronchiseptica* causes turbinate atrophy and pneumonic lesions characterized by necrosis, hemorrhage, neutrophil accumulation, and eventually fibrosis. Thus, retarded clearance mechanisms, increased accumulation of mucus, exposure of submucosal areas to which other bacteria may adhere, and increased nutrient availability could all play a role in generally increased colonization by other bacteria. *B. bronchiseptica* is also cytotoxic for alveolar macrophages in vitro which may result in decreased phagocytosis and clearance of bacteria which make it down to the lung. Therefore, there are many possible mechanisms by which *B. bronchiseptica* predisposes to infection with other bacteria.

METHODS OF TREATMENT

Treatment of PRDC varies with each individual production unit and system. Depending on the pathogens present, the age at which respiratory disease becomes a problem, and the severity of disease, the treatment to be used in each production system varies accordingly. There is a fundamental difference when discussing treatment options on a herd basis versus the individual person or pet animal which presents with a clinical problem. There is less emphasis on individual diagnostics and treatment, which may be expensive and labor-intensive, and more emphasis on herd diagnostics and preventative measures. Methods of treatment or prevention of respiratory disease in swine herds fall into the categories of management changes, vaccination, and antibiotic usage.

As can be seen from the previous discussion, there is great overlap in clinical signs and pathologic lesions in PRDC; therefore, diagnosis of the pathogens involved is imperative to develop a successful treatment approach. Identification of pathogens may be done by culture, immunohistochemical methods on collected tissue samples, PCR techniques, and serology. One must bear in mind that serology only implies that the animal was exposed at some time in the past or has maternally derived immunity; thus, paired samples showing a rise in titer are often recommended. Serology can be of benefit to gather information on what pathogens are circulating in a herd and the approximate times during production that the pigs are seroconverting. Another consideration is the choice of animals to examine. When practicing herd health, it is recommended to examine not only animals with end-stage disease but animals at different stages of production to get a clearer picture of the mixed disease process. Pathogens which initiate pneumonia may be difficult to find when the clinical signs with secondary pathogens are noticed.

Once the problem has been diagnosed, treatment and preventative options need to be discussed and implemented. Judicious and timely use of the appropriate antibiotics and vaccination protocols are typically used to control the respiratory disease within a system. Acute outbreaks may require antibiotic therapy to control. Treatment on an individual basis may be attempted if only a few animals or pens are affected; however, more often than not, therapy by addition of medication to feed or water is attempted when a whole facility is affected. Many studies have reported the efficacy of different antibiotics against selected microbial pathogens. Ultimately, the choice should be made based on several factors, such as approved label usage, antimicrobial susceptibility patterns, withdrawal times, cost, route of delivery, and whether the antibiotic can reach appropriate levels at the site of infection. Controversy has surrounded the use of antimicrobials on a herdwide basis, not so much for their use in treating outbreaks, as for their use with practices such as early weaning to decrease the transmission and carrier state of pigs as they are weaned. The outcome of the current debates as to whether this promotes antimicrobial resistance may influence future use of antibiotics in the agriculture industry.

Vaccination is another method by which to control disease in the herd. Once again, good diagnostics are needed to target the pathogens which are causing the most problems. The cost of vaccination and labor involved in administration must be weighed against the cost of decreased weight gains, increased days to market, and increased mortality. Vaccine choice can be critical, and there is a great deal of variation in the effectiveness of vaccination depending on the pathogens involved, cross-protection when multiple strains or serotypes exist, type of vaccine used (killed, attenuated, autogenous, subunit, or toxoid), and route of administration. Timing can also be critical and should be such that immunity is present at the time of expected exposure. Vaccination of the dam may provide maternal immunity to the preweaned or early-nursery pig, but vaccination or natural infection of the dam can also block an active immune response when trying to vaccinate the young pig. Vaccines may work very well in preventing clinical signs with certain pathogens, but rarely prevent colonization and thus may not completely block the ability of pathogens to contribute to secondary disease.

In addition to vaccination and antibiotic therapies, management changes to minimize disease are required. Without altering the management practices, the success of other therapeutic strategies fail. Identification of potential environmental or management problems may by themselves control the transmission or susceptibility to disease. Problems with overcrowding, ventilation, or temperature control need to be addressed because they cause stress or mechanical damage to the respiratory tract. Filling barns with pigs from a single source helps eliminate the introduction of new pathogens that often occurs when pigs from different sources are mixed. Optimally, herd management practices should be implemented that decrease the transmission of pathogens. Practices such as multisite production (separating pigs by stage of production), all-in/all-out production (moving pigs in and out of a building as a group with disinfection between groups), isolation, and acclimatization of new breeding stock (isolation to avoid bringing new diseases in and acclimatization to expose animals to agents already on the farm), segregated early weaning with or without the addition of medication to the feed (weaning at an early age, with or without antibiotics, to prevent transfer of agents from dam to offspring), and basics in biosecurity have helped control infectious disease outbreaks and led to the establishment of higher health herds. With all these management practices one must remember that the herd that is relatively free from pathogens may also be very vulnerable to the introduction of these diseases because of a general decrease in the immune status of the herd.

SUMMARY AND CONCLUSION

PRDC is a multifactorial complex of swine respiratory pathogens. It is considered one of the primary problems to the swine industry worldwide. However, the pathogens involved vary significantly among farms and production sites, making treatment and control frustrating to veterinarians and producers.

From the discussions above it is evident that there are a vast number of interactions that occur during mixed respiratory infections in pigs. The standard paradigm of primary virus infection followed by opportunistic bacterial infection certainly occurs, but the interactions can be much more complex involving multiple viruses, bacteria, and environmental factors. Pathogens can interfere with each other, be additive in their effects, or act synergistically. Because of the complicated nature of mixed infections, studying their interactions can be a daunting task. It is difficult to reproduce disease reliably, much less design experiments that examine the interactions among these pathogens. For this reason, the pathogenesis of mixed respiratory infections in swine are still largely speculative, based on research examining one or a few mechanisms, which are difficult to prove as the definitive cause of the disease.

Colonization of the mucosa requires that pathogens adhere, avoid clearance mechanisms, acquire nutrients, replicate, and resist defenses. Thus, when pathogens are able to induce changes to, or damage, epithelial surfaces exposing or upregulating receptors, inhibiting the mucociliary clearance mechanism, releasing nutrients such as iron, and allowing systemic invasion, it is most likely used by other pathogens to their advantage. Similarly, debilitation of alveolar macrophages by viruses or bacterial toxins is undoubtedly significant, since these phagocytes are responsible for clearance of bacteria that make it down to the lung. However, more subtle or indirect interactions may be just as important in promoting mixed infections. The use of adhesins secreted by other bacteria, or effects induced through intermediaries such as cytokines which alter the inflammatory and immune responses, may also play a role. Thus, there is much more work to be done before we fully understand the nature of mixed respiratory infections.

REFERENCES

1. **Albina, E., L. Piriou, E. Hutet, R. Cariolet, and R. L'Hospitalier.** 1998. Immune responses in pigs infected with porcine reproductive and respiratory syndrome virus (PRRSV). *Vet. Immunol. Immunopathol.* **61:**49–66.
2. **Allan, G. M., S. Kennedy, F. McNeilly, J. C. Foster, J. A. Ellis, S. J. Krakowka, B. M.** Meehan, and B. M. Adair. 1999. Experimental reproduction of severe wasting disease by co-infection of pigs with porcine circovirus and porcine parvovirus. *J. Comp. Pathol.* **121:**1–11.
3. **Allan, G. M., F. McNeilly, J. P. Cassidy, G. A. Reilly, B. Adair, W. A. Ellis, and M. S. McNulty.** 1995. Pathogenesis of porcine circovirus: experimental infections of colostrum deprived piglets and examination of pig foetal material. *Vet. Microbiol.* **44:**49–64.
4. **Allan, G. M., F. McNeilly, S. Kennedy, B. Meehan, J. Ellis, and S. Krakowka.** 2000. Immunostimulation, PCV-2 and PMWS. *Vet. Rec.* **147:**170–171.
5. **Amass, S. F., L. K. Clark, W. G. van Alstine, T. L. Bowersock, D. A. Murphy, K. E. Knox, and S. R. Albregts.** 1994. Interaction of *Mycoplasma hyopneumoniae* and *Pasteurella multocida* infections in swine. *J. Am. Vet. Med. Assoc.* **204:**102–107.
6. **Asai, T., M. Okada, M. Ono, T. Irisawa, Y. Mori, Y. Yokomizo, and S. Sato.** 1993. Increased levels of tumor necrosis factor and interleukin 1 in bronchoalveolar lavage fluids from pigs infected with *Mycoplasma hyopneumoniae*. *Vet. Immunol. Immunopathol.* **38:**253–260.
7. **Asai, T., M. Okada, M. Ono, Y. Mori, Y. Yokomizo, and S. Sato.** 1994. Detection of interleukin-6 and prostaglandin E2 in bronchoalveolar lavage fluids of pigs experimentally infected with *Mycoplasma hyponeumoniae*. *Vet. Immunol. Immunopathol.* **44:**97–102.
8. **Balasch, M., J. Segales, C. Rosell, M. Domingo, A. Mankertz, A. Urniza, and J. Plana-Duran.** 1999. Experimental inoculation of conventional pigs with tissue homogenates from pigs with post-weaning multisystemic wasting syndrome. *J. Comp. Pathol.* **121:**139–148.
9. **Benfield, D. A., J. Christopher-Hennings, E. A. Nelson, R. R. R. Rowland, J. K. Nelson, C. C. L. Chase, K. D. Rossow, and J. E. Collins.** 1997. Persistent fetal infection of porcine reproductive and respiratory syndrome (PRRS) virus. *Proc. Am. Assoc. Swine Pract.*, p. 455–458.
10. **Bertram, T. A.** 1990. *Actinobacillus pleuropneumoniae:* molecular aspects of virulence and pulmonary injury. *Can. J. Vet. Res.* **54:**S53–S56.
11. **Brockmeier, S. L., M. V. Palmer, and S. R. Bolin.** 2000. Effects of intranasal inoculation of porcine reproductive and respiratory syndrome virus, *Bordetella bronchiseptica,* or a combination of both organisms in pigs. *Am. J. Vet. Res.* **61:**892–899.
12. **Brockmeier, S. L., M. V. Palmer, S. R. Bolin, and R. B. Rimler.** 2001. Effects of intranasal inoculation with *Bordetella bronchiseptica,*

porcine reproductive and respiratory syndrome virus, or a combination of both organisms on subsequent infection with *Pasteurella multocida* in pigs. *Am. J. Vet. Res.* **62**:521–525.

13. **Brockmeier, S. L., and K. B. Register.** 2000. Effect of temperature modulation and bvg mutation of *Bordetella bronchiseptica* on adhesion, intracellular survival and cytotoxicity for swine alveolar macrophages. *Vet. Microbiol.* **73**:1–12.

14. **Brockmeier, S. L., K. B. Register, T. Magyar, A. J. Lax, G. D. Pullinger, and R. A. Kunkle.** 2002. Role of the dermonecrotic toxin of *Bordetella bronchiseptica* in the pathogenesis of respiratory disease in swine. *Infect. Immun.* **70**:481–490.

15. **Brown, G. B.** 1999. Streptococcus suis *Intranasal Challenge Model and Identification of a Potential Antiphagocytic Virulence Factor in* S. suis *Supernatant.* Ph.D. thesis. Iowa State University, Ames.

16. **Brown, I. H., D. J. Alexander, P. Chakraverty, P. A. Harris, and R. J. Manvell.** 1994. Isolation of an influenza A virus of unusual subtype (H1N7) from pigs in England, and the subsequent experimental transmission from pig to pig. *Vet. Microbiol.* **39**:125–134.

17. **Brown, I. H., P. Chakraverty, P. A. Harris, and D. J. Alexander.** 1995. Disease outbreaks in pigs in Great Britain due to an influenza A virus of H1N2 subtype. *Vet. Rec.* **136**:328–329.

18. **Brown, I. H., S. H. Done, Y. I. Spencer, W. A. Cooley, P. A. Harris, and D. J. Alexander.** 1993. Pathogenicity of a swine influenza H1N1 virus antigenically distinguishable from classical and European strains. *Vet. Rec.* **132**:598–602.

19. **Brown, I. H., S. Ludwig, C. W. Olsen, C. Hannoun, C. Scholtissek, V. S. Hinshaw, P. A. Harris, J. W. McCauley, I. Strong, and D. J. Alexander.** 1997. Antigenic and genetic analyses of H1N1 influenza A viruses from European pigs. *J. Gen. Virol.* **78**:553–562.

20. **Brown, I. H., R. J. Manvell, D. J. Alexander, P. Chakraverty, V. S. Hinshaw, and R. G. Webster.** 1993. Swine influenza outbreaks in England due to a new H1N1 virus. *Vet. Rec.* **132**:461–462.

21. **Callan, R. J., F. A. Hartmann, S. E. West, and V. S. Hinshaw.** 1997. Cleavage of influenza A virus H1 hemagglutinin by swine respiratory bacterial proteases. *J. Virol.* **71**:7579–7585.

22. **Caruso, J. P., and R. F. Ross.** 1990. Effects of *Mycoplasma hyopneumoniae* and *Actinobacillus* (*Haemophilus*) *pleuropneumoniae* infections on alveolar macrophage functions in swine. *Am. J. Vet. Res.* **51**:227–231.

23. **Carvalho, L. F., J. Segales, and C. Pijoan.** 1997. Effect of porcine reproductive and respiratory syndrome virus on subsequent *Pasteurella multocida* challenge in pigs. *Vet. Microbiol.* **55**:241–246.

24. **Castrucci, M. R., I. Donatelli, L. Sidoli, G. Barigazzi, Y. Kawaoka, and R. G. Webster.** 1993. Genetic reassortment between avian and human influenza A viruses in Italian pigs. *Virology* **193**:503–506.

25. **Cheung, A. K.** 1995. Investigation of pseudorabies virus DNA and RNA in trigeminal ganglia and tonsil tissues of latently infected swine. *Am. J. Vet. Res.* **56**:45–50.

26. **Chung, W. B., L. R. Backstrom, and M. T. Collins.** 1994. Experimental model of swine pneumonic pasteurellosis using crude *Actinobacillus pleuropneumoniae* cytotoxin and *Pasteurella multocida* given endobronchially. *Can. J. Vet. Res.* **58**:25–30.

27. **Ciprian, A., C. Pijoan, T. Cruz, J. Camacho, J. Tortora, G. Colmenares, R. Lopez-Revilla, and M. de la Garza.** 1988. *Mycoplasma hyopneumoniae* increases the susceptibility of pigs to experimental *Pasteurella multocida* pneumonia. *Can. J. Vet. Res.* **52**:434–438.

28. **Cooper, V. L., A. R. Doster, R. A. Hesse, and N. B. Harris.** 1995. Porcine reproductive and respiratory syndrome: NEB-1 PRRSV infection did not potentiate bacterial pathogens. *J. Vet. Diagn. Investig.* **7**:313–320.

29. **Cowart, R. P., L. Backstrom, and T. A. Brim.** 1989. *Pasteurella multocida* and *Bordetella bronchiseptica* in atrophic rhinitis and pneumonia in swine. *Can. J. Vet. Res.* **53**:295–300.

30. **De Bruin, M. G., J. N. Samsom, J. J. Voermans, E. M. van Rooij, Y. E. De Visser, and A. T. Bianchi.** 2000. Effects of a porcine reproductive and respiratory syndrome virus infection on the development of the immune response against pseudorabies virus. *Vet. Immunol. Immunopathol.* **76**:125–135.

31. **DeBey, M. C., and R. F. Ross.** 1994. Ciliostasis and loss of cilia induced by *Mycoplasma hyopneumoniae* in porcine tracheal organ cultures. *Infect. Immun.* **62**:5312–5318.

32. **Duan, X., H. J. Nauwynck, and M. B. Pensaert.** 1997. Virus quantification and identification of cellular targets in the lungs and lymphoid tissues of pigs at different time intervals after inoculation with porcine reproductive and respiratory syndrome virus (PRRSV). *Vet. Microbiol.* **56**:9–19.

33. **Dugal, F., M. Belanger, and M. Jacques.** 1992. Enhanced adherence of *Pasteurella multocida* to porcine tracheal rings preinfected with *Bordetella bronchiseptica*. *Can. J. Vet. Res.* **56**:260–264.

34. **Duncan, J. R., F. K. Ramsey, and W. P. Switzer.** 1966. Pathology of experimental *Bor-*

detella bronchiseptica infection in swine: pneumonia. *Am. J. Vet. Res.* **27**:467–472.

35. Duncan, J. R., R. F. Ross, W. P. Switzer, and F. K. Ramsey. 1966. Pathology of experimental *Bordetella bronchiseptica* infection in swine: atrophic rhinitis. *Am. J. Vet. Res.* **27**:457–466.

36. Ellis, J., L. Hassard, E. Clark, J. Harding, G. Allan, P. Willson, J. Strokappe, K. Martin, F. McNeilly, B. Meehan, D. Todd, and D. Haines. 1998. Isolation of circovirus from lesions of pigs with postweaning multisystemic wasting syndrome. *Can. Vet. J.* **39**:44–51.

37. Ellis, J., S. Krakowka, M. Lairmore, D. Haines, A. Bratanich, E. Clark, G. Allan, C. Konoby, L. Hassard, B. Meehan, K. Martin, J. Harding, S. Kennedy, and F. McNeilly. 1999. Reproduction of lesions of postweaning multisystemic wasting syndrome in gnotobiotic piglets. *J. Vet. Diagn. Investig.* **11**:3–14.

38. Fenwick, B. W. 1990. Virulence attributes of the liposaccharides of the HAP group organisms. *Can. J. Vet. Res.* **54**:S28–S32.

39. Frey, J., J. T. Bosse, Y. F. Chang, J. M. Cullen, B. Fenwick, G. F. Gerlach, D. Gygi, F. Haesebrouck, T. J. Inzana, R. Jansen, E. M. Kamp, J. Macdonald, J. I. Macinnes, K. R. Mittal, J. Nicolet, A. N. Rycroft, R. P. A. M. Segers, M. A. Smits, E. Stenbaek, D. K. Stuck, J. F. Van Den Bosch, P. J. Wilson, and R. Young. 1993. *Actinobacillus pleuropneumoniae* RTX toxins: uniform designation of haemolysins, cytolysins, pleurotoxin and their genes. *J. Gen. Microbiol.* **139**:1723–1728.

40. Fuentes, M., and C. Pijoan. 1986. Phagocytosis and intracellular killing of *Pasteurella multocida* by porcine alveolar macrophages after infection with pseudorabies virus. *Vet. Immunol. Immunopathol.* **13**:165–172.

41. Fuentes, M. C., and C. Pijoan. 1987. Pneumonia in pigs induced by intranasal challenge exposure with pseudorabies virus and *Pasteurella multocida*. *Am. J. Vet. Res.* **48**:1446–1448.

42. Galina, L., C. Pijoan, M. Sitjar, W. T. Christianson, K. Rossow, and J. E. Collins. 1994. Interaction between *Streptococcus suis* serotype 2 and porcine reproductive and respiratory syndrome virus in specific pathogen-free piglets. *Vet. Rec.* **134**:60–64.

43. Griffiths, I. B., S. H. Done, and B. W. Hunt. 1991. Pneumonia in a sow due to *Streptococcus suis* type II and *Bordetella bronchiseptica*. *Vet. Rec.* **128**:354–355.

44. Guan, Y., K. F. Shortridge, S. Krauss, P. H. Li, Y. Kawaoka, and R. G. Webster. 1996. Emergence of avian H1N1 influenza viruses in pigs in China. *J. Virol.* **70**:8041–8046.

45. Halbur, P. G., P. S. Paul, M. L. Frey, J. Landgraf, K. Eernisse, X. J. Meng, J. J. Andrews, M. A. Lum, and J. A. Rathje. 1996. Comparison of the antigen distribution of two US porcine reproductive and respiratory syndrome virus isolates with that of the Lelystad virus. *Vet. Pathol.* **33**:159–170.

46. Halbur, P. G., P. S. Paul, M. L. Frey, J. Landgraf, K. Eernisse, X. J. Meng, M. A. Lum, J. J. Andrews, and J. A. Rathje. 1995. Comparison of the pathogenicity of two US porcine reproductive and respiratory syndrome virus isolates with that of the Lelystad virus. *Vet. Pathol.* **32**:648–660.

47. Halbur, P., R. Thanawongnuwech, G. Brown, J. Kinyon, J. Roth, E. Thacker, and B. Thacker. 2000. Efficacy of antimicrobial treatments and vaccination regimens for control of porcine reproductive and respiratory syndrome virus and *Streptococcus suis* coinfection of nursery pigs. *J. Clin. Microbiol.* **38**:1156–1160.

48. Hamel, A. L., L. L. Lin, and G. P. Nayar. 1998. Nucleotide sequence of porcine circovirus associated with postweaning multisystemic wasting syndrome in pigs. *J. Virol.* **72**:5262–5267.

49. Harding, J. C. S., and E. G. Clark. 1997. Recognizing and diagnosing postweaning multisystemic wasting syndrome (PMWS). *Swine Health Prod.* **5**:201–203.

50. Harms, P. A., S. D. Sorden, P. G. Halbur, S. Bolin, K. Lager, I. Morozov, and P. S. Paul. 2001. Experimental reproduction of severe disease in CD/CD pigs concurrently infected with type 2 porcine circovirus and porcine reproductive and respiratory syndrome virus. *Vet. Pathol.* **38**:528–539.

51. Heinen, P. P., A. P. van Nieuwstadt, J. M. Pol, E. A. De Boer-Luijtze, J. T. Van Oirschot, and A. T. Bianchi. 2000. Systemic and mucosal isotype-specific antibody responses to pigs to experimental influenza virus infection. *Viral Immunol.* **13**:237–247.

52. Hines, R. K., and P. D. Lukert. 1994. Porcine circovirus as a cause of congenital tremors in newborn pigs. *Proc. Am. Assoc. Swine Pract.*, p. 344–345.

53. Iglesias, G., C. Pijoan, and T. Molitor. 1989. Interactions of pseudorabies virus with swine alveolar macrophages: effects of virus infection on cell functions. *J. Leukoc. Biol.* **45**:410–415.

54. Iglesias, G., C. Pijoan, and T. Molitor. 1992. Effects of pseudorabies virus infection upon cytotoxicity and antiviral activities of porcine alveolar macrophages. *Comp. Immunol. Microbiol. Infect. Dis.* **15**:249–259.

55. Iglesias, G. J., M. Trujano, J. Lokensgard, and T. Molitor. 1992. Study of the potential in-

volvement of pseudorabies virus in swine respiratory disease. *Can. J. Vet. Res.* **56**:74–77.

56. **Iglesias, J. G., M. Trujano, and J. Xu.** 1992. Inoculation of pigs with *Streptococcus suis* type 2 alone or in combination with pseudorabies virus. *Am. J. Vet. Res.* **53**:364–367.

57. **Inzana, T. J.** 1990. Capsules and virulence in the HAP group of bacteria. *Can. J. Vet. Res.* **54:** S22–S27.

58. **Jacques, M., M. Belanger, M. S. Diarra, M. Dargis, and F. Malouin.** 1994. Modulation of *Pasteurella multocida* capsular polysaccharide during growth under iron-restricted conditions and in vivo. *Microbiology* **140**:263–270.

59. **Karasin, A. I., C. W. Olsen, and G. A. Anderson.** 2000. Genetic characterization of an H1N2 influenza virus isolated from a pig in Indiana. *J. Clin. Microbiol.* **38**:2453–2456.

60. **Kennedy, S., D. Moffett, F. McNeilly, B. Meehan, J. Ellis, S. Krakowka, and G. M. Allan.** 2000. Reproduction of lesions of postweaning multisystemic wasting syndrome by infection of conventional pigs with porcine circovirus type 2 alone or in combination with porcine parvovirus. *J. Comp. Pathol.* **122**:9–24.

61. **Kielstein, P.** 1986. On the occurrence of toxin-producing *Pasteurella multocida* strains in atrophic rhinitis and in pneumonias of swine and cattle. *J. Vet. Med. Ser. B* **33**:418–424.

62. **Kiupel, M., G. W. Stevenson, S. K. Mittal, E. G. Clark, and D. M. Haines.** 1998. Circovirus-like viral associated disease in weaned pigs in Indiana. *Vet. Pathol.* **35**:303–307.

63. **Kluge, J. P., G. W. Beran, H. T. Hill, and K. B. Platt.** 1992. Pseudorabies (Aujeszky's disease), p. 312–323. *In* A. D. Leman, B. E. Straw, W. L. Mengeling, S. D'Allaire, and D. J. Taylor (ed.), *Diseases of Swine,* 7th ed. Iowa State University Press, Ames.

64. **Krakowka, S., J. A. Ellis, B. Meehan, S. Kennedy, F. McNeilly, and G. Allan.** 2000. Viral wasting syndrome of swine: experimental reproduction of postweaning multisystemic wasting syndrome in gnotobiotic swine by coinfection with porcine circovirus 2 and porcine parvovirus. *Vet. Pathol.* **37**:254–263.

65. **Lanza, I., I. H. Brown, and D. J. Paton.** 1992. Pathogenicity of concurrent infection of pigs with porcine respiratory coronavirus and swine influenza virus. *Res. Vet. Sci.* **53**:309–314.

66. **Larsen, D. L., A. Karasin, F. Zuckermann, and C. W. Olsen.** 2000. Systemic and mucosal immune responses to H1N1 influenza virus infection in pigs. *Vet. Microbiol.* **74**:117–131.

67. **Lee, B. W., R. F. Bey, M. J. Baarsch, and M. E. Larson.** 1995. Class specific antibody re-

sponse to influenza A H1N1 infection in swine. *Vet. Microbiol.* **43**:241–250.

68. **Meehan, B. M., F. McNeilly, D. Todd, S. Kennedy, V. A. Jewhurst, J. A. Ellis, L. E. Hassard, E. G. Clark, D. M. Haines, and G. M. Allan.** 1998. Characterization of novel circovirus DNAs associated with wasting syndromes in pigs. *J. Gen. Virol.* **79**:2171–2179.

69. **Messier, S., and R. F. Ross.** 1991. Interactions of *Mycoplasma hyopneumoniae* membranes with porcine lymphocytes. *Am. J. Vet. Res.* **52**:1497–1502.

70. **Molitor, T. W., E. M. Bautista, and C. S. Choi.** 1997. Immunity to PRRSV: double-edged sword. *Vet. Microbiol.* **55**:265–276.

71. **Molitor, T. W., J. Xiao, and C. S. Choi.** 1996. PRRS virus infection of macrophages: regulation by maturation and activation state. *Proc. Am. Assoc. Swine Pract.,* p. 563–569.

72. **Morin, M., C. Girard, Y. ElAzhary, R. Fajardo, R. Drolet, and A. Lagace.** 1990. Severe proliferative and necrotising pneumonia in pigs: a newly recognized disease. *Can. Vet. J.* **31**:837–839.

73. **Morozov, I., T. Sirinarumitr, S. D. Sorden, P. G. Halbur, M. K. Morgan, K. J. Yoon, and P. S. Paul.** 1998. Detection of a novel strain of porcine circovirus in pigs with postweaning multisystemic wasting syndrome. *J. Clin. Microbiol.* **36**:2535–2541.

74. **Narita, M., K. Kawashima, S. Matsuura, A. Uchimura, and Y. Miura.** 1994. Pneumonia in pigs infected with pseudorabies virus and *Haemophilus parasuis* serovar 4. *J. Comp. Pathol.* **110:** 329–339.

75. **National Animal Health Monitoring System.** 1996. *Swine '95: Grower/Finisher. Part II. Reference of 1995 U.S. Grower/Finisher Health and Management Practices,* p. 14–16. U.S. Department of Agriculture, Fort Collins, Colo.

76. **Nicolet, J.** 1990. Overview of the virulence attributes of the HAP-group of bacteria. *Can. J. Vet. Res.* **54:**S12–S15.

77. **Olsen, C. W., M. W. McGregor, A. J. Cooley, B. Schantz, B. Hotze, and V. S. Hinshaw.** 1993. Antigenic and genetic analysis of a recently isolated H1N1 swine influenza virus. *Am. J. Vet. Res.* **54**:1630–1636.

78. **Ottis, K., L. Sidoli, P. A. Bachmann, R. G. Webster, and M. M. Kaplan.** 1982. Human influenza A viruses in pigs: isolation of a H3N2 strain antigenically related to A/England/42/72 and evidence for continuous circulation of human viruses in the pig population. *Arch. Virol.* **73:** 103–108.

79. **Paul, P. S., P. G. Halbur, and E. M. Vaughn.** 1994. Significance of porcine respira-

tory coronavirus infection. *Comp. Cont. Educ. Pract. Vet.* **16**:1223–1233.

80. **Pijoan, C., R. B. Morrison, and H. D. Hilley.** 1983. Serotyping of *Pasteurella multocida* isolated from swine lungs collected at slaughter. *J. Clin. Microbiol.* **17**:1074–1076.

81. **Pol, J. M., L. A. van Leengoed, N. Stockhofe, G. Kok, and G. Wensvoort.** 1997. Dual infections of PRRSV/influenza or PRRSV/*Actinobacillus pleuropneumoniae* in the respiratory tract. *Vet. Microbiol.* **55**:259–264.

82. **Rappouli, R.** 1994. Pathogenicity mechanisms of Bordetella, p. 319–336. *In* J. L. Dangl (ed.), *Bacterial Pathogens of Plants and Animals.* Springer-Verlag, Berlin, Germany.

83. **Rasschaert, D., M. Duarte, and H. Laude.** 1990. Porcine respiratory coronavirus differs from transmissible gastroenteritis virus by a few genomic deletions. *J. Gen. Virol.* **71**:2599–2607.

84. **Rekik, M. R., D. J. Arora, and S. Dea.** 1994. Genetic variation in swine influenza virus A isolate associated with proliferative and necrotizing pneumonia in pigs. *J. Clin. Microbiol.* **32**:515–518.

85. **Rogers, D. G., A. A. Andersen, and B. D. Hunsaker.** 1996. Lung and nasal lesions caused by a swine chlamydial isolate in gnotobiotic pigs. *J. Vet. Diagn. Investig.* **8**:45–55.

86. **Rosell, C., J. Segales, J. Plana-Duran, M. Balasch, G. M. Rodriguez-Arrioja, S. Kennedy, G. M. Allan, F. McNeilly, K. S. Latimer, and M. Domingo.** 1999. Pathological, immunohistochemical, and in-situ hybridization studies of natural cases of postweaning multisystemic wasting syndrome (PMWS) in pigs. *J. Comp. Pathol.* **120**:59–78.

87. **Rosell, C., J. Segales, J. A. Ramos-Vara, J. M. Folch, G. M. Rodriguez-Arrioja, C. O. Duran, M. Balasch, J. Plana-Duran, and M. Domingo.** 2000. Identification of porcine circovirus in tissues of pigs with porcine dermatitis and nephropathy syndrome. *Vet. Rec.* **146**:40–43.

88. **Rycroft, A. N., and J. M. Cullen.** 1990. Complement resistance in *Actinobacillus (Haemophilus) pleuropneumoniae* infection of swine. *Am. J. Vet. Res.* **51**:1449–1453.

89. **Sakano, T., I. Shibata, Y. Samegai, A. Taneda, M. Okada, T. Irisawa, and S. Sato.** 1993. Experimental pneumonia of pigs infected with Aujeszky's disease virus and *Actinobacillus pleuropneumoniae. J. Vet. Med. Sci.* **55**:575–579.

90. **Schneider, J. D., and K.-J. Yoon.** 2001. Characterization of H3N2 swine influenza viruses in Iowa swine. *Proc. Am. Assoc. Swine Vet.,* p. 23–25.

91. **Segales, J., M. Domingo, M. Balasch, G. I. Solano, and C. Pijoan.** 1998. Ultrastructural study of porcine alveolar macrophages infected in vitro with porcine reproductive and respiratory syndrome (PRRS) virus, with and without *Haemophilus parasuis. J. Comp. Pathol.* **118**:231–243.

92. **Segales, J., M. Domingo, G. I. Solano, and C. Pijoan.** 1999. Porcine reproductive and respiratory syndrome virus and *Haemophilus parasuis* antigen distribution in dually infected pigs. *Vet. Microbiol.* **64**:287–297.

93. **Segales, J., M. Sitjar, M. Domingo, S. Dee, M. Del Pozo, R. Noval, C. Sacristan, A. De las Heras, A. Ferro, and K. S. Latimer.** 1997. First report of post-weaning multisystemic wasting syndrome in pigs in Spain. *Vet. Rec.* **141**:600–601.

94. **Shibata, I., M. Okada, K. Urono, Y. Samegai, M. Ono, T. Sakano, and S. Sato.** 1998. Experimental dual infection of cesarean-derived, colostrum-deprived pigs with *Mycoplasma hyopneumoniae* and pseudorabies virus. *J. Vet. Med. Sci.* **60**:295–300.

95. **Sirinarumitr, T., Y. Zhang, J. P. Kluge, P. G. Halbur, and P. S. Paul.** 1998. A pneumovirulent United States isolate of porcine reproductive and respiratory syndrome virus induces apoptosis in bystander cells both in vitro and in vivo. *J. Gen. Virol.* **79**:2989–2995.

96. **Solano, G. I., E. Bautista, T. W. Molitor, J. Segales, and C. Pijoan.** 1998. Effect of porcine reproductive and respiratory syndrome virus infection on the clearance of *Haemophilus parasuis* by porcine alveolar macrophages. *Can. J. Vet. Res.* **62**:251–256.

97. **Solano, G. I., J. Segales, J. E. Collins, T. W. Molitor, and C. Pijoan.** 1997. Porcine reproductive and respiratory syndrome virus (PRRSv) interaction with *Haemophilus parasuis. Vet. Microbiol.* **55**:247–257.

98. **Stevenson, G. W., M. Kiupel, S. K. Mittal, J. Choi, K. S. Latimer, and C. L. Kanitz.** 2001. Tissue distribution and genetic typing of porcine circoviruses in pigs with naturally occurring congenital tremors. *J. Vet. Diagn. Investig.* **13**:57–62.

99. **Thacker, E. L., P. G. Halbur, R. F. Ross, R. Thanawongnuwech, and B. J. Thacker.** 1999. *Mycoplasma hyopneumoniae* potentiation of porcine reproductive and respiratory syndrome virus-induced pneumonia. *J. Clin. Microbiol.* **37**:620–627.

100. **Thacker, E. L., B. J. Thacker, and B. H. Janke.** 2001. Interaction between *Mycoplasma hyopneumoniae* and swine influenza virus. *J. Clin. Microbiol.* **39**:2525–2530.

101. **Thacker, E. L., B. J. Thacker, M. Kuhn, P. A. Hawkins, and W. R. Waters.** 2000. Evaluation of local and systemic immune responses

induced by intramuscular injection of a *Mycoplasma hyopneumoniae* bacterin to pigs. *Am. J. Vet. Res.* **61**:1384–1389.

102. **Thanawongnuwech, R., G. B. Brown, P. G. Halbur, J. A. Roth, R. L. Royer, and B. J. Thacker.** 2000. Pathogenesis of porcine reproductive and respiratory syndrome virus-induced increase in susceptibility to *Streptococcus suis* infection. *Vet. Pathol.* **37**:143–152.

103. **Thanawongnuwech, R., P. G. Halbur, M. R. Ackermann, E. L. Thacker, and R. L. Royer.** 1998. Effects of low (modified-live virus vaccine) and high (VR-2385)-virulence strains of porcine reproductive and respiratory syndrome virus on pulmonary clearance of copper particles in pigs. *Vet. Pathol.* **35**:398–406.

104. **Thanawongnuwech, R., E. L. Thacker, and P. G. Halbur.** 1997. Effect of porcine reproductive and respiratory syndrome virus (PRRSV) (isolate ATCC VR-2385) infection on bactericidal activity of porcine pulmonary intravascular macrophages (PIMs): in vitro comparisons with pulmonary alveolar macrophages (PAMs). *Vet. Immunol. Immunopathol.* **59**:323–335.

105. **Thanawongnuwech, R., T. F. Young, B. J. Thacker, and E. L. Thacker.** 2001. Differential production of proinflammatory cytokines: in vitro PRRSV and *Mycoplasma hyopneumoniae* coinfection model. *Vet. Immunol. Immunopathol.* **79**:115–127.

106. **Tischer, I., H. Gelderblom, W. Vettermann, and M. A. Koch.** 1982. A very small porcine virus with circular single stranded DNA. *Nature* **295**:64–66.

107. **Tuomanen, E.** 1986. Piracy of adhesins: attachment of superinfecting pathogens to respiratory cilia by secreted adhesins of *Bordetella pertussis*. *Infect. Immun.* **54**:905–908.

108. **Vahle, J. L., J. S. Haynes, and J. J. Andrews.** 1995. Experimental reproduction of *Haemophilus parasuis* infection in swine: clinical, bacteriological, and morphologic findings. *J. Vet. Diagn. Investig.* **7**:476–80.

109. **Vahle, J. L., J. S. Haynes, and J. J. Andrews.** 1997. Interaction of *Haemophilus parasuis* with nasal and tracheal mucosa following intranasal inoculation of cesarean derived colostrum deprived (CDCD) swine. *Can. J. Vet. Res.* **61**:200–206.

110. **Van Alstine, W. G., G. W. Stevenson, and C. L. Kanitz.** 1996. Porcine reproductive and respiratory syndrome virus does not exacerbate *Mycoplasma hyopneumoniae* infection in young pigs. *Vet. Microbiol.* **49**:297–303.

111. **van Diemen, P. M., M. F. de Jong, G. de Vries Reilingh, P. van der Hel, and J. W.**

Schrama. 1994. Intranasal administration of *Pasteurella multocida* toxin in a challenge-exposure model used to induce subclinical signs of atrophic rhinitis in pigs. *Am. J. Vet. Res.* **55**:49–54.

112. **Van Reeth, K., G. Labarque, H. Nauwynck, and M. Pensaert.** 1999. Differential production of proinflammatory cytokines in the pig lung during different respiratory virus infections: correlations with pathogenicity. *Res. Vet. Sci.* **67**:47–52.

113. **Van Reeth, K., and H. Nauwynck.** 2000. Proinflammatory cytokines and viral respiratory disease in pigs. *Vet. Res.* **31**:187–213.

114. **Van Reeth, K., H. Nauwynck, and M. Pensaert.** 1996. Dual infections of feeder pigs with porcine reproductive and respiratory syndrome virus followed by porcine respiratory coronavirus or swine influenza virus: a clinical and virological study. *Vet. Microbiol.* **48**:325–335.

115. **Van Reeth, K., H. Nauwynck, and M. Pensaert.** 1998. Bronchoalveolar interferon-alpha, tumor necrosis factor-alpha, interleukin-1, and inflammation during acute influenza in pigs: a possible model for humans? *J. Infect. Dis.* **177**:1076–1079.

116. **Van Reeth, K., H. Nauwynck, and M. Pensaert.** 2000. A potential role for tumour necrosis factor-alpha in synergy between porcine respiratory coronavirus and bacterial lipopolysaccharide in the induction of respiratory disease in pigs. *J. Med. Microbiol.* **49**:613–620.

117. **Van Reeth, K., and M. Pensaert.** 1994. Prevalence of infections with enzootic respiratory and enteric viruses in feeder pigs entering fattening herds. *Vet. Rec.* **135**:594–597.

118. **Van Reeth, K., and M. B. Pensaert.** 1994. Porcine respiratory coronavirus-mediated interference against influenza virus replication in the respiratory tract of feeder pigs. *Am. J. Vet. Res.* **55**:1275–1281.

119. **Vecht, U., J. P. Arends, E. J. van der Molen, and L. A. van Leengoed.** 1989. Differences in virulence between two strains of *Streptococcus suis* type II after experimentally induced infection of newborn germ-free pigs. *Am. J. Vet. Res.* **50**:1037–1043.

120. **Vecht, U., H. J. Wisselink, J. E. van Dijk, and H. E. Smith.** 1992. Virulence of *Streptococcus suis* type 2 strains in newborn germfree pigs depends on phenotype. *Infect. Immun.* **60**:550–556.

121. **Wesley, R. D., W. L. Mengeling, and K. M. Lager.** 1998. Prior infection of nursery-age pigs with porcine reproductive and respiratory syndrome virus does not affect the outcome of

transmissible gastroenteritis virus challenge. *J. Vet. Diagn. Investig.* **10**:221–228.

122. **Wills, R. W., J. T. Gray, P. J. Fedorka-Cray, K. J. Yoon, S. Ladely, and J. J. Zimmerman.** 2000. Synergism between porcine reproductive and respiratory syndrome virus (PRRSV) and *Salmonella choleraesuis* in swine. *Vet. Microbiol.* **71**:177–192.

123. **Wills, R. W., J. J. Zimmerman, K.-J. Yoon, S. L. Swenson, M. J. McGinley, H. T. Hill, K. B. Platt, J. Christopher-Hennings, and E. A. Nelson.** 1997. Porcine reproductive and respiratory syndrome virus: a persistent infection. *Vet. Microbiol.* **55**:231–240.

124. **Yagihashi, T., T. Nunoya, T. Mitui, and M. Tajima.** 1984. Effect of *Mycoplasma hyopneumoniae* infection on the development of *Haemophilus pleuropneumoniae* pneumonia in pigs. *Nippon Juigaku Zasshi* **46**:705–713.

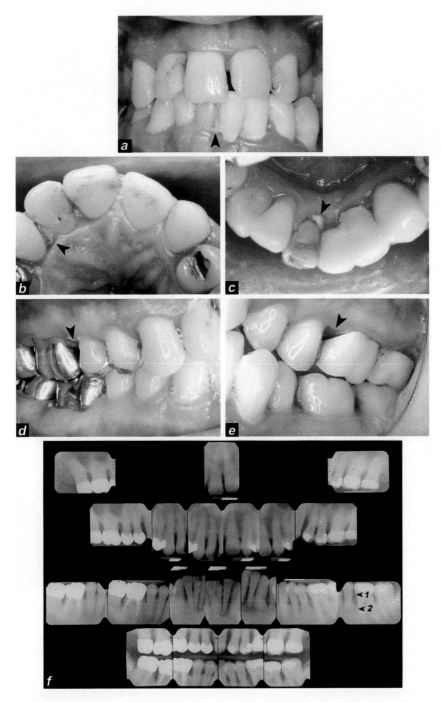

COLOR PLATE 1 (CHAPTER 8) Clinical and radiographic appearance of a 57-year-old patient with generalized advanced chronic periodontitis. (a) Bacterial plaque accumulation; (b) swelling and inflammation of gingival tissue; (c) mineralized plaque (calculus); (d and e) loss of interdental tissue due to bone loss; (f) generalized bone loss ranging from 15 to 100%. 1, expected location of alveolar bone height in health; 2, actual alveolar bone height demonstrating ~60% bone loss.

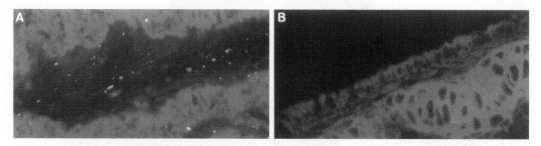

COLOR PLATE 2 (CHAPTER 14) Fluorescence photomicrograph composite of NTHI 1128 adhering to mucus present in the ET lumen before treatment with the mucolytic agent *N*-acetyl-L-cysteine (A) and the absence of fluorescent bacteria after treatment with *N*-acetyl-L-cysteine (B). Total magnification, ×162. (Reprinted from *Microbial Pathogenesis* [144] with permission of the publisher.)

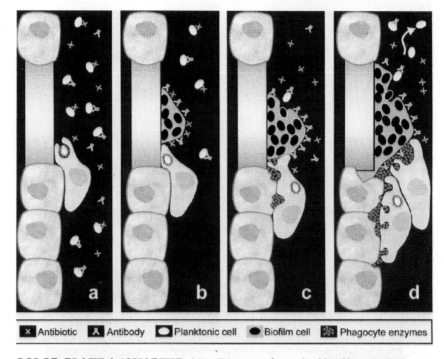

COLOR PLATE 3 (CHAPTER 14) Diagram of a medical biofilm. (a) Planktonic bacteria can be cleared by antibodies and phagocytes and are susceptible to antibiotics. (b) Adherent bacterial cells form biofilms preferentially on inert surfaces, and these sessile communities are resistant to antibodies, phagocytes, and antibiotics. (c) Phagocytes are attracted to the biofilms. Phagocytosis is frustrated, but phagocytic enzymes are released. (d) Phagocytic enzymes damage tissue around the biofilm, and planktonic bacteria are released from the biofilm. Release may cause dissemination and acute infection in neighboring tissue. (Reprinted from *Science* [49] with permission of the publisher. Copyright 1999, American Association for the Advancement of Science.)

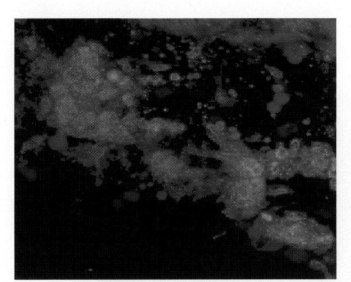

COLOR PLATE 4 (CHAPTER 14)
Confocal scanning laser micrograph of chinchilla middle ear mucosa after trans-bullar inoculation with *H. influenzae*. Starting on day 3, the animals were treated with antibiotics, at which point effusions in the middle ear were rendered culturally sterile. Unfixed specimens were obtained under general anesthesia, placed in buffer, and sent via overnight courier from the Center for Genomic Sciences (Allegheny Singer Research Institute, Pittsburgh, Pa.) to the Center for Biofilm Engineering (Montana State University, Bozeman, Mont.) for imaging. Specimens were stained with a Live/Dead BacLight bacterial viability kit (Molecular Probes, Eugene, Oreg.), which uses two dyes, SYTO 9 (green) and propidium iodide (red). Green indicates uncompromised bacterial cell membranes (live cells), while red indicates dead bacterial cells and is also taken up by the host cell nuclei. A mature biofilm with characteristic tower structure is shown.

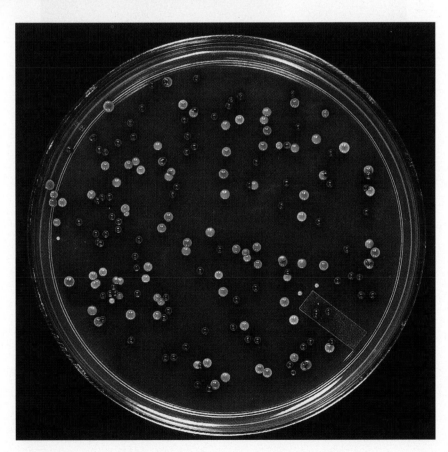

COLOR PLATE 5 (CHAPTER 17)   A mixed culture of *C. albicans* (green colonies), *C. tropicalis* (blue colonies), and *C. glabrata* (pink colonies) on CHROMagar.

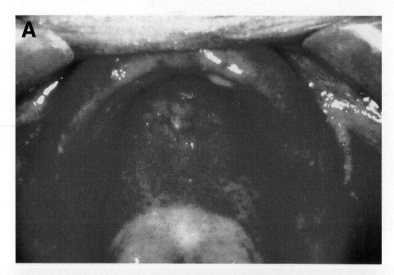

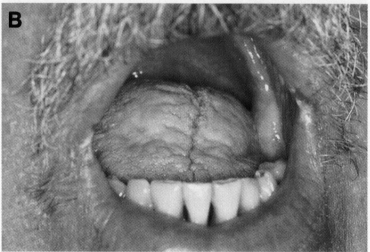

COLOR PLATE 6 (CHAPTER 18) Clinical presentation of oral candidiasis involving mixed infections of *Candida* and bacteria. (A) Denture-induced stomatitis, showing erythema of the mucosa that has been occluded by an upper denture. (B) Angular cheilitis, showing cracking and erythema at the commissure associated with leakage of *Candida*-infected saliva at the angles of the mouth. Photographs kindly provided by J. Luker.

OTITIS MEDIA

Lauren O. Bakaletz

14

It has long been recognized that secondary bacterial infections are a primary complication of viral respiratory tract infection (106). In all areas of the world, upper respiratory tract (URT) infections and their complicating sequelae are the leading causes of acute infectious morbidity (138). Moreover, these situations of mixed microbial superinfection often result in increased morbidity or mortality over that caused by the primary viral or bacterial infection and are founded on synergistic processes in which specific diseases exist only if several microbes are present (133). Prior to having an understanding of the exact mechanisms that contribute to such microbial synergy, evidence of the etiology of viral-bacterial superinfections could be discerned from close examination of epidemiological data. These data often depict regular, and sometimes seasonal, patterns of peak periods of viral isolation (or detection of viral infection diagnostically) preceding those of bacterial disease. Otitis media (OM), or inflammation of the middle ear, is one of these complicating sequelae of URT infections and is indeed a major health care concern of childhood.

OM, both acute and chronic, is highly prevalent worldwide (34, 105, 189). The most recently available statistics indicate that 24.5 million physician's office visits were made for OM in the United States alone in 1990, representing a >200% increase over those reported in the 1980s (23, 153). OM is the most frequently diagnosed illness in children younger than 15 years of age and is the primary cause for emergency room visits (34). It is estimated that 83% of all children will experience at least one episode of acute OM (AOM) by 3 years of age and that more than 40% of children will experience three or more episodes of AOM by this age (195). Although only very rarely associated with mortality any longer, the morbidity associated with OM is significant. Hearing loss is the most common complication of OM (19, 104) with behavioral, educational, and language development delays being additional consequences of early-onset OM with effusion (OME) (105, 194). The socioeconomic impact of OM is also great; direct and indirect costs of diagnosing and managing OM exceed $5 billion annually in the United States alone (3, 33, 114, 189). To date, use of antibiotics, both therapeutic and prophylactic, has been largely relied upon for medical management of the spectrum of clinical entities known collectively as OM (189). Widespread use of antimicrobials

Lauren O. Bakaletz, Division of Molecular Medicine, College of Medicine and Public Health, The Ohio State University, and Children's Research Institute, Columbus, OH 43205.

Polymicrobial Diseases, Edited by Kim A. Brogden and Janet M. Guthmiller,
© 2002 ASM Press, Washington, D.C.

for OM has met with controversy, however (189, 214), and the emergence of multiple-antibiotic resistant microorganisms is a sobering consequence of this well-established practice (46, 84, 139, 146). Surgical management of OM involves the insertion of tympanostomy tubes through the tympanic membrane (or eardrum) while a child is anesthetized. Although this procedure is commonplace (prevalence rates are ~13 per 1,000 children younger than 18 years of age) (24) and is highly effective in terms of relieving painful symptoms by draining the middle ear of accumulated fluids, it too has met with criticism because of the invasive nature of the procedure and the incumbent risks of putting a child under general anesthesia (21, 24, 153, 189).

Many environmental, anatomical, and other factors contribute to both the prevalence of middle ear infections in children and the chronicity or recurrent nature of OM. These factors include the immaturity of the pediatric immune system, existence of other ongoing infections, the anatomic positioning of the Eustachian tube in childhood, genetic predisposition, methods of feeding, smoking in the household, existence of allergies, and attendance at day care, among others (23, 32, 70). In addition, while children do mount an immune response both systemically as well as locally to the organism(s) present in their middle ears, due to the vast heterogeneity of the microorganisms that cause OM, this immune response does not confer protection against subsequent bouts of OM.

Whereas the multifactorial nature of middle ear infections is well acknowledged, it has only recently become fully appreciated that OM, both acute and chronic, is also a truly polymicrobial infection involving any of several URT viruses and one or more of three primary bacterial pathogens of the middle ear. This delayed understanding was partly due to difficulty in obtaining sequential samples from the middle ear for assay by culture and the fact that many middle ear fluids (or effusions) that were retrieved, in particular, from cases of chronic OM, were culture negative. Nevertheless, by

the late 1960s there were a few reports that several laboratories were beginning to isolate viruses from the middle ear (parainfluenza virus type 2, respiratory syncytial virus [RSV], adenovirus [AV], rhinovirus, and coxsackievirus B4) either alone or in association with bacteria. In 1971, Gwaltney (85) hypothesized that OM etiology could be purely viral, purely bacterial, or the result of a mixed viral-bacterial infection. However, not enough evidence existed at the time to accurately state which constituted the primary infection of the middle ear or if there was indeed a single primary etiologic agent, nor was it easily determined how often each etiologic possibility occurred.

INFECTION AND ETIOLOGIC AGENTS

Since then, an enormous amount of data has been amassed to indicate that, while one can indeed have a purely virus-induced inflammation of the middle ear or viral OM (118, 180), mixed bacterial and combined viral-bacterial infections of the tympanum are exceedingly common (36, 76, 107). With improved specimen collection and culture methodologies, even prior to the advent of powerful molecular detection methods, bacteria were cultured from 40 to 60% of middle ear fluids (MEFs) (76); virus alone could be isolated in approximately 6% of these fluids, and viruses plus bacteria could be cultured from approximately 17% of fluids recovered from the middle ear (5, 175). Moreover, at the time of OM diagnosis, more than 90% of patients were known to have signs of an URT infection, most likely viral in origin because 40 to 50% of these patients also had detectable virus in their nasopharynx (NP) (5).

A longitudinal study conducted by Henderson et al. (98) to determine the relative importance of viral respiratory tract infections or nasopharygeal colonization by *Streptococcus pneumoniae* or *Haemophilus influenzae* as factors influencing the occurrence of AOM with effusion (AOME) found a stronger association between infection with any of several viruses (RSV, influenza A or B virus, or AV) and

AOME (average relative risk, 3.2) than between NP colonization with either of the two cited bacterial species and AOME (average relative risk, 1.5). Infection with RSV, influenza A or B virus, and AV also correlated with an increased risk of recurrent middle ear disease. In 1985, Sarkkinen et al. (180) demonstrated that, during a natural epidemic of RSV infection, there was a concomitant and significant increase in occurrence of AOM. The authors of these studies thereby suggested that prevention of selected OM-associated viral URT infections could reduce the incidence of middle ear infections in childhood, a concept that is still widely held today.

Thus, ample epidemiological evidence and data were generated by direct-culture methodologies to support the association of URT viruses with acute bacterial infection of the middle ear (6, 98, 119, 122, 176, 181, 182). Peak incidence of OM occurred in concert with peak periods of isolation of many URT viruses (98, 176) (Fig. 1). In addition to culture and epidemiological data, the involvement of RSV, rhinovirus, AV, parainfluenza virus, influenza virus, coronavirus, enterovirus, and others was clearly demonstrated in children with OM by multiple immunoassays (5, 38, 39, 118, 123). By the late 1980s, the crucial role of the respiratory tract viruses in the pathogenesis of bacterial OM was firmly established and has been the subject of several excellent reviews (76, 87, 89, 91, 92, 94, 176, 177) despite our having an incomplete understanding of the mechanisms involved. Exposure to respiratory tract viruses (primarily via attendance at a day-care facility or association with siblings who act as transmitters of viral pathogens) has become established as a significant risk factor and/or predictor for early-onset, frequent, or recurrent OM in multiple studies (126, 154). In fact, in a prospective study of 596 infants from birth to 6 months of age, Daly and colleagues found that exposure to URT viruses is indisputably the most important predictor for early AOM, outweighing all others with an associated relative risk of 7.5 (52).

Whereas evidence has accumulated over time to demonstrate that multiple URT viruses can be involved in the pathogenesis of OM, only three primary bacterial agents are commonly associated with infections of the middle ear. These are the gram-positive microorganism *S. pneumoniae* and the two gram-negative microorganisms, nontypeable *H. influenzae* (NTHI) and *Moraxella catarrhalis*. While the distinctions sometimes blur, *S. pneumoniae*, or the pneumococcus, is most commonly associated with highly symptomatic acute OM (or AOM), whereas NTHI and *M. catarrhalis* are more commonly associated with cases of OM that are less symptomatic (or "silent") but of longer duration (i.e., chronic OM [COM] or OME). Regardless of the relative degree of symptoms associated with a case of OM, the presence of microorganisms and fluid in the middle ear space compromises the functions of the ear, both hearing and balance.

Because of growing acceptance of the increased role of both viruses and bacteria in OM, despite the fact that by traditional culture methods approximately 30% of MEFs collected from children with AOM and 30 to 50% of MEFs from cases of OME were considered sterile (76), much effort was made throughout the 1990s to develop improved detection methods to better understand the microbial etiology of OM. The advent of more sophisticated, specific, and sensitive assays for the detection of viral and bacterial DNA and/or RNA lent further support to the role of URT viruses as the predisposing agents or copathogens of bacterial OM. One of the first reports of the detection of genomic sequences of viruses in effusions collected from children with OME was published by Okamoto et al. (152). These investigators demonstrated that RSV sequences could be amplified in 62% of middle ear effusions assayed during and/or after a natural outbreak of RSV in the community.

Many laboratories subsequently developed and reported the use of molecular assays to detect one or more viral pathogens (151, 161, 184), a single bacterial species (102, 201, 208),

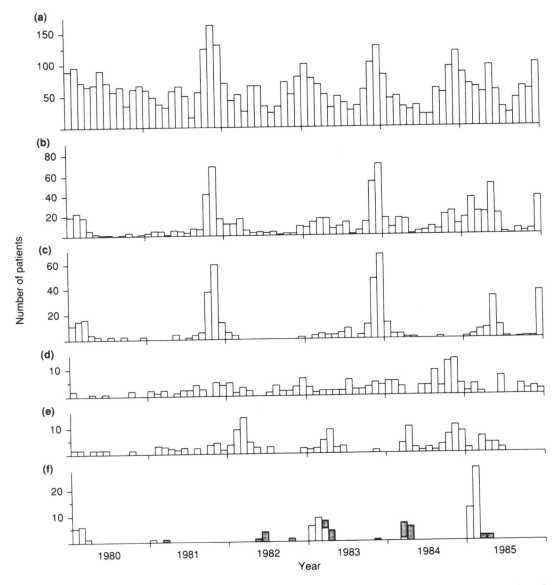

FIGURE 1 Number of patients per month with AOM ($n = 4,524$) (a) and respiratory virus infections (b to f) during a 6-year study in the Turku University Hospital (Turku, Finland). (b) All virus infections ($n = 961$); (c) respiratory syncytial virus ($n = 472$); (d) adenovirus ($n = 197$); (e) parainfluenza virus types 1, 2, and 3 ($n = 176$); (f) influenza A (unshaded) and influenza B (gray) viruses ($n = 116$). (Reprinted from *Pediatric Infectious Disease Journal* [176] with permission of the publisher.)

or mixed bacterial infections (99, 100, 167, 168) of the middle ear or their presence in NP secretions. The development and use of OM pathogen-specific multiplex assays to detect mixed viral-bacterial infections of the middle ear followed (18, 129). All of these assays have generated data that confirmed the commonality of mixed infections as the cause of OM, both acute and chronic, in animal models as well as in a clinical setting. Whereas by culture and immunodetection methods, viral involvement in OM has been reported to be between

30 and 50%, currently, by the use of PCR-based detection methods, the presence of at least one virus is detected in approximately 75% of children at the time of diagnosis of AOM, including positive viral detection in 48% of MEFs and in 62% of NP aspirates (162). Since bacterial superinfection of the middle ear, and the resultant effusion that develops, typically follow viral compromise, even this increase in reporting likely underrepresents viral involvement in OM.

ANIMAL MODELS

Several rodent hosts (gerbil, rat, mouse, guinea pig, and chinchilla) have been used to develop models of single pathogen-induced OM through the years, and each has its own inherent strengths and limitations (54, 58). However, the first laboratory to establish an animal model of OM based on a mixed microbial infection of the middle ear was the Giebink laboratory, which clearly demonstrated in 1980 that the incidence of culture-positive pneumococcal OM was significantly increased if the chinchilla host was coinoculated intranasally (i.n.) with any of several isolates of influenza A virus (78) (Fig. 2). Whereas only 4% of chinchillas (4% of ears) inoculated with influenza A virus alone or 21% of animals (13% of ears) inoculated with *S. pneumoniae* alone developed OM, this incidence was increased to 67% (52% of ears) when the animals were dually challenged.

Following the example of Giebink, we attempted to identify an appropriate viral co-partner for NTHI to better understand the pathogenesis of OM due to this gram-negative organism. An improved model was needed because NTHI alone was incapable of consistently inducing culture-positive OM from NP-colonized chinchillas when inoculated as the sole pathogen (187, 192). Moreover, existing transbullar models wherein NTHI was injected directly into the chinchilla middle ear, while resulting in severe OM in virtually all animals, did not represent the natural disease course in children. Attempts to partner the same strain of influenza A virus used by the

Giebink laboratory (influenza A/Alaska/6/77) with NTHI were unsuccessful; coinoculated animals had no greater incidence of OM than those receiving NTHI alone (author's unpublished observations). However, we later showed that a clinical isolate of AV (serotype 1) did indeed predispose juvenile chinchillas to culture-positive middle ear disease when partnered with NTHI (192). Animals that received NTHI by i.n. delivery 7 days after challenge with AV developed OM of greater severity than did cohorts that received either NTHI alone, AV alone, NTHI and AV at the same time, or NTHI 7 days prior to receiving AV. This dual challenge model resulted in the greatest incidence of culture-positive OM, the most prolonged presence of NTHI in the NP and middle ears, and the most severe damage to the middle ear mucosa and altered Eustachian tube function.

This study was followed by an investigation of the kinetics of development of this mixed infection, again in the chinchilla host (143). By using snap-frozen sections of Eustachian tube and middle ear mucosa to assay for adherent bacteria via fluorescent and transmission electron microscopy, we found that NTHI gradually ascended the Eustachian tube, in a retrograde fashion, from an NP colonization site to the middle ear cavity by adhering to mucus on the floor of the Eustachian tube (Fig. 3a and b). NTHI reaches the tympanum approximately 7 to 10 days after being introduced i.n. to AV-compromised chinchillas. Our ability to detect NTHI adhering to middle ear mucosa very close to the tympanic orifice of the Eustachian tube coincided with the onset of signs of OM in these animals (192) (Fig. 3c).

Thus, it became evident that the partnering of virus with bacterium and the timing of this interaction in the chinchilla host represented a highly specific interrelationship. Moreover, OM pathogenesis was clearly not predicated solely on general viral compromise of the uppermost airway. Whereas influenza A virus did indeed predispose to pneumococcal OM and AV similarly sets the stage for invasion of the middle ear by NTHI, we found, as stated

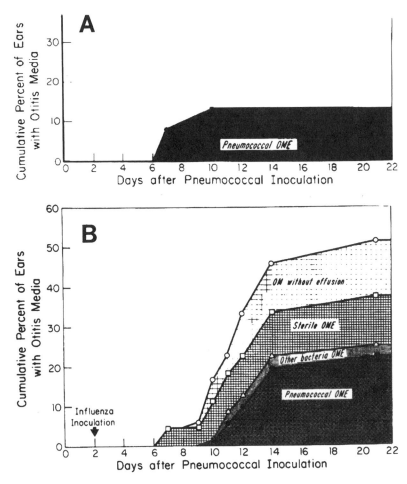

FIGURE 2 (A) Cumulative percentage of 38 ears (19 chinchillas) developing OME after i.n. inoculation of type 7F *S. pneumoniae*. All ears with effusion yielded pneumococci on culture. (B) Cumulative percentage of 72 ears (36 chinchillas) developing OME and without effusion after i.n. inoculation of type 7F *S. pneumoniae* and influenza A virus. Symbols: ●, animals with pneumococcal OME; △, animals with pneumococcal and other culture-positive OME (other bacteria included *S. aureus* [1 ear] and *Pseudomonas* species [1 ear]); □, animals with culture-positive as well as sterile OME; ○, animals with all types of OME and OM without effusion. (Both panels are reprinted from *Infection and Immunity* [78] with permission of the publisher.)

above, that influenza A virus does not predispose the chinchilla host to NTHI-induced OM. Nor does AV predispose to either *M. catarrhalis*-induced OM (17) or that caused by *S. pneumoniae* (197). Recent data from my laboratory (unpublished data) suggest that, in *M. catarrhalis*-induced OM, the etiology of the in-fection may require more than a single viral or bacterial copathogen and thus, the situation is more complex than what we currently believe to be the case for at least some infections of the middle ear due to *S. pneumoniae* or NTHI. Similar specificity of virus/bacterium synergy appears to be maintained in adults and children.

The oropharynges of 15% of adults with experimental influenza A virus infection became heavily colonized with *S. pneumoniae* 6 days after challenge (209), whereas isolation rates for other middle ear pathogens were not affected by infection with this virus. In children, *S. pneumoniae* is cultured significantly more often from MEFs that contain influenza A virus than those that are culture positive for either RSV or parainfluenza virus (97).

Although other rodents have not yet been used to model OM of mixed microbial etiology as has been done with the chinchilla, all the rodent models cited earlier have contributed a tremendous amount of information regarding the mechanisms by which the URT viruses predispose to bacterial invasion of the middle ear (reviewed below). Thereby, the importance of developing and utilizing relevant animal models cannot be overstated even in light of their inherent limitations. In fact, contributing greatly to the relative lack of progress made to date in our understanding of the pathogenesis of *M. catarrhalis*-induced OM, and consequently methods to prevent it, is the lack of a good animal model of middle ear dis-

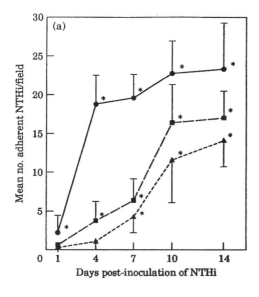

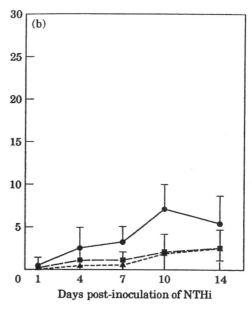

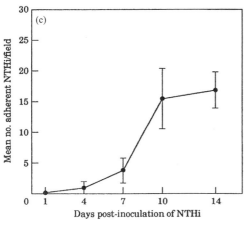

FIGURE 3 Adherence of NTHI to chinchilla eustachian tube floor (a) or roof (b) mucus during AV infection. Symbols: ●, pharyngeal; ■, mid-Eustachian tube; ▲, tympanic portion; *, significant difference compared with same day, same portion of ET roof, $P < 0.05$.) (c) Adherence of NTHI to chinchilla middle ear mucosal epithelium during adenovirus infection. (All panels are reprinted from *Microbial Pathogenesis* [143] with permission of the publisher.) Error bars indicate deviations.

ease induced by this pathogen. Models established to date for *M. catarrhalis* in mice, chinchillas, and rats lack many of the hallmark signs of an ongoing disease process and all demonstrate unequivocally the rapid clearance of *M. catarrhalis* from the airway and/or middle ears of these hosts (42, 58, 103, 204, 212).

MECHANISMS OF PATHOGENESIS

Multiple mechanisms have been identified that serve as contributing factors in the synergistic relationship between the URT viruses and the primary bacterial pathogens of OM, and while each of these is a highly specific effect, all fall within the general category of compromise of airway defenses. In most cases, it is highly likely that more than one of these mechanisms is operational at any given time and quite possibly varies depending on the time point within the multifactorial disease course of OM (12). Again, we have a better understanding of these processes as they relate to *S. pneumoniae* and NTHI to date than we do for *M. catarrhalis,* due in part to the absence of a useful model to help us define the pathogenic mechanisms of infection of the middle ear with this latter group of microorganisms. Some of these mechanisms are reviewed below.

Viral Effects on Bacterial Adherence and/or Colonization

In the late 70s, a hypothesis was put forth that one explanation for the commonly observed association between virus infection (specifically, influenza virus) and subsequent bacterial superinfection could be that cells infected with certain viruses might be more permissive to adherence of bacteria, which in turn could promote bacterial colonization and ultimately lead to infection and disease (179). Testing of this hypothesis was directly relevant to the study of the pathogenesis of OM when several investigators demonstrated that some of the URT viruses did indeed augment adherence by the bacterial pathogens of OM. Influenza A virus increases the adherence of type I *S. pneumoniae* to mouse tracheal epithelial cells (163) but not that of NTHI to chinchilla tracheal ep-

ithelium in an organ culture system (14). Hakansson et al. (86) showed in vitro that infection with AV types 1, 2, 3, and 5 significantly enhances the binding of adherent strains of *S. pneumoniae* that had been isolated from the NP of children with frequent episodes of AOM, to human lung epithelial cells. Their data suggest that AV upregulates the expression of receptors for *S. pneumoniae* on the surface of these respiratory epithelial cells. Jiang and colleagues (108) later demonstrated that RSV infection of A549 cells similarly significantly enhances attachment of NTHI that express outer membrane protein P5-homologous fimbriae but not the attachment of an isogenic mutant that does not express this adhesin (Fig. 4). This increase in adherence does not correlate with the relative amount of RSV antigen expressed by these human lung epithelial cells. However, UV-irradiated supernatants collected from RSV-infected cells also significantly enhances the attachment of fimbriated NTHI to A549 cells suggesting the presence of a preformed soluble precursor in these supernatants that enhances expression of a receptor for this NTHI adhesin.

With use of flow cytometry to detect bacteria adhering to influenza A virus-infected Hep-2 cells, El Ahmer et al. (61) recently showed that viral infection significantly increased adherence by all three groups of microorganisms most commonly associated with both AOM and COM. In their studies, 8 of 8 *M. catarrhalis* isolates, 5 of 5 respiratory tract isolates of *S. pneumoniae,* and 2 of 2 NTHI isolates showed significantly increased adherence to this particular target cell. By using a series of monoclonal antibodies to assay for potential changes in expression of cell surface antigens that could act as receptors for bacterial adherence, these investigators also found that infection of Hep-2 cells with influenza A virus resulted in a significant increase in binding of antibodies specific for both CD14 and CD18 but not Lewis[b], Lewis[x], or H type 2 markers. CD14 and CD18 have been shown to serve as a receptor site for adherence of several gram-negative bacteria, and thus virus-induced up-

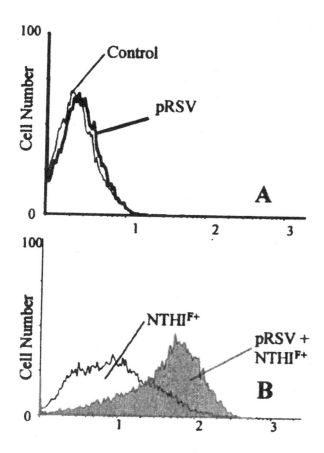

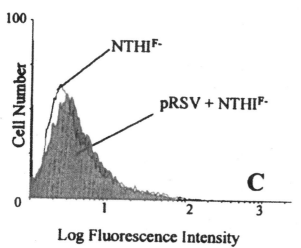

FIGURE 4 Histographic representation of number of A549 cells (y axis) expressing red fluorescence of PKH-26-labeled NTHI (x axis), as determined by flow cytometry (A549:NTHI = 1:100). (A) Background fluorescence of RSV-exposed (multiplicity of infection = 1, 24 h) or control A549 cells; (B and C) fluorescence of NTHI^{F+} and NTHI^{F-} attached to control or pRSV-exposed A549 cells. (Reprinted from *Infection and Immunity* [108] with permission of the publisher.)

regulation of host cell surface antigens that can act as bacterial receptor sites appears to be a common theme in the pathogenesis of OM and other diseases of the respiratory tract.

Since the origin of bacterial invaders of the middle ear are those microorganisms that colonize the NP, the finding that viral infection promotes bacterial adherence to airway epithelial cells has enormous implications for the disease course of OM. Early studies by Fainstein et al. (69) had shown that more type I pneumococci and *H. influenzae* adhere to pharyngeal cells collected from human volunteers experimentally infected with influenza A/USSR/77 after infection than to pharyngeal cells collected prior to challenge. Surprisingly, individuals with natural URT infection did not similarly demonstrate this enhanced adherence. More recently, Patel and colleagues (156) showed that colonization of respiratory tract epithelium by NTHI is increased upon exposure of cotton rats to RSV. Colonization of the NP by NTHI is significantly greater 4 days after RSV infection than in RSV-negative controls. However, thereafter, NTHI is cleared more rapidly from the NP of RSV-infected animals than from controls, and adherence of NTHI to cells collected from RSV-infected cotton rats at the time of maximal virus replication is not different than in these control animals. These data suggested that, whereas infection with RSV does temporarily induce significantly augmented colonization of the NP in the host, the exact mechanism(s) by which this occurs is not yet clear. With use of a chinchilla host, influenza A virus (but not AV) has similarly been found to enhance nasopharyngeal colonization by *S. pneumoniae,* and particularly by a strain with an opaque versus a transparent phenotype (197, 198). Hirano et al. (101) reported that influenza A virus infection of mice results in increased colonization by both NTHI and *S. pneumoniae;* however, the increase in recovery of NTHI was found to be significant only on day 5 after challenge when compared with controls. Conversely, a significant increase occurred in recovery of *S. pneu-*

moniae in nasal lavage fluids on days 5, 9, and 14 after influenza A virus challenge.

The positive correlation between viral URT infection and NP colonization has also been shown in human challenge models (209) wherein influenza A virus infection promotes colonization with *S. pneumoniae.* Moreover, NP colonization alone has been positively correlated with an increased incidence of OM in children (66, 67). In fact, even in the absence of a viral URT infection, children are colonized with the organisms that induce OM very soon after birth. Faden and colleagues (63) have shown that, at 6 months of age, 26% of infants are already colonized with *M. catarrhalis,* 24% with *S. pneumoniae,* and 9% with NTHI. By 1 year of age, these percentages increase to 72, 54, and 33%, respectively. These investigators have also shown that early colonization is associated with early initial episodes of AOM and that colonization with either *S. pneumoniae* or *H. influenza* in the first year of life increases the risk of becoming otitis prone fourfold compared with the absence of colonization with these microorganisms (Fig. 5). In addition, there is a direct relationship between the frequency of colonization and the frequency of AOM.

Despite their prevalence as colonizers of the pediatric NP, all three bacterial species associated with AOM and COM typically behave as benign commensals (or normal flora) and as such are largely ignored by the host. However, when children are also infected with a URT virus and thus experiencing compromise of their Eustachian tubes, these organisms often act as opportunistic pathogens. During URT viral infection, because of the temporary inability of the Eustachian tube to prevent their ascent (see the next section), bacterial commensals of the NP can gain access to the middle ear and begin to multiply, sometimes causing severe pain and/or long-term infection of the middle ear. These infections of the middle ear, and particularly those that occur very early in life, can induce pathological changes in the middle ear that set the stage for subsequent recurrent or chronic OM.

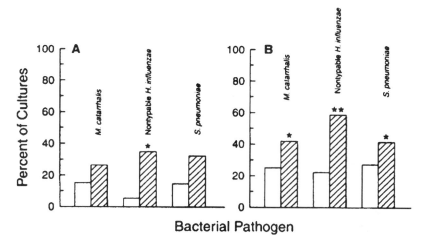

FIGURE 5 Comparison of nasopharyngeal carriage of *S. pneumoniae,* nontypeable *H. influenza,* and *M. catarrhalis* in normal (☐) and otitis-prone (▨) children during health (A) and during upper respiratory tract illness (B). ★, $P < 0.05$; ★★, $P < 0.001$ (15). (Reprinted from the *European Journal of Pediatrics* [63] with permission of the publisher.)

Viral Compromise of Eustachian Tube Function

Virus-induced damage to the mucosal epithelium lining the uppermost airway and the effect of this pathology on airway function, particularly that of the Eustachian tube, has also been shown to contribute significantly to bacterial superinfection of the middle ear (23, 142). In children, the Eustachian tube is shorter and more horizontal in orientation than in adults. The immature Eustachian tube is also more compliant (or "floppy") and the mechanisms for active opening of the tubal lumen, largely via the action of the tensor veli palatini muscle, are not yet fully effective (Fig. 6). These attributes make the pediatric Eustachian tube naturally more susceptible to invasion by microbes from the NP; however, this susceptibility is significantly enhanced during times of viral compromise.

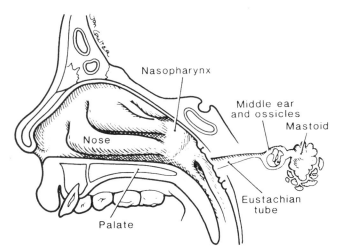

FIGURE 6 Anatomy of the Eustachian tube and middle ear system. (Reprinted from *The Pediatric Infectious Disease Journal* [23] with permission of the publisher.)

The effect of influenza A virus on the chinchilla Eustachian tube after i.n. inoculation was investigated by Giebink et al. (80) in an attempt to understand the mechanisms underlying the negative pressure recorded in the middle ears of these animals when infected with various strains of this virus. Inflammation of the tympanic membrane and an underpressured state of the middle ear mirrors both epithelial damage in the Eustachian tube and the accumulation of mucus and cellular debris in the tubal lumen (Fig. 7). Epithelial damage was found to be greatest in the proximal two-thirds of the Eustachian tube, whereas goblet cell metaplasia and increased secretory activity was greatest in the distal, tympanic one-third of the tube after i.n. challenge with influenza A/Alaska/6/77 virus. These data thus provided the first morphologic correlate for the development of negative middle ear pressure and contributed to our understanding of the basis for purulent OM that occurred during viral respiratory tract infection. Ohashi et al. (150) later reported similar findings in a guinea pig model following intratympanic inoculation of influenza A virus. However, whereas the character of the histopathology noted was highly reminiscent of that shown in the chinchilla, in their study, virus-induced damage was greatest more proximal to the tympanic bulla because of the direct challenge of the middle ear in this latter model.

The overall finding that URT viruses compromise Eustachian tube function in guinea pigs and chinchillas correlates well with virus-induced changes that occur in human volunteers challenged with rhinovirus or influenza A virus. Rhinovirus-induced effects on middle ear pressure status and nasal patency was measured in sequestered human volunteers challenged i.n. with this virus (26, 137). Abnormal middle ear pressures, decreased nasal patency,

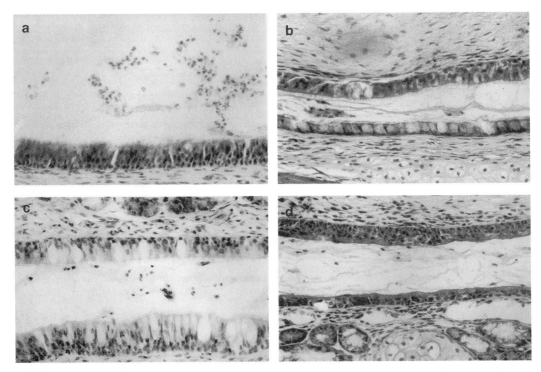

FIGURE 7 Eustachian tube lumen on day 5 (a and b) and day 10 (c and d) after i.n. influenza virus inoculation showing mucoid secretions and cellular debris (hematoxylin and eosin stain; original magnification, ×400). (Reprinted from *Annals of Otology, Rhinology & Laryngology* [80] with permission of the publisher.)

and depressed tubal function occur in 50% or more of the ears of subjects that developed a clinical illness (or "cold") due to rhinovirus. In another study, volunteers were inoculated with influenza A virus. More than 80% developed Eustachian tube dysfunction and middle ear underpressures of less than -100 mm H_2O on days 4 and 5 after challenge (59). Five of 21 subjects with low prechallenge antibody titers to influenza A virus also developed OME. These data thereby collectively support a causal relationship between viral URT infection, Eustachian tube obstruction, abnormal middle ear pressure, and OM.

The degree to which a particular virus compromises the airway, particularly the Eustachian tube, has a tremendous influence on whether or not OM is induced and, if so, how severe the disease course is. Giebink and Wright (81) clearly demonstrated this influence when they showed that different strains of influenza A virus had markedly altered levels of virulence in the chinchilla host when the outcome measures were: the development of a negative middle ear pressure, neutrophil dysfunction, and increased susceptibility to pneumococcal OM. These data thus supported epidemiological evidence that had shown a striking difference in prevalence of AOM associated with different influenza A outbreaks. Whereas 41% of children with A/Texas influenza had associated AOM, only 10% of those with A/USSR or 18% of those who were not infected with either virus strain had OM.

These data are in keeping with the general principle that, although nearly all respiratory tract viruses can predispose to bacterial OM, there does seem to be both intra- and inter-strain variability in their relative ability to do so. Uhari et al. (202) prospectively studied 658 children to analyze the etiology of respiratory tract infection with and without associated AOM. Of 197 children with AOM, the only virus that was more commonly isolated in these patients was RSV. While these investigators monitored children who were admitted to the hospital, and thus they studied a patient population that was more severely ill than the typical child with OM, many laboratories have reported the stronger association of RSV with AOM than many other URT viruses (92, 97, 98, 118, 119, 122, 162, 176, 180). Thus, those viral URT infections that are associated with more severe compromise of the uppermost airway appear to be those that enhance susceptibility to bacterial OM.

In animal models, the time between initial viral infection (or challenge) and bacterial invasion of the middle ear is approximately 9 days for the pneumococcus after influenza A virus inoculation (78) and 7 to 10 days for NTHI after AV inoculation (143). This time is similar to the interval between onset of symptoms of upper respiratory infection and AOM as shown epidemiologically. In a study of 204 cases of AOM that occurred in association with 412 episodes of URT infection, 75% of cases occurred during the first week after onset of symptoms and 85% occurred during the first 9 days (93). Koivunen et al. (121) recently examined 250 episodes of AOM in children and similarly found that 63% of AOM complicating URT infection occurred in the first week and 89% occurred by the end of the second week after onset of URT infection (Fig. 8). The greatest incidence of AOM was observed 2 to 5 days after the onset of respiratory symptoms. This interval between viral infection and bacterial superinfection of the ears was directly documented by Buchman et al. (27), who demonstrated the invasion of the middle ear of one subject by *S. pneumoniae* by PCR amplification of pneumococcal DNA from a middle ear effusion recovered 5 days after challenge with influenza A virus. These observations thereby fit well with the physician- and parent-described impression that ". . . a child gets a cold and a week later has an ear infection" (76).

Viral Effects on Antibiotic Efficacy
Both Arola et al. (7) and Chonmaitree et al. (37) first suggested the association between viruses and antibiotic treatment failure in patients with OM. Because OM is generally considered to be a "bacterial disease," antibiotic therapy was at one time recommended for all

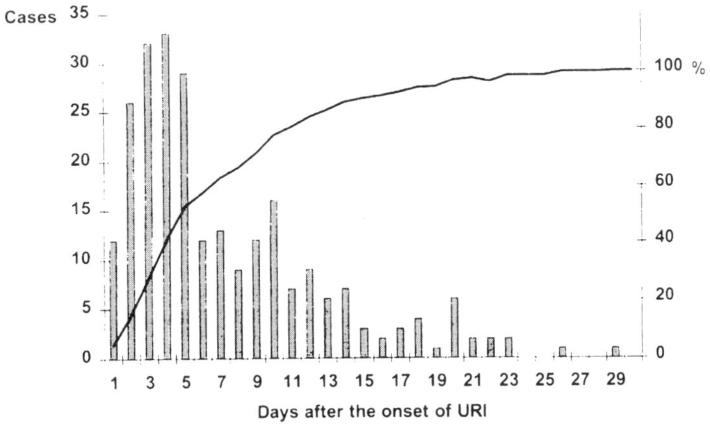

FIGURE 8 Occurrence of AOM after the onset of URI in 250 episodes. Bar, number of cases on each day; line, cumulative force of morbidity. (Reprinted from *The Pediatric Infectious Disease Journal* [121] with permission of the publisher.)

patients with AOM. In 4 to 18% of these patients, however, the signs of infection persist despite the fact that in approximately 81% of these cases the microbes isolated from the middle ears are susceptible to the prescribed antimicrobial (7). Both groups observed that patients who were unresponsive to treatment with antibiotics also tended to have positive viral cultures of the middle ear (Table 1). In a later prospective study of 271 infants and children with AOM, Chonmaitree et al. (38) found evidence of viral infection in 46% of these patients, 76% of whom also had bacteria present in their MEFs. More of the patients with this combined bacterial-viral infection (51%) had persistent OM 3 to 12 days after institution of antibiotic therapy than either those with bacterial OM (35%) or patients with OM due to a viral pathogen alone (19%). Other prospective studies corroborated the linkage between viral involvement in OM and antibiotic treatment failure (88, 157, 190). Collectively, these data suggested that the presence of viruses in the MEFs might be interfering either directly or indirectly with the clinical response to antibiotics. The exact mechanisms by which concomitant viral infection might be a determinant of treatment outcome in some AOM episodes (despite the susceptibility of the bacterial pathogen cultured from the middle ear to the antibiotic prescribed) thus became the subject of several investigations.

TABLE 1 Comparison of clinical and bacteriologic outcome of patients with AOM caused by bacteria alone or bacteria and virus[a]

Outcome at visit 2	No. (%) of patients infected with:	
	Bacteria alone ($n = 31$)	Bacteria and virus ($n = 12$)
Cured or improved	24 (77)	6 (50)
Failure		
Clinical[b]	3 (10)	0
Bacteriologic[c]	4 (13)	6 (50)
Resistant bacteria	3 (10)	2 (17)
Susceptible bacteria[d]	1 (3)	4 (33)

[a] Reprinted from *The Journal of Infectious Diseases* (37) with permission of the publisher.
[b] Negative cultures for virus and bacteria.
[c] With or without clinical symptoms, bacteria-alone group vs. bacteria-and-virus group ($P < 0.01$ by χ^2).
[d] Bacteria-alone group vs. bacteria-and-virus group ($P < 0.05$ by χ^2).

One explanation for the commonality of treatment failure in cases of viral-bacterial OM may lie in the combined effect of viral and bacterial invasion of the middle ear on penetration of antimicrobials from the bloodstream into the tympanum. With a diffusion model developed in chinchillas, Jossart et al. (111) compared middle ear elimination rates for three antimicrobials in four groups of animals: (i) controls that were not challenged with any microbe, (ii) those inoculated with influenza A virus alone i.n., (iii) those infected with both influenza A virus and *S. pneumoniae* by direct inoculation into the middle ear, and (iv) those inoculated directly into the middle ear with *S. pneumoniae* alone. After infection was established, a solution of amoxicillin, sulfamethoxazole, and trimethoprim was first instilled into the middle ear, then removed 4 h later. The authors of this study present the argument that, because passive diffusion occurs in both directions, and there is no evidence of an active transport mechanism for antibiotics into or from the environment of the middle ear, the model assumes that the rate of antibiotic elimination from the MEFs equals the rate of antibiotic penetration from the bloodstream, through the middle ear mucosa into the middle ear. Thereby, the rate constant of elimination and half-life of the antimicrobials were calculated from drug concentrations at the stated time points, and these values were used as a marker for antimicrobial penetration into the middle ear.

These investigators found that *S. pneumoniae* infection alone significantly shortened the middle ear elimination half-life of all three antimicrobials compared with the control group; the combined influenza A virus plus pneumococcus infection significantly lengthened the half-life of all three antimicrobials compared with the pneumococcal infection alone; and influenza A virus itself resulted in the longest half-lives for all three antimicrobials. Thus, the decreased penetration of antimicrobials into the middle ear that they theorized would occur in infections of combined viral-bacterial etiology, compared with those due to bacteria alone,

supported the clinical observation that patients with infections of mixed etiology may have decreased middle ear antimicrobial concentrations which in turn leads to treatment failure.

A subsequent study of 34 children with AOM was conducted by Canafax et al. (29) to prospectively evaluate whether viral coinfection in AOM reduced antibacterial efficacy of antibiotics by determining the penetration and pharmacokinetics of amoxicillin in either bacterial or combined bacterial and viral AOM. Middle ear fluids, nasal wash fluids, and serum were collected from all 34 children at selected times between 0.5 and 4 h after oral dosing (40 mg/kg/day) and geometric mean amoxicillin concentrations were determined. Lowest values were associated with children infected with the virus only (2.7 μg/ml in MEFs) and these values were similar to those obtained in children that yielded culture-negative effusions (2.9 μg/ml in MEFs). Geometric mean amoxicillin concentrations were higher in children with combined bacterial and viral infection (4.1 μg/ml in MEFs) and were highest in those with bacterial-only infections of the middle ear (5.7 μg/ml in MEFs). Thus, there was indeed lesser penetration of amoxicillin from serum into MEFs when virus was also present in the middle ear, providing additional evidence for a mechanism whereby a higher incidence of antibiotic treatment failure occurs in these individuals.

A potential link between treatment failure, the presence of virus in the middle ear, and levels of specific inflammatory mediators in MEFs was investigated by Chonmaitree et al. (41), who measured levels of interleukin-8 (IL-8), a polymorphonuclear neutrophil (PMN) chemotactic cytokine, and leukotriene B4 (LTB4), a potent inflammatory product of PMNs, in 271 MEFs collected from 196 children with AOM. Forty-two percent of these children had evidence of respiratory viral infection as well. Levels of both LTB4 and IL-8 were significantly higher at the time of diagnosis in children with either bacterial AOM or mixed bacterial-viral infection than levels in MEFs from culture-negative children. No virus-related effect was observed for IL-8 when bacteria were absent; however, these levels were significantly higher in MEFs that contained both bacteria and viruses than in all other groups. Moreover, in children who had both bacteria and virus isolated from one MEF but were virus-negative in the contralateral MEF, levels of both IL-8 and LTB4 were higher in the MEFs that contained both bacteria and virus in all but one case wherein the LTB4 level was greater in the MEF that was virus negative. Bacteriologic failure after 2 to 5 days of treatment with either of two antibiotic regimens was significantly associated with high LTB4 levels in initial MEFs, whereas recurrence of AOM within 1 month was associated with high IL-8 levels in these effusions. These findings suggest that both of these PMN-related inflammatory substances are produced during acute infections of the middle ear and may play an important role in delayed recovery and/or recurrence of disease.

Viral Effects on Host Immune Functions

Another topic of enormous interest as it relates to the pathogenesis of OM is the effect of URT viruses on host immune function. The global effect of viral infection on neutrophil (2) and alveolar macrophage (211) function has been appreciated for some time and transient peripheral PMN dysfunction has been reported in children with recurrent OM (79). Neutrophil dysfunction has also been linked with influenza A virus infection in a chinchilla model (1). Abramson et al. (1) reported significantly depressed chemotactic, chemiluminescent, and bactericidal activities 4 to 8 days after inoculation of virus when compared with controls. Although they did not directly test this, the authors suggested that the known increased susceptibility of chinchillas to pneumococcal OM after inoculation with influenza A virus (78) might be due, in part, to these impaired chemotactic and oxidative microbicidal activities of the neutrophils.

Viral-mediated release of cytokines and inflammatory mediators in the respiratory tract is also likely involved in the pathogenesis of OM. Cytokine activity in nasopharyngeal secretions collected during the course of a primary RSV infection shows the local production of IL-6 and tumor necrosis factor alpha (TNF-α) in 100% and 67% of infants and children, respectively (136, 147). Similarly, experimental influenza A virus infection in 17 adult volunteers led to significantly increased levels of IL-6, but not IL-4, in lavage fluids of all 12 subjects who shed virus (75). Increased levels of this pleotropic cytokine were not found in the five subjects who did not shed virus. Noah et al. (136, 147) examined children in a day care setting during acute upper respiratory infection, including children with OM, and also found markedly elevated levels of IL-1β, IL-6, IL-8, and TNF-α in nasal lavage fluids that were not dependent on the specific virus isolated. In addition, nasal mucosal biopsies showed increased transcripts for IL-1β, IL-6, and IL-8 in the epithelial cells of seven of nine subjects, thus suggesting that epithelial cells are a source of these proinflammatory cytokines in the nasal cavity. In these children, the levels of all cytokines, but not TNF-α, decreased significantly within 2 to 4 weeks.

The enhancing effect of combined bacterial-viral infections on production of inflammatory mediators in the middle ear by the host has also been shown (40). Histamine levels were measured in 677 MEF samples collected from 248 children with AOM, of which 47% had a documented viral infection as well. Histamine content was found to be significantly higher in either bacteria-positive or virus-positive fluids versus samples that were negative by culture, and together, bacteria and viruses have an additive effect on histamine content in MEFs. Thus histamine production is induced by infection of the middle ear and most markedly in situations of mixed microbial infections. High levels of histamine, cytokines, and other inflammatory mediators in MEFs can lead to increased inflammation in the middle ear and this enhancement of the host's immune response is, in essence, a double-edged sword. While an inflammatory response is essential for microbial clearance, it is also believed to contribute to both the pathogenesis and prolongation of OM via disease-associated tissue destruction and interference with penetration of antimicrobials into the site, among other mechanisms (94). For example, histamine also causes impaired ciliary activity and induces mucosal swelling in the tubotympanum thus prolonging mucociliary clearance time from the tympanic cavity. In fact, because of these known compromising effects, intratympanic instillation of histamine is now used to predispose to pneumococcal disease in a recently developed rat model of OM (207).

Viral Effects on Rheological Properties of Mucus and Mucociliary Transport

Many URT viruses, including those commonly associated with OM, are known to induce ciliary ultrastructural abnormalities or selective destruction of ciliated cells in airway epithelium (31, 163). Both of these mechanisms can compromise mucociliary clearance mechanisms throughout the respiratory tract, including in the nasal cavity of children with acute viral infection (31). Park et al. (155) studied influenza A virus-induced histopathology in chinchillas, including suppression of ciliary activity of the mucosa lining the Eustachian tube, and the subsequent impaired ability of this organ to move a small bolus of fluid from an inferior aspect of the middle ear cavity to the back of the throat where it can be swallowed. In this study, and in another by Chung et al. (43), influenza A virus induced pronounced damage to cilia and ciliated cells in addition to causing an extensive infiltration of PMNs into the subepithelial space. There were minimal changes to goblet cells.

Concurrent with these morphological changes was compromise of chinchilla Eustachian tube functions with maximal effects observed approximately 7 to 14 days after challenge (155). Ciliary beat frequency decreased from a normal rate of 19.2 ± 0.1 to 15.9 ± 0.3 Hz at the tympanic portion and 18.3 ± 0.1 Hz at the pharyngeal portion of the Eustachian

tube on day 7 after transbullar inoculation (Fig. 9A). Interestingly, 10 days after i.n. inoculation of influenza A virus, ciliary beat frequency values were significantly decreased at both the tympanic and pharyngeal portions of the Eustachian tube (14.6 ± 2.6 or 14.8 ± 2.3 Hz, respectively) (Fig. 9B). This slowing of ciliary beating, combined with the discoordinated activity among ciliated cells that also occurs as a result of viral infection, leads to compromised clearance function. Thus, the ability of the mucociliary escalator of the Eustachian tube to transport fluid out of the middle ear space was similarly maximally diminished on days 7 to 14 after transbullar challenge. Transport times increased from a normal time of approximately 150 s to a situation in which there was no appearance of dye at the pharyngeal orifice of the Eustachian tube even 15 min after its instillation into the middle ear (Table 2). Ohashi et al. (150) reported similar decreased ciliary activity and increased time to clearance (from 68.3 ± 7.5 s to a maximum of 155 ± 19 s on day 14) in guinea pigs inoculated with influenza A virus intratympanically.

AV also compromises Eustachian tube function in chinchillas (13); however, for this virus, maximal compromise occurs 10 to 21 days after i.n. inoculation or 7 to 14 days after transbullar inoculation of this host. Subepithelial hemorrhage and edema, intense PMN infiltration, and clumping and shortening or loss of cilia were observed in addition to focal necrosis and sloughing of epithelium to reveal the basal cell layer in sections of Eustachian tube recovered from these animals. The presence of intranuclear inclusions and marked hyperplasia of goblet cells were consistent with AV infection.

Whereas the exact nature of the induced histopathology in both the Eustachian tube and middle ear is indeed virus specific in these models of influenza A virus or AV infection, the net effect in all cases is a severe compromise of Eustachian tube function. This compromise results in a temporal loss of ability of this organ to function as a primary defense mechanism of the middle ear, keeping bacteria and/or additional viruses from invading the

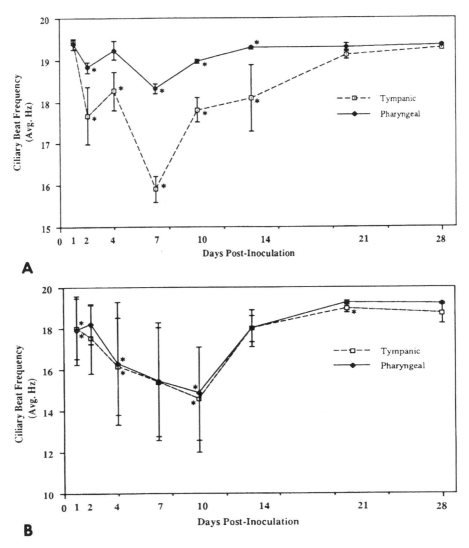

FIGURE 9 Ciliary beat frequency of chinchilla Eustachian tube epithelium at sites near the tympanic or pharyngeal orifice following inoculation of influenza A virus. *, significant difference ($P \leq 0.01$) from control. Error bars indicate standard deviations. (A) Transbullar inoculation; (B) i.n. inoculation. (Reprinted from *Annals of Otology, Rhinology & Laryngology* [155] with permission of the publisher.)

middle ear from the NP. At the point of maximal compromise of the epithelium lining the Eustachian tube, as measured by reduced ciliary beat frequency and significantly ameliorated ability to move a bolus of dye from the middle ear to the pharynx, the ascension of the Eustachian tube by bacteria colonizing the NP can be detected (192). Return to normal epithelial organization, ciliary morphology, and

mucociliary clearance function after virus-induced damage can take 28 days after experimental influenza A virus infection in guinea pigs (150) or chinchillas (43, 155) (Fig. 10), approximately 35 days in chinchilla models of AV infection (43, 192) (Fig. 11) and 2 to 10 weeks in children (31). Thus, the middle ear is most susceptible to ascending bacterial infection during these periods of recovery after

TABLE 2 Dye transport values for chinchillas injected transbullarly with influenza A/Alaska/6/77 virus[a]

Day postinoculation	Dye transport rate (s) (mean ± SD)[b]	
	Control ear	Test ear
1	180 ± 27 (4)	459 ± 31[c] (2)
2	130 ± 40 (3)	636 ± 142[c] (2)
4	151 ± 29 (4)	670 ± 325[c] (2)
7	160 ± 55 (4)	900 ± 0[c,d] (2)
14	134 ± 31 (4)	900 ± 0[c,d] (2)
21	139 ± 27 (4)	655 ± 346[c] (2)
28	155 (1)	147 ± 23 (2)

[a] Reprinted from *Annals of Otology, Rhinology & Laryngology* (155) with permission of the publisher.
[b] Values in parentheses are numbers of ears.
[c] Significant difference from control ($P \leq 0.01$).
[d] Fifteen minutes (900 s) was arbitrarily selected as the upper limit for these studies. No appearance of dye at nasopharyngeal orifice within 15 min yielded a transport value of 900.

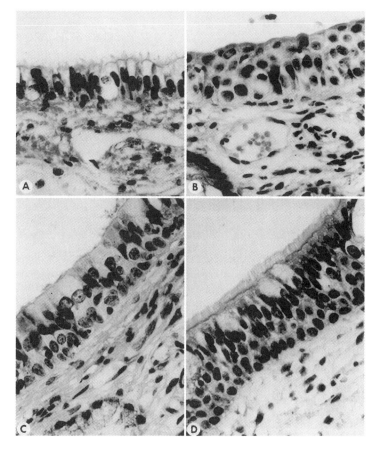

FIGURE 10 Light micrographs of chinchilla Eustachian tube epithelium after i.n. inoculation of influenza A virus (original magnification, ×64). (A) Two days postinoculation, tympanic site. (B) At 4 days, pharyngeal site. Note focal loss of ciliated cells. (C) At 10 days, pharyngeal site. Note short, regenerating cilia. (D) At 28 days, pharyngeal site. Note normal appearance of epithelium. (Reprinted from *Annals of Otology, Rhinology & Laryngology* [155] with permission of the publisher.)

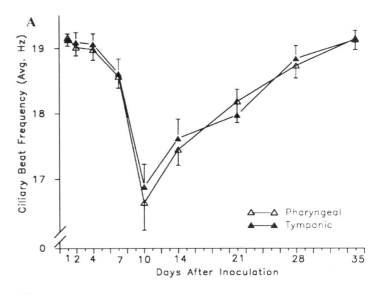

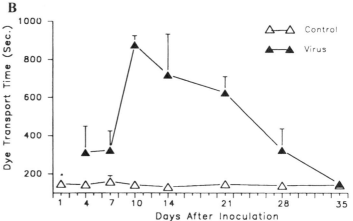

FIGURE 11 (A) Change over time in ciliary activity of Eustachian tube mucosal epithelium after i.n. inoculation of AV type 1. Data represent means and standard deviations of at least 30 readings. (B) Change over time in ability of Eustachian tube to transport dye after i.n. inoculation of AV type 1. (Both panels are reprinted from *The Journal of Infectious Diseases* [13] with permission of the publisher.)

URT infection. Given the variety of viruses a child is exposed to annually and the time it takes for the middle ear to recover after each bout of viral URT infection, one can easily imagine the scenarios that lead to AOM, recurrent OM, and chronic OME.

The specificity of the interrelationship between the viral and bacterial pathogens of OM was discussed above. One possible explanation for the specificity of this synergy resides in the fact that several viruses are known to have a distinct effect on the character of mucus secreted into the uppermost airway. For example, AV leads to both an increase in relative

amount and viscosity of NP secretions in chinchillas challenged with a serotype 1 isolate (13); however, the biochemistry of these secretions is not altered (192). By using a panel of 15 lectins with a broad range of specificity for labeling of cell surface carbohydrates, we found that there was no marked change in either labeling intensity or distribution of label between AV-infected chinchillas and control animals. The goblet cell hyperplasia noted to occur in the mucosa that lines the Eustachian tube is a hallmark of AV infection in chinchillas and provides a possible mechanism for the noted hypersecretion of mucus in these animals (Fig. 12). This hypersecretion phenomenon combined with an inability to adequately hydrate this increased amount of "normal" mucus likely accounts for the changes in the rheological properties of airway secretions that we have reported. This situation seems to favor ascension of the Eustachian tube and initiation of OM due to NTHI. In fact, NTHI adheres to mucus within the Eustachian tube lumen of AV-infected chinchillas rather than adhering to any particular cell type in this site (144) (Color Plate 2 [see color insert]).

Influenza A virus, on the other hand, also leads to an increased production of respiratory secretions in the first week after exposure of human volunteers (60). However, these secretions are not more viscous than normal and, unlike the situation with AV, there is a con-

comitant change in the biochemical character of the mucus blanket and epithelial cell surface carbohydrates attributed to the action of viral neuraminidase. Hirano et al. (101) inoculated mice with influenza A virus and examined their NP mucosa for changes in labeling patterns using a battery of lectins. Staining of the mucus blanket and epithelial cell surface with lectins (PNA, succWGA, and BSL-II) specific for either GlcNAc or Gal residues was significantly increased compared with controls, whereas labeling with lectins (WGA or MAA) with specificity for terminal sialic acid residues was only moderately enhanced in virus-infected animals and only on days 5 and 9 after virus inoculation. Because terminal glycosylation sequences of epithelial cell surface and mucus carbohydrates mediate adherence by

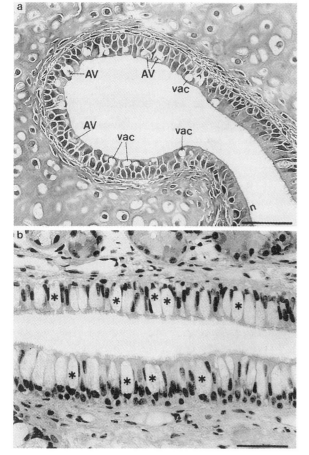

FIGURE 12 Cross-sections in mid-Eustachian tube 14 days after intranasal inoculation. (a) Note many vacuolated epithelial cells (vac) and those demonstrating late stages of intranuclear inclusions typical of AV. (b) Note marked goblet cell (*) hyperplasia. Bars = 50 μm. (Reprinted from *The Journal of Infectious Diseases* [13] with permission of the publisher.)

microorganisms, the effects of viral infection on these structures has important implications for the pathogenesis of OM.

Effects of Bacteria and Their Products on Airway Physiology and Function

While the URT viruses have been studied more extensively in terms of their synergistic relationship with bacteria in causing OM, the influence of the exact bacterial pathogen (or pathogens) present in MEFs on the course and severity of OM has also been a topic of some investigation. Bacteria, like viruses, elicit the production of inflammatory mediators in the middle ear, and several investigators (8, 9, 44, 55, 95, 109, 110, 112, 140, 145, 149, 183, 193, 196, 213, 215) have reported the elicitation of many proinflammatory cytokines, growth factors, and products of complement activation in MEFs in response to invasion of the middle ear by the bacterial pathogens of OM. However, to date, the inflammatory mediators elicited by each of these microorganisms and the effect they have on subsequent superinfection have not been fully elucidated. Nevertheless, a few studies have looked at the effect of bacterial products, particularly endotoxin (lipooligosaccharide [LOS] or lipopolysaccharide [LPS]) or extracellular enzymes, on the epithelium that lines the uppermost respiratory tract.

Ohashi et al. (149) found that LPS isolated from *Klebsiella pneumoniae* induces a marked decrease in ciliary beat frequency in guinea pig tubotympanal mucosa. Likewise, Bakaletz et al. (11) showed that either LOS isolated from *Salmonella enterica* serovar typhimurium or whole formalin-fixed NTHI, but not formalin-fixed *S. pneumoniae,* had a significant suppressive effect on the ability of the chinchilla Eustachian tube to transport fluid. Injection of purified LOS or a killed gram-negative (and thus endotoxin-containing) organism (NTHI) into the middle ear cavity results in an early production of an MEF, capillary leakage, and slowing of mucociliary transport.

Bacterial enzymes also likely play a role in the pathogenesis of OM. Neuraminidase purified from *S. pneumoniae* is known to alter chinchilla middle ear mucosa by removing sialic acid residues and exposing galactose residues of cell surface carbohydrates expressed on mucosal epithelial cells (128). Linder et al. (130, 131) further investigated the effects of pneumococcal extracellular enzymes, particularly neuraminidase, on the biochemistry of the tubotympanum-using chinchilla models. They found that inoculation with *S. pneumoniae* either via a transbullar or i.n. route induced a change in lectin-labeling pattern from that obtained with use of naive or control tissues, which demonstrates, like Doyle et al. (128), that terminal sialic acid residues had been removed and N-acetylglucosamine residues had been exposed. There was a marked increase in labeling with lectins (PNA, succWGA, BSL II or ECL) specific for either GlcNAc or Gal, whereas there was a decrease in labeling with lectins (SNA and WGA) specific for terminal sialic acid residues. Thus the pneumococcus, through the action of one of its extracellular enzymes, can induce the exposure of its own host cell receptor site, specifically Galβ1-4GlcNAcβ1-3Galβ. As discussed above, influenza A virus neuraminidase affects lectin labeling patterns in the uppermost airway in a similar manner which also likely contributes significantly to the specific association between this URT virus and pneumococcal OM (101).

Some evidence shows that the presence of one bacterial species in an MEF may alter the survival of others in these fluids (188). Viable *M. catarrhalis* appears to prolong the survival of both *S. pneumoniae* and *H. influenzae* when coincubated in sterile mucoid effusions collected from patients with ongoing secretory OM, whereas nonviable *M. catarrhalis* enhanced the growth of *S. pneumoniae* only. Conversely, both the pneumococcus and *H. influenzae* suppressed the growth of *M. catarrhalis* when coincubated in these mucoid MEFs. Although the exact mechanism for these variable effects on survivability are not known, the authors suggested that these phenomena are also likely in play in the middle ear during natural disease.

Thus, the course of disease development and resolution that occurs in the middle ear can be highly variable and largely depends on which microbe, or combination of microbes, initiates the infection as well as those that contribute to the superinfection.

Biofilms and OM

Despite the culture-negative status of 40 to 60% of MEFs, PCR-based assays consistently suggested a much higher incidence of bacterial involvement in OM. Due to the manyfold greater sensitivity of PCR, however, the early PCR-generated data were viewed somewhat skeptically and there were concerns as to whether these data were more reflective of false-positive results than an actual increased involvement of bacteria in COM or OME. Thereby, to determine whether the PCR-generated data were truly indicative of the existence of viable but not culturable bacteria in the middle ear or merely due to the persistence of residual "fossilized" DNA in the absence of viable bacteria, Post et al. (165) and later Aul and colleagues (10) designed a series of studies to address these concerns specifically and systematically. They found that purified DNA and DNA from intact but nonviable (heat-killed) bacteria do not persist for more than a day in effusions present in the middle ear cleft, even after inoculation with more than 10^8 genomic equivalents. In contrast, DNA from bacteria that were injected in a viable state is detectable by PCR for weeks. These data thus supported previous studies suggesting that PCR-positive but culture-negative effusions did indeed contain viable bacteria that were not readily cultured (or more likely, were not available for retrieval by lavage). Further, a subsequent report by this same group showing their ability to detect bacterial messenger RNA (which has a half-life measured in seconds to minutes) in culture-negative effusions by reverse transcriptase-PCR (RT-PCR) provided compelling evidence of the existence of metabolically active bacteria in these "sterile" effusions (170).

So the questions remaining were: Where are these viable microbes? Why are they not readily cultured from MEFs? In response, Garth Ehrlich, Chris Post, Bill Costerton, and their colleagues have recently put forth the hypothesis that OM is likely a true "biofilm disease" (49, 165, 166). Biofilms are by nature polymicrobial, they are inherently highly resistant to the action of antibodies and antimicrobials, and they are commonly associated with infections of a persistent nature (Color Plate 3 [see color insert]) (48, 49, 134, 169). This description fits well with that of chronic OM. Post et al. (166) have now demonstrated that a minimally passaged clinical isolate of NTHI can indeed make the transition between planktonic and sessile growth in the environment of the middle ear following transbullar inoculation of a chinchilla. This NTHI strain produced a biofilm on the mucosa lining of the middle ear as observed by scanning electron and confocal scanning laser microscopy (Color Plate 4 [see color insert]). This group continues to investigate the nature, mechanisms, and implications of biofilm production in the middle ear as a contributing factor to both the disease course as well as to the sequelae of OM.

The mechanisms by which biofilm communities resist antimicrobials and antibodies are replete (134); however, one mechanism that is likely to play a role in biofilm persistence in the middle ear is the ability of one microbe to confer antibiotic resistance to other members of the biofilm community because of their close physical association with one another. This phenomenon has been better studied for many of the classic quorum-sensing bacteria to date; however, Budhani et al. (28) showed that, when grown in a continuous culture biofilm system, β-lactamase production by *M. catarrhalis* protected *S. pneumoniae* from the action of exogenous β-lactam antibiotics. These microbes are clearly associated with infections of the middle ear and thus the data suggest how synergistic behavior in a mixed microbial biofilm such as this between *M. catarrhalis* and *S. pneumoniae* might lead to treatment failure in OM.

METHODS OF TREATMENT

We are continually adapting our treatment regimens for OM on the basis of newly acquired information and our improved understanding of the molecular mechanisms behind the pathogenesis of middle ear infections. Some of the ways this increased understanding has led to changes in our approaches to treat and/or prevent OM are reviewed below.

Use of Antimicrobials and Changing Treatment Paradigms

The prescribing of broad-spectrum antibiotics for OM, while still widely used as a treatment regimen, is no longer recommended for use prophylactically in otitis-prone children (73) because of the alarmingly rapid evolution of multiple-antibiotic-resistant bacteria in all three genera of bacteria responsible for OM (25, 56, 64, 65, 74, 84, 160, 172). Nevertheless, antibiotic use in children younger than age 15 for OM remains at a level that is more than 3 times that in any other age group (210). Moreover, approximately 40% of all antibiotic use in children younger than 5 years of age is for treatment of OM (34).

In addition to leading to the emergence of antibiotic resistant organisms, our treatment methods may actually be exacerbating the clinical course of OM. In a recent study by Dagan and colleagues (51), of 19 culture-positive patients in which an organism susceptible to the drug prescribed for treatment was isolated from the initial MEF (*H. influenzae, S. pneumoniae,* or both) but who also had a resistant *S. pneumoniae* strain in the NP, they showed that within a few days of treatment, the resistant NP organism had replaced the susceptible middle ear isolate in 47% of these patients. This phenomenon may constitute yet another important mechanism for bacterial superinfection of an ongoing case of OM that is already of mixed microbial etiology. Antibiotic treatment may also exacerbate inflammation in the middle ear. Kawana et al. (116) reported that penicillin treatment seems to augment inflammation in the middle ear during experimental pneumococcal OM

while effectively killing *S. pneumoniae*. Thus, decreasing antibiotic-induced bacterial lysis and the resulting accumulation of cell debris that leads to an increased inflammatory response, an approach that has been used in the treatment of bacterial meningitis, should perhaps be an additional goal for revised treatment paradigms for OM.

As a result of both this rapid emergence of multiple-antibiotic-resistant microbes and many reports that question the efficacy of *any* antibiotic treatment for chronic OM (50, 72, 214), there has been a call for a change in the overall treatment paradigm for OM (35, 57, 124, 159). Curtailed and more judicious use of antimicrobials for AOM (57), shorter courses of treatment when antibiotic use is warranted (47, 83, 124, 206), deferring antibiotic use in cases of OME or COM, and reserving the use of antibiotics prophylactically for only well-documented cases of recurrent AOM are all measures that have been advocated (35, 159).

Recent studies of 4,860 children in The Netherlands have shown that the vast majority of cases of AOM (>90%) can be managed with only nose drops and analgesics for the first 3 to 4 days. Thereafter, the minority of patients who do not show satisfactory recovery (4 to 5%) can be treated with antimicrobials. In fact guidelines issued by the Dutch College of General Practitioners for the treatment of AOM have recommended since 1990 that for patients 2 years of age or older, treatment should be for symptoms only for the first 3 days (83, 206). Thereafter, patients are reevaluated if symptoms continue and can be treated with a 7-day course of either amoxicillin or erythromycin when indicated. In children 6 months to 2 years of age, the treatment guidelines are the same, except that contact by phone or office visit is mandatory after 24 h. Any child in this latter age group who is acutely ill, or has not improved after 24 h with antimicrobials, is to be referred to an ear, nose, and throat specialist. In the above-cited study of 4,860 children, only two cases of antibiotic-responsive mastoiditis developed and there were no cases of bacterial meningitis; thus, concerns about the risk of serious complications occurring as a result of not treating AOM with antimicrobials appeared to be unfounded. While guidelines such as these may never be adopted globally, the Dutch experience is having an influence on how we think about antimicrobial use for OM. Further changes in treatment paradigms for OME and COM that include the use of antimicrobials may come about as a result of recent discussions about OM as a polybacterial biofilm disease.

Surgical Management of OM

Our increased understanding of the mixed microbial nature of OM as well as information suggesting biofilms involvement in COM also has implications for the surgical management of middle ear infections. For children with chronic or recurrent OM, tympanostomy tubes are often inserted through the tympanic membrane to reduce the symptoms of OM. These tubes do not prevent OM but rather relieve the pressure in the middle ear (and thus most of the painful symptoms of OM) created by the presence of pus and fluid in the middle ear cleft by draining these materials into the auditory canal. Tympanostomy tubes, however, may actually foster the chronicity of OM by providing an inert surface on which an antibiotic-resistant biofilm can form. Biofilms present in the lumen of tympanostomy tubes could serve as a constant source of bacterial cells that can invade the middle ear as well as provide a stimulus for the induction of inflammatory mediators in that site. Saidi et al. (178) recently used a guinea pig model of OM to assay the relative resistance of various silicone- or plastic-based tympanostomy tubes to the formation of a bacterial biofilm. All tympanostomy tubes tested, with the exception of an ion-bombarded silicone tube, showed an accumulated adherent bacterial biofilm by scanning electron microscopy. Thereby, how we design new, or select among available, indwelling devices such as tympanostomy tubes will likely be affected by the contribution of biofilms to the pathogenesis and sequelae of OM.

Treatment of Inflammation Associated with OM

Treatment of the inflammation associated with OM, by targeting the inflammatory mediators involved, has also been discussed as an alternative approach to medical management of OM. However, to date, little efficacy has been shown for decongestants, antihistamines, or specific prostaglandin inhibitors in this regard (30, 70, 112, 113, 135, 191). The use of steroids to ameliorate the inflammatory process in the middle ear has also been tried. Oral prednisolone is only modestly effective as an adjuvant therapy for cases of AOM that have associated discharge through tympanostomy tubes (173). In another study of 210 children with URT infection of 48 h duration or less, wherein half were treated with a placebo and half were treated for 7 days with fluticasone, AOM developed in 38.1% of children in the fluticasone group compared with 28.2% in the placebo group. In children with rhinovirus infection, however, AOM developed significantly more often in children treated with fluticasone (45.7%) than in the placebo group (14.7%). Thus, i.n. fluticasone propionate does not prevent AOM during viral URI in children and may actually *increase* the incidence of AOM during rhinovirus infection (174). Finally, since most of the proinflammatory cytokines elicited in OM serve as very early markers of infection of the middle ear, several investigators believe that intervention strategies that target these cytokines for pharmacological therapy are unlikely to be successful (140).

Use of Antiviral Agents and Viral Vaccines

Certainly one approach with a great likelihood of success, given the plethora of evidence demonstrating that without the URT viruses bacterial OM is unlikely to develop, is the prevention of OM by treating or immunizing against the viruses associated with bacterial middle ear infections. This could be accomplished by delivery of effective antiviral agents (89) or by vaccination (4, 82, 97). In studies conducted to date, whereas oral rimantadine treatment has not been found to reduce the otological manifestations of influenza in adults or children, i.n. zanamivir and oral oseltamivir were found to significantly reduce the middle ear pressure abnormalities associated with experimental influenza virus infection in adults (89, 90). Preliminary results from a study of oseltamivir treatment in children (171) suggest that this neuraminidase inhibitor also reduces the likelihood of influenza A virus-associated AOM. Other antiviral agents such as tremacamra (a recombinant soluble intercellular adhesion molecule, ICAM-1) (200), AG7088 (a 3C protease inhibitor) (199) or oral pleconaril (a capsid-binding agent) (199) have not been studied in children as effective therapies against OM; however, due to their efficacy in vitro and/or in clinical trials in adults, these studies appear warranted (89).

Some of the strongest evidence in support of both this approach and the critical role of the primary viral predisposing agent in bacterial OM has come as a result of data generated in clinical trials of influenza A virus vaccines. Three trials conducted to date have clearly shown that immunizing children against influenza A decreases the incidence of associated OM. A study conducted in Finland showed that of 187 vaccines, 1 to 3 years of age, and an identical number of matched controls, the incidence of AOM associated with influenza A virus was reduced by 83% in vaccinees (96). The total number of children in the vaccine group with AOM was 35 compared with 55 children in the control group, thus showing a 36% reduction among the vaccinees. Similarly, in a study conducted in eight day care centers in North Carolina with 186 children aged 6 to 30 months, Clements et al. (45) reported that episodes of both AOM and secretory OM were reduced by 32% and 28% in vaccinees, respectively (Tables 3 and 4). In a third study involving 288 children aged 15 to 71 months, receipt of a live, attenuated, cold-adapted, trivalent influenza A virus vaccine i.n. resulted in a vaccine efficacy of 93% against culture confirmed influenza (20). In this study, the vaccinated children also had 30% fewer episodes of febrile OM than the controls.

Despite these results and their predicted cost-effectiveness (132), widespread use of available influenza A vaccines in healthy children has not occurred. Nevertheless, many hope that the anticipated increased acceptability of the i.n. delivered influenza A vaccine will lead to broader use in the targeted pediatric population pending the resolution of a few remaining concerns regarding the safety of

TABLE 3 Demographic information on 186 participants in influenza-OM trial[a]

Characteristic	Group (no. of subjects)[b]					
	1 (94)	Non-1 (92)	2 (11)	3 (55)	4 (26)	Total
Males, %	45	51	36	55	50	89
Race, %						
White	91	83				163
Black	5	11				14
Other	4	6				9
Avg age at start, mo	20.2	19.3	25.7	18.4	18.1	19.7
Avg age past OM, mo	4.7[c]	3.5[c]	2.9	3.5	3.8	4.1
No. of myringotomy tubes						
At beginning	19	14				33
At end	25	22				47

[a] Reprinted from *Archives of Pediatric and Adolescent Medicine* (45) with permission of the publisher. Copyright 1995, American Medical Association.

[b] Group 1 was randomized to receive influenza vaccine, group 2 was randomized to receive hepatitis B vaccine, group 3 received ear examinations only by request of the parent, group 4 was randomized to receive ear examinations only, and group non-1 was not randomized to receive influenza vaccine.

[c] $P = 0.53$ (paired student t test), comparing group 1 with groups 2, 3, and 4 together.

TABLE 4 Percentage of infants with AOM and SOM infections before, during, and after influenza season[a]

Period studied	% of infants with infection in group[b]				
	1	Non-1	2	3	4
1 (before influenza season)					
AOM	28.0	22.8	27.3	16.4	34.6
SOM	45.2	40.2	36.4	34.5	53.8
2 (during influenza season)					
AOM	21.5[c]	36.4[c]	54.5	30.2	41.7
SOM	38.7[d]	53.4[d]	63.6	50.9	54.2
3 (after influenza season)					
AOM	24.7	16.5	18.2	13.5	22.7
SOM	30.3	27.1	36.4	25.0	27.3

[a] Reprinted from *Archives of Pediatric and Adolescent Medicine* (45) with permission of the publisher. Copyright 1995, American Medical Association. SOM, serous OM.
[b] Groups are defined in Table 1.
[c] $P = 0.02$ (OR = 0.47, 95%, CI 0.24–0.91), χ^2 statistic.
[d] $P = 0.04$ (OR = 0.54, 95% CI 0.29–0.97), χ^2 statistic.

delivery of a live vaccine such as this to infants and toddlers. Finally, passive transfer of human immune globulin, enriched with RSV-neutralizing antibodies (RSVIG), has also been shown to confer protection against AOM (186). Children that received high doses of RSVIG developed significantly fewer episodes of AOM than controls. Thus, immunization against the URT viral pathogens that predispose to bacterial OM promises to have a significant impact on the incidence of OM. However, developing effective vaccines for all of the URT viruses predominantly associated with bacterial OM and doing so for a pediatric population (185, 205) are not without many remaining challenges (4, 77).

Use of Vaccines That Target the Bacterial Pathogens of OM

Another approach that is being actively developed in many laboratories is an attempt to immunize (either parenterally or via a mucosal route) against the bacterial pathogens of OM (53, 71, 77, 115, 125, 127, 141, 164). Although many investigators favor the development of mucosal delivery routes for vaccines that target diseases of the upper airway (148), including OM (114, 116, 120), this approach has not yet been fully developed for pediatric

diseases to date. This is largely due to some remaining obstacles such as the substantial dilution phenomenon that occurs in the gastrointestinal tract for orally delivered immunogens; the need for mucosally delivered vaccines to be in a particulate form to foster uptake by M cells; the need to protect orally delivered immunogens to ensure their transit through the gut; and when involving replicating agents, overcoming the perceived potential inherent risks, among others (203). Nevertheless, many investigators are working on methods to bypass each of these obstacles for development of mucosally delivered vaccines; this approach may ultimately prove to be the most efficacious for prevention of OM.

In the meantime, however, vaccine candidates designed for a more traditional parenteral delivery route have been or are being developed. These too have a tremendous likelihood of success given that the track record to date for using this approach to prevent other infectious diseases of the respiratory tract has been extremely good. A review of the efficacy of many licensed vaccines currently in use and their ability to act, often via the induction of "herd immunity," is beyond the scope of this chapter; however, Underdown and Plotkin (203) provide an excellent review of the topic. With

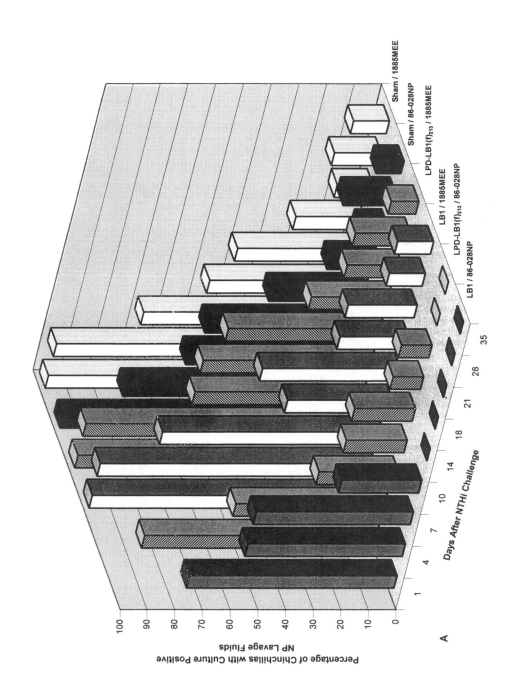

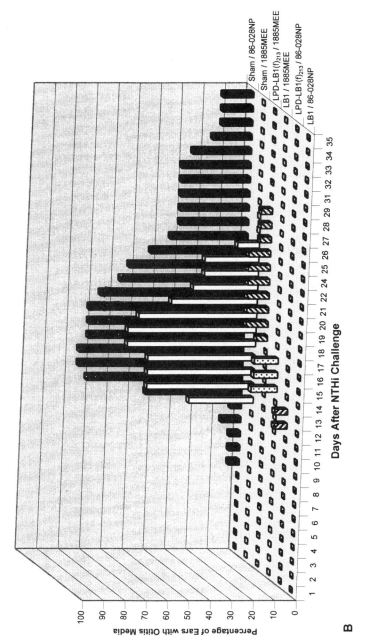

FIGURE 13 (A) Percentage of nasal lavage specimens that were culture positive for NTHI in AV-compromised chinchillas that received either saline (sham-immunized) or antisera directed against one of two adhesin-based immunogens [LB1 or LPD-LB1 (f)$_{2,1,3}$] by passive transfer prior to i.n. challenge with either of two strains of NTHI (86-028NP or 1885MEE). (B) Percentage of ears that developed OM within each cohort of animals depicted in A. (Both panels are reprinted from *Infection and Immunity* [117] with permission of the publisher.)

the goal of preventing OM, the parenteral immunization approach could actually utilize the polymicrobial etiology of OM to its advantage, particularly with regard to the predisposing viral infection-induced inflammation. Serum antibodies transude onto the surface of mucous membranes (15, 68, 158), including into the microenvironment of the middle ear (15, 68) and the NP (203). This transudation of serum components is particularly notable during inflammation. Since viral URT infections typically precede ascending bacterial infection of the middle ear, we can take advantage of the associated inflammation to promote the transudation of specific and protective antibodies (induced by immunization) onto the mucosal surface of the NP, thereby helping to eradicate or reduce the colonizing bacterial load. Antibodies that transude into the middle ear cleft could also be potentially instrumental in eradicating the typically low infecting dose of bacteria that might initially gain access to the middle ear before multiplying to the much higher concentrations that exist in active disease.

This approach has shown tremendous promise in chinchilla models (16, 117) wherein the incidence and severity of OM induced upon challenge with any of several isolates of NTHI could be significantly reduced or eliminated completely by immunization against colonization of the NP using vaccine candidates designed after one of several known NTHI adhesins (Fig. 13). We found that early eradication of NTHI from the NP or even reduction of the bacterial load in that anatomic site by several logs was associated with significant protection against development of OM. Whether or not similar protective efficacy will be induced in children with use of a parenteral approach to target NTHI-induced OM remains to be shown. In this regard, the recent approval and recommendation for use of a polyvalent pneumococcal capsular conjugate vaccine is encouraging. This parenterally delivered heptavalent conjugate vaccine was approximately 97% effective against invasive disease but was also associated with a 6 to 7% reduction in number of episodes of AOM in

vaccine recipients compared with controls (22, 62). In a follow up study, efficacy against OM caused by vaccine serotypes of *S. pneumoniae* was 57% (22, 62).

SUMMARY AND CONCLUSION

It is now widely accepted that many of the URT viruses play a pivotal role in predisposing to infections of the middle ear by either one or more of the three primary bacterial pathogens of OM. The mechanisms by which the viruses mediate their synergistic effect are replete; however, the common theme is compromise or dysregulation of protective functions of the host airway. Many of the methods we have developed to date to medically and/or surgically manage acute and chronic infections of the middle ear have inadvertently contributed to the persistence and recurrence of these infections due to both our lack of complete understanding of the disease process and the incredible adaptability of the microorganisms involved. However, many of these methods have heretofore not necessarily taken into account the polymicrobial nature of the disease, an understanding that is dramatically changing the way that we are currently approaching novel treatment and/or prevention methodologies for OM.

Good clinical evidence exists to believe that by eradicating the predisposing viral infection, one could have a significant effect on prevention of bacterial OM. This goal will not be accomplished easily because of the number of potential viral agents involved, in addition to many other inherent difficulties associated with developing effective viral vaccines; however, progress is clearly being made. Direct blockade of viral attachment and/or uptake via the use of specific antiviral agents is another goal, as is the approach of developing vaccines that target the bacterial commensals residing in the pediatric NP and thus essentially attempting to immunize against colonization. The recent suggestion that the microbes responsible for OM might be inducing the formation of biofilms that are likely to be polybacterial in nature further emphasizes the need to develop novel treatment regimens and vaccines to prevent OM. Vaccine or treatment strategies that effectively inhibit the initial establishment of infection in the middle ear cleft will be particularly important in this regard.

REFERENCES

1. **Abramson, J. S., G. S. Giebink, E. L. Mills, and P. G. Quie.** 1981. Polymorphonuclear leukocyte dysfunction during influenza virus infection in chinchillas. *J. Infect. Dis.* **143:**836–845.
2. **Abramson, J. S., and J. G. Wheeler.** 1994. Virus-induced neutrophil dysfunction: role in the pathogenesis of bacterial infections. *Pediatr. Infect. Dis. J.* **13:**643–652.
3. **Alsarraf, R., C. J. Jung, J. Perkins, C. Crowley, N. W. Alsarraf, and G. A. Gates.** 1999. Measuring the indirect and direct costs of acute otitis media. *Arch. Otolaryngol. Head Neck Surg.* **125:**12–18.
4. **Anderson, L. J.** 2000. Respiratory syncytial virus vaccines for otitis media. *Vaccine* **19**(Suppl. 1):S59–S65.
5. **Arola, M., O. Ruuskanen, T. Ziegler, J. Mertsola, K. Nanto-Salonen, A. Putto-Laurila, M. K. Viljanen, and P. Halonen.** 1990. Clinical role of respiratory virus infection in acute otitis media. *Pediatrics.* **86:**848–855.
6. **Arola, M., T. Ziegler, H. Puhakka, O. P. Lehtonen, and O. Ruuskanen.** 1990. Rhinovirus in otitis media with effusion. *Ann. Otol. Rhinol. Laryngol.* **99:**451–453.
7. **Arola, M., T. Ziegler, and O. Ruuskanen.** 1990. Respiratory virus infection as a cause of prolonged symptoms in acute otitis media. *J. Pediatr.* **116:**697–701.
8. **Arva, E., and B. Andersson.** 1999. Induction of phagocyte-stimulating and Th1-promoting cytokines by *in vitro* stimulation of human peripheral blood mononuclear cells with *Streptococcus pneumoniae.* *Scand. J. Immunol.* **49:**417–423.
9. **Arva, E., and B. Andersson.** 1999. Induction of phagocyte-stimulating cytokines by *in vitro* stimulation of human peripheral blood mononuclear cells with *Haemophilus influenzae.* *Scand. J. Immunol.* **49:**411–416.
10. **Aul, J. J., K. W. Anderson, R. M. Wadowsky, W. J. Doyle, L. A. Kingsley, J. C. Post, and G. D. Ehrlich.** 1998. Comparative evaluation of culture and PCR for the detection and determination of persistence of bacterial strains and DNAs in the *Chinchilla laniger* model of otitis media. *Ann. Otol. Rhinol. Laryngol.* **107:** 508–513.
11. **Bakaletz, L., S. R. Griffith, and D. J. Lim.** 1988. Effect of prostaglandin E2 and bacterial endotoxin on the rate of dye transport in the chinchilla eustachian tube, p. 99–102. *In* D. J. Lim, C. D. Bluestone, J. O. Klein, and J. D. Nelson (ed.), *Proceedings of the Fourth International Symposium on Recent Advances in Otitis Media.* B. C. Decker Inc., Toronto, Ontario, Canada.
12. **Bakaletz, L. O.** 1995. Viral potentiation of bacterial superinfection of the respiratory tract. *Trends Microbiol.* **3:**110–114.
13. **Bakaletz, L. O., R. L. Daniels, and D. J. Lim.** 1993. Modeling adenovirus type 1-induced otitis media in the chinchilla: effect on ciliary activity and fluid transport function of eustachian tube mucosal epithelium. *J. Infect. Dis.* **168:**865–872. (Erratum, **168:**1605, 1993.)
14. **Bakaletz, L. O., T. M. Hoepf, T. F. DeMaria, and D. J. Lim.** 1988. The effect of antecedent influenza A virus infection on the adherence of *Hemophilus influenzae* to chinchilla tracheal epithelium. *Am. J. Otolaryngol.* **9:**127–134.
15. **Bakaletz, L. O., and K. A. Holmes.** 1997. Evidence for transudation of specific antibody into the middle ears of parenterally immunized chinchillas after an upper respiratory tract infection with adenovirus. *Clin. Diagn. Lab. Immunol.* **4:**223–225.
16. **Bakaletz, L. O., B. J. Kennedy, L. A. Novotny, G. Dequesne, J. Cohen, and Y. Lobet.** 1999. Protection against development of otitis media induced by nontypeable *Haemophilus influenzae* by both active and passive immunization in a chinchilla model of virus-bacterium superinfection. *Infect. Immun.* **67:**2746–2762.
17. **Bakaletz, L. O., D. M. Murwin, and J. M. Billy.** 1995. Adenovirus serotype 1 does not act synergistically with *Moraxella (Branhamella) catarrhalis* to induce otitis media in the chinchilla. *Infect. Immun.* **63:**4188–4190.
18. **Bakaletz, L. O., G. J. White, J. C. Post, and G. D. Ehrlich.** 1998. Blinded multiplex PCR analyses of middle ear and nasopharyngeal fluids from chinchilla models of single- and mixed-pathogen-induced otitis media. *Clin. Diagn. Lab. Immunol.* **5:**219–224.
19. **Baldwin, R. L.** 1993. Effects of otitis media on child development. *Am. J. Otol.* **14:**601–604.
20. **Belshe, R. B., P. M. Mendelman, J. Treanor, J. King, W. C. Gruber, P. Piedra, D. I. Bernstein, F. G. Hayden, K. Kotloff, K. Zangwill, D. Iacuzio, and M. Wolff.** 1998. The efficacy of live attenuated, cold-adapted, trivalent, intranasal influenza virus vaccine in children. *N. Engl. J. Med.* **338:**1405–1412.
21. **Berman, S., R. Roark, and D. Luckey.** 1994. Theoretical cost effectiveness of management options for children with persisting middle ear effusions. *Pediatrics* **93:**353–363.
22. **Black, S., H. Shinefield, B. Fireman, E. Lewis, P. Ray, J. R. Hansen, L. Elvin, K. M. Ensor, J. Hackell, G. Siber, F. Malinoski, D.**

Madore, I. Chang, R. Kohberger, W. Watson, R. Austrian, K. Edwards, and the Northern California Kaiser Permanente Vaccine Study Center Group. 2000. Efficacy, safety and immunogenicity of heptavalent pneumococcal conjugate vaccine in children. *Pediatr. Infect. Dis. J.* **19**:187–195.

23. Bluestone, C. D. 1996. Pathogenesis of otitis media: role of eustachian tube. *Pediatr. Infect. Dis. J.* **15**:281–291.

24. Bright, R. A., R. M. Moore, Jr., L. L. Jeng, C. M. Sharkness, S. E. Hamburger, and P. M. Hamilton. 1993. The prevalence of tympanostomy tubes in children in the United States, 1988. *Am. J. Public Health* **83**:1026–1028.

25. Brook, I., and A. E. Gober. 1999. Resistance to antimicrobials used for therapy of otitis media and sinusitis: effect of previous antimicrobial therapy and smoking. *Ann. Otol. Rhinol. Laryngol.* **108**:645–647.

26. Buchman, C. A., W. J. Doyle, D. Skoner, P. Fireman, and J. M. Gwaltney. 1994. Otologic manifestations of experimental rhinovirus infection. *Laryngoscope* **104**:1295–1299.

27. Buchman, C. A., W. J. Doyle, D. P. Skoner, J. C. Post, C. M. Alper, J. T. Seroky, K. Anderson, R. A. Preston, F. G. Hayden, P. Fireman, et al. 1995. Influenza A virus-induced acute otitis media. *J. Infect. Dis.* **172**:1348–1351.

28. Budhani, R. K., and J. K. Struthers. 1998. Interaction of *Streptococcus pneumoniae* and *Moraxella catarrhalis*: investigation of the indirect pathogenic role of beta-lactamase-producing moraxellae by use of a continuous-culture biofilm system. *Antimicrob. Agents Chemother.* **42**: 2521–2526.

29. Canafax, D. M., Z. Yuan, T. Chonmaitree, K. Deka, H. Q. Russlie, and G. S. Giebink. 1998. Amoxicillin middle ear fluid penetration and pharmacokinetics in children with acute otitis media. *Pediatr. Infect. Dis. J.* **17**:149–156.

30. Cantekin, E. I., E. M. Mandel, C. D. Bluestone, H. E. Rockette, J. L. Paradise, S. E. Stool, T. J. Fria, and K. D. Rogers. 1983. Lack of efficacy of a decongestant-antihistamine combination for otitis media with effusion ("secretory" otitis media) in children. Results of a double-blind, randomized trial. *N. Engl. J. Med.* **308**:297–301.

31. Carson, J. L., A. M. Collier, and S. S. Hu. 1985. Acquired ciliary defects in nasal epithelium of children with acute viral upper respiratory infections. *N. Engl. J. Med.* **312**:463–468.

32. Casselbrant, M. L., E. M. Mandel, P. A. Fall, H. E. Rockette, M. Kurs-Lasky, C. D. Bluestone, and R. E. Ferrell. 1999. The heritability of otitis media: a twin and triplet study. *JAMA* **282**:2125–2130.

33. Cassell, G. H. 1997. *New and Reemerging Infectious Diseases: a Global Crisis and Immediate Threat to the Nation's Health: the Role of Research.* American Society for Microbiology, Washington, D.C.

34. Cassell, G. H., G. L. Archer, T. R. Beam, M. J. Gilchrist, D. Goldmann, D. C. Hooper, R. N. Jones, S. H. Kleven, J. Lederberg, S. B. Levy, D. H. Lein, R. C. Moellering, T. F. O'Brien, B. Osburn, M. Osterholm, D. M. Shlaes, M. Terry, S. A. Tolin, and A. Tomasz. 1994. *Report of the ASM Task Force on Antibiotic Resistance.* American Society for Microbiology, Washington, D.C.

35. Chartrand, S. A., and A. Pong. 1998. Acute otitis media in the 1990s: the impact of antibiotic resistance. *Pediatr. Ann.* **27**:86–95.

36. Chonmaitree, T., V. M. Howie, and A. L. Truant. 1986. Presence of respiratory viruses in middle ear fluids and nasal wash specimens from children with acute otitis media. *Pediatrics* **77**: 698–702.

37. Chonmaitree, T., M. J. Owen, and V. M. Howie. 1990. Respiratory viruses interfere with bacteriologic response to antibiotic in children with acute otitis media. *J. Infect. Dis.* **162**:546–549.

38. Chonmaitree, T., M. J. Owen, J. A. Patel, D. Hedgpeth, D. Horlick, and V. M. Howie. 1992. Effect of viral respiratory tract infection on outcome of acute otitis media. *J. Pediatr.* **120**:856–862.

39. Chonmaitree, T., M. J. Owen, J. A. Patel, D. Hedgpeth, D. Horlick, and V. M. Howie. 1992. Presence of cytomegalovirus and herpes simplex virus in middle ear fluids from children with acute otitis media. *Clin. Infect. Dis.* **15**:650–653.

40. Chonmaitree, T., J. A. Patel, M. A. Lett-Brown, T. Uchida, R. Garofalo, M. J. Owen, and V. M. Howie. 1994. Virus and bacteria enhance histamine production in middle ear fluids of children with acute otitis media. *J. Infect. Dis.* **169**:1265–1270.

41. Chonmaitree, T., J. A. Patel, T. Sim, R. Garofalo, T. Uchida, V. M. Howie, and M. J. Owen. 1996. Role of leukotriene B4 and interleukin-8 in acute bacterial and viral otitis media. *Ann. Otol. Rhinol. Laryngol.* **105**:968–974.

42. Chung, M. H., R. Enrique, D. J. Lim, and T. F. De Maria. 1994. *Moraxella (Branhamella) catarrhalis*-induced experimental otitis media in the chinchilla. *Acta Otolaryngol.* **114**:415–422.

43. Chung, M. H., S. R. Griffith, K. H. Park, D. J. Lim, and T. F. DeMaria. 1993. Cytological and histological changes in the middle ear after inoculation of influenza A virus. *Acta Otolaryngol.* (Stockholm) **113**:81–87.

44. Clemans, D. J., R. J. Bauer, J. A. Hanson, M. V. Hobbs, J. W. St. Geme III, C. F. Marrs, and J. R. Gilsdorf. 2000. Induction of proinflammatory cytokines from human respiratory epithelial cells after stimulation by nontypeable *Haemophilus influenzae*. *Infect. Immun.* 68:4430–4440.

45. Clements, D. A., L. Langdon, C. Bland, and E. Walter. 1995. Influenza A vaccine decreases the incidence of otitis media in 6- to 30- month-old children in day care. *Arch. Pediatr. Adolesc. Med.* 149:1113–1117.

46. Cohen, R., E. Bingen, E. Varon, F. de La Rocque, N. Brahimi, C. Levy, M. Boucherat, J. Langue, and P. Geslin. 1997. Change in nasopharyngeal carriage of *Streptococcus pneumoniae* resulting from antibiotic therapy for acute otitis media in children. *Pediatr. Infect. Dis. J.* 16:555–560.

47. Cohen, R., C. Levy, M. Boucherat, J. Langue, E. Autret, P. Gehanno, and F. de La Rocque. 2000. Five vs. ten days of antibiotic therapy for acute otitis media in young children. *Pediatr. Infect. Dis. J.* 19:458–463.

48. Costerton, J. W. 1999. Introduction to biofilm. *Int. J. Antimicrob. Agents* 11:217–221, 237–239.

49. Costerton, J. W., P. S. Stewart, and E. P. Greenberg. 1999. Bacterial biofilms: a common cause of persistent infections. *Science* 284:1318–1322.

50. Culpepper, L., and J. Froom. 1997. Routine antimicrobial treatment of acute otitis media: is it necessary? *JAMA* 278:1643–1645.

51. Dagan, R., E. Leibovitz, G. Cheletz, A. Leiberman, and N. Porat. 2001. Antibiotic treatment in acute otitis media promotes superinfection with resistant *Streptococcus pneumoniae* carried before initiation of treatment. *J. Infect. Dis.* 183:880–886.

52. Daly, K. A., J. E. Brown, B. R. Lindgren, M. H. Meland, C. T. Le, and G. S. Giebink. 1999. Epidemiology of otitis media onset by six months of age. *Pediatrics* 103:1158–1166.

53. De, B. K., J. S. Sampson, E. W. Ades, R. C. Huebner, D. L. Jue, S. E. Johnson, M. Espina, A. R. Stinson, D. E. Briles, and G. M. Carlone. 2000. Purification and characterization of *Streptococcus pneumoniae* palmitoylated pneumococcal surface adhesin A expressed in *Escherichia coli*. *Vaccine* 18:1811–1821.

54. DeMaria, T. F. 1989. Animal models for nontypable *Haemophilus influenzae* otitis media. *Pediatr. Infect. Dis. J.* 8:S40–S42.

55. DeMaria, T. F., J. M. Billy, and D. G. Danahey. 1996. Growth factors during endotoxin-induced otitis media. *Acta Otolaryngol. (Stockholm)* 116:854–856.

56. Derecola, A., D. L. Butler, R. L. Kaplan, L. A. Miller, and J. A. Poupard. 1999. A 5-year surveillance study of 44,691 isolates of *Haemophilus influenzae* project Beta-Alert 1993–1997. *Antimicrob. Agents Chemother.* 43:185–186.

57. Dowell, S. F., S. M. Marcy, W. R. Phillips, M. A. Gerber, and B. Schwartz. 1998. Otitis media: principles of judicious use of antimicrobial agents. *Pediatrics* 101:165–171.

58. Doyle, W. J. 1989. Animal models of otitis media: other pathogens. *Pediatr. Infect. Dis. J.* 8:S45–S47.

59. Doyle, W. J., D. P. Skoner, F. Hayden, C. A. Buchman, J. T. Seroky, and P. Fireman. 1994. Nasal and otologic effects of experimental influenza A virus infection. *Ann. Otol. Rhinol. Laryngol.* 103:59–69.

60. Doyle, W. J., D. P. Skoner, M. White, F. Hayden, A. P. Kaplan, M. A. Kaliner, Y. Shibayama, and P. Fireman. 1996. Pattern of nasal secretions during experimental influenza virus infection. *Rhinology* 34:2–8.

61. El Ahmer, O. R., M. W. Raza, M. M. Ogilvie, D. M. Weir, and C. C. Blackwell. 1999. Binding of bacteria to HEp-2 cells infected with influenza A virus. *FEMS Immunol. Med. Microbiol.* 23:331–341.

62. Eskola, J., T. Kilpi, A. Palmu, J. Jokinen, J. Haapakoski, E. Herva, A. Takala, H. Kayhty, P. Karma, R. Kohberger, G. Siber, and P. H. Makela. 2001. Efficacy of a pneumococcal conjugate vaccine against acute otitis media. *N. Engl. J. Med.* 344:403–409.

63. Faden, H. 2001. The microbiologic and immunologic basis for recurrent otitis media in children. *Eur J Pediatr.* 160:407–413.

64. Faden, H., J. Bernstein, L. Brodsky, J. Stanievich, and P. L. Ogra. 1992. Effect of prior antibiotic treatment on middle ear disease in children. *Ann. Otol. Rhinol. Laryngol.* 101:87–91.

65. Faden, H., G. Doern, J. Wolf, and M. Blocker. 1994. Antimicrobial susceptibility of nasopharyngeal isolates of potential pathogens recovered from infants before antibiotic therapy: implications for the management of otitis media. *Pediatr. Infect. Dis. J.* 13:609–612.

66. Faden, H., L. Duffy, R. Wasielewski, J. Wolf, D. Krystofik, Y. Tung, and Tonawanda/Williamsville Pediatrics. 1997. Relationship between nasopharyngeal colonization and the development of otitis media in children. *J. Infect. Dis.* 175:1440–1445.

67. Faden, H., L. Duffy, A. Williams, D. A. Krystofik, and J. Wolf. 1995. Epidemiology of nasopharyngeal colonization with nontypeable *Haemophilus influenzae* in the first 2 years of life. *J. Infect. Dis.* 172:132–135.

68. **Faden, H. S.** 1997. Immunology of the middle ear: role of local and systemic antibodies in clearance of viruses and bacteria. *Ann. N. Y. Acad. Sci.* **830:**49–60.

69. **Fainstein, V., D. M. Musher, and T. R. Cate.** 1980. Bacterial adherence to pharyngeal cells during viral infection. *J. Infect. Dis.* **141:** 172–176.

70. **Fireman, P.** 1990. The role of antihistamines in otitis. *J. Allergy Clin. Immunol.* **86:**638–641.

71. **Foxwell, A. R., J. M. Kyd, and A. W. Cripps.** 1998. Nontypeable *Haemophilus influenzae:* pathogenesis and prevention. *Microbiol. Mol. Biol. Rev.* **62:**294–308.

72. **Froom, J., L. Culpepper, M. Jacobs, R. A. DeMelker, L. A. Green, L. van Buchem, P. Grob, and T. Heeren.** 1997. Antimicrobials for acute otitis media? A review from the International Primary Care Network. *BMJ* **315:**98–102.

73. **Gates, G. A.** 1999. Otitis media: the pharyngeal connection. *JAMA* **282:**987–989.

74. **Gazagne, L., C. Delmas, E. Bingen, and H. Dabernat.** 1998. Molecular epidemiology of ampicillin-resistant non-beta-lactamase-producing *Haemophilus influenzae. J. Clin. Microbiol.* **36:** 3629–3635.

75. **Gentile, D., W. Doyle, T. Whiteside, P. Fireman, F. G. Hayden, and D. Skoner.** 1998. Increased interleukin-6 levels in nasal lavage samples following experimental influenza A virus infection. *Clin. Diagn. Lab. Immunol.* **5:** 604–608.

76. **Giebink, G. S.** 1989. The microbiology of otitis media. *Pediatr. Infect. Dis. J.* **8:**S18–S20.

77. **Giebink, G. S.** 1997. Vaccination against middle-ear bacterial and viral pathogens. *Ann. N. Y. Acad. Sci.* **830:**330–352.

78. **Giebink, G. S., I. K. Berzins, S. C. Marker, and G. Schiffman.** 1980. Experimental otitis media after nasal inoculation of *Streptococcus pneumoniae* and influenza A virus in chinchillas. *Infect. Immun.* **30:**445–450.

79. **Giebink, G. S., E. L. Mills, J. S. Huff, K. L. Cates, S. K. Juhn, and P. G. Quie.** 1979. Polymorphonuclear leukocyte dysfunction in children with recurrent otitis media. *J. Pediatr.* **94:** 13–18.

80. **Giebink, G. S., M. L. Ripley, and P. F. Wright.** 1987. Eustachian tube histopathology during experimental influenza A virus infection in the chinchilla. *Ann. Otol. Rhinol. Laryngol.* **96:** 199–206.

81. **Giebink, G. S., and P. F. Wright.** 1983. Different virulence of influenza A virus strains and susceptibility to pneumococcal otitis media in chinchillas. *Infect. Immun.* **41:**913–920.

82. **Glezen, W. P.** 2000. Prevention of acute otitis media by prophylaxis and treatment of influenza virus infections. *Vaccine* **19**(Suppl. 1):S56–S58.

83. **Gooch, W. M., 3rd, E. Blair, A. Puopolo, R. Z. Paster, R. H. Schwartz, H. C. Miller, H. L. Smyre, R. Yetman, G. G. Giguere, and J. J. Collins.** 1996. Effectiveness of five days of therapy with cefuroxime axetil suspension for treatment of acute otitis media. *Pediatr. Infect. Dis. J.* **15:**157–164.

84. **Green, M., and Wald, E. R.** 1996. Emerging resistance to antibiotics: impact on respiratory infections in the outpatient setting. *Ann. Allergy Asthma Immunol.* **77:**167–173.

85. **Gwaltney, J. M., Jr.** 1971. Virology of middle ear. *Ann. Otol. Rhinol. Laryngol.* **80:**365–370.

86. **Hakansson, A., A. Kidd, G. Wadell, H. Sabharwal, and C. Svanborg.** 1994. Adenovirus infection enhances in vitro adherence of *Streptococcus pneumoniae. Infect. Immun.* **62:**2707–2714.

87. **Hament, J. M., J. L. Kimpen, A. Fleer, and T. F. Wolfs.** 1999. Respiratory viral infection predisposing for bacterial disease: a concise review. *FEMS Immunol. Med. Microbiol.* **26:**189–195.

88. **Harsten, G., K. Prellner, B. Lofgren, and O. Kalm.** 1991. Serum antibodies against respiratory tract viruses in episodes of acute otitis media. *J. Laryngol. Otol.* **105:**337–340.

89. **Hayden, F. G.** 2000. Influenza virus and rhinovirus-related otitis media: potential for antiviral intervention. *Vaccine* **19**(Suppl. 1):S66–S70.

90. **Hayden, F. G., J. J. Treanor, R. S. Fritz, M. Lobo, R. F. Betts, M. Miller, N. Kinnersley, R. G. Mills, P. Ward, and S. E. Straus.** 1999. Use of the oral neuraminidase inhibitor oseltamivir in experimental human influenza: randomized controlled trials for prevention and treatment. *JAMA* **282:**1240–1246.

91. **Heikkinen, T.** 2000. The role of respiratory viruses in otitis media. *Vaccine* **19**(Suppl. 1): S51–S55.

92. **Heikkinen, T.** 2000. Role of viruses in the pathogenesis of acute otitis media. *Pediatr. Infect. Dis. J.* **19:**S17–S22, S22–S23.

93. **Heikkinen, T.** 1994. Temporal development of acute otitis media during upper respiratory tract infection. *Pediatr. Infect. Dis. J.* **13:**659–661.

94. **Heikkinen, T., and T. Chonmaitree.** 2000. Viral-bacterial synergy in otitis media: implications for management. *Curr. Infect. Dis. Rep.* **2:**154–159.

95. **Heikkinen, T., F. Ghaffar, A. O. Okorodudu, and T. Chonmaitree.** 1998. Serum interleukin-6 in bacterial and nonbacterial acute otitis media. *Pediatrics* **102:**296–299.

96. **Heikkinen, T., O. Ruuskanen, M. Waris, T. Ziegler, M. Arola, and P. Halonen.** 1991. Influenza vaccination in the prevention of acute otitis media in children. *Am. J. Dis. Child.* **145:** 445–448.

97. **Heikkinen, T., M. Thint, and T. Chonmaitree.** 1999. Prevalence of various respiratory viruses in the middle ear during acute otitis media. *N. Engl. J. Med.* **340:**260–264.

98. **Henderson, F. W., A. M. Collier, M. A. Sanyal, J. M. Watkins, D. L. Fairclough, W. A. Clyde, Jr., and F. W. Denny.** 1982. A longitudinal study of respiratory viruses and bacteria in the etiology of acute otitis media with effusion. *N. Engl. J. Med.* **306:**1377–1383.

99. **Hendolin, P. H., A. Markkanen, J. Ylikoski, and J. J. Wahlfors.** 1997. Use of multiplex PCR for simultaneous detection of four bacterial species in middle ear effusions. *J. Clin. Microbiol.* **35:**2854–2858.

100. **Hendolin, P. H., L. Paulin, and J. Ylikoski.** 2000. Clinically applicable multiplex PCR for four middle ear pathogens. *J. Clin. Microbiol.* **38:** 125–132.

101. **Hirano, T., Y. Kurono, I. Ichimiya, M. Suzuki, and G. Mogi.** 1999. Effects of influenza A virus on lectin-binding patterns in murine nasopharyngeal mucosa and on bacterial colonization. *Otolaryngol. Head Neck Surg.* **121:** 616–621.

102. **Hotomi, M., T. Tabata, H. Kakiuchi, and M. Kunimoto.** 1993. Detection of *Haemophilus influenzae* in middle ear of otitis media with effusion by polymerase chain reaction. *Int. J. Pediatr. Otorhinolaryngol.* **27:**119–126.

103. **Hu, W. G., J. Chen, F. M. Collins, and X. X. Gu.** 1999. An aerosol challenge mouse model for *Moraxella catarrhalis. Vaccine* **18:**799–804.

104. **Hunter, L. L., R. H. Margolis, and G. S. Giebink.** 1994. Identification of hearing loss in children with otitis media. *Ann. Otol. Rhinol. Laryngol. Suppl.* **163:**59–61.

105. **Infante-Rivard, C., and A. Fernandez.** 1993. Otitis media in children: frequency, risk factors, and research avenues. *Epidemiol. Rev.* **15:** 444–465.

106. **Jakab, G. J.** 1982. Viral-bacterial interactions in pulmonary infection. *Adv. Vet. Sci. Comp. Med.* **26:**155–171.

107. **Jero, J., and P. Karma.** 1997. Bacteriological findings and persistence of middle ear effusion in otitis media with effusion. *Acta Oto-Laryngol. Suppl.* **529:**22–66.

108. **Jiang, Z., N. Nagata, E. Molina, L. O. Bakaletz, H. Hawkins, and J. A. Patel.** 1999. Fimbria-mediated enhanced attachment of nontypeable *Haemophilus influenzae* to respiratory syncytial virus-infected respiratory epithelial cells. *Infect. Immun.* **67:**187–192.

109. **Johnson, I. J., T. Brooks, D. A. Hutton, J. P. Birchall, and J. P. Pearson.** 1997. Compositional differences between bilateral middle ear effusions in otitis media with effusion: evidence for a different etiology? *Laryngoscope* **107:** 684–689.

110. **Johnson, M., G. Leonard, and D. L. Kreutzer.** 1997. Murine model of interleukin-8-induced otitis media. *Laryngoscope* **107:**1405–1408.

111. **Jossart, G. H., D. M. Canafax, G. R. Erdmann, M. J. Lovdahl, H. Q. Russlie, S. K. Juhn, and G. S. Giebink.** 1994. Effect of *Streptococcus pneumoniae* and influenza A virus on middle ear antimicrobial pharmacokinetics in experimental otitis media. *Pharm. Res.* **11:** 860–864.

112. **Jung, T. T.** 1988. Arachidonic acid metabolites in otitis media pathogenesis. *Ann. Otol. Rhinol. Laryngol.* **132**(Suppl.):14–18.

113. **Jung, T. T., D. M. Smith, S. K. Juhn, and J. M. Gerrard.** 1980. Effect of prostaglandin on the composition of chinchilla middle ear effusion. *Ann. Otol. Rhinol. Laryngol.* **89**(Suppl.): 153–160.

114. **Kaplan, B., T. L. Wandstrat, and J. R. Cunningham.** 1997. Overall cost in the treatment of otitis media. *Pediatr. Infect. Dis. J.* **16:** S9–S11.

115. **Karalus, R., and A. Campagnari.** 2000. *Moraxella catarrhalis:* a review of an important human mucosal pathogen. *Microb. Infect.* **2:**547–559.

116. **Kawana, M., C. Kawana, and G. S. Giebink.** 1992. Penicillin treatment accelerates middle ear inflammation in experimental pneumococcal otitis media. *Infect. Immun.* **60:** 1908–1912.

117. **Kennedy, B. J., L. A. Novotny, J. A. Jurcisek, Y. Lobet, and L. O. Bakaletz.** 2000. Passive transfer of antiserum specific for immunogens derived from a nontypeable *Haemophilus influenzae* adhesin and lipoprotein D prevents otitis media after heterologous challenge. *Infect. Immun.* **68:**2756–2765.

118. **Klein, B. S., F. R. Dollete, and R. H. Yolken.** 1982. The role of respiratory syncytial virus and other viral pathogens in acute otitis media. *J. Pediatr.* **101:**16–20.

119. **Klein, J. O., and D. W. Teele.** 1976. Isolation of viruses and mycoplasmas from middle ear effusions: a review. *Ann. Otol. Rhinol. Laryngol.* **85:**140–144.

120. **Kodama, S., S. Suenaga, T. Hirano, M. Suzuki, and G. Mogi.** 2000. Induction of specific immunoglobulin A and Th2 immune responses to P6 outer membrane protein of nontypeable *Haemophilus influenzae* in middle ear mucosa by intranasal immunization. *Infect. Immun.* **68:**2294–2300.

121. **Koivunen, P., T. Kontiokari, M. Niemela, T. Pokka, and M. Uhari.** 1999. Time to development of acute otitis media during an upper respiratory tract infection in children. *Pediatr. Infect. Dis. J.* **18:**303–305.

122. **Korppi, M., M. Leinonen, M. Koskela, P. H. Makela, and K. Launiala.** 1989. Bacterial coinfection in children hospitalized with respiratory syncytial virus infections. *Pediatr. Infect. Dis. J.* **8:**687–692.

123. **Korppi, M., M. Leinonen, P. H. Makela, and K. Launiala.** 1991. Mixed infection is common in children with respiratory adenovirus infection. *Acta Paediatr. Scand.* **80:**413–417.

124. **Kozyrskyj, A. L., G. E. Hildes-Ripstein, S. E. Longstaffe, J. L. Wincott, D. S. Sitar, T. P. Klassen, and M. E. Moffatt.** 1998. Treatment of acute otitis media with a shortened course of antibiotics: a meta-analysis. *JAMA* **279:**1736–1742.

125. **Kurono, Y., M. Yamamoto, K. Fujihashi, S. Kodama, M. Suzuki, G. Mogi, J. R. McGhee, and H. Kiyono.** 1999. Nasal immunization induces *Haemophilus influenzae*-specific Th1 and Th2 responses with mucosal IgA and systemic IgG antibodies for protective immunity. *J. Infect. Dis.* **180:**122–132.

126. **Kvaerner, K. J., P. Nafstad, J. Hagen, I. W. Mair, and J. J. Jaakkola.** 1997. Early acute otitis media: determined by exposure to respiratory pathogens. *Acta Otolaryngol. Suppl.* **529:**14–18.

127. **Kyd, J. M., and A. W. Cripps.** 1999. Killed whole bacterial cells, a mucosal delivery system for the induction of immunity in the respiratory tract and middle ear: an overview. *Vaccine* **17:**1775–1781.

128. **LaMarco, K. L., W. F. Diven, and R. H. Glew.** 1986. Experimental alteration of chinchilla middle ear mucosae by bacterial neuraminidase. *Ann. Otol. Rhinol. Laryngol.* **95:**304–308.

129. **Liederman, E. M., J. C. Post, J. J. Aul, D. A. Sirko, G. J. White, C. A. Buchman, and G. D. Ehrlich.** 1998. Analysis of adult otitis media: polymerase chain reaction versus culture for bacteria and viruses. *Ann. Otol. Rhinol. Laryngol.* **107:**10–16.

130. **Linder, T. E., R. L. Daniels, D. J. Lim, and T. F. DeMaria.** 1994. Effect of intranasal inoculation of *Streptococcus pneumoniae* on the structure of the surface carbohydrates of the chinchilla eustachian tube and middle ear mucosa. *Microb. Pathog.* **16:**435–441.

131. **Linder, T. E., D. J. Lim, and T. F. DeMaria.** 1992. Changes in the structure of the cell surface carbohydrates of the chinchilla tubotympanum following *Streptococcus pneumoniae*-induced otitis media. *Microb. Pathog.* **13:**293–303.

132. **Luce, B. R., K. M. Zangwill, C. S. Palmer, P. M. Mendelman, L. Yan, M. C. Wolff, I. Cho, S. M. Marcy, D. Iacuzio, and R. B. Belshe.** 2001. Cost-effectiveness analysis of an intranasal influenza vaccine for the prevention of influenza in healthy children. *Pediatrics* **108:**E24.

133. **Mackowiak, P. A.** 1978. Microbial synergism in human infections (first of two parts) *N. Engl. J. Med.* **298:**21–26.

134. **Mah, T. F., and G. A. O'Toole.** 2001. Mechanisms of biofilm resistance to antimicrobial agents. *Trends Microbiol.* **9:**34–39.

135. **Mandel, E. M., H. E. Rockette, C. D. Bluestone, J. L. Paradise, and R. J. Nozza.** 1987. Efficacy of amoxicillin with and without decongestant-antihistamine for otitis media with effusion in children. Results of a double-blind, randomized trial. *N. Engl. J. Med.* **316:**432–437.

136. **Matsuda, K., H. Tsutsumi, Y. Okamoto, and C. Chiba.** 1995. Development of interleukin 6 and tumor necrosis factor alpha activity in nasopharyngeal secretions of infants and children during infection with respiratory syncytial virus. *Clin. Diagn. Lab. Immunol.* **2:**322–324.

137. **McBride, T. P., W. J. Doyle, F. G. Hayden, and J. M. Gwaltney, Jr.** 1989. Alterations of the eustachian tube, middle ear, and nose in rhinovirus infection. *Arch. Otolaryngol. Head Neck Surg.* **115:**1054–1059.

138. **McIntosh, K., P. Halonen, and O. Ruuskanen.** 1993. Report of a workshop on respiratory viral infections: epidemiology, diagnosis, treatment, and prevention. *Clin. Infect. Dis.* **16:**151–164.

139. **McLinn, S., and D. Williams.** 1996. Incidence of antibiotic-resistant *Streptococcus pneumoniae* and beta-lactamase-positive *Haemophilus influenzae* in clinical isolates from patients with otitis media. *Pediatr. Infect. Dis. J.* **15:**S3–S9.

140. **Melhus, A., and A. F. Ryan.** 2000. Expression of cytokine genes during pneumococcal and nontypeable *Haemophilus influenzae* acute otitis media in the rat. *Infect. Immun.* **68:**4024–4031.

141. **Michon, F., P. C. Fusco, C. A. Minetti, M. Laude-Sharp, C. Uitz, C. H. Huang, A. J. D'Ambra, S. Moore, D. P. Remeta, I. Heron, and M. S. Blake.** 1998. Multivalent pneumococcal capsular polysaccharide conjugate vaccines employing genetically detoxified

pneumolysin as a carrier protein. *Vaccine* **16:** 1732–1741.

142. **Miura, M., H. Takahashi, I. Honjo, S. Hasebe, and M. Tanabe.** 1997. Influence of the upper respiratory tract infection on tubal compliance in children with otitis media with effusion. *Acta Otolaryngol.* **117:**574–577.

143. **Miyamoto, N., and L. O. Bakaletz.** 1997. Kinetics of the ascension of NTHi from the nasopharynx to the middle ear coincident with adenovirus-induced compromise in the chinchilla. *Microb. Pathog.* **23:**119–126.

144. **Miyamoto, N., and L. O. Bakaletz.** 1996. Selective adherence of non-typeable *Haemophilus influenzae* (NTHi) to mucus or epithelial cells in the chinchilla eustachian tube and middle ear. *Microb. Pathog.* **21:**343–356.

145. **Narkio-Makela, M., J. Jero, and S. Meri.** 1999. Complement activation and expression of membrane regulators in the middle ear mucosa in otitis media with effusion. *Clin. Exp. Immunol.* **116:**401–409.

146. **Nelson, C. T., E. O. Mason, Jr., and S. L. Kaplan.** 1994. Activity of oral antibiotics in middle ear and sinus infections caused by penicillin-resistant *Streptococcus pneumoniae*: implications for treatment. *Pediatr. Infect. Dis. J.* **13:**585–589.

147. **Noah, T. L., F. W. Henderson, I. A. Wortman, R. B. Devlin, J. Handy, H. S. Koren, and S. Becker.** 1995. Nasal cytokine production in viral acute upper respiratory infection of childhood. *J. Infect. Dis.* **171:**584–592.

148. **Ogra, P. L., H. Faden, and R. C. Welliver.** 2001. Vaccination strategies for mucosal immune responses. *Clin. Microbiol. Rev.* **14:**430–445.

149. **Ohashi, Y., Y. Nakai, Y. Esaki, H. Ikeoka, and H. Koshimo.** 1988. Effects of bacterial endotoxin on ciliary activity in the tubotympanum. *Ann. Otol. Rhinol. Laryngol.* **97:**298–301.

150. **Ohashi, Y., Y. Nakai, Y. Esaki, Y. Ohno, Y. Sugiura, and H. Okamoto.** 1991. Influenza A virus-induced otitis media and mucociliary dysfunction in the guinea pig. *Acta Otolaryngol. Suppl.* **486:**135–148.

151. **Okamoto, Y., K. Kudo, K. Ishikawa, E. Ito, K. Togawa, I. Saito, I. Moro, J. A. Patel, and P. L. Ogra.** 1993. Presence of respiratory syncytial virus genomic sequences in middle ear fluid and its relationship to expression of cytokines and cell adhesion molecules. *J. Infect. Dis.* **168:**1277–1281.

152. **Okamoto, Y., K. Kudo, K. Shirotori, M. Nakazawa, E. Ito, K. Togawa, J. A. Patel, and P. L. Ogra.** 1992. Detection of genomic sequences of respiratory syncytial virus in otitis

media with effusion in children. *Ann. Otol. Rhinol. Laryngol.* **157**(Suppl.)**:**7–10.

153. **Paap, C. M.** 1996. Management of otitis media with effusion in young children. *Ann. Pharmacother.* **30:**1291–1297.

154. **Paradise, J. L., H. E. Rockette, D. K. Colborn, B. S. Bernard, C. G. Smith, M. Kurs-Lasky, and J. E. Janosky.** 1997. Otitis media in 2253 Pittsburgh-area infants: prevalence and risk factors during the first two years of life. *Pediatrics* **99:**318–333.

155. **Park, K., L. O. Bakaletz, J. M. Coticchia, and D. J. Lim.** 1993. Effect of influenza A virus on ciliary activity and dye transport function in the chinchilla eustachian tube. *Ann. Otol. Rhinol. Laryngol.* **102:**551–558.

156. **Patel, J., H. Faden, S. Sharma, and P. L. Ogra.** 1992. Effect of respiratory syncytial virus on adherence, colonization and immunity of non-typable *Haemophilus influenzae*: implications for otitis media. *Int. J. Pediatr. Otorhinolaryngol.* **23:**15–23.

157. **Patel, J. A., B. Reisner, N. Vizirinia, M. Owen, T. Chonmaitree, and V. Howie.** 1995. Bacteriologic failure of amoxicillin-clavulanate in treatment of acute otitis media caused by nontypeable *Haemophilus influenzae*. *J. Pediatr.* **126:**799–806.

158. **Persson, C. G., I. Erjefalt, U. Alkner, C. Baumgarten, L. Greiff, B. Gustafsson, A. Luts, U. Pipkorn, F. Sundler, C. Svensson, and P. Wollmer.** 1991. Plasma exudation as a first line respiratory mucosal defence. *Clin. Exp. Allergy* **21:** 17–24.

159. **Pichichero, M. E.** 1998. Changing the treatment paradigm for acute otitis media in children *JAMA* **279:**1748–1750.

160. **Pichichero, M. E., and C. L. Pichichero.** 1995. Persistent acute otitis media: I. Causative pathogens. *Pediatr. Infect. Dis. J.* **14:**178–183.

161. **Pitkaranta, A., J. Jero, E. Arruda, A. Virolainen, and F. G. Hayden.** 1998. Polymerase chain reaction-based detection of rhinovirus, respiratory syncytial virus, and coronavirus in otitis media with effusion. *J. Pediatr.* **133:**390–394.

162. **Pitkaranta, A., A. Virolainen, J. Jero, E. Arruda, and F. G. Hayden.** 1998. Detection of rhinovirus, respiratory syncytial virus, and coronavirus infections in acute otitis media by reverse transcriptase polymerase chain reaction. *Pediatrics* **102:**291–295.

163. **Plotkowski, M. C., E. Puchelle, G. Beck, J. Jacquot, and C. Hannoun.** 1986. Adherence of type I *Streptococcus pneumoniae* to tracheal epithelium of mice infected with influenza A/PR8 virus. *Am. Rev. Respir. Dis.* **134:**1040–1044.

164. Poolman, J. T., L. Bakaletz, A. Cripps, P. A. Denoel, A. Forsgren, J. Kyd, and Y. Lobet. 2000. Developing a nontypeable *Haemophilus influenzae* (NTHi) vaccine. *Vaccine* 19(Suppl 1):S108–S115.

165. Post, J. C., J. J. Aul, G. J. White, R. M. Wadowsky, T. Zavoral, R. Tabari, B. Kerber, W. J. Doyle, and G. D. Ehrlich. 1996. PCR-based detection of bacterial DNA after antimicrobial treatment is indicative of persistent, viable bacteria in the chinchilla model of otitis media. *Am. J. Otolaryngol.* 17:106–111.

166. Post, J. C., M. Ehrlich, and G. D. Ehrlich. 2000. Otitis media with effusion as a bacterial biofilm disease, p. 1–37. *In New Paradigms in Infectious Disease: Applications to Otitis Media, October 13–15, 2000, Pittsburgh, Pa.*

167. Post, J. C., R. A. Preston, J. J. Aul, M. Larkins-Pettigrew, J. Rydquist-White, K. W. Anderson, R. M. Wadowsky, D. R. Reagan, E. S. Walker, L. A. Kingsley, et al. 1995. Molecular analysis of bacterial pathogens in otitis media with effusion. *JAMA* 273:1598–1604.

168. Post, J. C., G. J. White, J. J. Aul, T. Zavoral, R. M. Wadowsky, Y. Zhang, R. A. Preston, and G. D. Ehrlich. 1996. Development and validation of a multiplex PCR-based assay for the upper respiratory tract bacterial pathogens *Haemophilus influenzae, Streptococcus pneumoniae,* and *Moraxella catarrhalis. Mol. Diagn.* 1:29–39.

169. Potera, C. 1999. Forging a link between biofilms and disease. *Science* 283:1837–1839.

170. Rayner, M. G., Y. Zhang, M. C. Gorry, Y. Chen, J. C. Post, and G. D. Ehrlich. 1998. Evidence of bacterial metabolic activity in culture-negative otitis media with effusion. *JAMA* 279:296–299.

171. Reisinger, K., F. Hayden, R. Whitley, R. Dutkowski, D. Ipe, R. Mills, and P. Ward. 2000. Oral oseltamivir is effective and safe in the treatment of children with acute influenza. *Clin. Microbiol. Infect.* 6(Suppl. 1):250.

172. Richter, S. S., P. L. Winokur, A. B. Brueggemann, H. K. Huynh, P. R. Rhomberg, E. M. Wingert, and G. V. Doern. 2000. Molecular characterization of the beta-lactamases from clinical isolates of *Moraxella (Branhamella) catarrhalis* obtained from 24 U.S. medical centers during 1994–1995 and 1997–1998. *Antimicrob. Agents Chemother.* 44: 444–446.

173. Ruohola, A., T. Heikkinen, J. Jero, T. Puhakka, T. Juven, M. Narkio-Makela, H. Saxen, and O. Ruuskanen. 1999. Oral prednisolone is an effective adjuvant therapy for acute otitis media with discharge through tympanostomy tubes. *J. Pediatr.* 134:459–463.

174. Ruohola, A., T. Heikkinen, M. Waris, T. Puhakka, and O. Ruuskanen. 2000. Intranasal fluticasone propionate does not prevent acute otitis media during viral upper respiratory infection in children. *J. Allergy Clin. Immunol.* 106:467–471.

175. Ruuskanen, O., M. Arola, T. Heikkinen, and T. Ziegler. 1991. Viruses in acute otitis media: increasing evidence for clinical significance. *Pediatr. Infect. Dis. J.* 10:425–427.

176. Ruuskanen, O., M. Arola, A. Putto-Laurila, J. Mertsola, O. Meurman, M. K. Viljanen, and P. Halonen. 1989. Acute otitis media and respiratory virus infections. *Pediatr. Infect. Dis. J.* 8:94–99.

177. Ruuskanen, O., and T. Heikkinen. 1994. Viral-bacterial interaction in acute otitis media. *Pediatr. Infect. Dis. J.* 13:1047–1049.

178. Saidi, I. S., J. F. Biedlingmaier, and P. Whelan. 1999. *In vivo* resistance to bacterial biofilm formation on tympanostomy tubes as a function of tube material. *Otolaryngol. Head Neck Surg.* 120:621–627.

179. Sanford, B. A., A. Shelokov, and M. A. Ramsay. 1978. Bacterial adherence to virus-infected cells: a cell culture model of bacterial superinfection. *J. Infect. Dis.* 137:176–181.

180. Sarkkinen, H., O. Ruuskanen, O. Meurman, H. Puhakka, E. Virolainen, and J. Eskola. 1985. Identification of respiratory virus antigens in middle ear fluids of children with acute otitis media. *J. Infect. Dis.* 151:444–448.

181. Sarkkinen, H. K., P. E. Halonen, P. P. Arstila, and A. A. Salmi. 1981. Detection of respiratory syncytial, parainfluenza type 2, and adenovirus antigens by radioimmunoassay and enzyme immunoassay on nasopharyngeal specimens from children with acute respiratory disease. *J. Clin. Microbiol.* 13:258–265.

182. Sarkkinen, H. K., O. Meurman, T. T. Salmi, H. Puhakka, and E. Virolainen. 1983. Demonstration of viral antigens in middle ear secretions of children with acute otitis media *Acta Paediatr. Scand.* 72:137–138.

183. Sato, K., C. L. Liebeler, M. K. Quartey, C. T. Le, and G. S. Giebink. 1999. Middle ear fluid cytokine and inflammatory cell kinetics in the chinchilla otitis media model. *Infect. Immun.* 67:1943–1946.

184. Shaw, C. B., N. Obermyer, S. J. Wetmore, G. A. Spirou, and R. W. Farr. 1995. Incidence of adenovirus and respiratory syncytial virus in chronic otitis media with effusion using the polymerase chain reaction. *Otolaryngol. Head Neck Surg.* 113:234–241.

185. Siegrist, C. A. 2000. Vaccination in the neonatal period and early infancy. *Int. Rev. Immunol.* **19:**195–219.

186. Simoes, E. A., J. R. Groothuis, D. A. Tristram, K. Allessi, M. V. Lehr, G. R. Siber, and R. C. Welliver. 1996. Respiratory syncytial virus-enriched globulin for the prevention of acute otitis media in high risk children. *J. Pediatr.* **129:**214–219.

187. Sirakova, T., P. E. Kolattukudy, D. Murwin, J. Billy, E. Leake, D. Lim, T. DeMaria, and L. Bakaletz. 1994. Role of fimbriae expressed by nontypeable *Haemophilus influenzae* in pathogenesis of and protection against otitis media and relatedness of the fimbrin subunit to outer membrane protein A. *Infect. Immun.* **62:**2002–2020.

188. Stenfors, L. E., and S. Raisanen. 1989. Presence of *Branhamella catarrhalis* alters the survival of *Streptococcus pneumoniae* and *Haemophilus influenzae* in middle ear effusion: an *in vitro* study. *J. Laryngol. Otol.* **103:**1030–1033.

189. Stool, S. E., A. O. Berg, S. Berman, C. J. Carney, J. R. Cooley, L. Culpepper, R. D. Eavey, L. V. Feagans, T. Finitzo, E. M. Friedman, J. A. Goertz, A. J. Goldstein, K. M. Grundfast, D. G. Long, L. L. Macconi, L. Melton, J. E. Roberts, J. L. Sherrod, and J. E. Sisk. 1994. *Otitis Media with Effusion in Young Children. Clinical Practice Guideline,* vol. 12. Agency for Health Care Policy and Research, Public Health Service, U.S. Department of Health and Human Services, Rockville, Md.

190. Sung, B. S., T. Chonmaitree, L. D. Broemeling, M. J. Owen, J. A. Patel, D. C. Hedgpeth, and V. M. Howie. 1993. Association of rhinovirus infection with poor bacteriologic outcome of bacterial-viral otitis media. *Clin. Infect. Dis.* **17:**38–42.

191. Sutbeyaz, Y., B. Yakan, H. Ozdemir, M. Karasen, F. Doner, and I. Kufrevioglu. 1996. Effect of SC-41930, a potent selective leukotriene B4 receptor antagonist, in the guinea pig model of middle ear inflammation. *Ann. Otol. Rhinol. Laryngol.* **105:**476–480.

192. Suzuki, K., and L. O. Bakaletz. 1994. Synergistic effect of adenovirus type 1 and nontypeable *Haemophilus influenzae* in a chinchilla model of experimental otitis media. *Infect. Immun.* **62:**1710–1718.

193. Swarts, J. D., J. Y. Westcott, and K. H. Chan. 1997. Eicosanoid synthesis and inactivation in healthy and infected chinchilla middle ears. *Acta Otolaryngol.* (Stockholm) **117:** 845–850.

194. Teele, D. W., J. O. Klein, C. Chase, P. Menyuk, B. A. Rosner, and the Greater Boston Otitis Media Study Group. 1990. Otitis media in infancy and intellectual ability, school achievement, speech, and language at age 7 years. *J. Infect. Dis.* **162:**685–694.

195. Teele, D. W., J. O. Klein, and B. Rosner. 1989. Epidemiology of otitis media during the first seven years of life in children in greater Boston: a prospective, cohort study. *J. Infect. Dis.* **160:**83–94.

196. Tejani, N. R., T. Chonmaitree, D. K. Rassin, V. M. Howie, M. J. Owen, and A. S. Goldman. 1995. Use of C-reactive protein in differentiation between acute bacterial and viral otitis media. *Pediatrics* **95:**664–669.

197. Tong, H. H., L. M. Fisher, G. M. Kosunick, and T. F. DeMaria. 2000. Effect of adenovirus type 1 and influenza A virus on *Streptococcus pneumoniae* nasopharyngeal colonization and otitis media in the chinchilla. *Ann. Otol. Rhinol. Laryngol.* **109:**1021–1027.

198. Tong, H. H., J. N. Weiser, M. A. James, and T. F. DeMaria. 2001. Effect of influenza A virus infection on nasopharyngeal colonization and otitis media induced by transparent or opaque phenotype variants of *Streptococcus pneumoniae* in the chinchilla model. *Infect. Immun.* **69:** 602–606.

199. Turner, R. B. 2001. The treatment of rhinovirus infections: progress and potential. *Antivir. Res.* **49:**1–14.

200. Turner, R. B., M. T. Wecker, G. Pohl, T. J. Witek, E. McNally, R. St George, B. Winther, and F. G. Hayden. 1999. Efficacy of tremacamra, a soluble intercellular adhesion molecule 1, for experimental rhinovirus infection: a randomized clinical trial. *JAMA* **281:** 1797–1804.

201. Ueyama, T., Y. Kurono, K. Shirabe, M. Takeshita, and G. Mogi. 1995. High incidence of *Haemophilus influenzae* in nasopharyngeal secretions and middle ear effusions as detected by PCR. *J. Clin. Microbiol.* **33:**1835–1838.

202. Uhari, M., J. Hietala, and H. Tuokko. 1995. Risk of acute otitis media in relation to the viral etiology of infections in children. *Clin. Infect. Dis.* **20:**521–524.

203. Underdown, B. J., and S. A. Plotkin. 1999. The induction of mucosal protection by parenteral immunization: a challenge to the mucosal immunity paradigm, p. 719–728, *Mucosal Immunology.* Academic Press, Inc., New York, N.Y.

204. Unhanand, M., I. Maciver, O. Ramilo, O. Arencibia-Mireles, J. C. Argyle, G. H. McCracken, Jr., and E. J. Hansen. 1992. Pul-

monary clearance of *Moraxella catarrhalis* in an animal model. *J. Infect. Dis.* **165:**644–650.

205. **Valiante, N. M., R. Rappuoli, R. A. Insel, P. McInnes, and A. Hoeveler.** 1999. The challenges of vaccinating the very young: lessons from a very old system of host defense. *Vaccine.* **17:**2757–2762.

206. **van Buchem, F. L., M. F. Peeters, and M. A. van't Hof.** 1985. Acute otitis media: a new treatment strategy. *Br. Med. J.* **290:**1033–1037.

207. **van der Ven, L. T., G. P. van den Dobbelsteen, B. Nagarajah, H. van Dijken, P. M. Dortant, J. G. Vos, and P. J. Roholl.** 1999. A new rat model of otitis media caused by *Streptococcus pneumoniae:* conditions and application in immunization protocols. *Infect. Immun.* **67:**6098–6103.

208. **Virolainen, A., P. Salo, J. Jero, P. Karma, J. Eskola, and M. Leinonen.** 1994. Comparison of PCR assay with bacterial culture for detecting *Streptococcus pneumoniae* in middle ear fluid of children with acute otitis media. *J. Clin. Microbiol.* **32:**2667–2670.

209. **Wadowsky, R. M., S. M. Mietzner, D. P. Skoner, W. J. Doyle, and P. Fireman.** 1995. Effect of experimental influenza A virus infection on isolation of *Streptococcus pneumoniae* and other aerobic bacteria from the oropharynges of allergic and nonallergic adult subjects. *Infect. Immun.* **63:**1153–1157.

210. **Wang, E. E., T. R. Einarson, J. D. Kellner, and J. M. Conly.** 1999. Antibiotic prescribing for Canadian preschool children: evidence of overprescribing for viral respiratory infections. *Clin. Infect. Dis.* **29:**155–160.

211. **Warshauer, D., E. Goldstein, T. Akers, W. Lippert, and M. Kim.** 1977. Effect of influenza viral infection on the ingestion and killing of bacteria by alveolar macrophages. *Am. Rev. Respir. Dis.* **115:**269–277.

212. **Westman, E. B., A. Hermansson, K. Prellner, A. Melhus, and S. Hellstrom.** 1994. *Moraxella catarrhalis*-induced purulent otitis media in the rat middle ear, p. 193–195. *In* G. Mogi, I. Honjo, T. Ishii, and T. Takasaka (ed.), *Second Extraordinary International Symposium on Recent Advances in Otitis Media.* Kugler Publications, Amsterdam, The Netherlands.

213. **Willett, D. N., R. P. Rezaee, J. M. Billy, M. B. Tighe, and T. F. DeMaria.** 1998. Relationship of endotoxin to tumor necrosis factor-alpha and interleukin-1 beta in children with otitis media with effusion. *Ann. Otol. Rhinol. Laryngol.* **107:**28–33.

214. **Williams, R. L., T. C. Chalmers, K. C. Stange, F. T. Chalmers, and S. J. Bowlin.** 1993. Use of antibiotics in preventing recurrent acute otitis media and in treating otitis media with effusion. A meta-analytic attempt to resolve the brouhaha. *JAMA* **270:**1344–1351. (Erratum, **271:**430, 1994.)

215. **Yellon, R. F., W. J. Doyle, T. L. Whiteside, W. F. Diven, A. R. March, and P. Fireman.** 1995. Cytokines, immunoglobulins, and bacterial pathogens in middle ear effusions. *Arch. Otolaryngol. Head Neck Surg.* **121:**865–869. (Erratum, **121:**1402.)

MIXED INFECTIONS OF INTESTINAL VIRUSES AND BACTERIA IN HUMANS

John A. Marshall

15

A range of viruses and bacteria (as well as parasites) can infect the human alimentary canal. Mixed infections of viruses and bacteria are not uncommon, and quite complex physiological changes can result from such infections. This chapter documents the main viruses and bacteria involved in mixed gastroenteritis infections and then surveys the frequency and nature of mixed viral-bacterial infections in humans. The literature on the possible mechanisms of such mixed infections is then examined under four headings: (i) the occurrence of asymptomatic infections by viral and bacterial enteropathogens; (ii) the clinical features of natural mixed infections in humans; (iii) the nature of mixed infections in animal models; (iv) relevant in vitro studies of viral-bacterial interaction.

BACTERIAL AGENTS OF GASTROENTERITIS IN HUMANS

Ten main bacterial groups associated with human gastroenteritis have been identified in mixed viral-bacterial infections in humans or used in experiments to study such mixed infections. A brief description of their classification and sites of action follows.

Escherichia coli

Six main groups of pathogenic *E. coli* are now known: enteropathogenic *E. coli* (EPEC), enteroinvasive *E. coli* (EIEC), enterotoxigenic *E. coli* (ETEC), enterohaemorrhagic *E. coli* (EHEC), enteroaggregative *E. coli* (EaggEC), and diffusely adherent *E. coli* (DAEC) (67). Some pathogenic *E. coli* strains show a particular pattern of adherence to HEp-2 cells referred to as "localized adherence" (66). Many, but not all, of these strains fall into the EPEC category (21) so that strains classified as locally adherent cannot at this stage be further categorized. In this chapter, the classification of *E. coli* is based on the information given in the particular report.

The pathogenesis of different strains of *E. coli* can vary; e.g., EIEC tends to invade epithelial cells and damage them through multiplication in the cytoplasm, whereas other strains such as ETEC and EHEC do not invade the cell (66). Toxin production is particularly important in the pathogenesis of noninvasive *E. coli* such as ETEC (66). Different strains of *E. coli* may also affect different parts of the intestine, e.g., ETEC tends to colonize the small intestine whereas EIEC and EPEC tend to infect both the small intestine and colon (25).

John A. Marshall, Victorian Infectious Diseases Reference Laboratory, Locked Bag 815, Carlton South, Victoria 3053, Australia.

Polymicrobial Diseases, Edited by Kim A. Brogden and Janet M. Guthmiller,
© 2002 ASM Press, Washington, D.C.

Shigella spp.

Four main species of shigellae are commonly recognized in humans: *Shigella dysenteriae, Shigella flexneri, Shigella boydii,* and *Shigella sonnei.* Shigellae normally infect colonic epithelial cells. Shigellae can produce a toxin which contributes to their pathogenic effect (55).

Salmonella spp.

Salmonella spp., which are all considered to be potentially pathogenic, currently number more than 2,370 recognized serological types. These bacteria bind to and penetrate the wall of the small intestine. Salmonellae produce toxins which contribute to their pathogenic effect (46).

Vibrio spp.

Common species of *Vibrio* associated with food-borne infections include *Vibrio cholerae, Vibrio parahaemolyticus,* and *Vibrio vulnificus. V. cholerae,* the most studied of this group, colonizes the small intestine, where pathogenesis of several strains is assisted by the production of toxins (24).

Campylobacter spp.

The genus *Campylobacter* includes a number of species which can cause gastroenteritis, notably *Campylobacter jejuni. C. jejuni* principally infects the colon, but infection may also involve the small intestine. Bacterial toxin production may facilitate cell damage (67, 99).

Yersinia enterocolitica

Bacteria related to *Yersinia enterocolitica* include many species which are usually referred to as the *Yersinia enterocolitica* group. These bacteria bind to and penetrate the small intestinal mucosa; they then colonize the Peyer's patches and can then spread to other organs. The pathogenesis of *Y. enterocolitica* is related in part to production of a toxin. *Y. enterocolitica* infection can cause a wide range of clinical symptoms, including diarrhea (3).

Aeromonas spp.

Infection with many species of the genus *Aeromonas* can be associated with gastroenteri-tis, particularly in children. Pathogenesis of the bacteria appears to be related to several factors, including toxin production in the host gut (50).

Clostridium spp.

Three main species are commonly associated with human disease: *Clostridium difficile, Clostridium perfringens,* and *Clostridium botulinum* (4, 67, 84). *C. difficile* can colonize the colon and induce diarrhea following the production of toxins (67). *C. perfringens* is a common cause of food poisoning; these bacteria can secrete a toxin during the process of sporulation within the intestine (4). *C. botulinum* is also an important cause of food poisoning. This bacterium can multiply and produce a neurotoxin in the intestine (84).

Bacillus spp.

Some species of the genus *Bacillus* are occasionally associated with outbreaks of food-borne illness. *Bacillus cereus* infection can involve either the small intestine or the colon (89). *B. cereus* produces a number of toxins which may contribute to the development of diarrhea (47).

Listeria spp.

Two species of the genus *Listeria, Listeria monocytogenes* and *Listeria ivanovii,* are considered pathogenic in humans and can affect the gastrointestinal tract (83).

VIRAL AGENTS OF GASTROENTERITIS IN HUMANS

Nine main virus groups associated with human gastroenteritis have been identified in mixed viral-bacterial infections or have been used in studies of such mixed infections. A brief description of the classification and site of action of human gastroenteritis viruses follows.

Rotaviruses

Rotaviruses are a major cause of gastroenteritis, particularly in children (9). The virus, which measures about 70 nm in diameter, is classified in the genus *Rotavirus* in the family *Reoviridae* (9). Rotavirus infects villus epithelial cells in the small intestine (9), although recent evidence indicates rotavirus can also produce a toxin (30).

"Norwalk-like" Viruses

"Norwalk-like" viruses (NLV) are an important cause of gastroenteritis in humans and are currently classified in the genus "Norwalk-like viruses" in the family *Caliciviridae* (38, 49). The particles measure about 35 nm in diameter (16). The virus appears to infect the epithelium of the small intestine (18).

Adenoviruses

Adenoviruses, particularly serotypes 40 and 41, are an important cause of gastroenteritis in humans, especially in children. These viruses are classified in the genus *Mastadenovirus* in the family *Adenoviridae* and measure about 70 to 90 nm in diameter (6, 98). The viruses appear to infect the duodenal mucosa (98).

Astroviruses

Astroviruses are a major cause of gastroenteritis in humans, particularly children. These viruses, which measure about 27 nm in diameter, are classified in the genus *Astrovirus* in the family *Astroviridae*. Astroviruses appear to infect the duodenal epithelium in the lower third of the villi (53, 65).

"Sapporo-like" Viruses

The "Sapporo-like" viruses comprise a genus within the family *Caliciviridae* and represent an important cause of illness, particularly in children (23, 38). They measure about 31 nm in diameter (58). The term "human calicivirus" has also been applied to this group (23), although the term is now often used to collectively describe the Norwalk-like viruses and Sapporo-like viruses (35). The pathogenesis of this virus does not appear to have been described in detail.

Toroviruses

Toroviruses are pleomorphic particles, about 100 to 140 nm in diameter, often with surface projections about 10 nm in length. These viruses are classified in the genus *Torovirus* in the family *Coronaviridae* (29, 45). The pathogenesis of toroviruses in humans is not well established, but the animal torovirus, Breda virus, replicates in intestinal epithelial cells (101). Toroviruses have been detected in children with gastroenteritis (45).

Coronaviruses

"Coronavirus-like particles" (CVLP), i.e., the fringed membranous particles sometimes detected in human feces, may be neither pathogenic in humans nor viral in nature (17, 60). The occasional identification of true coronaviruses in humans with gastroenteritis appears to be the exception rather than the rule (105).

Picornaviruses

A series of studies by Yamashita and colleagues has established that Aichi virus, a member of the family *Picornaviridae,* is a cause of gastroenteritis in humans (103, 104). Reports have also linked infections with viruses of the genus *Parechovirus* within the family *Picornaviridae* with gastrointestinal symptoms in humans (80).

Herpesviruses

Herpesviruses, notably cytomegalovirus (CMV), have been found in humans with gastroenteritis, particularly patients infected with the human immunodeficiency virus (HIV). CMV can infect the human gastrointestinal tract with resultant gastrointestinal symptoms (71).

INCIDENCE AND CHARACTERISTICS OF GASTROINTESTINAL MIXED VIRAL-BACTERIAL INFECTIONS IN HUMANS

A huge literature now documents the incidence of mixed viral-bacterial infections in gastroenteritis populations. Studies which give a clear categorization of cases of mixed infection are surveyed below. Most studies have focused on rotavirus (Table 1), adenovirus (Table 2), NLV (Table 3), and astrovirus

TABLE 1 Reports of mixed infections of rotavirus and bacteria in gastroenteritis populations

Other pathogen(s)	Gastroenteritis population	No. (%) positive	Population type	Population location	Reference
EPEC	67	2 (3.0)	Children	Brazil	81
	416	10 (2.4)	Children	Sweden	94
	814	16 (2.0)	Children	Bangladesh	1
	621	11 (1.8)	Children	Kuwait	75
	63	1 (1.6)	Children	Singapore	54
ETEC	70	5 (7.1)	Children	Malaysia	73
	62	4 (6.4)	Children	Mexico	31
	17	1 (5.9)	NS[a]	Jordan	62
	82	4 (4.9)	Children	Philippines	28
	345	15 (4.3)	Children	Costa Rica	61
	814	28 (3.4)	Children	Bangladesh	1
	80	2 (2.5)	Children	Mexico	33
	338	8 (2.4)	Children	Indonesia	79
	63	1 (1.6)	Children	Singapore	54
	416	3 (0.7)	Children	Sweden	94
	1,218	8 (0.7)	NS	Bangladesh	96
EaggEC	1,218	16 (1.3)	NS	Bangladesh	96
DAEC	1,218	2 (0.2)	NS	Bangladesh	96
E. coli localized adherent	1,218	3 (0.2)	NS	Bangladesh	96
Shigella	345	10 (2.9)	Children	Costa Rica	61
	338	5 (1.5)	Children	Indonesia	79
	130	1 (0.8)	Children and adults	Singapore	54
	5,810	29 (0.50)	NS	Bangladesh	96
	621	2 (0.3)	Children	Kuwait	75
	814	2 (0.2)	Children	Bangladesh	1
	3,785	5 (0.13)	Children	Australia	2
Salmonella	621	37 (6.0)	Children	Kuwait	75
	345	11 (3.2)	Children	Costa Rica	61
	30	1 (3)	Adults	Thailand	85
	338	2 (0.6)	Children	Indonesia	79
	3,785	18 (0.48)	Children	Australia	2
	NS	42	Children and adults	Hong Kong	56
V. cholerae	814	9 (1.1)	Children	Bangladesh	1
	5,810	28 (0.48)	NS	Bangladesh	96
Campylobacter	NS	22	Children and adults	Hong Kong	56
C. jejuni	814	25 (3.1)	Children	Bangladesh	1
	621	8 (1.3)	Children	Kuwait	75
	3,785	14 (0.37)	Children	Australia	2
Aeromonas	814	15 (1.8)	Children	Bangladesh	1
C. difficile	814	2 (0.2)	Children	Bangladesh	1
EPEC and *Salmonella*	621	7 (1.1)	Children	Kuwait	75
ETEC and *Shigella*	62	1 (1.6)	Children	Mexico	31
	338	2 (0.6)	Children	Indonesia	79
	345	1 (0.3)	Children	Costa Rica	61
ETEC and adenovirus	62	1 (1.6)	Children	Mexico	31
Salmonella and *Campylobacter*	NS	1	Children and adults	Hong Kong	56
Aeromonas and adenovirus	150	1 (0.7)	NS	United States	20

[a] NS, not stated.

TABLE 2 Reports of mixed infections of adenovirus and bacteria in gastroenteritis populations

Other pathogen(s)	Gastroenteritis population	No. (%) positive	Population type	Population location	Reference
EPEC	416	1 (0.2)	Children	Sweden	94
ETEC	62	2 (3.2)	Children	Mexico	31
	80	1 (1.2)	Children	Mexico	33
	130	1 (0.8)	Children and adults	Singapore	54
Shigella	3,785	1 (0.03)	Children	Australia	2
Salmonella	3,785	10 (0.26)	Children	Australia	2
C. jejuni	416	2 (0.5)	Children	Sweden	94
	3,785	2 (0.05)	Children	Australia	2

(Table 4), although occasional reports have linked other viruses with bacteria, e.g., CMV and *Campylobacter* in a HIV-positive patient with gastroenteritis (95), torovirus with *C. jejuni* in a child with gastroenteritis (45), and torovirus with EaggEC in a group of children with gastroenteritis in Brazil (52).

The frequency of cases of mixed infections with rotavirus or adenovirus and some bacteria (e.g., ETEC, *Salmonella, C. jejuni,* and EIEC) may simply reflect the relative importance of these bacteria as a cause of gastroenteritis in the setting studied and not any special interaction between the viruses and bacteria. The numerous reports of rotavirus or adenovirus with ETEC (Tables 1 and 2) and the tendency for the proportion of mixed infections with ETEC to be higher in developing countries than in developed countries (Singapore and Sweden [Table 1]) are probably related to the particular importance of ETEC as a cause of gastroenteritis in children in developing countries (66). The proportion of mixed infections with *Salmonella* or *C. jejuni* also tended to be lower in children from developed countries, such as Australia (Table 1), perhaps because of an improved standard of hygiene. Similarly, the absence of reports of mixed infections involving EIEC may be related to a relatively low incidence of EIEC gastroenteritis (66).

TABLE 3 Reports of mixed infections of NLV and bacteria in gastroenteritis populations

Other pathogen(s)	Gastroenteritis population	No. (%) positive	Population type	Population location	Reference
ETEC	47	2 (4.3)	Adults	Shipboard U.S. troops	69
EHEC	8	1 (12.5)	Adults	Australia	8
	NS[a]	1	NS	Australia	7
Shigella	NS	1	NS	Australia	J. A. Marshall, unpublished work
Salmonella	47	2 (4.3)	Adults	Shipboard U.S. troops	69
V. parahaemolyticus	47	1 (2.1)	Adults	Shipboard U.S. troops	69
Campylobacter	47	4 (8.5)	Adults	Shipboard U.S. troops	69
Aeromonas sobria	8	1 (12.5)	Adults	Australia	8
Bacillus thuringiensis	18	1 (5.6)	NS	Canada	44
Salmonella and *Campylobacter*	47	1 (2.1)	Adults	Shipboard U.S. troops	69

[a] NS, not stated.

TABLE 4 Reports of mixed infections of astrovirus and bacteria in gastroenteritis populations

Other pathogen(s)	Gastroenteritis population	No. (%) positive	Population type	Population location	Reference
EPEC	90	3 (3.3)	Children	Chile	34
ETEC	90	2 (2.2)	Children	Chile	34
	510	4 (0.8)	Children	Mexico	39
Shigella	510	1 (0.2)	Children	Mexico	39
Salmonella	510	1 (0.2)	Children	Mexico	39
Campylobacter	510	2 (0.4)	Children	Mexico	39
C. difficile	267	4 (1.5)	Children	United States	76
Shigella and *Campylobacter*	510	1 (0.2)	Children	Mexico	39

For mixed astrovirus-bacterial infections, again for some bacteria the frequency of mixed infections may reflect the relative importance of these bacteria as a cause of gastroenteritis. For example, the proportions of mixed infections involving astrovirus and *Shigella* or *Salmonella* were within the ranges observed for rotavirus and adenovirus (compare Table 4 with Tables 1 and 2). The data available are not sufficient to permit a comparison between the proportions of mixed infections with astrovirus and ETEC and the proportions of mixed infections with the other viruses (rotavirus, adenovirus, and NLV) and ETEC. A study in Guatemala for which exact quantitative data were not available found astrovirus in combination with EaggEC, DAEC, and localized adherent *E. coli,* and in combination with bacteria listed in Table 4 (EPEC, ETEC) (22).

Mixed NLV-bacterial infections (Table 3) differed from mixed viral-bacterial infections involving rotaviruses, adenoviruses, or astroviruses in two respects. The proportions of NLV cases with associated bacteria were high (particularly for *Campylobacter*) even in a developed community (shipboard U.S. troops) and bacteria observed included EHEC, which was not found in any mixed viral-bacterial infections involving the other three major viruses. The NLV database is small, and since it relates to adults rather than children, which predominate in Tables 1, 2, and 4, the difference between NLV and the other viruses may be due to a difference between children and adults.

Specific interactions between NLV and bacteria cannot be excluded, however.

Mixed infections with more than two enteropathogens have also occasionally been documented in gastroenteritis populations (Tables 1, 3, and 4), although these are relatively uncommon.

Some of the differences noted above may vanish as more data become available, but they may point to differences in the interactions of different viruses with bacteria and in the reaction of adults and children to mixed infections. The observations, mainly in animal and in vitro studies, which have an impact on these questions are discussed below.

MECHANISMS OF MIXED VIRAL-BACTERIAL INFECTIONS IN THE GASTROINTESTINAL TRACT

Excretion of Known Human Viral and Bacterial Enteropathogens in Asymptomatic Individuals or Individuals without Symptoms of Diarrhea

An important complicating factor in the interpretation of data on mixed viral-bacterial infections is the fact that in many individuals, infections with known viral (Table 5), bacterial (Table 6), or mixed viral-bacterial enteropathogens (Table 7) need not be associated with diarrhea. Thus, in many mixed infections one of the potential enteropathogens may make no contribution to the gastroenteritis. However, as shown below, evidence from human, animal, and in vitro studies shows that in

TABLE 5 Reports of the detection of known viral enteropathogens in individuals without diarrhea

Virus(es)	Reference(s)
Rotavirus	1, 10, 28, 43, 48, 61, 74, 75, 77, 81, 87, 94, 97
NLV	32, 37, 59, 70, 87
Adenovirus	40, 77, 81, 87
Astrovirus	10, 22, 87
Sapporo-like viruses	32, 58, 87
Rotavirus and astrovirus	22

some cases a mixed viral-bacterial infection has more or less serious consequences than infection with either the virus or the bacterium separately.

Studies of the Clinical Symptoms Following Mixed Viral-Bacterial Infections in Humans

Despite a considerable literature (Tables 1 to 4) documenting the ubiquitous nature of mixed infections in human gastroenteritis, very little information exists on how such mixed enteropathogens may interact and whether they may affect clinical symptoms. Three studies on mixed infections in humans have shown that three situations can occur: mixed infections may exacerbate clinical symptoms, produce the same symptoms as one of the infectious

agents, or give less severe symptoms than one of the agents alone. Hori et al. (42), who were studying enteric pathogens in gastroenteritis cases in Ghanaian children, observed that mixed pathogens (rotavirus and various bacteria) were found significantly more often in severe gastroenteritis cases than in either mild gastroenteritis cases or in controls. The mixed infections involved combinations of rotavirus with various bacteria, including ETEC, EPEC, and *Campylobacter* spp. Koopmans et al. (52) noted indications of more severe illness resulting from mixed torovirus-EaggEC infections than from infections with either pathogen alone in Brazilian children with gastroenteritis. On the other hand, Unicomb et al. (96), who were studying enteropathogens in gastroenteritis cases in Bangladeshi children, found that mixed rotavirus-*E. coli* infections were similar in severity to infections with rotavirus alone or *E. coli* alone. Mixed rotavirus-*V. cholerae* infections were similar in severity to infections with *V. cholerae* alone. These authors speculated that because *V. cholerae* infections and rotavirus infections both take place in the small intestine,

TABLE 6 Reports of the detection of known bacterial enteropathogens in individuals without diarrhea

Bacterium	Reference(s)
EPEC	1, 43, 74, 75, 81, 87, 97
EIEC	48, 97
ETEC	1, 27, 28, 48, 61, 74, 97
EHEC	48
EaggEC	1, 87
DAEC	1, 87
Shigella	1, 27, 43, 61, 74, 79, 97
Salmonella	1, 40, 43, 48, 61, 75, 85, 87, 97
Campylobacter	1, 40, 43, 48, 87, 97
Yersinia	48, 87
Aeromonas	1, 48, 85, 87, 97
C. difficile toxin	1, 81, 87
C. perfringens enterotoxin	87
Bacillus	87

TABLE 7 Mixed viral-bacterial enteropathogens in individuals without diarrhea

Mixed enteropathogens	Reference
Rotavirus and EPEC	81
Astrovirus and EPEC	22
Astrovirus and ETEC	22
Astrovirus and EaggEC	22
Astrovirus and DAEC	22
Astrovirus and *E. coli* localized adherent	22
Astrovirus and *C. jejuni*	22

the *V. cholerae* may have a competitive advantage from the rapid action of cholera toxin and hence lessen the pathogenic effect of the rotavirus infection. These authors also noted that *Shigella* infections alone were more severe than infections with *Shigella* and rotavirus in two ways. In infections with *Shigella* alone, there were more loose bowel movements in the 24 h before presentation and diarrhea lasted longer than in mixed infections. This finding indicates that in this situation there is a complex interaction in mixed infection to reduce the severity of the illness.

Animal Models of the Effects of Mixed Viral-Bacterial Enteropathogens

Enteropathogens in many animals, e.g., rotavirus and *E. coli,* are similar to those found in humans, so animal studies can provide useful information on the nature of mixed viral-bacterial infections in humans. Numerous studies with mice, rabbits, pigs, cattle, sheep, and horses, chiefly using rotavirus and *E. coli,* emphasize the many variables that can influence the clinical outcome of such mixed infections.

MICE

Newsome and Coney (68) found a synergistic effect between rotavirus and ETEC in infected mice. Four-day-old mice infected simultaneously with rotavirus and ETEC showed a higher mortality rate than those infected with either rotavirus or ETEC alone. Furthermore, mice with subclinical infections of rotavirus had a significant increase in mortality compared with rotavirus-free mice when challenged with the ETEC. The authors suggested this observed synergy might be related to a breakdown in the normal balance between intestinal secretion and absorption. They speculated that the increased intestinal secretion caused by the ETEC enterotoxin A could not be counteracted by adequate resorption because of damage caused to the villus epithelial cells by the rotavirus.

RABBITS

Thouless et al. (86) found a synergistic effect between rotavirus and EPEC in infected weanling (aged 10 to 16 weeks) rabbits; mixed infections caused more severe diarrheal disease in the rabbits than either pathogen alone. However, mixed inoculation of rabbits 28 to 38 weeks old with similar doses of rotavirus and EPEC caused infection but failed to produce diarrhea, indicating the synergistic effect of the two agents was related to the age of the animal.

PIGS

Tzipori et al. (90) found that 4-week-old pigs infected with rotavirus, and some days later with EHEC, developed a diarrheal disease that was more severe than that produced by each agent separately.

Benfield et al. (5) found that 3-day-old pigs inoculated with rotavirus, and 24 h later with ETEC, all died or were moribund within 6 days, whereas there was no natural mortality among pigs inoculated with one agent alone. Laboratory studies showed that lesions produced by ETEC in the dually inoculated pigs were no more severe than those in ETEC-only-inoculated pigs. Rotavirus did not consistently enhance the growth of ETEC in the small intestine of the dually inoculated pigs. The authors hypothesized that the more serious outcome of the combined agents was the outcome of the independent action of the two agents rather than being caused by some interaction between them.

In contrast to what has been observed for rotavirus and ETEC, there is evidence for a direct interaction between ETEC and other gastroenteritis viruses. A possible mechanism for such an interaction is suggested by the work of Whipp et al. (100). They found that for pigs whose villus epithelium had been damaged by the coronavirus "transmissible gastroenteritis virus," the increase in secretion induced by ETEC toxins was less than in uninfected pigs. This suggestion is supported by the findings of Cox et al. (19). They noted that preinfection of pigs with transmissible gastroenteritis virus one day before infection with ETEC resulted in decreased adhesion of the bacteria to the villus-brush border. It is possible that this decreased adhesion could lead to the decreased secretion observed by Whipp et al. (100). The clinical significance of these findings is unclear.

CATTLE

Gouet et al. (36) found that combined infections of colostrum-deprived gnotobiotic calves aged 4 days or less with EPEC and rotavirus produced a synergistic effect. These authors noted that the combination of rotavirus and EPEC in doses not lethal in themselves produced severe diarrhea, dehydration, and death.

Many groups have investigated mixed infections of rotavirus and ETEC in calves. A survey of these experiments shows that, under some circumstances, clinical illness is definitely more severe after mixed infections than following infection with either of the pathogens. Further, it is clear that the age of the calves is an important factor, so that the studies have been arranged here in order of increasing age.

Evidence for the nature of the synergistic effects of ETEC and rotavirus in very young calves comes from the studies of Hess et al. (41) and Torres-Medina (88). Hess et al. (41) infected specific-pathogen-free but not gnotobiotic colostrum-deprived calves with either bovine rotavirus, ETEC, or a combination of both enteropathogens within the first 24 h of life. ETEC infection alone produced severe diarrhea when 10^{10} organisms were given, but the calves remained healthy when inoculated with a dose of 10^7 organisms. Rotavirus inoculation alone produced no diarrhea or a mild diarrhea after about 29 h. However, when 10^7 ETEC organisms were given 12 to 14 h after rotavirus or simultaneously with rotavirus, a synergistic effect was observed, with severe diarrhea beginning after about 22 h and more rotavirus excretion than from calves infected with rotavirus alone. Torres-Medina (88) examined the effect of combined rotavirus and *E. coli* (either ETEC or non-ETEC) infection in 24-h-old colostrum-deprived gnotobiotic

calves. Calves infected with rotavirus and ETEC had more severe lesions than calves sham-infected, infected with rotavirus only, or infected with ETEC only. However, rotavirus infection did not affect adherence of ETEC to the intestinal mucosa.

Tzipori et al. (92) examined the effect of simultaneous combined infections of rotavirus and ETEC in specific-pathogen-free calves aged 1 to 4 days. Small-intestinal mucosal damage was more severe in calves inoculated with both rotavirus and ETEC than in calves inoculated with ETEC or rotavirus alone.

Tzipori et al. (93), investigating infections in older calves, showed that mixed infections of rotavirus and ETEC could induce illness in gnotobiotic calves where rotavirus or ETEC given alone could not. Combinations of rotavirus and ETEC produced diarrhea in calves 1 to 2 weeks old, although rotavirus or ETEC alone did not induce illness in calves of this age. The results of Snodgrass et al. (78) for calves of similar age were different, perhaps because conventionally reared rather than gnotobiotic calves were used. They examined 6-day-old calves inoculated with rotavirus, or ETEC, or rotavirus and ETEC, or uninoculated controls. Rotavirus infection consistently produced diarrhea, whereas ETEC alone did not colonize the intestine. In dual infections both rotavirus and ETEC multiplied, but the severity of diarrhea was no greater than that caused by rotavirus alone.

Runnels et al. (72) attempted to clarify what actually determined the severity of mixed infection in calves by examining factors likely to influence the severity of symptoms following mixed infections of rotavirus and ETEC in gnotobiotic calves. Synergism between ETEC and rotavirus for dual infection of 5- to 8-day-old calves was confirmed, but results were variable, and at least two factors appeared to be important in such experiments: age and feeding regimen. Inoculation at a younger age increased the severity of clinical illness, whereas increased milk intake by the calves reduced the severity of symptoms of mixed infections.

SHEEP

Wray et al. (102) examined the effect of combined infections of EPEC and rotavirus in 1-day-old lambs. EPEC alone produced diarrhea as did rotavirus infection. When both agents were given, the mortality rate was higher.

HORSES

Tzipori et al. (91) inoculated foals with rotavirus and ETEC. Neither agent alone initially produced diarrhea. Inoculation with both agents always induced diarrhea in foals up to 16 days old, but never in foals more than 20 days old.

CONCLUSION

Animal studies clearly show that under certain conditions mixed viral-bacterial infections can induce more severe clinical illness in a range of animals. However the factors that influence these results are complex. There is no clear understanding of how synergistic effects are produced, although a range of variables such as animal age and feeding regimen can influence clinical symptoms.

In Vitro Studies of Mixed Enteropathogenic Viral-Bacterial Infections

The mechanisms of pathogenesis of enteropathogenic bacteria can be complex and diverse and have been discussed in a detailed review by Nataro and Levine (67). They classified the pathogenic mechanisms of these bacteria into three groups: those that belonged to the "adherence/toxin paradigm" (such as *V. cholerae* and ETEC), those that belonged to the "invasion paradigm" (such as *L. monocytogenes* [83], *Shigella, Salmonella, Yersinia, Campylobacter,* and EIEC), and those that did not appear to belong to either of these groups (such as EPEC, EHEC, EaggEC, DAEC, *Aeromonas,* and *C. difficile*).

There is a growing literature on how "invasion paradigm" bacteria adhere to or invade virus-infected cells in vitro. There have been studies in this area using *Salmonella enterica*

serovar Typhimurium (11–14), *S. flexneri* (11, 15, 57, 63, 64), *C. jejuni* (51), *Y. enterocolitica* and *Yersinia pseudotuberculosis* (26), *L. monocytogenes* (82), and EIEC (11). Some in vitro studies have also been carried out on the effect of viral infection on the invasiveness of normally noninvasive bacteria (11, 13, 51, 57).

The viruses used in these studies frequently have not been enteropathogens (e.g., coxsackie B viruses, echoviruses 6 and 7, poliovirus, and measles virus), although rotavirus has been used in some studies, often with similar results (11, 26, 82).

In Vitro Studies of *Salmonella* Infection of Virus-infected Cells

Bukholm and Degre (13) demonstrated that the invasiveness of *S. enterica* serovar Typhimurium was significantly increased in HEp-2 cells infected with coxsackie B1 virus compared with virus-uninfected controls. Furthermore, a relationship existed between invasiveness and the infective virus concentration used; for up to 3 h after virus infection more cells, with a higher concentration of bacteria, were detected in the higher-virus-dose-infected cells compared with the lower-virus-dose-infected cells. A relationship also existed between bacterial invasiveness and time of incubation of the virus with the cells, with more bacteria entering the cells the longer the cells were incubated with virus. The trypan blue exclusion test indicated increased invasiveness was unrelated to a breakdown of the cell membrane. The authors suggested the virus infection might somehow alter the cell membrane such that bacterial adhesion and/or invasiveness are enhanced.

These findings were supported in a subsequent study when Bukholm et al. (14) studied the invasiveness of *S. enterica* serovar Typhimurium using HEp-2 cells pretreated with UV-inactivated coxsackie B1 virus. Even UV-inactivated virus enhanced the invasiveness of *S. enterica* serovar Typhimurium and indeed during the first 3 h of virus infection there was no difference in the enhancement of invasiveness between noninactivated and UV-inactivated virus. (However, in subsequent periods, the noninactivated virus permitted greater invasiveness of the bacteria.) The authors speculated that since UV-inactivated virus could alter the cell membrane, the hypothesis that enhanced invasiveness was related to cell membrane alterations was supported.

Bukholm (11) was able to link these findings to mixed gastroenteritis infections by studying the effect of preinfection with a known viral enteropathogen (rotavirus) on the invasiveness of *S. enterica* serovar Typhimurium by using MA-104 cells. As with the previous studies utilizing the coxsackie B1 virus, *Salmonella* invasiveness was enhanced.

In Vitro Studies of *S. flexneri* Infection of Virus-Infected Cells

Bukholm et al. (15) demonstrated that measles virus infection had an effect on the invasiveness of *S. flexneri* in HEp-2 cell cultures similar to that found for *S. enterica* serovar Typhimurium infections of coxsackie B1 virus-infected cells (see above). Bacterial invasiveness was significantly enhanced in cell cultures incubated with virus prior to bacterial inoculation. As before, this effect was a function of the time interval between introduction of the virus and inoculation with the bacteria as well as of virus concentration. A similar enhancement of invasiveness was found in cell cultures pretreated with UV-inactivated measles virus.

Again, as with the *Salmonella* studies (above), preinfection of MA-104 cells with rotavirus enhanced the invasiveness of *S. flexneri* (11).

To better understand the mechanism by which virus infection enhances *S. flexneri* invasiveness in vitro, Modalsli et al. (63) examined whether there was a relationship between the effect of the viral infection on the invasiveness of the bacterium, the phagocytosis of latex particles, and the permeability of the cell membrane. Coxsackie B1 virus infection of HEp-2 cells enhanced all three parameters, i.e., invasiveness of bacteria, phagocytosis of latex particles, and membrane permeability. The au-

thors concluded that all three parameters might be related, i.e., enhanced bacterial invasiveness could be linked to enhanced phagocytotic capacity of the cell and to altered membrane permeability.

Marchetti et al. (57) further developed an understanding of the invasiveness of *S. flexneri* in virus-infected cells when they demonstrated that preinfection of HeLa cells with a number of enteroviruses (poliovirus 1, coxsackie B3 virus, and echovirus 6) enhanced invasiveness of the bacterium. UV-inactivation of the three viruses reduced but did not extinguish the effect on bacterial invasiveness. These authors suggested that virus infection altered cell membranes such that internalization of *S. flexneri* was facilitated. Virus-induced mobilization of clathrin may have also facilitated this internalization process.

Modalsli et al. (64) showed that when coxsackie B1 virus RNA was microinjected into HEp-2 cells, there was no effect on *S. flexneri* invasiveness, even though new virus was formed in the cells. However, when the cells were prestimulated with UV-inactivated virus, the microinjected RNA induced an additional enhancement of bacterial invasiveness compared with that in cells only treated with the UV-inactivated virus. The authors concluded that enhanced invasiveness was influenced by viral replication, although replication alone was insufficient to enhance bacterial invasiveness.

In Vitro Studies of *C. jejuni* Infection of Virus-Infected Cells

Konkel and Joens (51) showed that the invasiveness of *C. jejuni* (strain ATCC 33560) was significantly increased in HEp-2 cells preinfected with echovirus 7, coxsackie B3 virus, and UV-inactivated coxsackie B3 virus. However, poliovirus and porcine enterovirus had no effect on the adherence and invasiveness of this strain of *C. jejuni*. The authors argued that the enhancement of the bacterial invasiveness was the result of specific rather than nonspecific events, because different enteroviruses had different effects on the invasiveness of *C. jejuni*.

In Vitro Studies of *Y. enterocolitica* and *Y. pseudotuberculosis* Infection of Virus-Infected Cells

Di Biase et al. (26) examined adherence to and invasion of Caco-2 cells, preinfected with rotavirus, by *Y. enterocolitica* and *Y. pseudotuberculosis*. In both cases, adherence and invasiveness were enhanced. When *E. coli* harboring the *inv* gene of *Y. pseudotuberculosis*, a gene involved in the invasion process, was tested, it also showed increased invasiveness into the rotavirus-infected cells. Superinfection of the rotavirus-infected cells with *Y. enterocolitica* or *Y. pseudotuberculosis* decreased viral antigen synthesis.

These authors speculated that rotavirus-infection-enhanced bacterial invasiveness may have resulted from altered membrane permeability and fluidity. The authors suggested rotavirus infection may produce receptors, such that bacterial attachment and entry are facilitated. Conversely, the decrease in viral antigen synthesis observed in the rotavirus- and *Yersinia*-infected cells may have been the result of the breakdown of cellular organelles caused by the multiplication of intracellular bacteria.

In Vitro Studies of *L. monocytogenes* Infection of Virus-Infected Cells

Superti et al. (82) examined the effect of rotavirus or poliovirus infection of Caco-2 cells on *L. monocytogenes* internalization and replication. Although rotavirus infection increased *L. monocytogenes* internalization, poliovirus infection inhibited bacterial entry. Furthermore, rotavirus infection promoted bacterial replication, whereas poliovirus infection hampered bacterial replication. *L. monocytogenes* infection stimulated rotavirus replication but not poliovirus replication.

These authors suggested the enhanced invasiveness of *L. monocytogenes* in rotavirus-infected cells could have been due to the presence of virally synthesized membrane receptors or to changes in membrane receptors specific for *L. monocytogenes* as a result of the viral infection. They speculated that cytoskeletal changes occurring as a result of bacterial replication may have been responsible for the stimulation of rotavirus replication.

The finding that poliovirus infection failed to enhance *L. monocytogenes* invasiveness was in agreement with the work of Konkel and Joens (51), who found that poliovirus infection did not enhance *C. jejuni* adherence and invasiveness in vitro (see above). Superti et al. (82) speculated poliovirus infection may have affected the cell membrane such that bacterial entry was inhibited.

In Vitro Studies of EIEC Infection of Virus-Infected Cells

Bukholm (11) showed that when MA-104 cells were preinfected with human rotavirus, the invasiveness of EIEC was enhanced.

In Vitro Studies of the Effect of Viral Infection on the Invasiveness of Noninvasive Bacteria

A range of studies utilizing a number of noninvasive bacteria have all shown that viral infection in vitro does not enhance the invasiveness of these bacteria. Thus, Bukholm and Degre (13) showed that coxsackie B1 virus infection of HEp-2 cells did not enable two strains of noninvasive *E. coli* to enter the cells. Bukholm (11) showed that rotavirus infection of MA-104 cells did not enable nonenteropathogenic *E. coli* to enter the cells. Konkel and Joens (51) found that *Campylobacter hyointestinalis* and *Campylobacter mucosalis*, two noninvasive isolates, could not invade HEp-2 cells infected with coxsackie B3 virus.

Marchetti et al. (57) showed that a mutant form of *S. flexneri*, which lacked invasive properties, did not show any invasive ability in HeLa cells infected with poliovirus 1, coxsackie B3 virus, and echovirus 6.

Summary of in Vitro Studies

In general, viral infection enhances the bacterial invasiveness of a range of enteropathogenic bacteria which would normally enter a cell, but the viral infection does not enable bacteria which normally do not enter a cell to invade it.

Different viruses can exert different effects in such experiments; for example, rotavirus and poliovirus preinfection have opposite effects on *L. monocytogenes* invasiveness (82). Furthermore preinfection with a particular virus can have a range of effects for different bacteria. Poliovirus infection, for example, inhibited the invasiveness of *L. monocytogenes,* had no effect on the invasiveness of at least one strain of *C. jejuni,* and enhanced the invasiveness of *S. flexneri.*

The mechanism of enhanced bacterial invasiveness following viral infection is unknown. Apparently, changes to the cell membrane following viral infection are crucial, but subsequent stages of viral replication may also be important.

Under some circumstances bacterial infection (e.g., *L. monocytogenes*) stimulated viral replication (i.e., rotavirus), whereas in other circumstances bacterial infection (i.e., *Y. enterocolitica* and *Y. pseudotuberculosis*) decreased viral (i.e., rotavirus) antigen synthesis. The mechanism of these effects is unknown.

CONCLUSION

Mixed viral-bacterial infections are common in human gastroenteritis. Some evidence from both human and animal studies shows that there can be a range of effects on clinical symptoms, varying from increased pathogenicity to no effect to reduced pathogenicity. In vitro studies indicate viral infection can facilitate or hamper bacterial adhesion or invasiveness, thus explaining increased or decreased pathogenicity. However, it is difficult to make predictions for specific virus-bacterium combinations or even to maintain that the full range of possible mechanisms of joint effects has been explored. The precise interactions between bacteria and viruses in mixed infection in the gastrointestinal tract are still poorly understood.

ACKNOWLEDGMENTS

I thank S. Maunders for typing the manuscript and the staff of the Royal Melbourne Hospital Library for invaluable assistance in obtaining references.

REFERENCES

1. **Albert, M. J., A. S. G. Faruque, S. M. Faruque, R. B. Sack, and D. Mahalanabis.** 1999. Case-control study of enteropathogens associated with childhood diarrhea in Dhaka, Bangladesh. *J. Clin. Microbiol.* **37:**3458–3464.
2. **Barnes, G. L., E. Uren, K. B. Stevens, and R. F. Bishop.** 1998. Etiology of acute gastroenteritis in hospitalized children in Melbourne, Australia, from April 1980 to March 1993. *J. Clin. Microbiol.* **36:**133–138.
3. **Barton, M. D., V. Kolega, and S. G. Fenwick.** 1997. *Yersinia enterocolitica,* p. 493–519. *In* A. D. Hocking, G. Arnold, I. Jenson, K. Newton, and P. Sutherland (ed.), *Foodborne Microorganisms of Public Health Significance,* 5th ed. Australian Institute of Food Science and Technology Inc., NSW Branch, Food Microbiology Group, Sydney, New South Wales, Australia.
4. **Bates, J. R.** 1997. *Clostridium perfringens,* p. 407–427. *In* A. D. Hocking, G. Arnold, I. Jenson, K. Newton, and P. Sutherland (ed.), *Foodborne Microorganisms of Public Health Significance,* 5th ed. Australian Institute of Food Science and Technology Inc., NSW Branch, Food Microbiology Group, Sydney, New South Wales, Australia.
5. **Benfield, D. A., D. H. Francis, J. P. McAdaragh, D. D. Johnson, M. E. Bergeland, K. Rossow, and R. Moore.** 1988. Combined rotavirus and K99 *Escherichia coli* infection in gnotobiotic pigs. *Am. J. Vet. Res.* **49:**330–337.
6. **Benko, M., B. Harrach, and W. C. Russell.** 2000. Family *Adenoviridae,* p. 227–238. *In* M. H. V. van Regenmortel, C. M. Fauquet, D. H. L. Bishop, E. B. Carstens, M. K. Estes, S. M. Lemon, J. Maniloff, M. A. Mayo, D. J. McGeoch, C. R. Pringle, and R. B. Wickner (ed.), *Virus Taxonomy.* Academic Press, San Diego, Calif.
7. **Bettelheim, K. A., V. Bennett-Wood, D. Lightfoot, P. J. Wright, and J. A. Marshall.** 2001. Simultaneous isolation of verotoxin-producing strains of *Escherichia coli* O128: H2 and viruses in gastroenteritis outbreaks. *Comp. Immunol. Microbiol. Infect. Dis.* **24:**135–142.
8. **Bettelheim, K. A., D. S. Bowden, J. C. Doultree, M. G. Catton, D. Chibo, N. J. P. Ryan, P. J. Wright, I. C. Gunesekere, J. M. Griffith, D. Lightfoot, G. G. Hogg, V. Bennett-Wood, and J. A. Marshall.** 1999. Combined infection of Norwalk-like virus and verotoxin-producing bacteria associated with a gastroenteritis outbreak. *J. Diarrhoeal Dis. Res.* **17:** 34–36.
9. **Bishop, R. F.** 1994. Natural history of human rotavirus infections, p. 131–167. *In* A. Z. Kapikian (ed.), *Viral Infections of the Gastrointestinal Tract.* 2nd ed. Marcel Dekker Inc., New York, N.Y.

10. **Bon, F., P. Fascia, M. Dauvergne, D. Tenenbaum, H. Planson, A. M. Petion, P. Pothier, and E. Kohli.** 1999. Prevalence of group A rotavirus, human calicivirus, astrovirus and adenovirus type 40 and 41 infections among children with acute gastroenteritis in Dijon, France. *J. Clin. Microbiol.* **37:**3055–3058.

11. **Bukholm, G.** 1988. Human rotavirus infection enhances invasiveness of enterobacteria in MA-104 cells. *APMIS* **96:**1118–1124.

12. **Bukholm, G., K. Bjornland, H. Ellekjaer, B. P. Berdal, and M. Degre.** 1988. Vesicular stomatitis virus infection enhances invasiveness of *Salmonella typhimurium*. *APMIS* **96:**400–406.

13. **Bukholm, G., and M. Degre.** 1984. Invasiveness of *Salmonella typhimurium* in HEp-2 cell cultures preinfected with coxsackie B 1 virus. *Acta Pathol. Microbiol. Immunol. Scand. Sect. B* **92:**45–51.

14. **Bukholm, G., M. Holberg-Petersen, and M. Degre.** 1985. Invasiveness of *Salmonella typhimurium* in HEp-2 cell cultures pretreated with UV-inactivated coxsackie virus. *Acta Pathol. Microbiol. Immunol. Scand. Sect. B* **93:**61–65.

15. **Bukholm, G., K. Modalsli, and M. Degre.** 1986. Effect of measles-virus infection and interferon treatment on invasiveness of *Shigella flexneri* in HEp2-cell cultures. *J. Med. Microbiol.* **22:**335–341.

16. **Cauchi, M. R., J. C. Doultree, J. A. Marshall, and P. J. Wright.** 1996. Molecular characterization of Camberwell virus and sequence variation in ORF3 of small round-structured (Norwalk-like) viruses. *J. Med. Virol.* **49:**70–76.

17. **Caul, E. O.** 1994. Human coronaviruses, p. 603–625. *In* A. Z. Kapikian (ed.), *Viral Infections of the Gastrointestinal Tract,* 2nd ed. Marcel Dekker Inc., New York, N.Y.

18. **Caul, E. O.** 1996. Viral gastroenteritis: small round structured viruses, caliciviruses and astroviruses. Part I. The clinical and diagnostic perspective. *J. Clin. Pathol.* (London) **49:**874–880.

19. **Cox, E., V. Cools, H. Thoonen, J. Hoorens, and A. Houvenaghel.** 1988. Effect of experimentally-induced villus atrophy on adhesion of K88ac-positive *Escherichia coli* in just-weaned piglets. *Vet. Microbiol.* **17:**159–169.

20. **Cox, G. J., S. M. Matsui, R. S. Lo, M. Hinds, R. A. Bowden, R. C. Hackman, W. G. Meyer, M. Mori, P. I. Tarr, L. S. Oshiro, J. E. Ludert, J. D. Meyers, and G. B. McDonald.** 1994. Etiology and outcome of diarrhea after marrow transplantation: a prospective study. *Gastroenterology* **107:**1398–1407.

21. **Cravioto, A., A. Tello, A. Navarro, J. Ruiz, H. Villafan, F. Uribe, and C. Eslava.** 1991. Association of *Escherichia coli* HEp-2 adherence patterns with type and duration of diarrhoea. *Lancet* **337:**262–264.

22. **Cruz, J. R., A. V. Bartlett, J. E. Herrmann, P. Caceres, N. R. Blacklow, and F. Cano.** 1992. Astrovirus-associated diarrhea among Guatemalan ambulatory rural children. *J. Clin. Microbiol.* **30:**1140–1144.

23. **Cubitt, W. D.** 1994. Caliciviruses, p. 549–568. *In* A. Z. Kapikian (ed.), *Viral Infections of the Gastrointestinal Tract,* 2nd ed. Marcel Dekker Inc., New York, N.Y.

24. **Desmarchelier, P. M.** 1997. Pathogenic vibrios, p. 285–312. *In* A. D. Hocking, G. Arnold, I. Jenson, K. Newton, and P. Sutherland (ed.), *Foodborne Microorganisms of Public Health Significance,* 5th ed. Australian Institute of Food Science and Technology Inc., NSW Branch, Food Microbiology Group, Sydney, New South Wales, Australia.

25. **Desmarchelier, P. M., and F. H. Grau.** 1997. *Escherichia coli,* p. 231–264. *In* A. D. Hocking, G. Arnold, I. Jenson, K. Newton, and P. Sutherland (ed.), *Foodborne Microorganisms of Public Health Significance,* 5th ed. Australian Institute of Food Science and Technology Inc., NSW Branch, Food Microbiology Group, Sydney, New South Wales, Australia.

26. **Di Biase, A. M., G. Petrone, M. P. Conte, L. Seganti, M. G. Ammendolia, A. Tinari, F. Iosi, M. Marchetti, and F. Superti.** 2000. Infection of human enterocyte-like cells with rotavirus enhances invasiveness of *Yersinia enterocolitica* and *Y. pseudotuberculosis*. *J. Med. Microbiol.* **49:**897–904.

27. **Donta, S. T., R. B. Wallace, S. C. Whipp, and J. Olarte.** 1977. Enterotoxigenic *Escherichia coli* and diarrheal disease in Mexican children. *J. Infect. Dis.* **135:**482–485.

28. **Echeverria, P., N. R. Blacklow, J. L. Vollet III, C. V. Ulyangco, G. Cukor, V. B. Soriano, H. L. Du Pont, J. H. Cross, F. Orskov, and I. Orskov.** 1978. Reovirus-like agent and enterotoxigenic *Escherichia coli* infections in pediatric diarrhea in the Philippines. *J. Infect. Dis.* **138:**326–332.

29. **Enjuanes, L., D. Brian, D. Cavanagh, K. Holmes, M. M. C. Lai, H. Laude, P. Masters, P. J. M. Rottier, S. G. Siddell, W. J. M. Spaan, F. Taguchi, and P. Talbot.** 2000. Family *Coronaviridae,* p. 835–849. *In* M. H. V. van Regenmortel, C. M. Fauquet, D. H. L. Bishop, E. B. Carstens, M. K. Estes, S. M. Lemon, J. Maniloff, M. A. Mayo, D. J. McGeoch, C. R. Pringle, and R. B. Wickner (ed.), *Virus Taxonomy.* Academic Press, San Diego, Calif.

30. **Estes, M. K., G. Kang, C. Q.-Y. Zeng, S. E. Crawford, and M. Ciarlet.** 2001. Pathogenesis

of rotavirus gastroenteritis, p. 82–100. *In* D. Chadwick, and J. A. Goode (ed.), *Gastroenteritis Viruses.* John Wiley and Sons, Ltd., Chichester, United Kingdom.

31. **Evans, D. G., J. Olarte, H. L. Du Pont, D. J. Evans, E. Galindo, B. L. Portnoy, and R. H. Conklin.** 1977. Enteropathogens associated with pediatric diarrhea in Mexico City. *J. Pediatr.* **91:**65–68.

32. **Farkas, T., X. Jiang, M. L. Guerrero, W. Zhong, N. Wilton, T. Berke, D. O. Matson, L. K. Pickering, and G. Ruiz-Palacios.** 2000. Prevalence and genetic diversity of human caliciviruses (HuCVs) in Mexican children. *J. Med. Virol.* **62:**217–223.

33. **Flores-Abuxapqui, J. J., G. J. Suarez-Hoil, M. A. Puc-Franco, M. R. Heredia-Navarrete, and J. Franco-Monsreal.** 1993. Prevalencia de enteropatogenos en ninos con diarrea liquida. *Rev. Latinoam. Microbiol.* **35:**351–356.

34. **Gaggero, A., M. O'Ryan, J. S. Noel, R. I. Glass, S. S. Monroe, N. Mamani, V. Prado, and L. F. Avendano.** 1998. Prevalence of astrovirus infection among Chilean children with acute gastroenteritis. *J. Clin. Microbiol.* **36:**3691–3693.

35. **Glass, R. I., J. Noel, T. Ando, R. Fankhauser, G. Belliot, A. Mounts, U. D. Parashar, J. S. Bresee, and S. S. Monroe.** 2000. The epidemiology of enteric caliciviruses from humans: a reassessment using new diagnostics. *J. Infect. Dis.* **181**(Suppl. 2):S254–S261.

36. **Gouet, P., M. Contrepois, H. C. Dubourguier, Y. Riou, R. Scherrer, J. Laporte, J. F. Vautherot, J. Cohen, and R. L'Haridon.** 1978. The experimental production of diarrhoea in colostrum deprived axenic and gnotoxenic calves with enteropathogenic *Escherichia coli*, rotavirus, coronavirus and in a combined infection of rotavirus and *E. coli. Ann. Rech. Vet.* **9:**433–440.

37. **Graham, D. Y., X. Jiang, T. Tanaka, A. R. Opekun, H. P. Madore, and M. K. Estes.** 1994. Norwalk virus infection of volunteers: new insights based on improved assays. *J. Infect. Dis.* **170:**34–43.

38. **Green, K. Y., T. Ando, M. S. Balayan, I. N. Clarke, M. K. Estes, D. O. Matson, S. Nakata, J. D. Neill, M. J. Studdert, and H.-J. Thiel.** 2000. Family *Caliciviridae*, p. 725–735. *In* M. H. V. van Regenmortel, C. M. Fauquet, D. H. L. Bishop, E. B. Carstens, M. K. Estes, S. M. Lemon, J. Maniloff, M. A. Mayo, D. J. McGeoch, C. R. Pringle, and R. B. Wickner (ed.), *Virus Taxonomy.* Academic Press, San Diego, Calif.

39. **Guerrero, M. L., J. S. Noel, D. K. Mitchell, J. J. Calva, A. L. Morrow, J. Martinez, G.**

Rosales, F. R. Velazquez, S. S. Monroe, R. I. Glass, L. K. Pickering, and G. M. Ruiz-Palacios. 1998. A prospective study of astrovirus diarrhea of infancy in Mexico City. *Pediatr. Infect. Dis. J.* **17:**723–727.

40. **Hellard, M. E., M. I. Sinclair, G. G. Hogg, and C. K. Fairley.** 2000. Prevalence of enteric pathogens among community based asymptomatic individuals. *J. Gastroenterol. Hepatol.* **15:** 290–293.

41. **Hess, R. G., P. A. Bachmann, G. Baljer, A. Mayr, A. Pospischil, and G. Schmid.** 1984. Synergism in experimental mixed infections of newborn colostrum-deprived calves with bovine rotavirus and enterotoxigenic *Escherichia coli* (ETEC). *Zentbl. Vetmed. Reihe B* **31:**585–596.

42. **Hori, H., P. Akpedonu, G. Armah, M. Aryeetey, J. Yartey, H. Kamiya, and M. Sakurai.** 1996. Enteric pathogens in severe forms of acute gastroenteritis in Ghanaian children. *Acta Pediatr. Jpn.* **38:**672–676.

43. **Howard, P., N. D. Alexander, A. Atkinson, A. O. Clegg, G. Gerega, A. Javati, M. Kajoi, S. Lupiwa, T. Lupiwa, M. Mens, G. Saleu, R. C. Sanders, B. West, and M. P. Alpers.** 2000. Bacterial, viral and parasitic aetiology of paediatric diarrhoea in the highlands of Papua New Guinea. *J. Trop. Pediatr.* **46:**10–14.

44. **Jackson, S. G., R. B. Goodbrand, R. Ahmed, and S. Kasatiya.** 1995. *Bacillus cereus* and *Bacillus thuringiensis* isolated in a gastroenteritis outbreak investigation. *Lett. Appl. Microbiol.* **21:**103–105.

45. **Jamieson, F. B., E. E. L. Wang, C. Bain, J. Good, L. Duckmanton, and M. Petric.** 1998. Human torovirus: a new nosocomial gastrointestinal pathogen. *J. Infect. Dis.* **178:**1263–1269.

46. **Jay, S., F. H. Grau, K. Smith, D. Lightfoot, C. Murray, and G. R. Davey.** 1997. *Salmonella*, p. 169–229. *In* A. D. Hocking, G. Arnold, I. Jenson, K. Newton, and P. Sutherland (ed.), *Foodborne Microorganisms of Public Health Significance,* 5th ed. Australian Institute of Food Science and Technology Inc., NSW Branch, Food Microbiology Group, Sydney, New South Wales, Australia.

47. **Jenson, I., and C. J. Moir.** 1997. *Bacillus cereus* and other *Bacillus* species, p. 379–406. *In* A. D. Hocking, G. Arnold, I. Jenson, K. Newton, and P. Sutherland (ed.), *Foodborne Microorganisms of Public Health Significance,* 5th ed. Australian Institute of Food Science and Technology Inc., NSW Branch, Food Microbiology Group, Sydney, New South Wales, Australia.

48. **Kain, K. C., R. L. Barteluk, M. T. Kelly, H. Xin, G. D. Hua, G. Yuan, E. M. Proctor, S. Byrne, and H. G. Stiver.** 1991. Etiology of

childhood diarrhea in Beijing, China. *J. Clin. Microbiol.* **29**:90–95.

49. **Kapikian, A. Z.** 1994. Norwalk and Norwalk-like viruses, p. 471–518. *In* A. Z. Kapikian (ed.), *Viral Infections of the Gastrointestinal Tract,* 2nd ed. Marcel Dekker Inc., New York, N.Y.

50. **Kirov, S. M.** 1997. *Aeromonas,* p. 473–492. *In* A. D. Hocking, G. Arnold, I. Jenson, K. Newton, and P. Sutherland (ed.), *Foodborne Microorganisms of Public Health Significance,* 5th ed. Australian Institute of Food Science and Technology Inc., NSW Branch, Food Microbiology Group, Sydney, New South Wales, Australia.

51. **Konkel, M. E., and L. A. Joens.** 1990. Effect of enteroviruses on adherence to and invasion of HEp-2 cells by *Campylobacter* isolates. *Infect. Immun.* **58**:1101–1105.

52. **Koopmans, M. P. G., E. S. M. Goosen, A. A. M. Lima, I. T. McAuliffe, J. P. Nataro, L. J. Barrett, R. I. Glass, and R. L. Guerrant.** 1997. Association of torovirus with acute and persistent diarrhea in children. *Pediatr. Infect. Dis. J.* **16**:504–507.

53. **Kurtz, J. B.** 1994. Astroviruses, p. 569–580. *In* A. Z. Kapikian (ed.), *Viral Infections of the Gastrointestinal Tract,* 2nd ed. Marcel Dekker Inc., New York, N.Y.

54. **Lam, S., S. B. Lim, M. Yin-Murphy, and M. Nasir.** 1987. Aetiology of diarrhoea in Singapore. *Ann. Acad. Med. Singapore* **16**:571–576.

55. **Lightfoot, D.** 1997. *Shigella,* p. 465–472. *In* A. D. Hocking, G. Arnold, I. Jenson, K. Newton, and P. Sutherland (ed.), *Foodborne Microorganisms of Public Health Significance,* 5th ed. Australian Institute of Food Science and Technology Inc., NSW Branch, Food Microbiology Group, Sydney, New South Wales, Australia.

56. **Ling, J. M., and A. F. Cheng.** 1993. Infectious diarrhoea in Hong Kong. *J. Trop. Med. Hyg.* **96**:107–112.

57. **Marchetti, M., M. P. Conte, C. Longhi, M. Nicoletti, L. Seganti, and N. Orsi.** 1992. Effect of enterovirus infection on susceptibility of HeLa cells to *Shigella flexneri* invasivity. *Acta Virol.* **36**:443–449.

58. **Marshall, J. A., C. J. Birch, H. G. Williamson, D. K. Bowden, C. M. Boveington, T. Kuberski, P. H. Bennett, and I. D. Gust.** 1982. Coronavirus-like particles and other agents in the faeces of children in Efate, Vanuatu. *J. Trop. Med. Hyg.* **85**:213–215.

59. **Marshall, J. A., S. Salamone, L. Yuen, M. G. Catton, and P. J. Wright.** 2001. High level excretion of Norwalk-like virus following resolution of clinical illness. *Pathology* **33**:50–52.

60. **Marshall, J. A., W. L. Thompson, and I. D. Gust.** 1989. Coronavirus-like particles in adults in Melbourne, Australia. *J. Med. Virol.* **29**:238–243.

61. **Mata, L., A. Simhon, R. Padilla, M. D. M. Gamboa, G. Vargas, F. Hernandez, E. Mohs, and C. Lizano.** 1983. Diarrhea associated with rotaviruses, enterotoxigenic *Escherichia coli, Campylobacter* and other agents in Costa Rican children 1976–1981. *Am. J. Trop. Med. Hyg.* **32**:146–153.

62. **Meqdam, M. M. M., M. T. Youssef, M. O. Rawashdeh, and M. S. Al-khdour.** 1997. Non-seasonal viral and bacterial episode of diarrhoea in the Jordan Valley, West of Jordan. *FEMS Immunol. Med. Microbiol.* **18**:133–138.

63. **Modalsli, K., G. Bukholm, and M. Degre.** 1990. Coxsackie B1 virus infection enhances the bacterial invasiveness, the phagocytosis and the membrane permeability in HEp-2 cells. *APMIS* **98**:489–495.

64. **Modalsli, K. R., S.-O. Mikalsen, G. Bukholm, and M. Degre.** 1993. Microinjection of HEp-2 cells with coxsackie B1 virus RNA enhances invasiveness of *Shigella flexneri* only after prestimulation with UV-inactivated virus. *APMIS* **101**:602–606.

65. **Monroe, S. S., M. J. Carter, J. E. Herrmann, J. B. Kurtz, and S. M. Matsui.** 2000. Family *Astroviridae,* p. 741–745. *In* M. H. V. van Regenmortel, C. M. Fauquet, D. H. L. Bishop, E. B. Carstens, M. K. Estes, S. M. Lemon, J. Maniloff, M. A. Mayo, D. J. McGeoch, C. R. Pringle, and R. B. Wickner (ed.), *Virus Taxonomy.* Academic Press, San Diego, Calif.

66. **Nataro, J. P., and J. B. Kaper.** 1998. Diarrheagenic *Escherichia coli. Clin. Microbiol. Rev.* **11**:142–201.

67. **Nataro, J. P., and M. M. Levine.** 1994. Bacterial diarrheas, p. 697–752. *In* A. Z. Kapikian (ed.), *Viral Infections of the Gastrointestinal Tract,* 2nd ed. Marcel Dekker Inc., New York, N.Y.

68. **Newsome, P. M., and K. A. Coney.** 1985. Synergistic rotavirus and *Escherichia coli* diarrheal infection of mice. *Infect. Immun.* **47**:573–574.

69. **Oyofo, B. A., R. Soderquist, M. Lesmana, D. Subekti, P. Tjaniadi, D. J. Fryauff, A. L. Corwin, E. Richie, and C. Lebron.** 1999. Norwalk-like virus and bacterial pathogens associated with cases of gastroenteritis onboard a U.S. navy ship. *Am. J. Trop. Med. Hyg.* **61**:904–908.

70. **Parashar, U. D., L. Dow, R. L. Fankhauser, C. D. Humphrey, J. Miller, T. Ando, K. S. Williams, C. R. Eddy, J. S. Noel, T. Ingram, J. S. Bresee, S. S. Monroe, and R. I. Glass.** 1998. An outbreak of viral gastroenteritis associated with consumption of sandwiches: implications for the control of transmission by food handlers. *Epidemiol. Infect.* **121**:615–621.

71. **Pollok, R. C. G., and M. J. G. Farthing.** 2000. Enteric viruses in HIV-related diarrhoea. *Mol. Med. Today* **6:**483–487.

72. **Runnels, P. L., H. W. Moon, P. J. Matthews, S. C. Whipp, and G. N. Woode.** 1986. Effects of microbial and host variables on the interaction of rotavirus and *Escherichia coli* infections in gnotobiotic calves. *Am. J. Vet. Res.* **47:** 1542–1550.

73. **Samuel, S., J. Vadivelu, and N. Parasakthi.** 1997. Characteristics of childhood diarrhea associated with enterotoxigenic *Escherichia coli* in Malaysia. *Southeast Asian J. Trop. Med. Public Health* **28:**114–119.

74. **Schorling, J. B., C. A. Wanke, S. K. Schorling, J. F. McAuliffe, M. A. de Souza, and R. L. Guerrant.** 1990. A prospective study of persistent diarrhea among children in an urban Brazilian slum. *Am. J. Epidemiol.* **132:**144–156.

75. **Sethi, S. K., F. A. Khuffash, and W. Al-Nakib.** 1989. Microbial etiology of acute gastroenteritis in hospitalized children in Kuwait. *Pediatr. Infect. Dis. J.* **8:**593–597.

76. **Shastri, S., A. M. Doane, J. Gonzales, U. Upadhyayula, and D. M. Bass.** 1998. Prevalence of astroviruses in a children's hospital. *J. Clin. Microbiol.* **36:**2571–2574.

77. **Singh, P. B., M. A. Sreenivasan, and K. M. Pavri.** 1989. Viruses in acute gastroenteritis in children in Pune, India. *Epidemiol. Infect.* **102:** 345–353.

78. **Snodgrass, D. R., M. L. Smith, and F. L. Krautil.** 1982. Interaction of rotavirus and enterotoxigenic *Escherichia coli* in conventionally-reared dairy calves. *Vet. Microbiol.* **7:**51–60.

79. **Soenarto, Y., T. Sebodo, P. Suryantoro, Krisnomurti, S. Haksohusodo, Ilyas, Kusniyo, Ristano, M. A. Romas, Noerhajati, S. Muswiroh, J. E. Rohde, N. J. Ryan, R. K. J. Luke, G. L. Barnes, and R. F. Bishop.** 1983. Bacteria, parasitic agents and rotaviruses associated with acute diarrhoea in hospital in-patient Indonesian children. *Trans. Soc. R. Trop. Med. Hyg.* **77:**724–730.

80. **Stanway, G., P. Joki-Korpela, and T. Hyypia.** 2000. Human parechoviruses: biology and clinical significance. *Rev. Med. Virol.* **10:**57–69.

81. **Stewien, K. E., E. N. Mos, R. M. Yanaguita, J. A. Jerez, E. L. Durigon, C. M. Harsi, H. Tanaka, R. M. Moraes, L. A. Silva, M. A. A. Santos, J. M. G. Candeias, K. Tanaka, T. C. T. Peret, E. R. Baldacci, and A. E. Gilio.** 1993. Viral, bacterial and parasitic pathogens associated with severe diarrhoea in the city of Sao Paulo, Brazil. *J. Diarrhoeal Dis. Res.* **11:**148–152.

82. **Superti, F., G. Petrone, S. Pisani, R. Morelli, M. G. Ammendolia, and L. Seganti.** 1996. Superinfection by *Listeria monocytogenes* of cultured human enterocyte-like cells infected with poliovirus or rotavirus. *Med. Microbiol. Immunol.* **185:**131–137.

83. **Sutherland, P. S., and R. J. Porritt.** 1997. *Listeria monocytogenes,* p. 333–378. *In* A. D. Hocking, G. Arnold, I. Jenson, K. Newton, and P. Sutherland (ed.), *Foodborne Microorganisms of Public Health Significance,* 5th ed. Australian Institute of Food Science and Technology Inc., NSW Branch, Food Microbiology Group, Sydney, New South Wales, Australia.

84. **Szabo, E. A., and A. M. Gibson.** 1997. *Clostridium botulinum,* p. 429–464. *In* A. D. Hocking, G. Arnold, I. Jenson, K. Newton, and P. Sutherland (ed.), *Foodborne Microorganisms of Public Health Significance,* 5th ed. Australian Institute of Food Science and Technology Inc., NSW Branch, Food Microbiology Group, Sydney, New South Wales, Australia.

85. **Taylor, D. N., P. Echeverria, M. J. Blaser, C. Pitarangsi, N. Blacklow, J. Cross, and B. G. Weniger.** 1985. Polymicrobial aetiology of travellers' diarrhoea. *Lancet* **i:**381–383.

86. **Thouless, M. E., R. F. DiGiacomo, and B. J. Deeb.** 1996. The effect of combined rotavirus and *Escherichia coli* infections in rabbits. *Lab. Anim. Sci.* **46:**381–385.

87. **Tompkins, D. S., M. J. Hudson, H. R. Smith, R. P. Eglin, J. G. Wheeler, M. M. Brett, R. J. Owen, J. S. Brazier, P. Cumberland, V. King, and P. E. Cook.** 1999. A study of infectious intestinal disease in England: microbiological findings in cases and controls. *Commun. Dis. Public Health* **2:**108–113.

88. **Torres-Medina, A.** 1984. Effect of combined rotavirus and *Escherichia coli* in neonatal gnotobiotic calves. *Am. J. Vet. Res.* **45:**643–651.

89. **Tuazon, C. U.** 1995. Other *Bacillus* species, p. 1890–1894. *In* G. L. Mandell, J. E. Bennett, and R. Dolin (ed.), *Mandell, Douglas and Bennett's Principles and Practice of Infectious Diseases,* 4th ed. Churchill Livingstone, New York, N.Y.

90. **Tzipori, S., D. Chandler, T. Makin, and M. Smith.** 1980. *Escherichia coli* and rotavirus infections in four-week-old gnotobiotic piglets fed milk or dry food. *Aust. Vet. J.* **56:**279–284.

91. **Tzipori, S., T. Makin, M. Smith, and F. Krautil.** 1982. Enteritis in foals induced by rotavirus and enterotoxigenic *Escherichia coli*. *Aust. Vet. J.* **58:**20–23.

92. **Tzipori, S., M. Smith, C. Halpin, T. Makin, and F. Krautil.** 1983. Intestinal changes associated with rotavirus and enterotoxigenic *Escherichia coli* infection in calves. *Vet. Microbiol.* **8:**35–43.

93. **Tzipori, S. R., T. J. Makin, M. L. Smith, and F. L. Krautil.** 1981. Clinical manifestations of diarrhea in calves infected with rotavirus and enterotoxigenic *Escherichia coli. J. Clin. Microbiol.* **13:**1011–1016.

94. **Uhnoo, I., E. Olding-Stenkvist, and A. Kreuger.** 1986. Clinical features of acute gastroenteritis associated with rotavirus, enteric adenoviruses, and bacteria. *Arch. Dis. Child.* **61:**732–738.

95. **Ullrich, R., W. Heise, C. Bergs, M. L'age, E. O. Riecken, and M. Zeitz.** 1992. Gastrointestinal symptoms in patients infected with human immunodeficiency virus: relevance of infective agents isolated from gastrointestinal tract. *Gut* **33:**1080–1084.

96. **Unicomb, L. E., S. M. Faruque, M. A. Malek, A. S. G. Faruque, and M. J. Albert.** 1996. Demonstration of a lack of synergistic effect of rotavirus with other diarrheal pathogens on severity of diarrhea in children. *J. Clin. Microbiol.* **34:**1340–1342.

97. **Vergara, M., M. Quiroga, S. Grenon, E. Pegels, P. Oviedo, J. Deschutter, M. Rivas, N. Binsztein, and R. Claramount.** 1996. Prospective study of enteropathogens in two communities of Misiones, Argentina. *Rev. Inst. Med. Trop. Sao Paulo* **38:**337–347.

98. **Wadell, G., A. Allard, M. Johansson, L. Svensson, and I. Uhnoo.** 1994. Enteric adenoviruses, p. 519–547. *In* A. Z. Kapikian (ed.), *Viral Infections of the Gastrointestinal Tract,* 2nd ed. Marcel Dekker Inc., New York, N.Y.

99. **Wallace, R. B.** 1997. *Campylobacter,* p. 265–284. *In* A. D. Hocking, G. Arnold, I. Jenson, K. Newton, and P. Sutherland (ed.), *Foodborne Microorganisms of Public Health Significance,* 5th ed. Australian Institute of Food Science and Technology Inc., NSW Branch, Food Microbiology Group, Sydney, New South Wales, Australia.

100. **Whipp, S. C., H. W. Moon, L. J. Kemeny, and R. A. Argenzio.** 1985. Effect of virus-induced destruction of villous epithelium on intestinal secretion induced by heat-stable *Escherichia coli* enterotoxins and prostaglandin E_1 in swine. *Am. J. Vet. Res.* **46:**637–642.

101. **Woode, G. N.** 1994. The toroviruses: bovine (Breda virus) and equine (Berne virus) and the torovirus-like agents of humans and animals, p. 581–602. *In* A. Z. Kapikian (ed.), *Viral Infections of the Gastrointestinal Tract,* 2nd ed. Marcel Dekker Inc., New York, N.Y.

102. **Wray, C., M. Dawson, A. Afshar, and M. Lucas.** 1981. Experimental *Escherichia coli* and rotavirus infection in lambs. *Res. Vet. Sci.* **30:**379–381.

103. **Yamashita, T., K. Sakae, S. Kobayashi, Y. Ishihara, T. Miyake, A. Mubina, and S. Isomura.** 1995. Isolation of cytopathic small round virus (Aichi virus) from Pakistani children and Japanese travelers from Southeast Asia. *Microbiol. Immunol.* **39:**433–435.

104. **Yamashita, T., K. Sakae, H. Tsuzuki, Y. Suzuki, N. Ishikawa, N. Takeda, T. Miyamura, and S. Yamazaki.** 1998. Complete nucleotide sequence and genetic organization of Aichi virus, a distinct member of the *Picornaviridae* associated with acute gastroenteritis in humans. *J. Virol.* **72:**8408–8412.

105. **Zhang, X. M., W. Herbst, K. G. Kousoulas, and J. Storz.** 1994. Biological and genetic characterization of a hemagglutinating coronavirus isolated from a diarrhoeic child. *J. Med. Virol.* **44:**152–161.

INTERACTIONS BETWEEN HERPESVIRUSES AND BACTERIA IN HUMAN PERIODONTAL DISEASE

Jørgen Slots

16

Destructive periodontal diseases are infectious disorders, but the specific mechanisms by which tooth-supportive tissue is lost remain obscure. This chapter proposes an infectious disease model for severe periodontitis in which herpesviral-bacterial interactions assume a major etiopathogenic role. Herpesviruses, especially cytomegalovirus (HCMV), Epstein-Barr virus type 1 (EBV-1), and HCMV/EBV-1 dual infection, have recently been identified in most of the advanced periodontitis lesions of children, adolescents, and adults. Herpes simplex virus (HSV) type 1, human herpesvirus 6 (HHV-6), HHV-7, and HHV-8 (individuals infected with the human immunodeficiency virus [HIV]) can also be detected in some periodontitis lesions. Evidence suggests that herpesvirus-infected periodontitis lesions harbor elevated levels of periodontopathic bacteria, including *Actinobacillus actinomycetemcomitans*, *Porphyromonas gingivalis*, *Dialister pneumosintes*, *Prevotella intermedia*, *Prevotella nigrescens*, and *Treponema denticola*. Conceivably, periodontal active herpesvirus infection impairs periodontal defenses, thereby permitting subgingival overgrowth of periodontopathic bacteria. It is further hypothesized that gingival tissue plays a role in the maintenance of herpesvirus load in vivo and that the shedding of herpesviruses from periodontal sites during reactivation plays a role in virus transmission. Understanding the significance of herpesviruses in human periodontitis may allow for improved diagnosis and, ultimately, disease prevention.

PERIODONTAL DISEASE

The term periodontal disease represents a variety of clinical manifestations of infectious disorders affecting the tooth-supporting tissues. Traditionally, periodontal disease is divided into gingivitis and periodontitis. Gingivitis indicates an inflammatory disease that is limited to gingiva with no clinical evidence of loss of periodontal ligament fibers or alveolar bone. Gingivitis sites show pocket depths typically ranging from 2 to 4 mm. The disease is reversible after instituting proper oral hygiene.

Periodontitis denotes an inflammatory destruction of the periodontal ligament and supporting bone. The course of periodontitis is characterized by intermittent exacerbations of the disease. Some periodontitis patients remain stable for many years, while other patients have a history of sporadic or gradually advancing disease that eventually may lead to tooth mobility and tooth loss. Although periodontitis

Jørgen Slots, School of Dentistry, MC 0641, University of Southern California, Los Angeles, CA 90089-0641.

Polymicrobial Diseases, Edited by Kim A. Brogden and Janet M. Guthmiller, © 2002 ASM Press, Washington, D.C.

has been found to be reversible, its reversibility is difficult to achieve and limited in degree, often requiring surgical regenerative procedures that may carry high financial costs.

Periodontitis is the major cause of tooth mortality in many developed countries, and most developing nations (59). Periodontitis, as measured by the presence of periodontal pockets exceeding 4-mm depth on an average of three to four teeth, affects approximately 30% of the U.S. population (58). Periodontal pockets of depths of 7 mm or more are present in less than 5% of the U.S. adult population (58) and in 2 to 28% of adults in Western European countries (90).

Periodontitis can be classified by type of patient (child, adolescent, adult, compromised host), by etiology (bacterial, fungal, or viral infection), by rate of progression (stable, aggressive), by extent of affected dentition (localized, generalized), by size of lesions (initial, moderate, or advanced breakdown), by morphology of lesions (angular or horizontal defect), by type of associated gingivitis (chronic, necrotizing), and by effectiveness of treatment (responsive, recalcitrant). Classification of periodontitis based on specific infectious agent etiology would facilitate treatment decisions, but such a classification system is presently unavailable.

PERIODONTAL INFECTIONS

Since the mid-1970s, significant inroads have been made into the microbiology and immunology of periodontal diseases. We can now feel confident that periodontitis represents several infectious disease entities with different pathogenic mechanisms (78).

The significance of bacteria in the development of virtually all types of periodontal disease is undisputable. While it is clear that approximately 500 bacterial species can be identified in periodontal pockets (64), it is also clear that relatively few species are considered legitimate pathogens of periodontitis. The bacterial mass is critical for the development of gingivitis and some types of chronic periodontitis ("nonspecific" infection), while the type of bacteria seems to be of greater importance in the initiation of aggressive periodontitis ("specific" infection). Colonization of specific microbial pathogens together with microbial synergy, the host immune response, and various environmental risk factors are major determinants of the probability of acquiring destructive periodontal disease (78).

Important periodontopathic bacteria include gram-negative facultative (*A. actinomycetemcomitans*) and anaerobic rods (*P. gingivalis, Bacteroides forsythus, D. pneumosintes*) (76). Organisms of probable periodontopathic significance are *P. intermedia, P. nigrescens, Campylobacter rectus, Peptostreptococcus micros, Fusobacterium* species, *Eubacterium* species, β-hemolytic streptococci, *Treponema* species, and perhaps yeasts, staphylococci, enterococci, pseudomonads, and various enteric rods (76).

During the past 5 years, herpesviruses have emerged as putative pathogens in destructive periodontal disease (17, 62). In particular, HCMV and EBV-1 seem to play important roles in the etiopathogenesis of severe types of periodontitis. Genomes of the two herpesviruses are frequently detected in aggressive periodontitis of children, adolescents, and adults, in periodontitis of immunocompromised hosts, and in necrotizing types of gingivitis (77). Genomes of HSV type 1 (3, 18, 23) and HHV-6 and HHV-7 (14) have also been identified in periodontitis lesions. Kaposi's sarcoma-associated virus (HHV-8) has been detected in HIV-related periodontitis (49).

This chapter reviews the continually evolving field of herpesviral infections of the human periodontium and proposes a model for aggressive periodontitis that is based on a combined herpesviral-bacterial causation of the disease. Emphasis is placed on the possible role of HCMV and EBV in the development of human periodontitis.

HERPESVIRUSES

For a general introduction to herpesviruses, the reader is referred to several authoritative reviews (2, 10, 40, 70). Herpesviral characteristics of potential importance in the pathogenesis of periodontitis are outlined below. Members of the herpesvirus family are composed of a double-stranded DNA genome contained within a nucleocapsid surrounded by a lipid envelope. To date, eight human viruses of the family *Herpesviridae* have been identified, namely, HSV types 1 and 2, varicella-zoster virus, EBV, HCMV, HHV-6, HHV-7, and HHV-8.

Most individuals become infected with herpesviruses early in life, and depending on the geographic location, between 60 and 100% of adults are carriers of HCMV and EBV (10, 40). A notable exception is HHV-8, which is contracted in adulthood. Primary herpesviral infections proceed with no signs of clinical disease in most individuals. The clinical manifestations of herpesvirus infections are very diverse and range in immunocompetent individuals from mild or subclinical disease to encephalitis, pneumonia, and other potentially lethal infections and to various types of cancer including lymphoma, sarcoma, and carcinoma (17). Herpesviral infections show a tendency to cell and tissue tropism, but the molecular basis for herpesviral tropism remains obscure.

HCMV infection is of great clinical significance in pregnant women, newborn infants with congenital infection, immunosuppressed transplant patients, and individuals with HIV infection (32). HCMV is the most common life-threatening infection in transplant and HIV-infected patients (32). HCMV has been also associated with cervical carcinoma and adenocarcinomas of the prostate and colon (22).

EBV is the causative agent of infectious mononucleosis and is implicated in the etiology of EBV-associated hemophagocytic syndrome, chronic active EBV infection lymphomas, inflammatory pseudotumor, lymphomatoid granulomatosis, Hodgkin's disease, nasopharyngeal carcinoma, and gastric carcinoma (46, 57). EBV was recently implicated in recurrent tonsillitis and tonsillar hypertrophy (24, 36). EBV is also associated with oral hairy leukoplakia and may show some relationship with rheumatoid arthritis and chronic fatigue syndrome.

Herpesviruses occur in a prolonged state of latency and in an active state. Latent viral genomes are almost entirely transcriptionally quiescent (71). Reactivating from latency results in renewed general viral gene expression (71). Herpesviruses are dependent on immune activating mechanisms for reactivation from viral latency to the production of a new viral progeny (82). Reactivation may occur spontaneously or as a result of concurrent infection, fever, drugs, tissue trauma, emotional stress, exposure to ultraviolet light, or other factors impairing the host immune defense.

Herpesviruses reside in and may functionally alter cells of central importance for regulating the immune system. HCMV infects most cell types and establishes latency in macrophage-granulocyte progenitors (41) and peripheral blood mononuclear cells (81). During symptomatic infection, HCMV DNA can be detected in polymorphonuclear leukocytes probably as a result of phagocytosis, although active viral replication may occasionally occur (53). EBV infects B lymphocytes, where it establishes latency (9), and may also infect monocytes (74) and polymorphonuclear leukocytes (43). Immunosuppression is the cardinal feature of herpesvirus-active infections.

Control of viral replication and prevention of pathology depend on both innate and adaptive immune mechanisms (66). Herpesvirus infections induce a strong antiviral immune response that nonetheless is incapable of eradicating the infection. The cellular immune response plays an important role in controlling resident herpesviral infections by means of major histocompatibility complex class I-restricted cytotoxic CD8$^+$ T lymphocytes that recognize viral peptides on the surface of infected cells (71). Infants and children infected with HCMV/EBV dual infection may experience more severe disease and markedly stronger T-lymphocyte responses than children infected with HCMV or EBV alone (89). On the other hand, herpesviruses also encode several genes that interfere with the activation of major histocompatibility complex class I-

and class II-restricted T lymphocytes and natural killer (NK) cells, modify the function of cytokines and their receptors, interact with complement factors, and modulate signal transduction and transcription factor activity as well as other cellular functions, thereby providing evasion strategies against antiviral specific immune responses (45).

Molecular testing is increasingly important in the diagnosis and monitoring of patients affected by viral diseases (4). PCR-based detection has revolutionized diagnostic virology by providing a sensitive and specific tool to detect and quantify viral DNA and RNA in clinical specimens (12). Use of PCR for detection of HCMV DNA can show HCMV in blood of almost all patients with overt HCMV disease, but low viral load can also be detected in a substantial number of patients with asymptomatic infections that never progress to disease. PCR techniques are also valuable in detecting chronic EBV infection in tissue and B lymphocytes, and are considerably faster and more sensitive than conventional tissue culture methods. Quantitative PCR may aid in differentiating a clinically significant herpesvirus burden from a latent one.

HERPESVIRUSES IN PERIODONTAL DISEASE

The occurrence of HCMV and EBV-1 and selected periodontal pathogenic bacteria in disease-active and disease-inactive early-onset periodontitis lesions has been studied (38). In 16 patients, who each contributed samples from two progressing and two stable periodontitis sites of similar pocket depth, HCMV, EBV-1, and HCMV/EBV-1 coinfection were significantly associated with disease-active periodontitis (Table 1). Significant associations were also found between the presence of *D. pneumosintes, P. gingivalis,* and *D. pneumosintes/ P. gingivalis* coinfection, and disease-active periodontitis (Table 1). Each periodontitis site that demonstrated HCMV/EBV-1 coinfection and all but one site showing *D. pneumosintes/P. gingivalis* coinfection revealed bleeding upon probing, a clinical sign of increased risk of progressive disease (42).

Localized juvenile periodontitis debuts at puberty, is confined to permanent incisors and first molars, affects mainly black individuals, and has a familial predisposition (44). Michalowics et al. (51) determined the occurrence of HCMV, EBV-1, *P. gingivalis,* and *A. actinomycetemcomitans* in subgingival plaque from 15 adolescents with localized juvenile periodontitis, 20 adolescents with incidental periodontal attachment loss, and 65 randomly selected healthy controls. All study subjects were Afro-Caribbeans living in Jamaica. The most parsimonious multivariate model for localized juvenile periodontitis included *P. gingivalis* (odds ratio, 8.7; 95% confidence limits,

TABLE 1 Occurrence of HCMV and EBV-1 in 32 progressing and 32 stable periodontitis sites of 16 early-onset periodontitis patients[a]

Item	32 disease-active periodontitis sites	32 disease-stable periodontitis sites	P value (χ^2 test)
Avg probing pocket (depth in mm)	5.9 ± 0.8	5.2 ± 1.0	Not significant
Teeth exhibiting bone loss (% of all teeth)	41.3 ± 6.3	43.9 ± 6.2	Not significant
Bleeding upon probing (no. [%] positive sites)	31 (96.9)	19 (59.4)	<0.001
No. (%) of HCMV-positive sites	19 (59.4)	4 (12.5)	<0.001
No. (%) of EBV-1-positive sites	14 (43.8)	4 (12.5)	0.01
HCMV-EBV-1 coinfection (no. [%] positive sites)	9 (28.7)	0 (0)	0.004
D. pneumosintes (no. [%] positive sites)	20 (62.5)	6 (18.8)	<0.001
P. gingivalis (no. [%] positive sites)	23 (71.9)	12 (37.5)	0.01
D. pneumosintes and *P. gingivalis* coinfection (no. [%] positive sites)	15 (46.9)	0 (0)	<0.001

[a] Adapted from reference 38.

TABLE 2 Occurrence of HCMV and EBV-1 in deep and shallow periodontal sites of 11 localized juvenile periodontitis patients[a]

Item	No. (%) of virus-positive sites		
	5 active, deep periodontal sites	4 stable, deep periodontal sites	11 stable, shallow periodontal sites
HCMV	5 (100)	2 (50)	2 (18)
HCMV-active infection	5 (100)	0 (0)	0 (0)
EBV-1	3 (60)	3 (75)	2 (18)
HCMV–EBV-1 coinfection	3 (60)	1 (25)	2 (18)
A. actinomycetemcomitans	5 (100)	0 (0)	Not done

[a] Adapted from reference 85.

1.7 and 44.2) and HCMV (odds ratio, 6.6; 95% confidence limits, 1.7 and 26.1). The odds of having localized juvenile periodontitis increased multiplicatively when both *P. gingivalis* and HCMV were present (odds ratio, 51.4; 95% confidence limits, 5.7 and 486.5), when compared with the odds associated with having neither of the two infectious agents. Apparently, *P. gingivalis* and HCMV are independently and strongly associated with localized juvenile periodontitis in Jamaican adolescents, and *P. gingivalis* and HCMV act synergistically to influence the risk for both the occurrence and the extent of disease. Electron microscopy studies have previously detected various types of virions in localized juvenile periodontitis lesions (11, 67).

Ting et al. (85) studied the relationship between HCMV activation and disease-active versus disease-stable periodontal sites in 11 localized juvenile periodontitis patients aged 10 to 23 years (Table 2). HCMV mRNA of the major capsid protein, indicative of viral activation, was detected in deep pockets of all five HCMV-positive patients with early disease (aged 10 to 14 years), but only in one of three HCMV-positive patients older than 14 years, and not in any shallow pocket tested. HCMV activation was found exclusively in periodontal sites having no visible radiographic crestal alveolar lamina dura, a sign of likely periodontal disease progression (68). HCMV activation has also been detected in severe periodontitis lesions of adults (16). Furthermore, periodontal sites with active HCMV infection were more

heavily infected with *A. actinomycetemcomitans* than sites with latent HCMV infection. Ting et al. (85) hypothesized that during root formation of permanent incisors and first molars at 3 to 5 years of age, primary HCMV infection in tissues surrounding the tooth germ might alter the root surface structure and increase the susceptibility to future periodontal breakdown. HCMV infections in infants are able to cause marked changes in tooth morphology (83; M. Wacinska, J. Janicha, A. Remiszewski, and A. Wal, *J. Dent. Res.* **80**:1294, abstr. 198, 2001), and teeth affected by localized juvenile periodontitis frequently show cemental hypoplasia (8). Subsequently, at the time of puberty, reactivation of periodontal HCMV or other herpesviruses due to hormonal changes may give rise to periodontal overgrowth of pathogenic bacteria and breakdown around teeth with damaged periodontium.

HCMV and EBV-1 have been detected in rare types of aggressive periodontitis in young individuals (Table 3). In a Hopi Indian population, a single adolescent showed generalized juvenile periodontitis and was the only study subject revealing periodontal HCMV/EBV-1 dual infection (F. B. Skrepcinski, S. Tetrev, T. E. Rams, B. Sutton, A. Contreras, and J. Slots, *J. Dent. Res.* **76**:439, abstr. 3406, 1997). One periodontitis patient with Papillon-Lefèvre syndrome also presented periodontal HCMV/EBV-1 dual infection (88). One patient with Fanconi's anemia periodontitis demonstrated periodontal HCMV-active infection and HSV (56).

TABLE 3 Occurrence of HCMV and in rare types of aggressive periodontitis in young individuals

Periodontal disease (reference)	HCMV and EMV-1 coinfection	HCMV active infection	*A. actinomycetemcomitans*
Generalized juvenile periodontitis, teenage patient (Skrepcinski et al., *J. Dent. Res.* **76:**439, 1997)[a]	Yes	No data	Yes
Papillon-Lefevre syndrome periodontitis, 11-year-old patient (88)	Yes	No data	Yes
Fanconi's anemia periodontitis, 11-year-old patient (56)	No	Yes	Yes

[a] Of 75 adolescent Hopi Indians, 8 showed various types of destructive periodontal disease. One Hopi Indian showed generalized periodontitis and was the only study subject who revealed HCM/EBV-1 periodontal coinfection.

Acute necrotizing ulcerative gingivitis (ANUG) affects immunocompromised, malnourished, and psychosocially stressed young individuals and may occasionally spread considerably beyond the periodontium and give rise to a life-threatening infection termed noma/cancrum oris (55). Table 4 shows the distribution of herpesviruses in ANUG-affected and non-ANUG-affected children 3 to 14 years of age from Nigeria. A significantly higher prevalence of HCMV and other herpesviruses was detected in ANUG lesions of malnourished children than in non-ANUG, normal, and malnourished children. In Europe and the United States, ANUG affects mainly adolescents, young adults, and HIV-infected individuals, and almost never affects young children. The earlier occurrence of ANUG in Africa may be due to acquisition of HCMV in

early childhood (63) and a generally impaired immune defense. ANUG in the African population studied may arise from increased rate of herpesvirus activation because of malnutrition (25) and periodontal presence of virulent bacteria (26).

Periodontitis in HIV-infected patients may resemble that of periodontitis of non-HIV-infected individuals, or be associated with profusely gingival bleeding or necrotic gingival tissue (35). HIV-induced immunosuppresion facilitates herpesvirus reactivation (27). Significantly more herpesviruses can be detected in gingival specimens from HIV-periodontitis lesions than from periodontitis lesions of non-HIV patients ($P < 0.001$) (14). HCMV occurred in 81% of the HIV-associated periodontitis lesions and in 50% of the non-HIV-periodontitis lesions; it was the most common

TABLE 4 Occurrence of HCMV and EBV-1 in ANUG sites and normal periodontal sites of Nigerian children suffering from malnutrition[a]

Herpesvirus(es)	No. (%) of virus-positive sites		P (χ^2 test)
	ANUG+ malnutrition (22 subjects)	Normal oral health malnutrition (20 subjects)	
HCMV	13 (59.0)	0 (0)	<0.001
EBV-1	6 (27.3)	1 (5.0)	0.13
HCMV/EBV-1 coinfection	8 (36.4)	0 (0)	0.009

[a] Adapted from reference 13.

herpesvirus identified. In HIV-positive individuals, HCMV has also been implicated in acute periodontitis (21), periodontal abscess formation and osteomyelitis (6), and refractory chronic sinusitis (86). EBV-2 was detected in 57% biopsies from HIV-periodontitis but was absent in non-HIV-periodontitis biopsies ($P = 0.002$). An unusually high incidence of EBV-2 in HIV-infected patients has been reported (75, 91). Loning et al. (47) found EBV DNA sequences in gingival epithelium of HIV-infected individuals, and Madinier et al. (48) detected EBV in gingival papilla specimens from 40% of HIV-infected patients and from 40% of non-HIV-infected individuals. Only one specimen of nasal, laryngeal, and oral mucosa, other than gingival mucosa, revealed EBV DNA, suggesting inflamed gingiva served as a reservoir for EBV (48). HHV-8 was detected in periodontitis lesions of 24% of HIV-infected individuals who, however, showed no clinical sign of Kaposi's sarcoma, but not in any periodontitis site of non-HIV-infected individuals. In HIV-infected patients, HCMV, EBV, HSV, and HHV-8 genomes are also generally found in saliva (7, 29) and have been related to ulcerative oral lesions (28, 37, 69, 84) and widespread gingival and mucosal inflammation (28). The clinical characteristics of HIV-associated periodontal diseases and the high rate of

oral herpesviruses in HIV patients are consistent with the involvement of herpesvirus infections in these diseases.

Herpesviruses may interfere with periodontal healing as well. In a periodontal regeneration study, four periodontal sites that showed either HCMV or EBV-1 experienced an average gain in clinical attachment of 2.3 mm compared with 16 viral-negative sites that showed a mean attachment gain of 5.0 mm ($P = 0.004$) (80). By infecting and altering the function of fibroblasts and other periodontal cells, herpesviruses may reduce the regenerative potential of the periodontal ligament. Unrecognized herpesviral infections of the periodontium may help explain why some individuals show little or no response to periodontal regenerative treatment.

The relationship between herpesviruses and putative periodontopathic bacteria was studied in 140 adults with gingivitis or periodontitis (19). As shown in Table 5, periodontal HCMV and EBV-1 were related to elevated occurrence of the pathogens *P. gingivalis, B. forsythus, P. intermedia, P. nigrescens,* and *T. denticola.* Periodontal HCMV is also closely associated with a high rate of occurrence of *D. pneumosintes* and progressive periodontitis (79). Moreover, as discussed above, localized juvenile periodontitis lesions exhibiting HCMV

TABLE 5 Associations between HCMV and EBV-1 and periodontopathic bacteria[a]

Virus	Bacteria or disease	Odds ratio	P
HCMV	Severe periodontitis	4.7	0.03
	P. gingivalis + *P. nigrescens*	3.2	0.01
	P. gingivalis + *P. nigrescens* + *T. denticola*	2.6	0.05
	P. gingivalis + *B. forsythus* + *P. nigrescens*	3.2	0.01
EBV-1	Severe periodontitis	5.1	0.05
	P. gingivalis	3.4	0.01
	P. gingivalis + *P. intermedia*	4.4	0.005
	P. gingivalis + *T. denticola*	4.2	0.004
	P. gingivalis + *B. forsythus*	3.8	0.006
	P. gingivalis + *P. nigrescens*	2.7	0.05
	P. gingivalis + *B. forsythus* + *T. denticola*	4.1	0.005
	P. gingivalis + *P. nigrescens* + *T. denticola*	3.3	0.03

[a] Adapted from reference 19.

infection tend to show elevated levels of *P. gingivalis* (51) and *A. actinomycetemcomitans* (85). The close association between periodontal herpesviruses and periodontopathic bacteria lends credence to the notion that both types of infectious agents are involved in the development of periodontitis. In the same way, evidence is emerging that otitis media (34), respiratory tract infections (5), and other nonoral infections (15) that previously were thought to be of bacterial origin might be caused by combined viral-bacterial infections (also see chapters 11 to 15). Abramson and Mills (1) suggested that viruses predispose the host to secondary infections by inducing abnormalities in adherence, chemotaxis, phagocytic, oxidative, secretory, and bactericidal activities of polymorphonuclear leukocytes, cells of major importance in controlling medical and periodontal bacterial infections (87).

PATHOGENIC MECHANISMS OF HERPESVIRUSES IN PERIODONTAL DISEASE

Herpesviruses may cause periodontal pathosis as a direct result of the virus infection and replication, or as a result of virally induced impairment of the host defense. Herpesvirus-mediated periodontopathogenicity may take place through at least five mechanisms, operating alone or in combination.

First, herpesviruses may cause direct cytopathic effects on fibroblasts, keratinocytes, endothelial cells, inflammatory cells such as polymorphonuclear leukocytes, lymphocytes, macrophages, and possibly bone cells (17). Since the cells above are key constituents of inflamed periodontal tissue, herpesvirus-induced cytopathic effects may hamper tissue turnover and repair.

Second, gingival herpesvirus infection may promote subgingival attachment and colonization of periodontopathic bacteria similar to the enhanced bacterial adherence to virus-infected cells observed in other infections. Viral proteins expressed on eukaryotic cell membranes can act as bacterial receptors and generate new bacterial binding sites (17). Also, loss of virus-

damaged epithelial cells may expose the basement membrane and the surface of regenerating cells, providing new sites for bacterial binding (17).

Third, HCMV and EBV can infect and alter functions of monocytes, macrophages, and lymphocytes in periodontitis lesions (20). As implied above, impairment of cells involved in the periodontal defense may predispose to overgrowth by periodontal pathogens.

Fourth, herpesvirus infections induce a proinflammatory response including expression of cytokines and chemokines (54). In periodontitis, herpesvirus-induced expression of cytokines is particularly intriguing. HCMV infection can up-regulate interleukin-1β and tumor necrosis factor alpha gene expression of monocytes and macrophages (17). In turn, interleukin-1β and tumor necrosis factor alpha may up-regulate matrix metalloproteinase, down-regulate tissue inhibitors of metalloproteinase, and mediate periodontal bone destruction (17). Increased production of these proinflammatory cytokines by macrophages and monocytes has been associated with enhanced susceptibility to destructive periodontal disease (61). EBV may act as a potent polyclonal B-lymphocyte activator, capable of inducing proliferation and differentiation of immunoglobulin-secreting cells, features associated with periodontal disease progression (17). Active EBV infection can also generate antineutrophil antibodies and neutropenia that may lead to increased bacterial pathogenicity and overgrowth (17).

Finally, herpesviruses can produce tissue injury as a result of immunopathologic responses (52), and immunopathologic reactions have been implicated in the pathogenesis of human periodontal disease (30). HCMV can induce cell-mediated immunosuppression by down-regulating cell surface expression of major histocompatibility complex class I molecules, thereby interfering with cytotoxic T-lymphocyte recognition (52). In addition, HCMV sequesters chemokines, induces Fc receptors, interferes with induction of major histocompatibility class II antigens, inhibits natural killer cell activity, and can efficiently block the presentation of immediate early antigens, the first viral proteins to be produced (52). Moreover, HCMV can suppress antigen-specific cytotoxic T-lymphocyte functions, resulting in decreases in circulating CD4$^+$ cells and increases in CD8$^+$ suppressor cells, which in turn may lead to global impairment of cell-mediated immunity (17). EBV may induce proliferation of cytotoxic T lymphocytes, the main purpose of which is to recognize and destroy virally infected cells, but may secondarily also hamper various aspects of the periodontal immune response (17). EBV can suppress T-lymphocyte functions as well (50). EBV-infected B lymphocytes may shed viral structural antigens that result in production of blocking antibodies, immune complex formation, and T-suppressor cell activation (39, 50). Together, these mechanisms probably contribute to the ability of herpesviruses to persist in their hosts and may play a role in immunopathology of herpesviral diseases.

HERPESVIRUS-BACTERIUM-HOST RESPONSE INTERACTIONS IN PERIODONTITIS

Figure 1 describes the possible role of herpesviruses in periodontal tissue destruction. Initially, gingival inflammation induced by dental plaque bacteria causes herpesvirus-infected inflammatory cells to enter the periodontium. Subsequent herpesvirus reactivation in the gingival tissue may then aggravate the disease. Herpesvirus reactivation may occur spontaneously or as a result of various types of impairment of the host immune defense including HIV infection, pregnancy, hormonal changes, and psychosocial and physical stress. Sarid el al. (73) showed that among female students who endured stress during academic examinations, a significant increase could be detected in EBV-specific IgG and IgA salivary antibody values as well as in salivary EBV activation as measured by salivary EBV DNA or infectious virus. Factors that activate herpesviruses are also recognized risk indicators of periodontitis (72). Indeed, the reason various

immunosuppressive events aggravate periodontal disease might be partially due to accompanying herpesvirus activation. Herpesvirus active infection may further diminish the resistance of periodontal tissues, thereby inducing subgingival overgrowth of periodontal pathogenic bacteria by one or more of the periodontopathic mechanisms described above. However, the interaction between herpesviruses and bacteria is most likely bidirectional, with bacterial enzymes or other inflammation-inducing products having the potential to activate periodontal herpesviruses (the vicious circle concept). In a recent study, experimental mice infected with *P. gingivalis* prior to infection with HCMV exhibited higher mortality rates than mice infected with *P. gingivalis* subsequent to HCMV infection, suggesting preexisting *P. gingivalis* infection increased the pathogenicity of HCMV (J. Stern, E. Shai, A. Halabi, Y. Houri-Haddad, L. Shapira, and A. Palmon, *J. Dent. Res.* **80:**1314, abstr. 46, 2001).

Herpesviral-bacterial interactions may help explain the disease characteristics of destructive periodontal disease. Alteration between prolonged periods of latency interrupted by periods of activation of herpesviral infections may be partly responsible for the burstlike episodes of periodontitis disease progression. Tissue tropism of herpesviral infections may help explain the localized pattern of tissue destruction in periodontitis. Frequent reactivation of periodontal herpesviruses may account for the rapid periodontal breakdown in some patients even in the presence of relatively little dental plaque. Absence of herpesviral infection or viral reactivation may clarify why some individuals carry periodontopathic bacteria while still maintaining periodontal health or minimal disease.

The recognition that periodontitis is a multifactorial disease involving herpesviruses, bacteria, and host defense may explain why aggressive periodontitis is relatively uncommon in most populations despite a high prevalence of individuals harboring both herpesviruses and bacterial pathogens. It might be that periodontal tissue breakdown is contingent upon

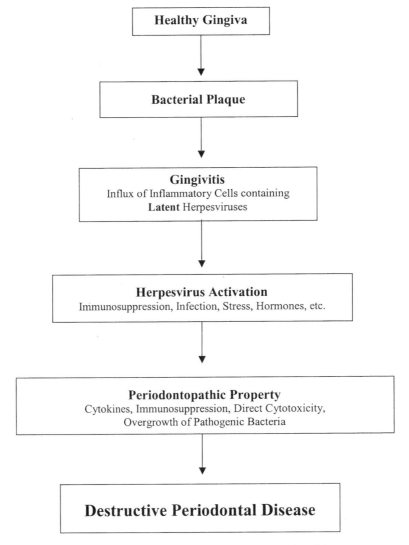

FIGURE 1. Herpesviruses in destructive periodontal disease.

the simultaneous occurrence of several infectious disease events, including (i) adequate herpesvirus load (gingivitis level) in periodontal sites, (ii) activation of herpesviruses in the periodontium, (iii) inadequate protective antiviral cytotoxic T-lymphocyte response, (iv) presence of specific periodontal pathogenic bacteria, and (v) inadequate protective antibacterial antibody response. In most individuals, these five suggested pathogenic determinants of periodontitis might come together in a detrimental constellation relatively infrequently and mainly during periods of suppressed immune response. Clearly, the importance of combined herpesviral-bacterial infections and associated host responses in the development of periodontitis needs to be studied further.

CONCLUSION AND PERSPECTIVES

Several lines of evidence implicate herpesvirus species in the etiology and/or pathogenesis of human periodontal disease. These include the following:

1. Presence of nucleic acid sequences of HCMV, EBV-1, and other herpesviruses in aggressive periodontitis lesions of children, adolescents, and adults

2. Association between herpesviruses and ANUG in malnourished African children

3. Detection of nucleic acid sequences of herpesviruses in inflammatory periodontal cells

4. Probable profound effect of herpesviral infection on periodontal defense cells

5. Potential of herpesviruses to augment the expression of tissue-damaging cytokines and chemokines in periodontal inflammatory cells

6. Increased frequency of periodontopathic bacteria in herpesvirus-positive periodontitis lesions

7. Association between periodontal HCMV-active infection and disease-active periodontitis

The notion of herpesviruses playing key roles in many types of severe periodontitis may have significant therapeutic implications. A new direction to prevent and treat periodontitis may focus on controlling disease-initiating herpesviruses. Reducing gingivitis by various antiplaque measures has been shown to diminish the herpesviral load in periodontal sites (33, 60). Future approaches to periodontal prophylaxis and treatment may include vaccination specific against herpesviruses. Thus, recent progress in studies of the importance of herpesviruses, herpesviral-bacterial interaction, and host inflammatory mechanisms in periodontitis holds great promise in leading to novel ways to prevent and cure the disease.

In addition, productive herpesviruses in inflamed gingival tissue may seed to other body sites or shed into saliva and subsequently infect other individuals. Pauk et al. (65) found that among 92 men who were HIV-seronegative but who had sex with HIV-positive men having Kaposi's sarcoma, deep kissing was an independent risk factor for infection with HHV-8. Pauk et al. (65) concluded that oral exposure to infectious saliva is a potential risk factor for the acquisition of HHV-8 among men who have sex with men and suggested that currently recommended safer sex practices may not protect against HHV-8 infection. Contreras et al. (14) detected HHV-8 in 24% of gingival biopsy samples from HIV-seropositive individuals. The data presented are consistent with the suggestion that gingival tissue is a site for herpesvirus replication, potential persistence, and a source of infective HHV-8 in saliva. Gingiva has also been proposed to constitute a reservoir for HSV (92). EBV has for decades been known to be transmitted by saliva, even among lay people who named infectious mononucleosis the "kissing disease" (31). If indeed inflamed gingiva constitutes a significant nidus for infectious herpesviruses, maintaining gingival health by professional periodontal therapy and oral hygiene measures may help reduce the risk of transmissible herpesvirus disease.

Basic research on herpesviruses may also benefit from the finding of herpesviruses in periodontal disease. During active HCMV and EBV diseases, cells of the myeloid lineage, including monocytes/macrophages and B lymphocytes, can disseminate reactivated viruses to a variety of cells and tissues. However, it is not known if epithelial cells, endothelial cells, fibroblasts, and vascular smooth muscle cells, themselves, contain latent HCMV and EBV that become reactivated or if these cells become infected de novo during active infection. One difficulty in herpesvirus research is the unavailability of readily accessible study material, especially in systemically healthy subjects having latent herpesviral infections. Since repeated viral samples can be collected from the periodontium in a noninvasive manner, herpesvirus-infected periodontal sites might constitute a valuable research model for studying the pathophysiology of herpesvirus latency and reactivation.

Clinical virology, as well, may take advantage of the frequent presence of herpesviruses in the diseased periodontium. Sampling the periodontal pocket or minor soft tissue curettage of the pocket epithelium and underlying connective tissue may help identify herpesvirus-infected individuals.

REFERENCES

1. **Abramson, J. S., and E. L. Mills.** 1988. Depression of neutrophil function induced by viruses and its role in secondary microbial infections. *Rev. Infect. Dis.* **10:**326–341.
2. **Ahmed, R., L. A. Morrison, and D. M. Knipe.** 1996. Persistence of viruses, p. 219–250. *In* B. N. Fields, D. M. Knipe, and P. M. Howley (ed.), *Fields Virology,* 3rd ed. Lippincott-Raven Publishers, Philadelphia, Pa.
3. **Amit, R., A. Morag, Z. Ravid, N. Hochman, J. Ehrlich, and Z. Zakay-Rones.** 1992. Detection of herpes simplex virus in gingival tissue. *J. Periodontol.* **63:**502–506.
4. **Arens, M.** 1999. Methods for subtyping and molecular comparison of human viral genomes. *Clin. Microbiol. Rev.* **14:**612–626.
5. **Bakaletz, L. O.** 1995. Viral potentiation of bacterial superinfection of the respiratory tract. *Trends Microbiol.* **3:**110–114.
6. **Berman, S., and J. Jensen.** 1990. Cytomegalovirus-induced osteomyelitis in a patient with the acquired immunodeficiency syndrome. *South. Med. J.* **83:**1231–1232.
7. **Blackbourn, D. J., E. T. Lennette, J. Ambroziak, D. V. Mourich, and J. A. Levy.** 1998. Human herpesvirus 8 detection in nasal secretions and saliva. *J. Infect. Dis.* **177:**213–216.
8. **Blomlöf, L., L. Hammarström, and S. Lindskog.** 1986. Occurrence and appearance of cementum hypoplasias in localized and generalized juvenile periodontitis. *Acta Odontol. Scand.* **44:**313–320.
9. **Bornkamm, G. W., and W. Hammerschmidt.** 2001. Molecular virology of Epstein-Barr virus. *Philos. Trans. R. Soc. Lond. B.* **356:**437–459.
10. **Britt, W. J., and C. A. Alford.** 1996. Cytomegalovirus, p. 2493–2524. *In* B. N. Fields, D. M. Knipe, and P. M. Howley (ed.), *Fields Virology,* 3rd ed. Lippincott-Raven Publishers, Philadelphia, Pa.
11. **Burghelea, B., and H. Serb.** 1990. Nuclear bodies and virus-like particles in gingival tissue of periodontopathic patients. *Arch. Roum. Pathol. Exp. Microbiol.* **49:**89–92.
12. **Clementi, M.** 2000. Quantitative molecular analysis of virus expression and replication. *J. Clin. Microbiol.* **38:**2030–2036.
13. **Contreras, A., W. A. Falkler, Jr., C. O. Enwonwu, E. O. Idigbe, K. O. Savage, M. B.** Afolabi, D. Onwujekwe, T. E. Rams, and J. Slots. 1997. Human *Herpesviridae* in acute necrotizing ulcerative gingivitis in children in Nigeria. *Oral Microbiol. Immunol.* **12:**259–265.
14. **Contreras, A., A. Mardirossian, and J. Slots.** 2001. Herpesviruses in HIV-periodontitis. *J. Clin. Periodontol.* **28:**96–102.
15. **Contreras, A., and J. Slots.** 1996. Mammalian viruses in human periodontitis. *Oral Microbiol. Immunol.* **11:**381–386.
16. **Contreras, A., and J. Slots.** 1998. Active cytomegalovirus infection in human periodontitis. *Oral Microbiol. Immunol.* **13:**225–230.
17. **Contreras, A., and J. Slots.** 2000. Herpesviruses in human periodontal disease. *J. Periodontal Res.* **35:**3–16.
18. **Contreras, A., and J. Slots.** 2001. Typing of herpes simplex virus from human periodontium. *Oral Microbiol. Immunol.* **16:**63–64.
19. **Contreras, A., M., Umeda, C. Chen, I. Bakker, J. L. Morrison, and J. Slots.** 1999. Relationship between herpesviruses and adult periodontitis and periodontopathic bacteria. *J. Periodontol.* **70:**478–484.
20. **Contreras, A., H. H. Zadeh, H. Nowzari, and J. Slots.** 1999. Herpesvirus infection of inflammatory cells in human periodontitis. *Oral Microbiol. Immunol.* **14:**206–212.
21. **Dodd, C. L., J. R. Winkler, G. S. Heinic, T. E. Daniels, K. Yee, and D. Greenspan.** 1993. Cytomegalovirus infection presenting as acute periodontal infection in a patient infected with the human immunodeficiency virus. *J. Clin. Periodontol.* **20:**282–285.
22. **Doniger, J., S. Muralidhar, and L. J. Rosenthal.** 1999. Human cytomegalovirus and human herpesvirus 6 genes that transform and transactivate. *Clin. Microbiol. Rev.* **12:**367–382.
23. **Ehrlich, J., G. H. Cohen, and N. Hochman.** 1983. Specific herpes simplex virus antigen in human gingiva. *J. Periodontol.* **54:**357–360.
24. **Endo, L. H., D. Ferreira, M. C. Montenegro, G. A. Pinto, A. Altemani, A. E. Bortoleto, Jr., and J. Vassallo.** 2001. Detection of Epstein-Barr virus in tonsillar tissue of children and the relationship with recurrent tonsillitis. *Int. J. Pediatr. Otorhinolaryngol.* **58:**9–15.
25. **Enwonwu, C. O., W. A. Falkler, Jr., E. O. Idigbe, B. M. Afolabi, M. Ibrahim, D. Onwujekwe, O. Savage, and V. I. Meeks.** 1999. Pathogenesis of cancrum oris (noma): confounding interactions of malnutrition with infection. *Am. J. Trop. Med. Hyg.* **60:**223–232.
26. **Falkler, W. A., Jr., C. O. Enwonwu, and E. O. Idigbe.** 1999. Microbiological understandings and mysteries of noma (cancrum oris). *Oral Dis.* **5:**150–155.

27. **Fauci, A. S.** 1993. Immunopathogenesis of HIV infection. *J. Acquir. Immune Defic Syndr.* **6:** 655–662.

28. **Flaitz, C. M., C. M. Nichols, and M. J. Hicks.** 1996. Herpesviridae-associated persistent mucocutaneous ulcers in acquired immunodeficiency syndrome. A clinicopathologic study. *Oral Surg. Oral Med. Oral Pathol. Oral Radiol. Endod.* **81:**433–441.

29. **Fons, M. P., C. M. Flaitz, B. Moore, B. S. Prabhakar, C. M. Nichols, and T. Albrecht.** 1994. Multiple herpesviruses in saliva of HIV-infected individuals. *J. Am. Dent. Assoc.* **125:**713–719.

30. **Gemmell, A., R. I. Marshall, and G. J. Seymour.** 1997. Cytokines and prostaglandins in immune homeostasis and tissue destruction in periodontal disease. *Periodontol. 2000* **14:**112–143.

31. **Giesbrecht, E.** 1972. Infectious mononucleosis—the kissing disease. *Can. Nurse* **68:**37–40.

32. **Griffiths, P. D., and V. C. Emery.** 1997. Cytomegalovirus, p. 445–470. *In* D. D. Richman, R. J. Whitley, and F. G. Hayden (ed.), *Clinical Virology.* Churchill Livingstone, New York, N.Y.

33. **Hanookai, D., H. Nowzari, A. Contreras, J. L. Morrison, and J. Slots.** 2000. Herpesviruses and periodontopathic bacteria in Trisomy 21 periodontitis. *J. Periodontol.* **71:**376–384.

34. **Heikkinen, T., and T. Chonmaitree.** 2000. Viral-bacterial synergy in otitis media: implications for management. *Curr. Infect. Dis. Rep.* **2:**154–159.

35. **Holmstrup, P., and J. Westergaard.** 1998. HIV infection and periodontal diseases. *Periodontol. 2000* **18:**37–46.

36. **Ikeda, T., R. Kobayashi, M. Horiuchi, Y. Nagata, M. Hasegawa, F. Mizuno, and K. Hirai.** 2000. Detection of lymphocytes productively infected with Epstein-Barr virus in nonneoplastic tonsils. *J. Gen. Virol.* **81:**1211–1216.

37. **Itin, P. H., and S. Lautenschlager.** 1997. Viral lesions of the mouth in HIV-infected patients. *Dermatology* **194:**1–7.

38. **Kamma, J. J., A. Contreras, and J. Slots.** 2001. Herpes viruses and periodontopathic bacteria in early-onset periodontitis. *J. Clin. Periodontol.* **28:**879–885.

39. **Khanna, R., S. R. Burrows, and D. J. Moss.** 1995. Immune regulation in Epstein-Barr virus-associated diseases. *Microbiol. Rev.* **59:**387–405.

40. **Kieff, E.** 1996. Epstein-Barr virus and its replication, p. 2343–2396. *In* B. N. Fields, D. M. Knipe, and P. M. Howley (ed.), *Fields Virology,* 3rd ed. Lippincott-Raven Publishers, Philadelphia, Pa.

41. **Kondo, K., H. Kaneshima, and E. S. Mocarski.** 1994. Human cytomegalovirus latent infection of granulocyte-macrophage progenitors. *Proc. Natl. Acad. Sci. USA* **91:**11879–11883.

42. **Lang, N. P., A. Joss, and M. S. Tonetti.** 1996. Monitoring disease during supportive periodontal treatment by bleeding on probing. *Periodontol. 2000* **12:**44–48.

43. **Larochelle, B., L. Flamand, P. Gourde, D. Beauchamp, and J. Gosselin.** 1998. Epstein-Barr virus infects and induces apoptosis in human neutrophils. *Blood* **92:**291–299.

44. **Lindhe, J., and J. Slots.** 1989. Periodontal disease in children and young adults, p. 193–220. *In* J. Lindhe (ed.), *Textbook of Clinical Periodontology,* 2nd ed. Munksgaard, Copenhagen, Denmark.

45. **Loenen, W. A., C. A. Bruggeman, and E. J. Wiertz.** 2001. Immune evasion by human cytomegalovirus: lessons in immunology and cell biology. *Semin. Immunol.* **13:**41–49.

46. **Longnecker, R.** 1998. Molecular biology of Epstein-Barr virus, p. 133–172. *In* D. McCance (ed.), *Human Tumor Viruses.* ASM Press, Washington, D.C.

47. **Loning, T., R. P. Henke, P. Reichart, and J. Becker.** 1987. In situ hybridization to detect Epstein-Barr virus DNA in oral tissues of HIV-infected patients. *Virchows Arch. A* **412:**127–133.

48. **Madinier, I., A. Doglio, L. Cagnon, J. C. Lefebvre, and R. A. Monteil.** 1992. Epstein-Barr virus DNA detection in gingival tissues of patients undergoing surgical extractions. *Br. J. Oral Maxillofac. Surg.* **30:**237–243.

49. **Mardirossian, A., A. Contreras, M. Navazesh, H. Nowzari, and J. Slots.** 2000. Herpesviruses 6, 7, and 8 in HIV- and non-HIV-associated periodontitis. *J. Periodontal Res.* **35:** 278–284.

50. **Menezes, J., S. K. Sundar, and C. A. Ahoronheim.** 1985. Immunosuppressive effects of Epstein-Barr virus infection, p. 115–134. *In* N. Gilmore and W. A. Wainberg (ed.), *Viral Mechanisms of Immunosuppression.* Liss, New York, N.Y.

51. **Michalowicz, B. S., M. Ronderos, R. Camara-Silva, A. Contreras, and J. Slots.** 2000. Human herpesviruses and *Porphyromonas gingivalis* are associated with early-onset periodontitis. *J. Periodontol.* **71:**981–988.

52. **Michelson, S.** 1999. Human cytomegalovirus escape from immune detection. *Intervirology* **42:** 301–307.

53. **Mocarsky, E. D., Jr.** 1996. Cytomegalovirus and their replication, p. 2447–2492. *In* B. N. Fields, D. M. Knipe, and P. M. Howley (ed.), *Fields Virology,* 3rd ed. Lippincott-Raven Publishers, Philadelphia, Pa.

54. **Mogensen, T. H., and S. R. Paludan.** 2001. Molecular pathways in virus-induced cytokine production. *Microbiol. Mol. Biol. Rev.* **65:**131–150.

55. **Murayama, Y., H. Kurihara, A. Nagai, D. Dompkowski, and T. E. Van Dyke.** 1994. Acute necrotizing ulcerative gingivitis: risk factors involving host defense mechanisms. *Periodontol. 2000* **6:**116–124.

56. **Nowzari, H., M. G. Jorgensen, T. T. Ta, A. Contreras, and J. Slots.** 2001. Aggressive periodontitis associated with Fanconi's anemia. A case report. *J. Periodontol.* **72:**1601–1606.

57. **Okano, M.** 1998. Epstein-Barr virus infection and its role in the expanding spectrum of human diseases. *Acta Paediatr.* **87:**11–8.

58. **Oliver, R. C., L. J. Brown, and H. Löe.** 1998. Periodontal diseases in the United States population. *J. Periodontol.* **69:**269–278.

59. **Ong, G.** 1998. Periodontal disease and tooth loss. *Int. Dent. J.* **48** (Suppl. 1):233–238.

60. **Pacheco, J. J., C. Coelho, F. Salazar, A. Contreras, J. Slots, and C. H. Velazco.** Treatment of Papillon-Lefèvre syndrome periodontitis. *J. Clin. Periodontol.,* in press.

61. **Page, R. C., S. Offenbacher, H. E. Schroeder, G. J. Seymour, and K. S. Kornman.** 1997. Advances in the pathogenesis of periodontitis: summary of developments, clinical implications and future directions. *Periodontol. 2000* **14:**216–248.

62. **Parra, B., and J. Slots.** 1996. Detection of human viruses in periodontal pockets using polymerase chain reaction. *Oral Microbiol. Immunol.* **11:**289–293.

63. **Pass, R. F.** 1985. Epidemiology and transmission of cytomegalovirus. *J. Infect. Dis.* **152:**243–248.

64. **Paster, B. J., S. K. Boches, J. L. Galvin, R. E. Ericson, C. N. Lau, V. A. Levanos, A. Sahasrabudhe, and F. E. Dewhirst.** 2001. Bacterial diversity in human subgingival plaque. *J. Bacteriol.* **183:**3770–3783.

65. **Pauk, J., M. L. Huang, S. J. Brodie, A. Wald, D. M. Koelle, T. Schacker, C. Celum, S. Selke, and L. Corey.** 2000. Mucosal shedding of human herpesvirus 8 in men. *N. Engl. J. Med.* **343:**1369–1377.

66. **Ploegh, H. L.** 1998. Viral strategies of immune evasion. *Science* **280:**248–253.

67. **Preus, H. R., I. Olsen, and E. Namork.** 1987. The presence of phage-infected Actinobacillus actinomycetemcomitans in localized juvenile periodontitis patients. *J. Clin. Periodontol.* **14:**605–609.

68. **Rams, T. E., M. A. Listgarten, and J. Slots.** 1994. Utility of radiographic crestal lamina dura for predicting periodontitis disease-activity. *J. Clin. Periodontol.* **21:**571–576.

69. **Regezi, J. A., L. R. Eversole, B. F. Barker, G. M. Rick, and S. Silverman, Jr.** 1996. Herpes simplex and cytomegalovirus coinfected oral ulcers in HIV-positive patients. *Oral Surg. Oral Med. Oral Pathol. Oral Radiol. Endod.* **81:**55–62.

70. **Rickinson, A., and E. Kieff.** 1996. Epstein-Barr virus, p. 2397–2446. *In* B. Fields, D. Knipe, and P. Howley (ed.), *Fields Virology,* 3rd ed. Lippincott-Raven Publishers, Philadelphia, Pa.

71. **Rickinson, A. B., and D. J. Moss.** 1997. Human cytotoxic T lymphocyte responses to Epstein-Barr virus infection. *Annu. Rev. Immunol.* **15:**405–431.

72. **Salvi, G. E., H. P. Lawrence, S. Offenbacher, and J. D. Beck.** 1997. Influence of risk factors on the pathogenesis of periodontitis. *Periodontol. 2000* **14:**173–201.

73. **Sarid, O., O. Anson, A. Yaari, and M. Margalith.** 2001. Epstein-Barr virus specific salivary antibodies as related to stress caused by examinations. *J. Med. Virol.* **64:**149–156.

74. **Savard, M., C. Belanger, M. Tardif, P. Gourde, L. Flamand, and J. Gosselin.** 2000. Infection of primary human monocytes by Epstein-Barr virus. *J. Virol.* **74:**2612–2619.

75. **Sculley, T. B., A. Apolloni, L. Hurren, D. J. Moss, and D. A. Cooper.** 1990. Coinfection with A- and B-type Epstein-Barr virus in human immunodeficiency virus-positive subjects. *J. Infect. Dis.* **162:**643–648.

76. **Slots, J., and C. Chen.** 1999. The oral microflora and human periodontal disease, p. 101–127. *In* G. W. Tannock (ed.), *Medical Importance of the Normal Microflora.* Kluwer Academic Publishers, London, England.

77. **Slots, J., and A. Contreras.** 2000. Herpesviruses: a unifying causative factor in periodontitis? *Oral Microbiol. Immunol.* **15:**276–279.

78. **Slots, J., and T. E. Rams.** 1992. Microbiology of periodontal disease, p. 425–443. *In* J. Slots and M. A. Taubman (ed), *Contemporary Oral Microbiology and Immunology.* Mosby-Year Book, Inc., St. Louis, Mo.

79. **Slots, J., C. Sugar, and J. J. Kamma.** Cytomegalovirus periodontal presence is associated with subgingival *Dialister pneumosintes* and alveolar bone loss. *Oral Microbiol Immunol.,* in press.

80. **Smith MacDonald, E., H. Nowzari, A. Contreras, J. Flynn, J. L. Morrison, and J. Slots.** 1998. Clinical and microbiological evaluation of a bioabsorbable and a nonresorbable barrier membrane in the treatment of periodontal intraosseous lesions. *J. Periodontol.* **69:**445–453.

81. **Söderberg-Nauclér, C., K. N. Fish, and J. A. Nelson.** 1997. Reactivation of latent human cytomegalovirus by allogeneic stimulation of blood cells from healthy donors. *Cell* **91:**119–126.

82. **Söderberg-Nauclér, C., and J. A. Nelson.** 1999. Human cytomegalovirus latency and reacti-

vation—a delicate balance between the virus and its host's immune system. *Intervirology* **42**:314–321.

83. **Stagno, S., R. F. Pass, J. P. Thomas, J. M. Navia, and M. E. Dworsky.** 1982. Defects of tooth structure in congenital cytomegalovirus infections. *Pediatrics* **69**:646–648.

84. **Syrjänen, S., R. Leimola-Virtanen, A. Schmidt-Westhausen, and P. A. Reichart.** 1999. Oral ulcers in AIDS patients frequently associated with cytomegalovirus (CMV) and Epstein-Barr virus (EBV) infections. *J. Oral Pathol. Med.* **28**:204–209.

85. **Ting, M., A. Contreras, and J. Slots.** 2000. Herpesviruses in localized juvenile periodontitis. *J. Periodontal Res.* **35**:17–25.

86. **Upadhyay, S., S. C. Marks, R. L. Arden, L. R. Crane, and A. M. Cohn.** 1995. Bacteriology of sinusitis in human immunodeficiency virus-positive patients: implications for management. *Laryngoscope* **105**:1058–1060.

87. **Van Dyke, T. E., and J. Vaikuntam.** 1994. Neutrophil function and dysfunction in periodontal disease. *Curr. Opin. Periodontol.* 19–27.

88. **Velazco, C. H., C. Coelho, F. Salazar, A. Contreras, J. Slots, and J. J. Pacheco.** 1999. Microbiological features of Papillon-Lefèvre syndrome periodontitis. *J. Clin. Periodontol.* **26**:622–627.

89. **Wakiguchi, H., H. Hisakawa, H. Kubota, and T. Kurashige.** 1999. Strong response of T cells in infants with dual infection by Epstein-Barr virus and cytomegalovirus. *Pediatr. Int.* **41**:484–489.

90. **World Health Organization.** *Global Oral Data Bank 1997.* World Health Organization, Geneva, Switzerland.

91. **Yao, Q. Y., R. J. Tierney, D. Croom-Carter, D. Dukers, G. M. Cooper, C. J. Ellis, M. Rowe, and A. B. Rickinson.** 1996. Frequency of multiple Epstein-Barr virus infections in T-cell immunocompromised individuals. *J. Virol.* **70**:4884–4894.

92. **Zakay-Rones, Z., J. Ehrlich, N. Hochman, and R. Levy.** 1986. Hypothesis: the gingival tissue as a reservoir for herpes simplex virus. *Microbiologica* **9**:367–371.

POLYMICROBIAL DISEASES INVOLVING FUNGI

MIXED MYCOTIC INFECTIONS

David R. Soll

17

As opportunistic pathogens, the infectious fungi lie in wait in the host or continually bombard the host until some aspect of the host physiology, usually related to the immune system, falters. They then overgrow body cavities, penetrate tissues, and alter further the immune system in the development of infection. In the case of *Candida* spp. (7, 56), cells grow in the normal microflora alongside bacteria as benign commensals causing no disease. The intensity of commensal carriage can be quite high and the body sites colonized in healthy individuals can be quite diverse (56, 83), demonstrating a high level of adaptation and pathogenic sophistication. Then, in response to a diverse variety of alterations in host physiology, not always identifiable, as in the case of vaginitis patients, commensals convert to pathogens. In severely immunocompromised patients, *Candida* spp. can enter the bloodstream and can thus disseminate to a variety of tissues and organs, leading to host death. Some *Candida* spp., notably *Candida glabrata* and *Candida krusei,* are naturally drug resistant, making treatment difficult (21, 24, 96). In the case of *Aspergillus fumigatus* and related species, airborne spores are continually inhaled and purged by healthy individuals (42).

Because *Aspergillus* spp. represent the dominant airborne fungal spore (53), it appears that they did not have to develop the commensal skills of *Candida* spp., which do not produce airborne spores, in order to function as opportunistic human pathogens (42). In the case of *Aspergillus* spp., when the mechanisms for purging inhaled spores are compromised, the organism infects tissue and penetrates the bloodstream, resulting in life-threatening infections. *A. fumigatus* and related species are highly refractile to drug treatment in systematic infections (42). Therefore, although the fungi represent a diverse group of pathogens, their common theme in pathogenesis is opportunism.

In considering the question of mixed mycotic infections, we are faced with a number of issues related to the specific pathogenic strategies that have developed in different species and related to the phylogenetic levels of unrelatedness. First, we must consider, where relevant, the issues of commensalism, opportunism, and infection. Second, we must consider exactly what we mean by mixed colonization, or mixed infection, as it relates to genetic relatedness. Mixing can occur between kingdoms (e.g., bacteria and fungi), between genera within a kingdom (e.g., *Aspergillus* spp. and *Candida* spp.), between species within a genus (e.g., *Candida albicans* and *Candida tropicalis*),

David R. Soll, Department of the Biological Sciences, University of Iowa, Iowa City, IA 52242.

Polymicrobial Diseases, Edited by Kim A. Brogden and Janet M. Guthmiller,

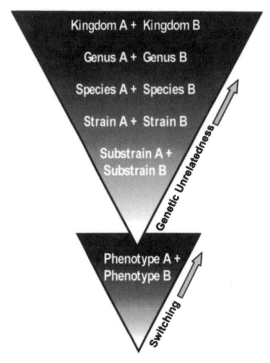

FIGURE 1 The levels of genetic relatedness (or unrelatedness) basic to mixed infections. In the scheme, mixing based on genetic differences (upper triangle) is separated from mixing due to epigenetic switching (lower triangle).

between strains within a species, and between substrains within a strain, a result of microevolution (Fig. 1). Each of these combinations is relevant since each involves combinations of genetically distinct organisms with potentially different phenotypes, even at the substrain level. In this context, colonizing populations can also contain mixed phenotypes that are quite stable but which may be the result of high-frequency phenotypic switching systems that involve epigenetic mechanisms rather than genetic change at the level of DNA sequence. The intention of this chapter is to consider all of the levels of genetic and phenotypic mixing outlined in Fig. 1.

CANDIDA SP. COMMENSALISM

Candida spp. live as commensals in the oral cavity, gastrointestinal tract, and anus of healthy men and women, in the vaginal canal

and vulva of healthy women, and in the groin of healthy men. The frequency of commensal colonization, or "carriage," is quite high. In his book *Candida and Candidosis: a Review and Bibliography* (56), Frank Odds reviewed the published literature on commensal carriage through 1988. He found that *C. albicans* had been reported as occurring in nine primates besides humans, including baboons, chimpanzees, and gorillas; in domesticated animals, including cattle, dogs, and horses; in other mammals, including marsupials; in amphibians; and in birds. He estimated from the extensive list of reviewed studies that the mean proportions of healthy humans and patients carrying a *Candida* sp. in the oral cavity were 26 and 34%, respectively, and that the mean proportions of healthy women and patients carrying *Candida* spp. in the vagina were 10 and 23%, respectively (56). The range of frequencies in the studies reviewed by Odds for a particular body location varied to an extreme. For instance, oral carriage estimates for studies in the United Kingdom varied from 9 to 50% for healthy adults, demonstrating most likely extreme differences between studies in the efficiency of the sampling methods. It seems quite possible that the higher frequencies obtained in such studies were the more accurate ones and that the values obtained in any one study were always underestimates. Unfortunately, it was rare that such studies provided an estimate of the relative intensity of carriage at an individual body location or involved sampling of more than one body location per individual, leading to several problems. First, information on intensities may have altered judgements on whether colonization of a particular individual represented carriage, infection, or chance encounters of yeasts passing through a body location. Second, sampling of one body location cannot be considered a measure of carriage in general, since it has been shown that healthy women can carry yeast in their oral cavity but not in their vagina, and vice versa (83). Therefore, sampling only one body location exacerbates the problem of underestimating commensal carriage. To obtain a more accurate estimate of carriage, we performed a study in which 52 healthy women were sampled at 17 anatomical locations, using a procedure that estimated the relative intensity of carriage (83). The results suggested that the true frequency of carriage in healthy women is high when all anatomical locations are sampled. The highest frequencies of carriage were in the oral cavity (56%), then in the vulvovaginal area (40%), and finally in the anorectal region (24%) (Table 1) (83). The general frequency of carriage for individuals, including carriage in all body locations, was 73%. This value, although seemingly high, must still be considered an under-

estimate for several reasons. First, the agar used for plating in this study supported growth of the majority of *Candida* spp., but it did not support *C. glabrata* growth (37). *C. glabrata* is now the second most common commensal *Candida* sp. (63). Second, carriage was measured only in young women, who may have very different frequencies of carriage in the oral cavity and vaginal areas than elderly women and different levels of carriage than children or males (37). A similar detailed study therefore needs to be performed on carriage in individuals in different age groups, given the changes observed in carriage as a function of age (37, 46). A similar study must also be performed on males. Finally, it should be noted that the most common sampling methods using cotton swabs are expedient but not the most efficient for assessing carriage (56).

The female carriage study by Soll et al. (83) demonstrated that body niches lined by mucosae and bathed in secreted fluids, such as the oral cavity and vagina, harbored *Candida* spp. far more frequently than the transiently damp areas lined with skin, such as the groin, underarm, under the breast, and between the toes, or drier areas, such as the pubic hair line, behind the knee, and the nipple (Table 1) (83). The vaginal wall, vaginal pool, and vulva, when colonized, had the highest carriage intensities, and anus, stool, and oral locations had lower intensities (Table 1). This study (83) revealed several aspects of commensalism that may impact future considerations of mixed carriage. First, when individuals carried a *Candida* sp., it was not always in all possible body locations. For instance, 62% of individuals with vulvovaginal carriage also carried yeast in the oral cavity. However, 52% of individuals without vulvovaginal carriage carried yeast in the oral cavity, and 35% of individuals without oral carriage carried yeast in the vulvovaginal region (83). Second, isolates obtained simultaneously from the oral cavity and the vaginal canal were different species, different strains, or different substrains (83). Results from a second study of healthy, nonpregnant women also revealed that in a majority of cases in which there

TABLE 1 Summary of carriage of *Candida* spp. in 17 body locations of 52 healthy young women[a]

Type of carriage	% Carriage	Intensity score[b]
In specific body locations[c]		
Vaginal wall	29	3.2
Vaginal pool	31	2.9
Vulva	31	2.7
Groin	10	1.6
Anus	22	1.9
Stool	15	1.4
Inner cheek	33	1.8
Under tongue	29	1.3
Back of tongue	46	1.9
Between toes	8	1.3
In general areas		
Oral	56	
Anorectal	24	
Vulvovaginal	40	
Any	73	

[a] Synopsized from reference 83. Of 52 women, 14 had no detectable carriage in any body location.
[b] Carriage was measured by rubbing each body location with a culturette, which was placed in a sterile culture tube, and the sterile dilute solution was then released to wet the very tip. The culturette was immediately transported to the microbiology laboratory, where it was immersed in 0.5 ml of sterile water and mixed, and 0.1 ml of the sample suspension was spread on each of three agar plates containing supplemented Lee's medium. The cultures were incubated for 7 days, and yeast colonies were counted. Scoring was as follows: 0 colonies per three plates, score of 0; 1 to 4 colonies per three plates, score of 1; 5 to 20 colonies per three plates, score of 2; 21 to 200 colonies per three plates, score of 3; over 200 colonies per three plates, score of 4. For details, see reference 83.
[c] No *Candida* sp. isolates were obtained from the underarm, nipple, or ear. *Candida* spp. were isolated in only one case from the navel, under the breast, and the back of the knee and in only two cases from the pubic hair line. These low-carriage body locations were not included in the table.

was simultaneous carriage in the vagina and the oral cavity, the isolates were unrelated (101). These studies together demonstrated that a single host could carry different *Candida* species, strains, or substrains, but in different body locations. On the basis of the entire host, this represents mixed infection, but on the basis of individual body locations, it does not. These results also suggested that different species, strains, and substrains adapt to the different environmental pressures of different body locations. One would expect such adaptation over long periods to result in single-strain carriage in a particular anatomical location in a healthy individual.

MIXED *CANDIDA* SP. AND BACTERIAL CARRIAGE

Mixed carriage, in the traditional sense, is that in which two or more organisms differing in kingdom, genus, or species can be found in the same body location, sharing an environment. It is obvious that commensal strains of *Candida* spp. share environments in the oral cavity with oral bacteria (90), in the gut with gastrointestinal bacteria (49), and in the vaginal canal with vaginal bacteria, most notably the lactobacilli (51). Galask and coworkers

compiled lists of organisms isolated from the vaginal canal of prehysterectomy (59) and posthysterectomy (14) patients. The latter list, synopsized in Table 2, is extensive and includes the proportions of patients that carried both bacteria and vaginal yeast (14). What is noteworthy in the list is the differences between the proportions of bacterial carriage with and without yeast for particular bacterial species. For instance, 18% of women carried both nonhemolytic streptococci (not group D) and yeast, but 0% carried these bacteria in the absence of yeast (Table 2), suggesting a requirement of yeast carriage for carriage of nonhemolytic streptococci. In contrast, other gram-negative rods (*Enterobacter*, *Citrobacter*, and *Pseudomonas* spp.) were isolated with yeast in 0% of women but without yeast in 33% of women (not in synopsized Table 2), suggesting that yeast carriage excluded carriage of other gram-negative rods. For the list in Table 2, in which findings for only the bacteria showing more than 10% cocolonization levels with yeast are synopsized, the mean percentages found with and without yeast were similar, but this is misleading, as noted above, on the basis of specific species. The results found by Galask and Ohm (14) therefore

TABLE 2 Proportions of posthysterectomy patients carrying bacteria and yeast[a]

Organism(s)	% of cultures:	
	Positive for a bacterium and positive for yeast	Positive for a bacterium and negative for yeast
Lactobacilli	27	9
Nonhemolytic non-group D streptococci	18	0
Group D streptococci	18	30
Staphylococcus epidermidis	18	15
Escherichia coli	36	36
Peptococcus asaccharolyticus	18	9
Peptococcus magnus	18	33
Unidentified anaerobic gram-positive cocci	18	6
Bacteroides fragilis	27	42
Bacteroides species	27	12
Mean ± SD	23 ± 6	19 ± 15

[a] Synopsized from reference 14. Positive bacterial cultures with yeast cocolonization of <10% are not listed; only the bacterial species showing the highest levels of cocolonization are shown.

suggest some very interesting cocarriage relationships between specific bacteria and yeast.

A balance between bacteria and *Candida* spp. in the microflora in healthy individuals is also suggested by the frequently reported increases in *Candida* sp. colonization and infections after treatment with antibacterial antibiotics, most notably tetracycline (see review in reference 56). Antibiotic-induced colonization and infection in the mouth, vagina, and feces have been reported (49, 51, 71, 90) and are believed to result from the reduction of bacteria assumed to normally suppress *Candida* sp. growth. It is believed that anaerobic bacteria are the major competitors of *Candida* sp. colonization (33, 34), and it has been demonstrated in vitro that anaerobic bacteria can release metabolites that suppress *C. albicans* growth in vitro (31). Although it therefore seems reasonable to conclude that the level of *C. albicans* carriage is regulated by associated bacteria in the microflora, Winner and Hurley, in their book *Candida albicans* (100), note problems in interpreting this balance from studies in which it is observed that the level of *Candida* sp. colonization increases in association with antibiotic therapy. Indeed, in studies of the growth kinetics of *C. albicans* and *Lactobacillus acidophilus* in mixed cultures in defined growth medium, we observed that each species attained the same final stationary-phase levels as monocultures of the respective organisms in the same medium, suggesting that the growth of each of the two species in mixed culture was regulated by a different growth-limiting component of the medium (D. R. Soll, unpublished observation). However, such in vitro analyses are not so much a test of bacterium-yeast interactions in general as they are a test of bacterium-yeast competition for respective growth-limiting components in the nutrient medium utilized. It therefore is still not clear whether bacteria that colonize a particular anatomical location regulate the growth dynamics of colonizing yeast or vice versa. To answer this question definitively, experiments that measure the effects of *Candida* spp. on bacteria and the effects of bacteria on *Candida*

spp. in natural body fluids will have to be designed.

In addition to observing the effects of bacteria on yeast growth, we have accumulated evidence that bacteria can affect the growth phenotype of yeast. *C. albicans* and related species grow in both budding and hyphal phenotypes (18, 75). The latter phenotype has been associated with infection and is presumed to play a role in tissue invasion (56). In primary cultures of vaginal samples, we have observed on several occasions effects of bacterial colonies on the growth morphologies of cells in *Candida* colonies (D. R. Soll and S. Lockhart, unpublished observations). In Fig. 2, the effects of a bacterial colony on the morphology of *C. albicans* colonies in proximity are apparent. The *C. albicans* colonies are wrinkled due to growth in the hyphal form. Colonies farther away from the bacterial colony have the normal smooth

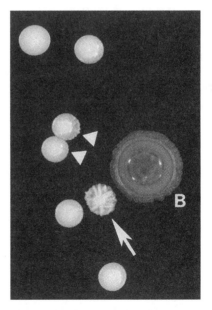

FIGURE 2 Primary culture from the vaginal canal in which the bacterial colony (B) alters the morphology of closely associated *C. albicans* colonies by inducing hypha and pseudohypha formation. Altered portions of colonies (arrowheads) and an entirely altered colony (arrow) are indicated. The changes are not hereditary (Soll and Lockhart, unpublished observation).

phenotype, as a result of growth in the budding-cell form.

CARRIAGE OF MULTIPLE *CANDIDA* SPECIES

Since *Candida* spp. other than *C. albicans* are carried as commensals in healthy individuals (see review in reference 56), there should be cases of *Candida* sp. cocarriage. Although methods for obtaining such information are readily available, there have been few attempts to address this question. The most common reason for this is that studies rarely employ collection methods that allow such discrimination. Standard methods of sample collection from a single body location, such as the mouth or vagina, usually involve rubbing a swab across the mucosa and then rubbing the sample swab across agar. If carriage is intense, the streak on the agar will grow confluently. If it is sparse, individual clonal colonies will arise. In the latter case, a single colony is usually picked, streaked, and analyzed. If a colonizing population is completely clonal (i.e., represents one genotype), then growth to confluency or selection of a single colony does not affect the genetic integrity of the sample. However, if a sample includes multiple yeast species, there will be enrichment in a confluent culture of the species that grows fastest on the particular medium used, and the enriched species may represent either the minor genotype at the site of colonization or the major genotype. Either way, the proportions of the species in the final confluent culture will not represent the proportions at the site of infection. Alternatively, if a single colony is selected from a primary culture, it may not be representative of the genetic heterogeneity of the infecting cell population. To ensure that in vitro cultures represent in vivo colonization, cells must be cloned directly from the colonized site by diluting the sample to the extent that individual colonies, each developing from a single cell, are generated for analysis, and agar medium that supports the growth of all expected species must be used. To discriminate between different *Candida* species in the original sample, CHROMagar can be used.

CHROMagar discriminates primarily by colony color, and in some cases by colony morphology, between a number of *Candida* spp., including *C. albicans, C. krusei, C. tropicalis,* and *C. glabrata,* the major *Candida* species (58, 62, 69). In Color Plate 5 (see color insert), an example of a mixed culture of *C. albicans, C. tropicalis,* and *C. glabrata* plated on CHROMagar and incubated for 7 days at 25°C is provided. The *C. albicans* colonies are green, the *C. tropicalis* colonies are blue, and the *C. glabrata* colonies are pink. The species tentatively identified by CHROMagar can then be verified by sugar assimilation patterns, using commercial kits such as the API 20C identification kit provided by BioMerieux-Vitek (5, 26). In an analysis of the frequency, intensity, and species and strains of *Candida* spp. in the oral cavity of healthy individuals from five different age groups, Kleinegger et al. (37) collected colonies from primary cultures with different colony morphologies and typed them, using the API 20C identification kit. They found that 7% of individuals carrying yeast in the oral cavity carried multiple species. The combinations were *C. albicans* and *C. parapsilosis, C. parapsilosis* and *C. zeylanoides, C. albicans* and *Saccharomyces cerevisiae,* and *C. albicans* and *Y. lipolytica.* In the last two cases, the following proportions were scored: 76% *C. albicans* and 24% *S. cerevisiae,* and 15% *C. albicans* and 85% *Yarrowia lipolytica.* In the study by Kleinegger et al. (37), an agar that did not support *C. glabrata* growth was used. Therefore, 7% mixed carriage is very likely an underestimate. The intensities of colonization of the multiple species indicated that mixed carriage in these instances represented substantial colonization. Lockhart et al. (46) performed a similar study in which they focused attention on the healthy elderly. They used CHROMagar in primary platings and verified interpreted species with the API 20C identification kit. The agar they used supported *C. glabrata* growth. They found that the oral cavity of 31% (*n* = 20) of test individuals was colonized with more than one yeast species. While 71% of yeast-positive subjects were colonized with *C. albicans,* 47% were colonized with that species alone and 24% were colonized with *C. albicans* plus one or two additional species. In contrast, while 29% of yeast-positive subjects were colonized with *C. glabrata,* only 8% were colonized with that species alone and 21% of yeast-positive subjects were colonized with *C. glabrata* plus one or more other species. Therefore, while 34% of *C. albicans* isolates were in mixed infections, 72% of *C. glabrata* isolates were in mixed infections. In Table 3, the species and intensity of carriage in mixed infections determined in the study of Lockhart et al. (46) are presented. It is clear from these results that in many cases the intensities of the cocolonizing species are both quite high.

Although the study by Lockhart et al. (46) suggests that mixed mycotic carriage is quite common in the elderly, one can take issue with the interpretation that mixed colonization in these cases truly represents carriage in healthy individuals, since a dramatic change was observed between the younger age groups (60 to 69 and 70 to 79 years) and the oldest age group

(≥80 years), as well as between individuals without and with dentures. The mean numbers of species per oral cavity (± standard deviations) in age groups 60 to 69, 70 to 79, and ≥80 years were 1.0 ± 0.0, 1.4 ± 0.7, and 1.5 ± 0.7, respectively. The mean numbers of species per oral cavity (± standard deviations) in individuals without dentures in age groups 70 to 79 and ≥80 years were 1.1 ± 0.3 and 1.4 ± 0.6, respectively, while those for individuals with dentures were 1.8 ± 0.8 and 1.7 ± 0.8, respectively. These results suggest that aging (i.e., ≥80 years) and denture wear are predisposing conditions for multiple mycotic carriage.

CARRIAGE OF MULTIPLE *CANDIDA* STRAINS AND SUBSTRAINS

If bacteria and fungi, and different fungal genera and species, all had the same phenotype, therapies would be singular, and information on mixed colonization would not affect therapy and would therefore not be very interesting. In fact, bacteria differ dramatically from

TABLE 3 Species and intensities of carriage in healthy individuals over 70 years of age[a]

Subject no.	Species (intensity of carriage)[b]
19	*C. albicans* (127), *C. parapsilosis* (1), *S. cerevisiae* (2)
21	*C. glabrata* (532), *C. parapsilosis* (36)
24	*C. albicans* (>1,000), *C. glabrata* (1,000), *C. tropicalis* (230)
25	*C. albicans* (663), *C. glabrata* (35)
26	*C. albicans* (>1,000), *C. glabrata* (>1,000)
28	*C. albicans* (>1,000), *C. glabrata* (>1,000)
29	*C. albicans* (1), *C. glabrata* (44)
30	*C. albicans* (554), *S. cerevisiae* (37)
38	*C. albicans* (49), *C. glabrata* (218)
39	*C. albicans* (79), *C. glabrata* (12), *S. cerevisiae* (12)
41	*C. albicans* (>1,000), *S. cerevisiae* (150)
44	*C. tropicalis* (>1,000), *S. cerevisiae* (2)
56	*C. tropicalis* (>1,000), *S. cerevisiae* (2)
58	*C. albicans* (345), *C. glabrata* (138)
64	*C. albicans* (334), *C. glabrata* (337), *C. tropicalis* (337)
65	*C. glabrata* (29), *C. tropicalis* (165)
67	*C. albicans* (7), *C. tropicalis* (15), *C. parapsilosis* (15)
68	*C. albicans* (>1,000), *S. cerevisiae* (2)
79	*C. glabrata* (43), *C. parapsilosis* (53)
86	*C. albicans* (21), *C. glabrata* (>1,000), *C. tropicalis* (>1,000)

[a] Synopsized from reference 46.
[b] Total number of CFU per 3 CHROMagar plates per oral cavity.

fungi in their methods of tissue invasion and in their drug susceptibility profiles, and different fungal species differ as well. We therefore are interested in mixed infections as a result of mixed phenotypes. Strains and substrains of a single species can also differ phenotypically, and for that reason, information on such mixed infections is also important from a therapeutic point of view. Because colony phenotypes on general agars and specialty agars like CHROM-agar usually do not discriminate between strains, more complicated molecular methods must be employed. To discriminate between strains and substrains of a species, a variety of genetic fingerprinting methods have been developed (78, 85; D. R. Soll, C. Pujol, and S. Lockhart, unpublished data, 2001), including Southern blot hybridization with species-specific complex probes, the random amplified polymorphic DNA (RAPD) technique, the multilocus enzyme electrophoresis (MLEE) technique, and a number of additional genetically based methods. RAPD and MLEE methods have been adapted to fingerprint the major infectious fungal species (78, 85; Soll et al., unpublished), and complex DNA fingerprinting probes have been developed for *C. albicans* (44, 68, 70), *C. tropicalis* (29), *C. glabrata* (45), *C. parapsilosis* (11), *Candida dubliniensis* (28), and *A. fumigatus* (15). For *C. albicans,* it has been demonstrated that MLEE, RAPD analysis, and the complex probe Ca3 are all highly effective in discriminating between completely unrelated strains, identifying the same strain, and discriminating microevolution in a single colonizing strain (65). For each of these DNA fingerprinting methods, one can calculate a similarity coefficient (S_{AB}) for every pair of isolates in a collection (78, 85; Soll et al., unpublished). The S_{AB} reflects relatedness. By characterizing a DNA fingerprinting method with a set of test isolates that represent all genetic relationships, one can estimate the S_{AB} ranges or thresholds that define genetic unrelatedness (i.e., that define different unrelated strains) and microevolution (i.e., that define different substrains) (78, 85; Soll et al., unpublished). This is demonstrated in a dendrogram generated from S_{AB}s computed for all pairs of a collection of isolates

that included (i) isolates that were genetically identical, (ii) isolates that were highly related but nonidentical (substrains), and (iii) isolates that were unrelated (Fig. 3). An S_{AB} of 1.00 represents identicalness and is obtained for those

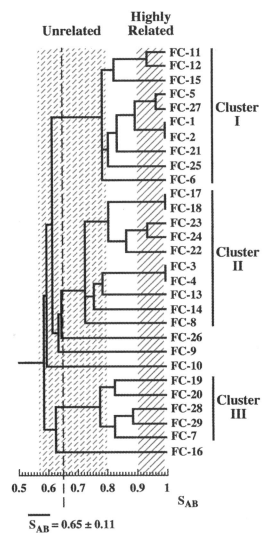

FIGURE 3 Dendrogram generated from the S_{AB}s computed for every pair in a set of test isolates that included identical, highly related, and unrelated isolates, originally analyzed by Pujol et al. (65). This set of isolates has been separated into three clusters and outliers (strains not in clusters). The unrelated and highly related ranges of S_{AB}s are arbitrarily set between 0.57 and 0.80 and between 0.90 and 0.99, respectively (78). Strains were fingerprinted by Southern blot analysis with the complex probe Ca3.

isolates expected to be identical. S_{AB}s between 0.90 and 0.99 represent substrains that have resulted from microevolution (44, 47, 98). One can also use the range of S_{AB}s between 0.57 and 0.80 as a measure of unrelatedness (Fig. 3). One can determine whether unrelated strains in a set of test isolates reside in the same genetic group or different genetic groups by generating a mixed dendrogram based on the S_{AB}s between all test isolates and a characterized control collection, by use of one of the available computer-assisted systems that have been developed for genetic fingerprinting (78). In the case of *C. albicans,* several different methods have identified three major groups for isolates collected in the United States (48, 65). These groups and outliers (isolates that do not cluster in the three major groups) are noted in Fig. 3.

Unfortunately, there have been very few studies of the genetic composition of commensal populations of infectious fungi in which multiple clones obtained from a primary sample were analyzed for genetic relatedness. Lockhart et al. (44) performed such an analysis on three commensal sets of isolates, one from

the back of the tongue and two from the vulva. They fingerprinted 12, 14, and 13 clones, respectively, from each of the three primary cultures, p1, p2, and p3, using the C1 fragment of the complex Ca3 probe, which is a hypersensitive indicator of microevolution (44). The results of this study are summarized in Table 4, and the collections of commensal isolates from individuals p2 and p3 are compared in Fig. 4 with a more general collection of unrelated *C. albicans* isolates by use of Ca3 fingerprinting to demonstrate the clustering of each collection at relatively high S_{AB}s. Although very limited, these data suggest that in the commensal state, a single body site is colonized by a single strain that is undergoing microevolution. The observation that two of the tested populations contained two patterns and one contained four patterns (44), in each case with very high S_{AB}s, indicated that microevolution occurred. Since changes in the Ca3 pattern occur at a rate in vitro of one band per 1,000 generations (66), the small microevolutionary differences observed within the commensal populations p2 and p3 in Fig. 4 can be explained by two alter-

TABLE 4 Microevolution in commensal and pathogenic populations revealed by C1 fingerprinting of *C. albicans*[a]

Individual	State of organism	Body location	No. of clones analyzed	Avg S_{AB}	% Isolates with:		No. of minor patterns	No. of band differences in minor patterns[b]
					Predominant pattern	Minor pattern		
p1	Commensal	Tongue	12	0.990	67	33	1	1 (+/−)
p2	Commensal	Vulva	14	0.997	93	7	1	1 (+)
p3	Commensal	Vulva	13	0.986	62	38	3	1 (+), 1 (+), 1 (+)
p4	Pathogenic	Vulva	12	1.000	92	8	1	1 (+)
p5	Pathogenic	Vulva	9	0.996	89	11	1	1 (−)
p6	Pathogenic	Vaginal wall	12	1.000	83	17	1	1 (−)
p7	Pathogenic	Vaginal wall	10	1.000	90	10	1	1 (−)
p8	Pathogenic	Vaginal wall	12	0.981	58	42	2	1 (+), 1 (+)
p9	Pathogenic	Vaginal wall	12	0.997	92	8	1	1 (+)

[a] Data are synopsized from reference 44.
[b] Each variant pattern was assessed according to the number of additional (+) or lost (−) bands relative to the predominant pattern.

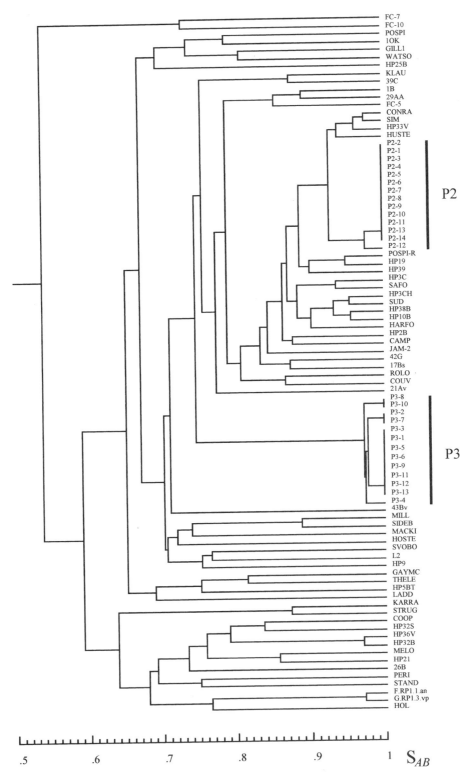

FIGURE 4 Collections of clonal *C. albicans* isolates, each from a primary sample from two patients (P2 and P3), were DNA fingerprinted with the complex probe Ca3 and incorporated into a mixed dendrogram that includes a more general collection of unrelated isolates. Note how the P2 and P3 collections cluster at very high S_{AB}s and exhibit microevolution in each case.

native scenarios. Either the commensal strains in the different body locations are frequently replaced or a single strain is maintained, but substrains compete for a body niche and the successful one enriches rapidly. The relative permanence of commensal strains suggests that the latter scenario occurs repeatedly. In a less direct analysis of microevolution, Soll et al. (83) compared pairs of vulva and vaginal canal isolates from the same healthy women, using the complex DNA fingerprinting probe Ca3. For seven of nine women, the S_{AB} was 1.00, and for the remaining two women the S_{AB}s were 0.98 and 0.96. Since the vaginal canal and vulva are contiguous, they can be considered a single body niche. The limited variability and high S_{AB}s reinforce the conclusion that single strains undergoing microevolution continuously colonize body niches in healthy individuals. However, there is really too little data to assess minor cocarriage of different *Candida* strains and substrains. The results of Kleinegger et al. (37) suggest 7% carriage of multiple species. Proof of cocarriage of multiple strains and substrains is made more difficult in the absence of an indicator agar such as that available for discriminating between species. To obtain a more accurate picture of carriage of multiple strains and substrains, far more detailed experiments must be performed in which (i) at least 20 additional healthy individuals with carriage are analyzed, (ii) CHROM-agar is utilized for identifying multiple-species carriage, and (iii) at least 30 individual yeast colonies are cloned from each species from the primary sample and DNA fingerprinted for genetic relatedness. This study should then be expanded as a function of age and gender.

RECURRENT *CANDIDA* SP. INFECTIONS

Candida spp. cause chronic infections, most notably in the vagina of otherwise apparently healthy women. For reasons not immediately apparent, these women present with recurrent infections interspersed with treatment periods in which the infection is suppressed. Genetic comparisons of isolates taken from sequential infections have demonstrated that the most frequent scenario is strain maintenance with or without microevolution. Lockhart et al. (47) used DNA fingerprinting with the complex probe Ca3 to assess the genetic relatedness of *C. albicans* isolates obtained from the oral cavity, vagina, and stools of 18 recurrent vaginitis patients over periods of up to 644 days. They found that in all test cases, the S_{AB}s of sequential isolates from the same individual were either identical or highly related. Two to six sequential isolates per patient were characterized. The combined number of comparisons for the 18 patients was 33, the range of S_{AB}s was 0.87 to 1.00, and the average S_{AB} for sequential pairwise comparisons ($\pm$ standard deviation) was 0.97 ± 0.03. Although longitudinal in design, these results support the conclusion that a single strain causes recurrent vaginal infections. The summed results revealed no mixed-strain or -species infections. In a more direct experiment, Lockhart et al. (44) assessed by DNA fingerprinting with the C1 fragment of the Ca3 probe between 9 and 12 independent clones obtained from each of six vaginitis patients. For the six collections, the lowest average S_{AB} was 0.97 (Table 4), well above the estimated threshold of 0.90 for variation due to microevolution (Fig. 3). On the other hand, in every collection, there were variants exhibiting microevolution (Table 4). This study therefore supports the conclusion that in recurrent vaginal infections, the populations usually are composed of a single strain. Variation stems from microevolution. However, just as in the case of commensal carriage, there have not been careful enough studies to test for minor cocolonizing by unrelated strains. To obtain a more accurate picture, far more detailed DNA fingerprinting experiments that include (i) a larger number of recurrent populations and (ii) more clones from primary samples must be performed. In an analysis of a large number of yeast isolates ($n = 389$) from vaginitis patients, Lisiak et al. (43) found that 7% of pregnant and delivering women were colonized with multiple *Candida species*, the same proportion of mixed-species carriage obtained by Kleinegger et al. (37). Although this study was not performed on recurrence patients and strain variability was not assessed, it suggests that with large samples, mixed-carriage infections that include both multiple species and multiple strains will very likely be identified.

MIXED FUNGAL AND BACTERIAL INFECTIONS

As we have discussed, yeast and bacteria live side by side as commensals in the natural microflora of healthy individuals. Since both bacteria and fungi are opportunistic pathogens, it is no surprise that they are frequently coisolated from sites of infection. In many cases, it is not always clear which organism is responsible for the initial infection and which organism represents a secondary infection or saprophytic interloper there for a free lunch. For instance, in the pathogenesis of genital white piedra, the majority of hair follicles contain both coryneform bacteria and yeast (10). The most common yeast is *Trichosporon beigelii*. In this case, it has been suggested that infection is caused by both organisms. In an individual suffering from adult T-cell leukemia, *Pneumocystis carinii* and *Legionella pneumophila* serogroup 1 were coisolated from cysts, which was interpreted as a mixed infection (88). In cases of corneal superinfections occurring after treatment of acute hemorrhagic conjunctivitis with corticosteroids, mixed infections have been demonstrated (91). Pneumonias have been ascribed to mixed infections of *Staphylococcus aureus* and *C. parapsilosis* (92). Mixed bacterial-fungal infections have been frequently described for endocarditis infections (6, 8, 17, 20, 23, 61), peritonitis infections (4, 12, 27), and liver abscesses (55). In postmenopausal women, mixed vaginal infections involving combinations of bacteria, *Trichomonas vaginalis,* and *C. albicans* have been reported (87). In an analysis of women with histories of recurrent bacterial vaginosis, approximately one-third were diagnosed with vulvovaginal candidiasis, which was considered a *Candida* sp. superinfection (67). In addition, in a study of vaginitis caused by *C. glabrata,* Sobel and Chaim (74) found that one-third of symptomatic patients had mixed infections of *C. glabrata* and bacteria.

MIXED FUNGAL SPECIES INFECTIONS

Mixed fungal infections that include fungal species from different genera have also been reported. For instance, de Doncker et al. (9) found that of 36 patients treated for onychomycosis of the toenail, 19 had mixed infections that included combinations of *Aspergillus* spp., *Fusarium* spp., *Scopulariopsis brevicaulis,* and *Alternis* spp.; Gugnani et al. (19) reported a case of otomycosis that included a mixture of *Aspergillus niger* and *C. albicans;* and Kimura et al. (35) reported mixed *Trichosporon* sp. and *Candida* sp. dissemination in an autopsy. Meyers (50) presented the extraordinarily high death rates of 75% for bone marrow transplant patients infected with *Aspergillus* spp. alone and 100% for patients infected with *Aspergillus* spp. and *Candida* spp. These examples and additional ones not reviewed here demonstrate that mixed fungal infections involving different genera occur in decaying tissue such as that around the toenail in onychomycosis infections and in fungemias in immunosuppressed patients. In the former types of infections, the decaying skin does not harbor an effective cellular immune system, and in the latter types of infections, the immune system is generally suppressed.

Mixed infections involving different species of the same genus have been reported in a variety of disease states. As noted above, Lisiak et al. (43) found that in pregnant and delivering women hospitalized in Bydgoszcz, 7% were colonized with two *Candida* species. Willinger and Manafi (99), in evaluating CHROMagar, found that 3% ($n = 40$) of 1,150 clinical samples contained multiple *Candida* species, and Kleinegger et al. (37) demonstrated simultaneous oral carriage of *C. albicans* and *C. parapsilosis* in two healthy toddlers and simultaneous oral carriage of *C. parapsilosis* and *C. zeylanoides* in one healthy child. In an analysis of 11 human immunodeficiency virus-positive subjects, Vargas (93) recently demonstrated combinations of *C. albicans* and *C. tropicalis* in one patient; *C. albicans, Candida guilliermondii, C. tropicalis,* and *C. glabrata* in a second patient; and *C. albicans* and *C. glabrata* in a third patient. As noted in the review of *Candida* sp. commensalism in the elderly (see "Carriage of Multiple *Candida* Species" above), Lockhart et al. (46) demonstrated mixed colonization that included *C. albicans* and a variety of *Candida* species (Table 3). Again, one might expect that increased frequencies of mixed-species infections result from compromising host conditions that affect the natural defenses that usually suppress growth or purge invaders, in the case of systemic or disseminated infections. One might expect that in cases of severely immunocompromised patients, such as bone marrow transplant recipients, the frequency of infections involving mixed fungal genera would be similar to that of infections involving mixed fungal species, since severe immunosuppression seems to be an "equal opportunity employer." In such cases, frequencies and combinations would be functions of exposure and the efficiency of colonization and of the capacity of each independent pathogen to penetrate tissue. In cases in which host defenses are compromised but not necessarily eradicated, particular body niches might still be selective in mixed infections. In these cases, mixed-species infections would be primarily those that include species that normally colonized that niche in the commensal state.

MIXED FUNGAL STRAIN AND SUBSTRAIN INFECTIONS

With the advent of DNA fingerprinting techniques (78, 85; Soll et al., unpublished), mixed infections that include unrelated strains of the same species have also been reported. In the review of *Candida* sp. commensalism above, methods that provide genetic resolution between unrelated strains of the same species were described, and they included restriction fragment length polymorphism with a probe, RAPD analysis, MLEE, and a number of additional methods, reviewed recently by Soll and coworkers (78, 85; Soll et al., unpublished).

Unfortunately, the methods used by many researchers for genetic fingerprinting have not been carefully characterized for genetic resolution (78), so when it is reported that two or more isolates of a particular species possess different genotypes, one cannot be sure if the differences reflect genetically unrelated strains or highly related substrains that recently diverged because of microevolution. This distinction is important from the standpoint of mixed infections, since one might assume that the phenotypic capabilities, and hence the virulence traits, of substrains are more similar than those of unrelated strains, a distinction that could affect therapeutic strategies.

The problem of identifying multiple-strain infections was reviewed above in the sections on *Candida* commensalism. As has been argued for commensal studies, discrimination between strains and substrains in infecting populations requires the immediate separation of clones in primary cultures. Since there is some likelihood that strains from the same species will form colonies with similar morphologies, a protocol in which 10 or more clones from the primary culture are genetically fingerprinted, as in the study of Lockhart et al. (44), is required. By use of this general protocol, there have been several reports of mixed-strain infections. For instance, Neuveglise et al. (54), using restriction fragment length polymorphism with a repeat sequence probe to assess *A. fumigatus* colonization of six cystic fibrosis patients, found that each patient was colonized simultaneously by multiple strains and that these strains were repeatedly isolated for 1 to several years. This is the first study suggesting that multiple strains can be simultaneously maintained for prolonged periods in the same individual.

Perhaps one of the most revealing studies of mixed-strain infection involved a *C. tropicalis* systemic infection in a bone marrow transplant patient (86). The patient was monitored during the course of the infection for colonization at several body locations, including the blood, and individual colonies from primary cultures were DNA fingerprinted with the *C. albicans* complex probe Ca3 and the *C. tropicalis* complex probe Ct 13-8. The sequence of isolates is presented in Fig. 5. On day 0, a *C. albicans* strain (C.alb-1) was isolated from urine, and on days 58 and 65, two additional, unrelated *C. albicans* strains were identified in throat cultures. However, the life-threatening infection in the blood involved two strains of *C. tropicalis,* C.trop-1 and C.trop-2, distinguished by Ct 13-8 fingerprinting. C.trop-1 first was isolated from a blood sample on day 2 and exhibited "irregular edge" colony morphology. C.trop-2 was then isolated from a skin blister on day 3. On day 6, C.trop.-1 and C.trop.-2 were both isolated from a blood sample. On day 2, a low dose of amphotericin B was administered intravenously, and on day 5 the dose was increased. From day 7 on, only the C.trop.-1 strain remained in the blood. On day 11, flucytosine was administered simultaneously with amphotericin B and continued for 3 weeks. From days 12 through 65, neither *C. tropicalis* strain was isolated from blood, but on days 58 and 64, a third *C. tropicalis* strain (C.trop.-3) was identified in throat and stool samples, respectively, by Ct 13-8 fingerprinting. In vitro growth cultures of C.trop.-1 and C.trop.-2 in 5×10^{-2} mg of amphotericin B per ml revealed that the former strain was far more resistant to amphotericin B over time than the latter strain, which was consistent with the disappearance of the latter but not the former after an increased dose of amphotericin B was applied. The former strain was removed from the blood by flucytosine treatment. This single detailed case study demonstrated that in a mixed systemic infection of two *C. tropicalis* strains, one responded to amphotericin B treatment and one did not, and their in vitro sensitivities to the drug were consistent with the in vivo results. What is so surprising about this single detailed case study is the sheer number of unrelated strains and species of *Candida* involved, three strains of *C. albicans* and three strains of *C. tropicalis*. It seems highly unlikely that all of these strains were original commensals and more likely that when the patient was immunosuppressed, new strains took up resi-

dence in the host. This single case study (86) demonstrates the extraordinary susceptibility of immunosuppressed patients to life-threatening multifungal infections.

Finally, we have discussed the microevolution of strains in infecting vulvovaginitis populations. Because recurrent episodes of vaginitis are in most cases due to a single infecting strain that is suppressed but not eradicated by therapies between episodes, the single strain continues to microevolve (47). Unfortunately, there is scant information on the microevolution of infecting populations over shorter periods, such as in blood infections. In the case of the *C. tropicalis* infection described in Fig. 5, a third strain of *C. tropicalis* appeared in the throat at 5 to 8 days and then in the stools at 64 days. The two isolates of this strain exhibited small changes in DNA fingerprinting patterns reflecting microevolution. What would be far more informative is an analysis of multiple isolates collected at very short intervals during drug therapy. Such information would shed light on the rate of genetic change associated with the emergence of drug resistance over the short periods that include drug therapy. Indeed, White and coworkers (98) documented the acquisition of azole resistance in a strain of *C. albicans* that was associated with microevolution identified by the complex DNA fingerprinting probe Ca3.

PHENOTYPIC HETEROGENEITY THROUGH SWITCHING: THE LAST FORM OF MIXED INFECTION

Traditionally, mixed colonization or a mixed infection refers to combinations of genera or species cohabiting the same host location. We first extended that definition to include combinations of strains and substrains. In this chapter, we will now extend the definition even further to include high-frequency phenotypic switching, which appears to arise epigenetically. The rationale for this extension is quite simple. The intent of examining mixed infections is to understand the expanded pathogenesis represented by multiple infecting species, since different organisms have different pathogenic

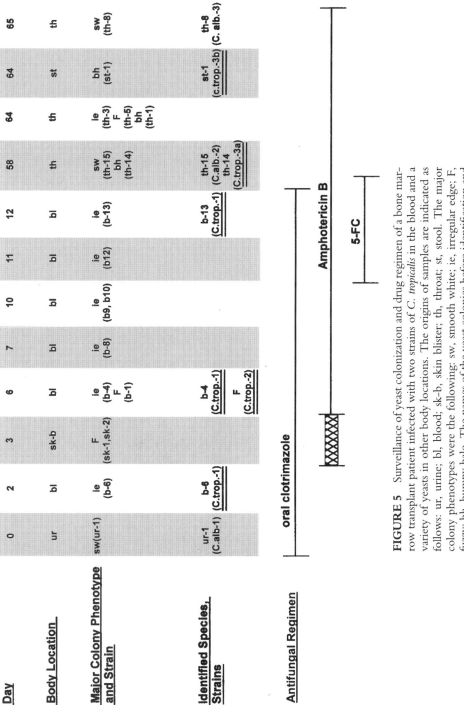

FIGURE 5 Surveillance of yeast colonization and drug regimen of a bone marrow transplant patient infected with two strains of *C. tropicalis* in the blood and a variety of yeasts in other body locations. The origins of samples are indicated as follows: ur, urine; bl, blood; sk-b, skin blister; th, throat; st, stool. The major colony phenotypes were the following: sw, smooth white; ie, irregular edge; F, fuzzy; bh, bumpy halo. The names of the yeast colonies before identification and DNA fingerprinting are presented under "Major Colony Phenotype and Strain" (in parentheses) and with the identified species and strains. The identified species and strain, for example, C.alb-1, refer to species and strain number in order of isolation. Low-dosage (hatched bar) and maximum-dosage (solid bars) drug regimens are indicated. 5–FC, flucytosine. Modified from reference 86.

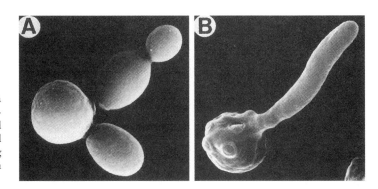

FIGURE 6 The basic bud-hypha transition in *C. albicans*. (A) A budding cell in which the mother and daughter cell have in turn budded and are separating; (B) a cell forming a germ tube. Note the bud scars on the mother cell.

potentials and different phenotypic characteristics that impact treatment. Different infecting species may differ in drug susceptibility, their capacity to cause tissue damage, their capacity to disseminate, and their capacity to alter the immune system. Therefore, it is not the genetic differences per se of cocolonizing organisms that ultimately engage us, but rather the differences in phenotype. Thus, we must finally consider epigenetic as well as genetic changes that alter phenotype and lead to phenotypically heterogeneous colonizing populations.

The infectious fungi have evolved extremely powerful mechanisms for generating phenotypic heterogeneity in a population. The first, the bud-hypha transition, allows *Candida* spp. to differentiate from a budding form (Fig. 6A) to a myceliated form (Fig. 6B) (18, 75) in order to penetrate tissue (56). Commensal populations usually express primarily the budding form, while infecting populations usually include mixed phenotypes (bud plus hyphae). In some cases, tissues are completely colonized by hyphae. Although the bud-hypha transition, or dimorphism, provides alternate growth forms, it never seemed to provide the degree of variability one would expect of an organism like *C. albicans*, which can live as both a commensal and a pathogen, can inhabit every damp or wet body niche in a healthy individual, and can invade virtually every tissue during infection. It was therefore no surprise to discover in 1985 (64, 72) that standard laboratory strains of *C. albicans* could switch between general phenotypes (Fig. 7) at relatively high frequencies in a spontaneous and reversible fashion, and subse-

quently that switching regulated a variety of virulence genes (76, 79, 80). Spontaneous frequencies of switching in commensal and infectious strains vary between 10^{-1} and 10^{-4}. Although most thoroughly studied in *C. albicans*,

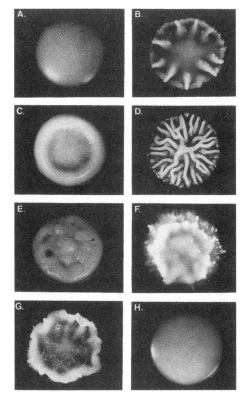

FIGURE 7 Colony morphologies in the switching system in *C. albicans* 3153A. (A) Original smooth; (B) star; (C) ring; (D) wrinkle; (E) mottled; (F) hat; (G) fuzzy; (H) revertant smooth. Reprinted from reference 72 with permission.

reversible, high-frequency switching has been demonstrated in *C. glabrata* (41), *C. tropicalis* (86), *C. parapsilosis* (11), and *Cryptococcus neoformans* (13, 16). Switching in *C. albicans* affects the secretion of aspartyl proteinases (25, 52, 93, 97), adhesion (32, 95), drug susceptibility (94), the bud–hypha transition (1), sensitivity to white blood cells and metabolites (28), antigenicity (2), and virulence in animal models (39, 40). It has been proposed that the capacity to switch is a strategy for rapid adaptation to environmental challenges (57, 77). Hence, each colonizing population includes variants with disparate phenotypes at frequencies of 10^{-1} to 10^{-4}, poised to enrich in response to a challenge that wipes out the dominant phenotype. In Fig. 8, an example of a primary culture of yeast colonies collected from the vagina of a healthy female is presented. The different colony morphologies reflect the switching repertoire (i.e., switch phenotypes) of a single colonizing strain.

The molecular basis of switching has not been elucidated, but there is growing evidence that it is rooted in alternate chromatin states (36, 89). Recently, it was demonstrated that the deacetylases Hda1 and Rpd3 (36, 89) and the NAD-dependent deacetylase Sir2 (60) play roles in suppressing switching in *C. albicans*. The switch event flips sets of phase-specific genes on and off through phase-specific *trans*-acting factors (79, 80). In some switching systems, like the white-opaque transition in *C. albicans* strain WO-1 (2, 73), which has evolved into a model experimental system for investigating the molecular basis of switching (79–81), the alternate phenotypes are so disparate that one would think they represented different species. In *C. glabrata,* all strains switch between "white," "light brown," "dark brown," and "very dark brown" phenotypes in which there is graded gene expression that follows color intensity (41). In this system, the expression of the hemolysin gene *HLP1* is also expressed in a graded fashion (41).

High-frequency phenotypic switching has been demonstrated at sites of commensalism (22) and at sites of infection (22, 30, 84, 94). In Fig. 8, colonies formed by isolates from succes-

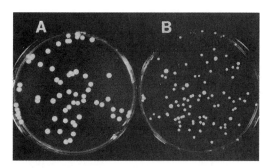

FIGURE 8 Isolates from sequential episodes of recurrent vaginal candidiasis caused by a single strain. (A) The original large-colony phenotype in episode 1. (B) The small- and medium-sized-colony phenotype in episode 2. DNA fingerprinting with probe Ca3 demonstrated that all colonies represented the same strain. Plating experiments demonstrated that small- and medium-sized-colony phenotype cells switched back to the large- colony phenotype. Reprinted from reference 82.

sive episodes of recurrent vaginal candidiasis have been plated at low density to assess colony morphologies (82). In the first recurrence episode, the isolated strain formed large colonies (Fig. 8A), while in the second episode the isolated strain formed small and medium-sized colonies (Fig. 8B). All isolates had the same Ca3 fingerprint pattern but differed in azole susceptibility (82). The smaller-colony phenotype was demonstrated to switch back to the original large-colony phenotype. Jones et al. (30) first demonstrated that the average isolate from deep mycoses switched more frequently than the average isolate from superficial mycoses, suggesting that an alteration in frequency preceded or followed the establishment of a severe infection. Hellstein et al. (22) then demonstrated that oral infection strains on average switched more frequently than oral commensal strains, and Vargas et al. (94) demonstrated that isolates from the oral cavity of AIDS patients switched on average at higher frequencies than isolates from healthy control individuals. Vargas et al. (94) also demonstrated that switching in fresh isolates from patients had remarkable effects both on drug susceptibility and on the secretion of acid proteinase. These results demonstrate that in addition to the phenotypic heterogeneity provided by cocolonizing organisms at the kingdom, genus, species, strain, and substrain levels of genetic relatedness, the heterogeneity provided by presumed epigenetic mechanisms such as high-frequency phenotypic switching must be recognized.

CONCLUSIONS

It has been argued here that limiting the definition of mixed infections to those involving different species is in fact far too restrictive. We have expanded the definition to include different strains of a single species and different substrains of a single strain. Since our interest in mixed infections stems from the differences attributed to the phenotypes of the cocolonizing organisms, we have argued that one must consider as well the different switch phenotypes generated by high-frequency phenotypic switching, since these phenotypes are relatively stable, leading to stable mixed phenotypes in colonizing populations. Methods that distinguish unrelated strains, substrains that have diverged due to recent microevolutionary events, and the same strain expressing different switch phenotypes, in particular DNA fingerprinting technologies, have been reviewed. In identifying mixed colonization, our challenge is first to identify genetic diversity. Identifying mixed bacterial-fungal infections means that both antibacterial and antifungal antibiotics may be required (i.e., combination therapy). In mixed fungal infections, we are confronted with mixtures that may include drug-sensitive and drug-resistant species and strains. Surprisingly, the same phenotypic combinations can be the result of microevolution or phenotypic switching. By understanding the pathogenic strategies, phenotypic characteristics, and switching capabilities of individual strains and by applying methods that identify both the genetic and the phenotypic complexity of a colonizing population, we will be in a far better position to treat infections or apply prophylactic treatments before infections occur. This information and the strategies that emerge from it are particularly critical in cases of immunosuppressed individuals.

ACKNOWLEDGMENTS

The most recent work from the Soll laboratory reviewed in this chapter was funded by Public Health Service grant AI3975.

I am indebted to S. Lockhart for unpublished observations reviewed here and to K. Daniels for assistance in generating figures.

REFERENCES

1. **Anderson, J., L. Cundiff, B. Schnars, M. Gao, I. Mackenzie, and D. R. Soll.** 1989. Hypha formation in the white-opaque transition of *Candida albicans*. *Infect. Immun.* **57:**458–467.
2. **Anderson, J., R. Mihalik, and D. R. Soll.** 1990. Ultrastructure and antigenicity of the unique cell wall pimple of the *Candida* opaque phenotype. *J. Bacteriol.* **172:**224–235.
3. **Anderson, J. M., T. Srikantha, B. Morrow, S. H. Miyasaki, T. C. White, N. Agabian, J. Schmid, and D. R. Soll.** 1993. Characterization and partial nucleotide sequence of the DNA fingerprinting probe Ca3 of *Candida albicans*. *J. Clin. Microbiol.* **31:**1472–1480.
4. **Bayle, E., B. Pelle, J. P. Halgrain, K. Tran-Ky, and K. Moussalier.** 1979. Perforation duodenal a *Candida albicans*. *Nouv. Presse Med.* **8:**3674.
5. **Bernal, S., E. Martin Mazuelos, M. Chavez, J. Coronilla, and A. Valverde.** 1998. Evaluation of the new API *Candida* system for identification of the most clinically important yeast species. *Diagn. Microbiol. Infect. Dis.* **32:**217–221.
6. **Boyce, J. M. H.** 1975. A case of prosthetic valve endocarditis caused by *Corynebacterium hogmanni* and *Candida albicans*. *Br. Heart J.* **37:**1195–1197.
7. **Calderone, R. (ed.).** 2002. Candida *and Candidiasis*. ASM Press, Washington, D.C.
8. **Case Records of the Massachusetts General Hospital.** 1975. Case 30-1975. *N. Engl. J. Med.* **293:**247–253.
9. **de Doncker, P. R., R. K. Scher, R. L. Baran, J. Decroix, H. J. Degreef, D. I. Roseeuw, V. Havu, T. Rosen, A. K. Gupta, and G. E. Pierard.** 1997. Itraconazole therapy is effective for pedal onychomycosis caused by some nondermatophyte molds and in mixed infection with dermatophytes and molds: a multicenter study with 36 patients. *J. Am. Acad. Dermatol.* **36:**173–177.
10. **Ellner, K. M., M. E. McBride, D. C. Kalter, J. A. Tschen, and J. E. Wolf, Jr.** 1990. White piedra: evidence for a synergistic infection. *Br. J. Dermatol.* **123:**355–363.
11. **Enger, L., S. Joly, C. Pujol, P. Simonson, M. A. Pfaller, and D. R. Soll.** 2001. Cloning and characterization of a complex DNA fingerprinting probe for *Candida parapsilosis*. *J. Clin. Microbiol.* **39:**658–669.

12. **Freund, U., Z. Gimmon, and S. Katz.** 1979. *Candida* infected ascites caused by perforated ulcer. *Mycopathologia* **66:**191–192.

13. **Fries, B. C., D. C. Goldman, R. Cherniak, R. Ju, and A. Casadevall.** 1999. Phenotypic switching in *Cryptococcus neoformans* results in changes in the cellular morphology and glucuronoxyomannan structure. *Infect. Immun.* **67:** 6076–6083.

14. **Galask, R. P., and M. J. Ohm.** 1978. Bacterial flora and mycotic infections of the vagina and cervix in post-hysterectomy patients. *Mykosen* **1**(Suppl. 1)**:** 236–245.

15. **Girardin, H., J.-P. Latge, T. Srikantha, B. Morrow, and D. R. Soll.** 1993. Development of DNA probes for fingerprinting *Aspergillus fumigatus*. *J. Clin. Microbiol.* **31:**1547–1554.

16. **Goldman, D., B. Fries, S. Franzot, L. Montella, and A. Casadevall.** 1998. Phenotypic switching in the human pathogenic fungus *Cryptococcus neoformans* is associated with changes in virulence and pulmonary inflammatory response in rodents. *Proc. Natl. Acad. Sci. USA* **95:**14967–14972.

17. **Gonzalez-Lavin, L., E. Scappatura, M. Lise, and D. N. Ross.** 1970. Mycotic aneurysms of the aortic root. *Ann. Thorac. Surg.* **9:**551–561.

18. **Gow, N. A.** 1997. Germ tube growth of *Candida albicans*. *Curr. Top. Med. Mycol.* **8:**43–55.

19. **Gugnani, H. C., B. C. Okafor, F. Nzelibe, and A. N. Njoku-Obi.** 1989. Etiological agents of otomycosis in Nigeria. *Mycoses* **32:**224–229.

20. **Hairston, P., and W. H. Lee, Jr.** 1970. Management of infected prosthetic heart valves. *Ann. Thorac. Surg.* **9:**229–237.

21. **Hazen, K. C.** 1995. New and emerging yeast pathogens. *Clin. Microbiol. Rev.* **8:**462–478.

22. **Hellstein, J., H. Vawter-Hugart, P. Fotos, J. Schmid, and D. R. Soll.** 1993. Genetic similarity and phenotypic diversity of commensal and pathogenic strains of *Candida albicans* isolated from the oral cavity. *J. Clin. Microbiol.* **31:**3190–3199.

23. **Henderson, J., and J. F. Nickerson.** 1964. Bacterial endocarditis with *Candida albicans* superinfection. *Can. Med. Assoc. J.* **90:**452–458.

24. **Hitchcock, C. A., G. Pye, P. F. Troke, E. M. Johnson, and D. W. Warnock.** 1993. Fluconazole resistance in *Candida glabrata*. *Antimicrob. Agents Chemother.* **37:**1962–1965.

25. **Hube, B., M. Monod, D. A. Schofield, A. J. Brown, and N. A. Gow.** 1994. Expression of seven members of the gene family encoding secretory aspartyl proteinases in *Candida albicans*. *Med. Microbiol.* **14:**87–99.

26. **Jabra-Rizk, M. A., W. A. Falker, W. G. Merz, A. A. Bagui, J. I. Kelley, and T. F. Meiller.** 2000. Retrospective identification and characterization of *Candida dubliniensis* isolates among *Candida albicans* clinical laboratory isolates from human immunodeficiency virus (HIV)-infected and non-HIV-infected individuals. *J. Clin. Microbiol.* **38:**2423–2426.

27. **Johnson, D. E., M. M. Conroy, J. E. Foker, P. Ferrieri, and T. R. Thompson.** 1980. *Candida* peritonitis in the newborn infant. *J. Pediatr.* **97:**298–300.

28. **Joly, S., C. Pujol, M. Rysz, K. Vargas, and D. R. Soll.** 1999. Development and characterization of complex DNA fingerprinting probes for the infectious agent *Candida dubliniensis*. *J. Clin. Microbiol.* **37:**1035–1044.

29. **Joly, S., C. Pujol, K. Schroppel, and D. R. Soll.** 1996. Development and verification of two species fingerprinting probes for *Candida tropicalis* amenable to computer analysis. *J. Clin. Microbiol.* **34:**3063–3071.

30. **Jones, S., G. White, and P. R. Hunter.** 1994. Increased phenotypic switching in strains of *Candida albicans* associated with invasive infections. *J. Clin. Microbiol.* **32:**2869–2870.

31. **Kennedy, M. J.** 1981. Inhibition of *Candida albicans* by the anaerobic oral flora of mice *in vitro*. *Sabouraudia* **19:**205–208.

32. **Kennedy, M. J., A. L. Rogers, L. R. Hanselman, D. R. Soll, and R. J. Yancey.** 1988. Variation in adhesion and cell surface hydrobicity in *Candida albicans* white and opaque phenotypes. *Mycopathologia* **102:**149–156.

33. **Kennedy, M. J., and P. A. Volz.** 1985. Effect of various antibiotics on gastrointestinal colonization and dissemination by *Candida albicans*. *Sabouraudia J. Med. Vet. Mycol.* **23:**265–273.

34. **Kennedy, M. J., and P. A. Volz.** 1985. Ecology of *Candida albicans* gut colonization: inhibition of *Candida* adhesion, colonization, and dissemination from the gastrointestinal tract by bacterial antagonism. *Infect. Immun.* **49:**654–663.

35. **Kimura, M., H. Takahashi, T. Satou, and S. Hashimoto.** 1989. An autopsy case of disseminated trichosporonosis with candidiasis of the urinary bladder. *Virchows Arch. A Pathol. Anat. Histopathol.* **416:**159–162.

36. **Klar, A., T. Srikantha, and D. R. Soll.** 2001. A histone deacetylation inhibitor and mutant promote colony-type switching of the human pathogen *Candida albicans*. *Genetics* **158:**919–924.

37. **Kleinegger, C., S. T. Lockhart, K. Vargas, and D. R. Soll.** 1996. Frequency, intensity, species, and strains of oral yeast vary as a function of host age. *J. Clin. Microbiol.* **34:**2246–2254.

38. **Kolotila, M. P., and R. D. Diamond.** 1990. Effects of neutrophils and in vitro oxidants on survival and phenotypic switching of *Candida albicans* WO-1. *Infect. Immun.* **58:**1174–1179.

39. **Kvaal, C., S. Lachke, T. Srikantha, K. Daniels, J. McCoy, and D. R. Soll.** 1999. Misexpression of the opaque phase-specific gene *PEP1* (*SAP1*) in the white phase of *Candida albicans* confers increased virulence in a mouse model of cutaneous infection. *Infect. Immun.* **67:**6652–6662.

40. **Kvaal, C. A., T. Srikantha, and D. R. Soll.** 1997. Misexpression of the white phase-specific gene *WH11* in the opaque phase of *Candida albicans* affects switching and virulence. *Infect. Immun.* **65:**4468–4475.

41. **Lachke, S., T. Srikantha, L. Tsai, K. Daniels, and D. R. Soll.** 2000. Phenotypic switching in *Candida glabrata* involves phase-specific regulation of the metallothionein gene *MT-II* and the newly discovered hemolysin gene *HLP*. *Infect. Immun.* **68:**884–895.

42. **Latgé, J. P.** 1999. *Aspergillus fumigatus* and aspergillosis. *Clin. Microbiol. Rev.* **12:**310–350.

43. **Lisiak, M., C. Klyszejko, Z. Marcinkowski, and Z. Gwiezdzinski.** 2000. Yeast species identification in vulvovaginal candidiasis: susceptibility to nystatin. *Ginekol. Pol.* **71:**959–963.

44. **Lockhart, S., J. J. Fritch, A. S. Meier, K. Schroppel, T. Srikantha, R. Galask, and D. R. Soll.** 1995. Colonizing populations of *Candida albicans* are clonal in origin but undergo microevolution through C1 fragment reorganization as demonstrated by DNA fingerprinting and C1 sequencing. *J. Clin. Microbiol.* **33:**1501–1509.

45. **Lockhart, S. R., S. Joly, C. Pujol, J. D. Sobel, M. A. Waller, and D. R. Soll.** 1997. Development and verification of fingerprinting probes for *Candida glabrata*. *Microbiology* **143:**3733–3746.

46. **Lockhart, S. R., S. Joly, K. Vargas, J. Swails-Wenger, L. Enger, and D. R. Soll.** 1999. Natural defenses against *Candida* colonization breakdown in the oral cavities of the elderly. *J. Dent. Res.* **78:**857–868.

47. **Lockhart, S. R., B. D. Reed, C. L. Pierson, and D. R. Soll.** 1996. Most frequent scenario for recurrent *Candida* vaginitis is strain maintenance with "substrain shuffling": demonstration by sequential DNA fingerprinting with probes Ca3, C1, and CARE2. *J. Clin. Microbiol.* **34:**767–777.

48. **Lott, T. J., D. A. Logan, B. P. Holloway, R. Fundyga, and J. Arnold.** 1999. Towards understanding the evolution of the human commensal yeast, *Candida albicans*. *Microbiology* **145:**1137–1143.

49. **Mehta, A. B., H. R. Mahajam, D. D. Vora, A. C. Shah, and A. B. Agarwala.** 1970. Comparative evaluation of antifungal agents in the prevention of tetracycline-induced candidiasis of gastrointestinal tract. *J. Assoc. Physicians India* **18:**621–626.

50. **Meyers, J. D.** 1990. Fungal infections in bone marrow transplant patients. *Semin. Oncol.* **17:**10–13.

51. **Mohapatra, L. N., K. Ramachandran, J. C. M. Shastry, and B. M. Tandon.** 1969. Prophylactic use of amphotericin B for *Candida* infection amongst patients on broad-spectrum antibiotic treatment. *Indian J. Med. Res.* **57:**128–132.

52. **Morrow, B., T. Srikantha, and D. R. Soll.** 1992. Transcription of the gene for a pepsinogen, PEP1, is regulated by white-opaque switching in *Candida albicans*. *Mol. Cell. Biol.* **12:**2997–3005.

53. **Mullins, J., P. Hutchinson, and R. G. Slavin.** 1984. *Aspergillus fumigatus* spore concentrations in outside air: Cardiff and St. Louis compared. *Clin. Allergy* **14:**251–254.

54. **Neuveglise, C., J. Sarfati, J. P. Debeaupuis, H. Vu Thien, J. Just, G. Tournier, and J. P. Latge.** 1997. Longitudinal study of *Aspergillus fumigatus* strains isolated from cystic fibrosis patients. *Eur. J. Clin. Microbiol. Infect. Dis.* **16:**747–750.

55. **Niebel, J., U. Farack, and V. Mursic.** 1984. Bacterial-mycotic liver abscess in nonimmunocompromised host. *Infection* **12:**256–257.

56. **Odds, F. C.** 1988. *Candida and Candidosis: a Review and Bibliography*. Bailliere Tindall, London, United Kingdom.

57. **Odds, F. C.** 1997. Switch of phenotype as an escape mechanism of the intruder. *Mycoses* **40:**S9–S12.

58. **Odds, F. C., and R. Bernaerts.** 1994. CHROMagar *Candida*, a new differential isolation medium for presumptive identification of clinically important *Candida* species. *J. Clin. Microbiol.* **32:**1923–1929.

59. **Ohm, M. J., and R. P. Galask.** 1975. Bacterial flora of the cervix from 100 prehysterectomy patients. *Am. J. Obstet. Gynecol.* **122:**683–687.

60. **Perez-Martin, J., J. A. Uria, and A. D. Johnson.** 1999. Phenotypic switching in *Candida albicans* is controlled by a SIR2 gene. *EMBO J.* **18:**2580–2592.

61. **Perrenoud, J. J., and G. Lanitis.** 1976. La septicemie a levures en chirurgie. *Rev. Med. Suisse Romande* **96:**923–930.

62. **Pfaller, M. A., A. Houston, and S. Coffmann.** 1996. Application of CHROMagar Candida for rapid screening of clinical specimens for *Candida albicans, Candida tropicalis,* and *Candida (Torulopsis) glabrata*. *J. Clin. Microbiol.* **34:**58–61.

63. **Pfaller, M. A., R. N. Jones, S. A. Messer, M. B. Edmond, R. P. Wenzel, and S. P. Group.** 1988. National surveillance of nosocomial blood stream infection due to species of *Candida albicans:* frequency of occurrence and antifungal susceptibility in the SCOPE Program. *Diagn. Microbiol. Infect. Dis.* **30:**121–129.

64. Pomes, R., C. Gil, and C. Nombela. 1985. Genetic analysis of Candida albicans morphological mutants. *J. Gen. Microbiol.* **131:**2107–2113.

65. Pujol, C., S. Joly, S. Lockhart, S. Noel, M. Tibayrenc, and D. R. Soll. 1997. Parity of MLEE, RAPD, and Ca3 hybridization as fingerprinting methods for *Candida albicans. J. Clin. Microbiol.* **35:**2348–2358.

66. Pujol, C., S. Joly, B. Nolan, T. Srikantha, S. Lockhart, and D. R. Soll. 1999. Microevolutionary changes in *Candida albicans* identified by the complex Ca3 probe involve insertions and deletions of RPS units at specific genomic sites. *Microbiology* **145:**2635–2646.

67. Redondo-Lopez, V., C. Meriwether, C. Schmitt, M. Opitz, R. Cook, and J. D. Sobel. 1990. Vulvovaginal candidiasis complicating recurrent bacterial vagnosis. *Sex Transm. Dis.* **17:**51–53.

68. Sadhu, C., M. J. McEachern, E. P. Rustchenko-Bulgac, J. Schmid, D. R. Soll, and J. Hicks. 1991. Telomeric and dispersed repeat sequences in *Candida* yeasts and their use in strain identification. *J. Bacteriol.* **173:**842–850.

69. San-Milian, R., L. Ribacoba, J. Ponton, and G. Quindos. 1996. Evaluation of a commercial medium for identification of *Candida* species. *J. Clin. Microbiol. Infect. Dis.* **15:**153–158.

70. Schmid, J., E. Voss, and D. R. Soll. 1990. Computer-assisted methods for assessing strain relatedness in *Candida albicans* by fingerprinting with the moderately repetitive sequence Ca3. *J. Clin. Microbiol.* **28:**1236–1243.

71. Shastry, J. C., K. Ramachandran, L. N. Mohapatra, and B. N. Tandon. 1969. A study of *Candida* in throat swabs and gastrointestinal tract of the patients on broad-spectrum antibiotic or steroid treatment. *Indian J. Med. Res.* **57:**133–140.

72. Slutsky, B., J. Buffo, and D. R. Soll. 1985. High frequency switching of colony morphology in *Candida albicans. Science* **230:**666–669.

73. Slutsky, B., M. Staebell, J. Anderson, L. Risen, M. Pfaller, and D. R. Soll. 1987. "White-opaque transition": a second high-frequency switching system in *Candida albicans. J. Bacteriol.* **169:**189–197.

74. Sobel, J. D., and W. Chaim. 1997. Treatment of *Torulopsis glabrata* vaginitis: retrospective review of boric acid therapy. *Clin. Infect. Dis.* **24:**649–652.

75. Soll, D. R. 1986. The regulation of cellular differentiation in the dimorphic yeast *Candida albicans. Bioessays* **5:**5–11.

76. Soll, D. R. 1992. High frequency switching in *Candida albicans. Clin. Microbiol. Rev.* **5:**188–203.

77. Soll, D. R. 1992. Switching and its possible role in *Candida* pathogenesis, p. 156–172. *In* J. E. Bennett, R. J. Hay, and P. K. Peterson (ed.), *New Fungal Strategies.* Churchill Livingstone, Edinburgh, Scotland.

78. Soll, D. R. 2000. The ins and outs of DNA fingerprinting the infectious fungi. *Clin. Microbiol. Rev.* **13:**332–370.

79. Soll, D. R. 2001. The molecular biology of switching in *Candida,* p. 161–182. *In* R. A. Calderone and R. L. Cihlar (ed.), *Fungal Pathogenesis: Principles and Clinical Application.* Marcel Dekker, New York, N.Y.

80. Soll, D. R. 2002. Phenotypic switching, p. 123–142. *In* R. Calderone (ed.), Candida *and* Candidiasis. ASM Press, Washington, D.C.

81. Soll, D. R., J. Anderson, and M. Bergen. 1991. The developmental biology of the white-opaque transition in *Candida albicans,* p. 20–45. *In* R. Prasad (ed.), *Candida albicans: Cellular and Molecular Biology.* Springer-Verlag KG, Berlin, Germany.

82. Soll, D. R., R. Galask, S. Isley, T. V. G. Rao, D. Stone, J. Hicks, J. Schmid, K. Mac, and C. Hanna. 1989. "Switching" of *Candida albicans* during successive episodes of recurrent vaginitis. *J. Clin. Microbiol.* **27:**681–690.

83. Soll, D. R., R. Galask, J. Schmid, C. Hanna, K. Mac, and B. Morrow. 1991. Genetic dissimilarity of commensal strains of *Candida* spp. carried in different anatomical locations of the same healthy women. *J. Clin. Microbiol.* **29:**1702–1710.

84. Soll, D. R., C. J. Langtimm, J. McDowell, J. Hicks, and R. Galask. 1987. High-frequency switching in *Candida* strains isolated from vaginitis patients. *J. Clin. Microbiol.* **25:**1611–1622.

85. Soll, D. R., S. R. Lockhart, and C. Pujol. Laboratory procedures for the epidemiological analysis of microorganisms. *In* P. R. Murray, E. J. Baron, M. A. Pfaller, F. C. Tenover, and R. H. Yolken (ed.), *Manual of Clinical Microbiology,* 8th ed., in press. American Society for Microbiology, Washington, D.C.

86. Soll, D. R., M. Staebell, C. J. Langtimm, M. Pfaller, J. Hicks, and T. V. G. Rao. 1988. Multiple *Candida* strains in the course of a single systemic infection. *J. Clin. Microbiol.* **26:**1448–1459.

87. Spinillo, A., A. M. Bernuzzi, C. Cevini, R. Gulminetti, S. Luzi, and A. De Santalo. 1997. The relationship of bacterial vaginosis, *Candida* and *Trichomonas* infection to symptomatic vaginitis in postmenopausal women attending a vaginitis clinic. *Maturitas* **27:**253–260.

88. Srakaki, F. M., M. Higa, M. Tateyama, Y. Yamozato, T. Ishimine, M. Toyama, T. Miyara, M. Koide, and A. Saito. 1999. Concurrent infection with *Legionella pneumophila* and

Pneumocystis carinii in a patient with T cell leukemia. *Intern. Med.* **38**:160–163.

89. **Srikantha, T., L. K. Tsai, A. Klar, and D. R. Soll.** 2001. The histone deacetylases *HDA1* and *RPD3* play distinct roles in the regulation of high-frequency phenotypic switching in *Candida albicans. J. Bacteriol.* **183**:4614–4625.

90. **Steelig, M. S.** 1996. Mechanisms by which antibiotics increase the incidence and severity of candidiasis and alter the immunological defenses. *Bacteriol. Rev.* **30**:442–459.

91. **Vajpayee, R. B., N. Sharma, M. Chand, G. C. Tabin, M. Vajpayee, and J. R. Anand.** 1998. Corneal superinfection in acute hemorrhagic conjunctivitis. *Cornea* **17**:614–617.

92. **Valenti, S., C. Vignolo, E. Benevolo, and F. Braido.** 1996. Mixed infection by *Staphylococcus* and *Candida,* and Wigener's granulomatosis. *Mon. Arch. Chest Dis.* **51**:387–390.

93. **Vargas, K.** 1998. Molecular epidemiology of *Candida albicans* in patients with AIDS. Ph.D. thesis. University of Iowa, Iowa City.

94. **Vargas, K. G., S. A. Messer, M. A. Pfaller, S. R. Lockhart, J. T. Stapleton, J. Hellstein, and D. R. Soll.** 2000. Elevated phenotypic switching and drug resistance of *Candida albicans* from human immunodeficiency virus-positive individuals prior to first thrush episode. *J. Clin. Microbiol.* **38**:3595–3607.

95. **Vargas, K., P. W. Wertz, D. Drake, B. Morrow, and D. R. Soll.** 1994. Differences in adhesion of *Candida albicans* 3153A cells exhibiting switch phenotypes to buccal epithelium and stratum corneum. *Infect. Immun.* **62**:1328–1335.

96. **White, T. C., K. A. Marr, and R. A. Bowden.** 1998. Clinical, cellular, and molecular factors that contribute to antifungal drug resistance. *Clin. Microbiol. Rev.* **11**:382–402.

97. **White, T. C., S. H. Miysaki, and N. Agabian.** 1993. Three distinct secreted aspartyl proteinases in *Candida albicans. J. Bacteriol.* **175**:6126–6133.

98. **White, T. C., M. A. Pfaller, M. G. Rinaldi, J. Smith, and S. W. Bedding.** 1997. Stable azole drug resistance associated with a substrain of *Candida albicans* from an HIV-infected patient. *Oral Dis.* **3**:S102–S109.

99. **Willinger, B., and M. Manafi.** 1999. Evaluation of CHROMagar Candida for rapid screening of clinical specimens for Candida species. *Mycoses* **42**:61–65.

100. **Winner, H. I., and R. Hurley.** 1964. *Candida albicans.* Churchill, London, United Kingdom.

101. **Xu, J., C. M. Boyd, E. Livingston, W. Meyer, J. F. Mudden, and T. G. Mitchell.** 1999. Species and genotypic diversity and similarities of pathogenic yeasts colonizing women. *J. Clin. Microbiol.* **37**:3835–3843.

INTERACTIONS BETWEEN *CANDIDA* SPECIES AND BACTERIA IN MIXED INFECTIONS

Howard F. Jenkinson and L. Julia Douglas

18

INTRODUCTION

Candida albicans is an opportunistic fungal pathogen found as part of the normal microflora in the human digestive tract. It is just one of approximately 200 species in the genus *Candida,* but accounts for up to 75% of all candidal infections. In general, innate and acquired host defense mechanisms act in concert with the resident bacterial flora such that *Candida* organisms grow and survive as commensals. However, even a slight modification of the host defense system, or host ecological environment, can assist the transformation of *C. albicans* into a pathogen capable of causing infections that may be lethal. The most common body sites showing asymptomatic colonization by *Candida* are the oral cavity, rectum, and vagina. Oral swabs or rinses are positive for *C. albicans* in up to 40% of healthy adult subjects, while 20 to 25% of healthy women carry *C. albicans* in the vagina. Colonization by *Candida* is thought to occur at an early age, with the organisms being acquired during passage through the birth canal, during nursing, or from food. Long-term colonization is probably responsible for eliciting the circulating immunoglobulin G (IgG) and mucosal secretory immunoglobulin A (S-IgA) antibodies to *C. albicans* that are detectable in most healthy individuals. It is these acquired host responses, in conjunction with the anti-*Candida* activities of polymorphonuclear leukocytes and macrophages, that probably play a significant part in normally restricting *C. albicans* to superficial growth at mucosal sites.

C. albicans (and the closely related yeast *Candida dubliniensis*) is a dimorphic fungus, growing as an oval-shaped budding yeast (blastospore), or as pseudohyphae or true hyphae; both yeast and hyphal forms are usually found in infected tissues. The dimorphic transition is one of many characteristic properties of *C. albicans* associated with virulence. Other virulence factors include adhesins, which promote binding of *Candida* to host cells and tissues, hydrolytic enzymes such as proteinases that enhance adhesion and tissue destruction (32), and molecules such as CR3-like receptor and HSP 90 that modulate immune cell functions (31, 49). The development of pathogenicity is facilitated by endogenous physiological modifications of host immunity, by immunodeficiency diseases, or by iatrogenic factors. The latter include chemical and physical therapeutic techniques that weaken the body defenses at various levels and allow *Candida* to invade.

Howard F. Jenkinson, Department of Oral and Dental Science, University of Bristol Dental School, Bristol BS1 2LY, United Kingdom. *L. Julia Douglas,* Division of Infection and Immunity, Institute of Biomedical and Life Sciences, University of Glasgow, Glasgow G12 8QQ, United Kingdom.

Polymicrobial Diseases, Edited by Kim A. Brogden and Janet M. Guthmiller,
© 2002 ASM Press, Washington, D.C.

Although recent evidence suggests that some hospital-acquired (nosocomial) *Candida* infections may behave like minor epidemics with selection of more virulent strains (47), it is often the commensal (endogenous) organisms that are believed to be the initial sources of infection. However, it is important to recognize that *C. albicans* has the ability to live in harmony with the host, for a lifetime, within the resident complex microflora present on mucosal surfaces. In the oral cavity, *C. albicans* grows and survives by competing and cooperating with an estimated 300 or more species of bacteria. There is compelling evidence that *C. albicans* and *C. dubliniensis* form tight associations with specific oral bacterial species, and that these promote adhesion and colonization by mixed-species communities (41). Thus, when *Candida* infections arise, they often occur in association with bacteria. On the other hand, there is also strong evidence to suggest that components of the resident microflora, present in the oral cavity and at other mucosal sites, perform to check *C. albicans* growth. This is why factors that perturb the normal microflora, such as antibiotic therapy, or changes in hormonal or mucosal secretions, may encourage *C. albicans* overgrowth.

This chapter considers the etiology and pathology of some disease conditions that arise from, or involve directly, *Candida* interactions with bacteria. The clinical manifestations, and processes of adhesion and biofilm formation, are described for mixed-species infections, in particular those involving colonization of oral tissues and dental or medical prostheses by mixed communities of *Candida* and bacteria. Knowledge gained from studies of microbial colonization mechanisms in the laboratory and in vivo, and of disease mechanisms from model systems, should assist in the development of more effective methods for controlling or preventing *Candida* infections.

Types of *Candida* Infection

Infections caused by *Candida* may be superficial or systemic. Superficial infections of the cutaneous or mucocutaneous tissues include oropharyngeal candidiasis (involving the buccal mucosa, palate, and tongue), vaginitis, conjunctivitis, esophagitis, or gastrointestinal candidiasis. Systemic infections, which can be fatal and may involve multiple organs, include endocarditis, pyelonephritis, esophagitis, meningitis, and disseminated candidiasis (*Candida* septicemia).

Mucocutaneous candidiasis is observed in subjects with cellular immune deficiencies or who are immunosuppressed, have anemia or diabetes, or whose normal microflora is disturbed or suppressed. Oral thrush, a disease recognized in infants by Hippocrates, appears as soft creamy-colored plaques on the tongue and buccal mucosa. Thrush in the newborn or elderly may be related to inefficiency of the thymus, while adult males who develop thrush may be suspected of being infected with human immunodeficiency virus (HIV). *Candida* vulvovaginitis is often associated with pregnancy or contraceptive use and may be linked to modification of T-cell and neutrophil functions by progesterone. Primary or secondary defects in myeloid or lymphoid lineages generally facilitate development of *Candida* infections, while neutropenia is one of the main causes of systemic *Candida* proliferation.

Predisposing Factors

The frequency of systemic *Candida* infections has grown steadily during the past decade, and *C. albicans,* together with a few closely related species such as *C. tropicalis, C. glabrata,* and *C. parapsilosis,* is now recognized as an important nosocomial pathogen. This is due, at least in part, to an increase in invasive surgical techniques, the growing use of prosthetic devices, particularly intravascular catheters, and the development of new drug therapies. Surgical procedures themselves, with their associated physical and psychological stresses, may promote breakthrough growth of *Candida*. Catheters and other prostheses provide novel sites for colonization by *C. albicans* and other microorganisms as biofilms. Corticosteroid therapy affects neutrophil, macrophage, and T-cell activities, chemotherapy with cytotoxic drugs leads to depletion of leukocytes, and polyantibiotic treatment perturbs or suppresses the mucosal microflora. All of these various drug regimens have the potential to result in *Candida* infections. On the other hand, surgical damage, catheterization or other prosthetic implantation, and the wearing of prosthetic appliances such as dentures, may lead to infections that are polymicrobial in nature, often comprising *C. albicans* in association with one or more defined species of endogenous host bacteria. In addition, it is apparent that many other oral disease conditions, including various forms of human periodontal disease afflicting the tooth roots, pulp, and gums (gingivitis), may involve mixed-species infections of *C. albicans* and bacteria.

CANDIDA–MIXED-SPECIES INFECTIONS

Denture-Induced Stomatitis

This condition is essentially a candidal infection of the oral mucosa that is promoted by a close-fitting upper denture. The upper denture cuts off the underlying mucosa from the normal lubricatory and protective functions of saliva. In susceptible patients, denture stomatitis is seen as a symptomless area of erythema, always sharply limited to the area of mucosa occluded by the upper denture (Color Plate 6A [see color insert]). Such inflammation is not seen under a more mobile lower denture because the salivary flow is less restricted. The clinical picture is usually quite clear and diagnosis is confirmed by microscopic analysis of smears taken from the inflamed mucosa or from the fitting surface of the denture. Gram-stained smears typically show *Candida* hyphal forms, as well as yeasts that have proliferated between the denture base and mucosa. Histologically, there is usually a mild chronic inflammatory infiltrate, probably in response to secreted *C. albicans* virulence factors such as phospholipases and proteinases. However, the presence of heavy oral bacterial growth on the palatal mucosa and fitting surface of the denture, and of bacteria not usually recognized as components of the oral microbiota, e.g., *Staphylococcus aureus* and *Escherichia coli*, are

likely to support inflammatory reactions in the palatal mucosa.

Angular Cheilitis

Angular cheilitis is a disease frequently associated with denture-induced stomatitis and is caused by leakage of *Candida*-infected saliva at the angles of the mouth. It is also a characteristic sign of oral candidosis in general and systemic disorders, including HIV infections; diabetes mellitus and skin diseases are common among recurrent angular cheilitis patients. In elderly patients with dentures, local factors, such as skin creased as a result of sagging of the facial tissues with age, promote fungal and bacterial growth in saliva-contaminated skin folds. Clinically, mild inflammation occurs at the angles of the mouth with cracking and erythema at the commissure (Color Plate 6B). The microflora in angular cheilitis usually involves *C. albicans* or other *Candida* species, and *S. aureus* that may act to preserve the cheilitis. Different species of bacteria including hemolytic streptococci, enterococci, *E. coli*, *Klebsiella,* and *Pseudomonas* may also play a role in the pathogenesis and maintenance of this labial lesion.

Gingivitis

Inflammation of the gingival tissues is usually related to plaque accumulation on the tooth surfaces and gingival margins caused by inadequate oral hygiene. Chronic gingivitis is considered to be antecedent to the loss of periodontal attachment (periodontitis) and involves a shift in the plaque microflora from predominantly gram-positive bacteria to a complex microflora comprising up to 50% gram-negative bacteria including *Fusobacterium, Prevotella,* and *Treponema* species. Other forms of gingivitis, that may involve acute inflammation with ulceration (acute ulcerative gingivitis [AUG]), are promoted by heavy cigarette smoking, emotional stress, or immunosuppression, e.g., HIV infection. Gingival disorders are also associated with infections with *S. aureus*, enteric bacteria, *Pseudomonas,* and *Candida,* and are usually related to suppression of the normal subgingival microflora by antibiotics. In addition, systemic conditions, e.g., immunosuppression, or locally compromised conditions, e.g., osseointegrated implants and membranes for guided tissue regeneration, may be predisposing factors for the establishment of these microorganisms that are not usually present at healthy sites around the teeth.

Periodontal Disease

Adult periodontitis is a condition in which few or all teeth in a dentition may be involved; individual teeth can show vertical or horizontal bone loss, and associated gingivitis can range from very slight inflammation to severe bleeding with pus formation. Adult periodontitis lesions show a high proportion of anaerobic bacteria, mainly gram-negative organisms and spirochetes. Within these populations, specific species complexes, e.g., *Porphyromonas gingivalis, Bacteroides forsythus,* and *Treponema denticola,* show especially strong relationships to active periodontitis (61). Cigarette smoking is a potential risk factor associated with progression of periodontal disease, and smokers with early-onset periodontitis harbor a greater number of pathogenic microorganisms in periodontal pockets (24). In addition to the common major periodontal pathogens, an increased incidence of *E. coli, S. aureus, C. albicans,* and *Aspergillus fumigatus* underlines the potentially damaging effects of cigarette smoking on host defenses (39).

Approximately 10% of adult periodontitis patients experience continued loss of periodontal attachment despite periodontal therapy. A wide range of anaerobic bacteria can be recovered from these refractory periodontitis cases, as well as staphylococci and *C. albicans.* Therapy may be unsuccessful because it is difficult to access pathogenic organisms that have invaded gingival tissues or root structures. In addition, *C. albicans* is most frequently isolated in mixed infections with oral streptococci, *Peptostreptococcus micros* and *Fusobacterium nucleatum* from endodontic samples of root canals in persistent endodontic infections. Thus, *Candida* probably has an important role in therapy-resistant apical periodontitis (66) and in polymicrobial infections of root canals with pulp necrosis (42).

Periodontitis in HIV-infected patients often exhibits rapid onset and progression, particularly if patients have experienced AUG, with attachment loss within 9 months for up to 75% of patients. Leukemia patients on immunosuppressive therapies and broad spectrum antibiotics are susceptible to rapidly progressive periodontitis and colonization by staphylococci, enteric rods, *Pseudomonas,* and *Candida.* In patients with acute leukemia these agents may seed from periodontal pockets into the bloodstream and induce life-threatening septicemia.

Prosthetic Implant Infections

Several implant systems are now being used to replace missing teeth. Most implants osseointegrate without problems, and when surrounded by healthy tissue they carry microflora associated with periodontal health (44). However, implants may be lost because of excessive occlusal loading forces (traumatic failures) or as a result of microbial infections (infectious failures). Infectious failures are associated with complex microbial etiologies, either with periodontal pathogens such as *P. micros, Campylobacter recta,* and *Prevotella* spp., or with overgrowth of atypical periodontal microflora such as staphylococci, *E. coli, Pseudomonas,* and *Candida,* particularly after prolonged use of systemic antimicrobial agents or chlorhexidine mouth washes.

In patients with surgical laryngectomies, rehabilitation of the voice is accomplished with a voice prosthesis, which acts as a shunt valve between the trachea and esophagus (Fig. 1). Voice prostheses are usually made of medical-grade silicone rubber and, like other prostheses, are subject to microbial contamination. Indwelling voice prostheses often fail within several months of placement, because a polymicrobial biofilm forms on the esophageal side causing malfunction of the valve mechanism (65). The formation of a mixed biofilm is promoted because in laryngectomized patients salivary flow rates are often reduced (as a side effect of radiotherapy) and the antimicrobial properties of saliva are therefore subdued. The biofilms that

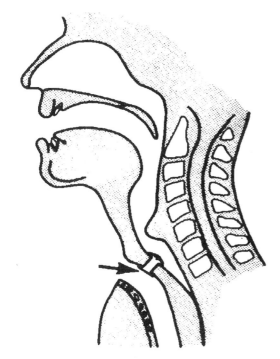

FIGURE 1 Diagrammatic representation of positioning of partially implanted silicone rubber voice prosthesis (arrow). Diagram kindly provided by G. J. Elving.

form contain a variety of oral streptococci (e.g., *S. gordonii, S. anginosus, S. salivarius*), staphylococci (e.g., *S. epidermidis*), enterococci, and *Candida* spp., mainly *C. albicans*. Although adhesion of bacteria may be a prerequisite for *Candida* colonization, as it may also be for denture-induced stomatitis (51, 65), it is thought that *Candida* growing into the silicone rubber is responsible mainly for the deterioration of the prostheses.

Endotracheal tubes, nasogastric tubes, and urinary catheters are continually exposed to a range of microorganisms and thus, like oral and voice prostheses, tend to become colonized by mixed-species biofilms. These biofilms, containing different combinations of organisms and often encased within a mass of extracellular polymeric material, can be readily demonstrated by use of electron microscopy (48). Catheter-associated urinary tract infection is the most common nosocomial infection in hospitals and nursing homes; nosocomial bacteriuria or candiduria develops in up to 25% of patients requiring a urinary catheter for 7 days or more (46). However, in devices totally implanted into the body, such as prosthetic heart valves, cardiac pacemakers, and joint replacements (hip, knee, etc.), the risk of contamination occurs essentially at the time of surgical placement. Infections of such devices are usually by single microbial species, most frequently coagulase-negative staphylococci or *S. aureus,* although polymicrobial infections of orthopedic prostheses have been reported (11). The most commonly infected, surgically implanted device is the central venous catheter, which is used to administer fluids and nutrients as well as cytotoxic drugs. Infusion therapy carries a substantial risk of producing iatrogenic sepsis, either bacteremia or fungemia. Infections can arise in a variety of ways and at any time during the use of the catheter, which may be prolonged. Sometimes the infusion fluid itself or the catheter hub is contaminated. More commonly, organisms are introduced from the patient's skin microflora, from the hands of medical personnel or even from contaminated antiseptics used to swab the insertion site. The distal tip of the catheter may be contaminated at the time of insertion, or organisms may migrate down the interface between the catheter surface and the skin (i.e., down the catheter wound). Alternatively, if some other portal of entry exists, perhaps from the gut, then microorganisms may seed the catheter tip from the bloodstream. The range of microbes encountered in these infections is wide, including components of the skin microflora, some from the environment, and some of enteric origin. Most commonly, infections are caused by coagulase-negative staphylococci, *S. aureus,* enterococci, and *Candida,* predominantly involving only a single species. However, mixed-species infections of *S. epidermidis* and *C. albicans,* for example, have been reported (17). Overall, *Candida* spp. are currently responsible for 8% of all hospital-acquired infections and are the fourth most common cause of septicemia.

MIXED-SPECIES COLONIZATION

Microbial Colonization of the Oral Cavity

The oral cavity and nasopharynx harbor diverse and complex microbial communities. Microorganisms accumulate on the hard (dental) and softer (mucosal) tissues, or on prostheses, as sessile biofilms. These organisms engage the host in a cellular and molecular dialogue that usually serves to constrain the commensal microflora. However, under certain circumstances, components of the resident microflora become directly, or indirectly, responsible for disease. Microbial adhesion is the underlying process that drives oral colonization and ultimately disease progression.

The warm, moist, and generally nutrient-rich environment of the mouth favors microbial colonization of the available surfaces, but the mechanical shearing forces of salivary flow and tongue movement tend to dislodge and expel microorganisms. The importance of salivary flow in controlling colonization is well illustrated by the finding that individuals with xerostomia (dry mouth), who have reduced salivary flow for a variety of reasons, suffer from an overgrowth of dental plaque, a high incidence of dental decay, and an increased susceptibility to mucosal lesions. Successful colonizers are able to adhere to the surfaces available and resist, not only the innate host defense components present in saliva, but also the cleansing action of shear forces. In general, adhesion processes involve physicochemical (thermodynamic) forces providing surface-surface interactions, and higher-affinity adhesin-receptor interactions involving complementary molecules that act stereospecifically (41). This specificity of adhesion bestows specificity of colonization of the tissue site (15) and specificity of microbial community composition. Microorganisms that lack specific adhesive mechanisms are either lost from the oral cavity, or are found only at sites that are highly retentive.

Salivary fluid continually bathes and coats the oral tissues and microorganisms present.

Molecules within saliva, such as lysozyme, lactoferrin, salivary peroxidase, and the host defense peptides of the histatin and cystatin families, all have the potential to inhibit microbial growth and metabolic activities of susceptible organisms. Other components such as salivary mucins, glycoprotein agglutinins, and S-IgA agglutinate microorganisms and facilitate their removal by expectoration or swallowing (35). These components, together with the proline-rich proteins (PRPs), statherin and α-amylase, also function as receptors for microbial adhesion when they are deposited onto oral surfaces. Thus, initial microbial adhesion to tooth or other hard surfaces, e.g., denture acrylic, and to a lesser extent epithelial cell surfaces, is mediated by interactions with deposited salivary molecules (Fig. 2). The epithelial surfaces support microflorae that are

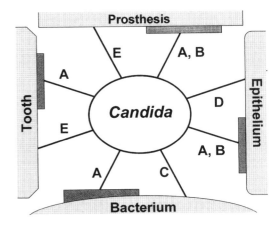

FIGURE 2 *Candida* multiple interactions with oral surfaces, salivary components, host components and bacteria in oral biofilms. Interactions designated A through E are as follows: A, adhesion of *C. albicans* to the surfaces of teeth or prostheses coated with an acquired pellicle of salivary proteins and glycoproteins or to epithelial cells or bacteria via adsorbed salivary components (different salivary components may be adsorbed to the different surfaces); B, adhesion of *C. albicans* to the surfaces of prostheses or epithelial cells via adsorbed or attached tissue matrix proteins; C, adhesion of *C. albicans* to bacteria via protein-carbohydrate and protein-protein reactions; D, adhesion of *C. albicans* to epithelial cell receptors; E, physicochemical interaction of yeast cells with unmodified tooth enamel or prosthetic material.

distinct from those formed on hard surfaces, partly because of retention effects (epithelia desquamate) but also because epithelial cells present unique receptor molecules including glycolipids and extracellular matrix proteins. Thus, it is logical to propose that the ability of microorganisms to grow and survive at colonizing sites depends primarily on their repertoire of functional adhesins. Adhesion favors community development within which nutritional interrelationships, and concerted resilience and resistance to innate and acquired host defenses, are fostered.

Mechanisms of Bacterial and Candidal Adhesion

In general, it is accepted that the buildup of plaque in the oral cavity starts with the adsorption of salivary proteins to a surface, thus forming an acquired pellicle. Bacteria that have high affinities of adhesion to salivary pellicle, such as species of *Streptococcus* and *Actinomyces,* are primary colonizers of teeth. Their deposition onto a surface provides a linking film onto which further attachment and accumulation of cells can occur. Every new organism that binds to the linking film presents a new surface and therefore forms a basis for the accretion of defined microbial groupings. Oral microorganisms such as *Fusobacterium, Porphyromonas,* and *Candida,* are not generally considered to be primary colonizers, but they do have the ability to bind avidly to experimental salivary pellicles. These organisms may therefore have become adapted to bind preferentially to salivary components that have become deposited on primary colonizers. While specific components of saliva are recognized as receptors by microorganisms, the nature of the components deposited depends on the physicochemical properties of the surface. Thus, acidic PRPs and statherin become readily deposited onto enamel and provide high-affinity receptors for *S. gordonii* and *A. naeslundii* (19, 20). In addition, human salivary mucin MG1, α-amylase, and S-IgA may also be deposited onto denture acrylic surfaces and provide additional receptors for a range of microorganisms. In some in-

stances the molecular mechanisms of cell adhesion are well understood. Adhesion of various oral streptococci to salivary glycoprotein agglutinin gp-340 (56) is mediated by high-molecular-mass cell wall-anchored proteins of the antigen I/II family (34). These are Ca^{2+}-dependent proteins with lectin-like activities recognizing glycosidic structures present within host glycoproteins and glycolipids. Adhesion of *A. naeslundii* and *P. gingivalis* to PRPs and statherin is mediated by adhesins located on the fimbriae of these organisms (20, 40). However, the adhesins present on the *C. albicans* cell surface that mediate binding to various salivary pellicle components, such as statherin (14, 38) and basic PRPs (54), have not yet been identified.

Multiple adherent interactions occur between microbial cells and salivary pellicle, epithelial cells, other microbial cells, host matrix proteins such as fibronectin and collagen, and platelets. Such a plethora of adhesion mechanisms involve production by the microbial cells of a wide range of adhesins. Multimodal adhesion facilitates diversity in colonization, enabling organisms to attach to a variety of surfaces presenting different receptors, and increases the avidity of binding to individual substrates. *C. albicans* exhibits a wide range of adhesion capabilities (Fig. 2) and is especially predisposed to forming mixed-species communities with bacteria. In addition to its high capacity to bind to salivary pellicle components adsorbed to enamel or acrylic surfaces, it also exhibits electrostatic and hydrophobic properties that enhance adhesion of cells to charged or hydrophobic surfaces (60), and that are positively correlated with adhesion levels to host tissues. *Candida* binds to a variety of host-cell receptors through lectin-like or protein-protein-type interactions, including galactosyl (37) or fucosyl (12, 64) receptors, also to fibronectin, laminin, fibrinogen, and collagen (reviewed in reference 13) (see Fig. 2). Because many species of oral bacteria bind similar components, they therefore compete with *C. albicans* for these receptors (52). A special adhesive mechanism of *C. albicans* involves hypha-specific protein Hwp1. This serves as a substrate for epithelial cell transglutaminase which effectively cross-links *Candida* to the epithelial cell surface (62). However, of particular relevance to the formation of mixed-species biofilms is the property of *C. albicans* (and *C. dubliniensis*) to bind a range of bacteria. It is this property, together with the spectrum of other adhesive interactions as portrayed in Fig. 2, that enables *Candida* to persist so successfully as a commensal on mucosal surfaces, and within denture plaque biofilms that act as protective reservoirs (1).

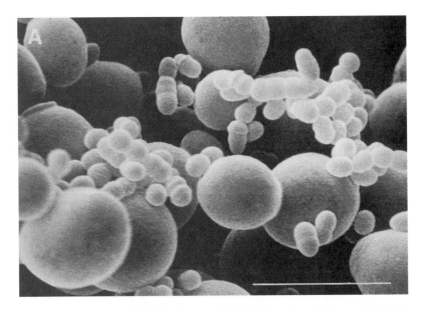

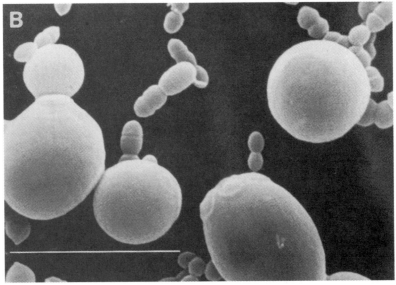

FIGURE 3   Coaggregation and coadhesion of *C. albicans* and oral streptococci. (A) Coaggregation of *C. albicans* in suspension with *Streptococcus gordonii*. (B) Adhesion of *C. albicans* cells to *S. gordonii* cells immobilized onto polystyrene. Bars, 5 μm. Reproduced with permission from reference 29.

Mechanisms of Mixed Community Development

Coaggregation and coadhesion reactions of microorganisms are significant colonization factors because they enable development, stabilization, and maintenance of complex communities. The ability of an organism, such as *Candida,* to adhere to preattached organisms is an obvious advantage if it is not present in sufficiently high numbers, or lacks a sufficiently high affinity for adhesion sites, to compete with the primary colonizers. Coaggregation, or intermicrobial adhesion reactions, involve principally protein-carbohydrate or protein-protein interactions between complementary molecules present on the microbial cell surfaces. *C. albicans* has the ability to coaggregate with several oral streptococcal species (36), with *S. gordonii* having one of the highest affinities for *C. albicans* in suspension. Scanning electron micrographs of in vitro coaggregates show that streptococci attach singly, or in short chains, to yeast cells, effectively forming cross-bridges (Fig. 3A). When streptococcal cells are deposited onto a surface, *C. albicans* cells appear to localize specifically onto the streptococci (Fig. 3B). This interaction depends on at least three adhesin-receptor pairs (30): the recognition by an unidentified *C. albicans* surface protein of streptococcal cell wall linear polysaccharide; the binding activities of streptococcal antigen I/II proteins SspA and SspB to a *C. albicans* receptor; and the activity of *S. gordonii* high-molecular-mass cell wall adhesin CshA, that confers surface hydrophobicity. The fluid phase coaggregation reaction is blocked effectively by addition of soluble streptococcal polysaccharide (29), but the multimodal adhesion of *C. albicans* to immobilized streptococcal cells is not. *Candida* coadhesion with streptococci is thus a complex multimodal interaction by which mixed-species colonization would be promoted. *C. albicans* also coaggregates with *A. naeslundii* (23), while *C. albicans* and *C. dubliniensis* both coaggregate with *Fusobacterium* species (22, 33). These latter interactions, which are inhibitable by mannose, are thought to involve a *Fusobacterium* adhesin binding to a *Candida* cell surface mannan receptor (33). These kinds of intergeneric associations are believed to be responsible, at least in part, for the development of defined communities of yeast and oral bacteria (Fig. 4). The ability of *Candida* to interact with streptococci, actinomyces, and fusobacteria enables them to become enmeshed within more complex communities at different oral cavity sites. These interplays are consistent with the findings of *C. albicans* in associations with *P. gingivalis* and *T. denticola* in periodontitis, with *F. nucleatum* in gingivitis, and with streptococci in plaque formed on teeth or dentures. Evidence shows that in groups with higher susceptibility to caries there is a higher incidence of *Candida* (63). The ability of *C. albicans* to cocolonize with streptococci (10, 28) and to grow and survive at low pH (<4.5) suggests that active carious lesions may harbor *C. albicans.*

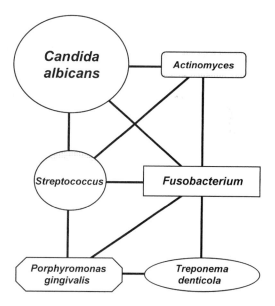

FIGURE 4 Intergeneric coaggregation reactions and coadhesion of *Candida* with oral bacteria in mixed-species biofilms. Interactions between *Candida, Streptococcus, Actinomyces,* and *Fusobacterium* involve multiple adhesin-receptor reactions and promote retention of these organisms in defined relationships within oral biofilms. The abilities of *P. gingivalis* and *T. denticola* to bind streptococci and fusobacteria contribute to their success as secondary colonizers, especially within subgingival communities.

The formation and maintenance of these *Candida*-bacteria communities are subject to modification by extrinsic factors. Interactions of *Candida* with bacterial biofilms may be modified by environmental parameters such as pH and nutrient supply (7), and by host factors such as salivary components (28, 51). The adsorption of salivary proteins, such as basic PRPs, to the *S. gordonii* cell surface promotes adhesion of *C. albicans* (55), while S-IgA and salivary mucin MG2 might act to destabilize such associations (45, 50). Understanding the complex mechanisms by which *Candida* and bacteria cocolonize will assist development of new protocols to block adhesive reactions and control the formation of biofilms.

Structure and Properties of *Candida* Biofilms Formed In Vitro

As an alternative to adhesion and coaggregation studies, *Candida* biofilms can be grown on plastic surfaces in vitro, either in the presence or absence of bacteria. Although investigation of mixed-species biofilms is still at an early stage, several model systems have been used to characterize the properties and drug susceptibilities of single-species *Candida* biofilms (4). The simplest system involves growing adher-ent populations on the surfaces of small discs cut from catheters. Growth is monitored quantitatively by a colorimetric assay that depends on the reduction of a tetrazolium salt, or by [³H]leucine incorporation; both methods give excellent correlation with biofilm dry weight (25). Biofilm growth by different *Candida* species and strains, and on different catheter materials, can be compared with this protocol. A recent modification of the method to study *C. albicans* biofilm formation on strips of denture acrylic (polymethylmethacrylate) has shown that biofilm growth, as measured by the tetrazolium reduction procedure, is stimulated by pretreating the acrylic strips with saliva (16). Similar results have been reported (53) with use of a bioluminescent ATP assay based on the firefly luciferase-luciferin system.

Scanning electron microscopy has revealed that *C. albicans* biofilms on catheter discs, or denture acrylic, consist of yeasts, hyphae, and pseudohyphae. The organisms are arranged in a bilayer structure (5); there is a dense, basal yeast layer which appears to anchor the biofilm to the surface, and an overlying but more open, hyphal layer (Fig. 5A). When appropriate preparative techniques are used, a matrix of extracellular polymeric material can be visual-

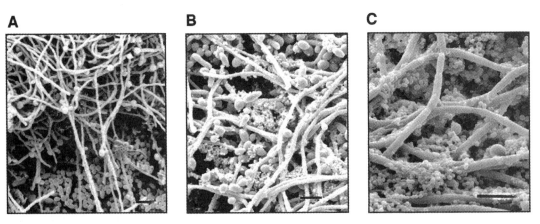

FIGURE 5 *C. albicans* and mixed-species biofilms formed in vitro. (A) *C. albicans* biofilm showing bilayer structure of germ-tube-forming cells and hyphae growing above layers of yeast cells (blastospores). (B) Mixed-species biofilm of *C. albicans* (yeast and hyphal forms) and *S. gordonii* (smaller cocci with individual cells and clusters adhering predominantly to blastospores). (C) Mixed-species biofilm of *C. albicans* (mainly hyphal forms) and *Streptococcus salivarius*. Bars, 10 μm.

ized around the biofilm cells. The synthesis of this material increases markedly if developing biofilms are subjected to a liquid flow (27). Production of an extracellular matrix has also been reported for *C. albicans* biofilms formed on human premolar teeth (58).

Candida biofilms are, like bacterial biofilms, more resistant to the action of antimicrobial agents, including clinically important antifungal drugs such as amphotericin B, fluconazole, and nystatin, as well as the antiseptic chlorhexidine that is used in the treatment of patients with denture stomatitis (16, 26). The mechanisms of resistance are not known but may include drug exclusion by the biofilm matrix, phenotypic changes resulting from nutrient limitation or a low growth rate, or surface-induced gene expression. Drug exclusion seems unlikely in view of experiments in which susceptibility profiles of biofilms incubated statically (which have relatively little matrix) were compared with those for biofilms incubated with gentle shaking (which produce much greater amounts of matrix material). Biofilms grown with or without shaking failed to exhibit significant differences in susceptibility to any of the drugs tested, suggesting that drug resistance is unrelated to the extent of matrix formation (6). To investigate possible phenotypic changes resulting from decreased growth rate, *C. albicans* biofilms were generated at different growth rates in a perfused biofilm fermentor, and susceptibility of biofilm cells to amphotericin B was compared with that of planktonic organisms grown at the same growth rate in a chemostat. The results showed that biofilms were resistant to the drug at all growth rates tested, whereas planktonic cells were resistant only at low growth rates (2). A separate study using a different model system demonstrated that glucose- and iron-limited biofilms grown at the same low rate were equally resistant to amphotericin B (3).

Overall, it seems unlikely that drug exclusion or decreased growth rate are factors of major importance in determining the drug resistance of *Candida* biofilms. In support of the notion that *Candida* responds to a surface-growth-associated signal, evidence has been obtained that biofilms formed on two different types of polyvinyl chloride catheter, produced by different manufacturers, show significant differences in susceptibilities to amphotericin B (6). This suggests that decreased antifungal drug sensitivity may be related to highly specific, surface-induced gene expression. Such a mechanism would be directly analogous to bacterial biofilm systems in which contact-induced gene expression is now well established (57).

Mixed *Candida*-Bacterial Biofilms

There is mounting interest in the study of *Candida*-bacteria biofilms formed in vitro. Preliminary work indicates the likelihood of extensive interspecies interactions in these adherent populations. For example, the catheter disc model system has been used to investigate mixed-species biofilms consisting of *C. albicans* and *Staphylococcus epidermidis,* a common agent of catheter-related infections. Two strains of *S. epidermidis* were used: a slime-producing wild type and a slime-negative mutant derived from it by chemical mutagenesis. Scanning electron microscopy revealed numerous physical interactions between the staphylococci and both yeasts and hyphae in these mixed species biofilms (B. Adam, G. S. Baillie, and L. J. Douglas, unpublished results). Drug susceptibility studies further indicated that fungal cells may modulate the action of antibiotics and that, conversely, bacteria can affect antifungal activity. For example, the presence of *Candida* in a biofilm increased the resistance of slime-negative staphylococci to vancomycin. On the other hand, *Candida* resistance to fluconazole was enhanced in the presence of slime-producing staphylococci, but was unaffected by the presence of the slime-negative mutant (Adam et al., unpublished).

Similar observations have been made with mixed-species biofilms consisting of *C. albicans* and oral streptococci on denture acrylic. Physical interactions between yeasts, hyphae, and either *S. gordonii* or *S. salivarius* were apparent

368 ■ JENKINSON AND DOUGLAS

by the use of scanning electron microscopy (Fig. 5B and C). Moreover, in results analogous to those obtained with *Candida-Staphylococcus* biofilms, the presence of oral streptococci enhanced the resistance of *C. albicans* to amphotericin B and nystatin (N. J. S. Henderson, B. Adam, and L. J. Douglas, unpublished results). Clearly, understanding the molecular basis of this decreased drug sensitivity will assist in the future development of more powerful ways to eliminate *Candida* from biofilm-related infections.

TREATMENT AND MANAGEMENT

No effective means is yet available of simply preventing adhesion of *C. albicans* and bacteria to plastic materials in situ. Good hygiene measures applied to teeth and dentures, and removal of pseudomembranous and plaque layers on mucosal membranes, are fundamental to antimicrobial prophylaxis and treatment of denture stomatitis. It is important to first reduce the numbers of biofilm microorganisms by mechanical measures, and then to administer an effective concentration of antimicrobial agent at the site of the lesion. *C. albicans* adheres tenaciously with oral bacteria to methylmethacrylate denture base, and so provides a reservoir of organisms that may continually detach and reinfect the mucosa. Elimination of the microbial biofilm from the denture base is thus crucial and can be achieved by careful scrubbing and then cleansing by soaking the denture in 0.1% hypochlorite solution. Another means of inhibiting growth and retention of *C. albicans* on the denture is to coat the fitting surface of the denture, while it is being worn, with a gel containing an antifungal compound, usually miconazole. It takes between 1 and 2 weeks for *C. albicans* to be eliminated and for the inflammation to clear. The inflamed mucosa responds to topical application of antifungal drugs, but agents such as nystatin and amphotericin can only gain access to the palate mucosa if the patient removes the denture while the antifungal tablets are allowed to dissolve in the mouth. Combinations of *Candida* and staphylococci, or enteric bacteria, are usually adequately controlled by starting patient treatment with an antifungal agent. Lack of response to the antifungal treatment may be due to reduced antifungal sensitivity in the mixed-species biofilm, poor patient compliance, or an underlying disorder such as iron or immune deficiency. If there is immune deficiency, the candidal infection is usually florid or associated with patches of thrush, in which case a blood analysis is recommended. Resistant cases may be treated with oral itraconazole or fluconazole, both of which have systemic effects. Antifungal treatment of patients with intraoral *Candida* infection often causes an associated angular cheilitis condition to resolve. However, since angular cheilitis may result from a mixed infection of *Candida* with *S. aureus* or enteric bacteria, local application of fusidic acid or metronidazole creams may also be required to eliminate this condition.

While polyene and azole antifungals are still the principal compounds used to treat patients with *Candida* infections, widespread use of azoles has resulted in an increase in the prevalence of azole-resistant *C. albicans* and *C. dubliniensis,* and a shift to infections caused by other species such as *C. krusei*. It is imperative, therefore, that new anti-*Candida* agents be developed. Accordingly, there is much interest at present in the family of histidine-rich proteins, designated histatins, which are usually found in human saliva and are capable of killing and inhibiting the germination of a wide range of microorganisms, especially *Candida* (43). The major members of this family, constituting about 80% of all histatins present in parotid and submandibular secretions, are histatins 1, 3, and 5, comprising 38, 32, and 24 amino acid residues, respectively. Histatin 5 appears to be the most effective at killing *Candida*. The mechanism of killing by histatins is not fully understood (67), but uptake of histatin into the cytoplasm appears to be necessary. Histatins, being host-derived antimicrobial peptides, are unlikely to promote the emergence of resistant *Candida* strains or provoke adverse host reactions, so they may be very suitable for treatment of fungal infections. Although it should be feasible to use histatin preparations in local delivery, it is also suggested that to augment salivary histatin concentrations in patients with refractory candidiasis, it may be possible to use gene therapy. Experiments have shown that delivery of the *HIS2* gene (encoding histatin 3) into salivary gland cells results in functional overexpression of histatin 3 (8). The efficiency of histatin expression in animal models of oropharyngeal candidiasis is currently being tested as a prelude to possible human applications.

Salivary antimicrobial peptides, such as histatins, or synthetic antimicrobial peptides with sufficiently broad specificity to cover a range of microorganisms are suggested as possible agents for controlling biofilm formation on voice prostheses (18). Interestingly though, the application of probiotic microorganisms in combination with a modified diet may assist in the control of *Candida* on voice box prostheses (65). Thus, strains of *Lactobacillus fermentum* and *L. acidophilus* have been found to produce antifungal substances, hydrogen peroxide, and antiadhesive biosurfactants that may all interfere with colonization of silicone rubber prostheses by *Candida*. For other surgically implanted prostheses, impregnation of the materials with antiseptic agents may render them less likely to be colonized by bacteria (9). For example,

gram-positive cocci and fungi are more likely to colonize central venous catheters made of standard polyurethane than catheters impregnated with antiseptic (59).

SUMMARY AND CONCLUSIONS

Roughly 40% of the healthy adult population carries *C. albicans* in their oral cavities, with the organism being present in dental plaque and on mucosal surfaces, the tongue, and denture surfaces. It may be isolated from healthy sites, but often greater numbers are isolated from diseased sites, such as those associated with gingivitis, periodontitis, infected root canals, and denture stomatitis. In normal circumstances the yeast is found in relatively low numbers within commensal communities, but if changes in host physiology or environmental conditions favor its numerical dominance, it may then be able to outcompete the resident bacterial flora (Fig. 6). Specific perturbations that promote *Candida* outgrowth include disruption of the bacterial components of the commensal microflora (e.g., by the application of broad-spectrum antibiotics), dampening of the host innate defenses (e.g., reduction of salivary flow), and compromising the function of the cellular immune system (e.g., through viral infection or pharmaceutical intervention). The interactions between

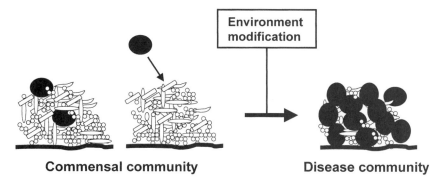

Commensal community   **Disease community**

FIGURE 6   The critical effect of perturbation of host environmental conditions in the shift from commensal to pathogenic microflora. *Candida* cells (black) are present in low numbers within the oral microflora or are acquired from other individuals. A major disruption of the host physiology, e.g., reduced salivary flow or immune cell function, or of bacterial flora, e.g., following antibiotic treatment, provides conditions for *Candida* to outcompete the numerically dominant members of the microflora and cause disease.

Candida and bacteria are especially important in the establishment of oral microbial communities and in the etiology of candidiasis. There are few other examples of cooperative interactions between bacteria and unicellular eukaryotic microorganisms.

Adhesion processes are the defining events in establishing these polymicrobial biofilms. As the physiological and molecular processes that occur during biofilm formation are studied in greater detail, it is becoming apparent that organisms within biofilms acquire properties that are quite different from those of their free-living counterparts. Biofilm formation involves activation of genes, the products of which are essential for survival and confer biofilm-related properties, such as increased resistance to immune cell detection, to environmental trauma, and to antimicrobial compounds. The key mechanisms and molecules that are involved in biofilm formation and in enhanced resistance will provide novel targets for strategies designed to control and prevent *Candida* biofilm-associated diseases.

Antifungal therapy may be effective in controlling an individual *Candida* infection, but it does not, of course, provide immunity. It is also vitally important to improve the understanding of the immunological mechanisms that promote susceptibility to *Candida* infection. It will only be by enhancing the immune status of subjects at risk, as well as by introducing new antifungal therapies, that the incidence of candidal infections will be reduced.

ACKNOWLEDGMENTS

We thank J. Luker for helpful comments on the manuscript. We also acknowledge the invaluable contributions of G. Baillie, R. Cannon, S. Hawser, A. Holmes, and J. O'Sullivan to research in our laboratories.

Our research is financially supported by the Wellcome Trust, Sir Jules Thorn Charitable Trust, Health Research Council of New Zealand, and New Zealand Dental Research Foundation.

REFERENCES

1. **Arendorf, T. M., and D. M. Walker.** 1980. The prevalence and intra-oral distribution of *Candida albicans* in man. *Arch. Oral Biol.* **25:**1–10.
2. **Baillie, G. S., and L. J. Douglas.** 1998. Effect of growth rate on resistance of *Candida albicans* biofilms to antifungal agents. *Antimicrob. Agents Chemother.* **42:**1900–1905.
3. **Baillie, G. S., and L. J. Douglas.** 1998. Iron-limited biofilms of *Candida albicans* and their susceptibility to amphotericin B. *Antimicrob. Agents Chemother.* **42:**2146–2149.
4. **Baillie, G. S., and L. J. Douglas.** 1999. *Candida* biofilms and their susceptibility to antifungal agents. *Methods Enzymol.* **310:**644–656.
5. **Baillie, G. S., and L. J. Douglas.** 1999. Role of dimorphism in the development of *Candida albicans* biofilms. *J. Med. Microbiol.* **48:**671–679.
6. **Baillie, G. S., and L. J. Douglas.** 2000. Matrix polymers of *Candida* biofilms and their possible role in biofilm resistance to antifungal agents. *J. Antimicrob. Chemother.* **46:**397–403.
7. **Basson, N. J.** 2000. Competition for glucose between *Candida albicans* and oral bacteria grown in mixed culture in a chemostat. *J. Med. Microbiol.* **49:**969–975.
8. **Baum, B. J., and B. C. O'Connell.** 1999. In vivo gene transfer to salivary glands. *Crit. Rev. Oral Biol. Med.* **10:**276–283.
9. **Bayston, R.** 2000. Biofilms and prosthetic devices, p. 295–307. *In* D. G. Allison, P. Gilbert, M. H. Lappin-Scott, and M. Wilson (ed.), *Community Structure and Cooperation in Biofilms.* Cambridge University Press, Cambridge, England.
10. **Branting, C., M. L. Sund, and L. E. Linder.** 1989. The influence of *Streptococcus mutans* on adhesion of *Candida albicans* to acrylic surfaces in vitro. *Arch. Oral Biol.* **34:**347–353.
11. **Brause, B. D.** 1989. Infected orthopedic prostheses, p. 111–127. *In* A. L. Bisno and F. A. Waldvogel (ed.), *Infections Associated with Indwelling Medical Devices.* American Society for Microbiology, Washington, D.C.
12. **Cameron, B. J., and L. J. Douglas.** 1996. Blood group glycolipids as epithelial cell receptors for *Candida albicans. Infect. Immun.* **64:**891–896.
13. **Cannon, R. D., and W. L. Chaffin.** 1999. Oral colonization by *Candida albicans. Crit. Rev. Oral Biol. Med.* **10:**359–383.
14. **Cannon, R. D., A. K. Nand, and H. F. Jenkinson.** 1995. Adherence of *Candida albicans* to human salivary components adsorbed to hydroxylapatite. *Microbiology* **141:**213–219.
15. **Carlen, A., P. Bratt, C. Stenudd, J. Olsson, and N. Stromberg.** 1998. Agglutinin and acid proline-rich protein receptor patterns may modulate bacterial adherence and colonization on tooth surfaces. *J. Dent. Res.* **77:**81–90.
16. **Chandra, J., P. K. Mukherjee, S. D. Leidich, F. F. Faddoul, L. L. Hoyer, L. J. Douglas, and M. A. Ghannoum.** 2001. Antifungal resis-

tance of candidal biofilms formed on denture acrylic in vitro. *J. Dent. Res.* **80**:903–908.

17. **Costerton, J. W., T. J. Marrie, and K.-J. Cheng.** 1985. Phenomena of bacterial adhesion, p. 3–43. *In* D. C. Savage and M. Fletcher (ed.), *Bacterial Adhesion Mechanisms and Physiological Significance.* Plenum Press, New York, N.Y.

18. **Elving, G. J., H. C. van der Mei, H. J. Busscher, A. Amerongen, E. C. I. Veerman, R. van Weissenbruch, and F. W. J. Albers.** 2000. Antimicrobial activity of synthetic salivary peptides against voice prosthetic microorganisms. *Laryngoscope* **110**:321–324.

19. **Gibbons, R. J., and D. I. Hay.** 1988. Human salivary acidic proline-rich proteins and statherin promote the attachment of *Actinomyces viscosus* LY7 to apatitic surfaces. *Infect. Immun.* **56**:439–445.

20. **Gibbons, R. J., D. I. Hay, J. O. Cisar, and W. B. Clark.** 1988. Adsorbed salivary proline-rich protein 1 and statherin: receptors for type 1 fimbriae of *Actinomyces viscosus* T14V-J1 on apatitic surfaces. *Infect. Immun.* **56**:2990–2993.

21. **Gibbons, R. J., D. I. Hay, and D. H. Schlesinger.** 1991. Delineation of a segment of adsorbed salivary acidic proline-rich proteins which promotes adhesion of *Streptococcus gordonii* to apatitic surfaces. *Infect. Immun.* **59**:2948–2954.

22. **Grimaudo, N. J., and W. E. Nesbitt.** 1997. Coaggregation of *Candida albicans* with oral *Fusobacterium* species. *Oral Microbiol. Immunol.* **12**:168–173.

23. **Grimaudo, N. J., W. E. Nesbitt, and W. B. Clark.** 1996. Coaggregation of *Candida albicans* with *Actinomyces* species. *Oral Microbiol. Immunol.* **11**:59–61.

24. **Haffajee, A. D., and S. S. Socransky.** 2001. Relationship of cigarette smoking to the subgingival microbiota. *J. Clin. Periodontol.* **28**:377–388.

25. **Hawser, S. P., and L. J. Douglas.** 1994. Biofilm formation by *Candida* species on the surface of catheter materials in vitro. *Infect. Immun.* **62**:915–921.

26. **Hawser, S. P., and L. J. Douglas.** 1995. Resistance of *Candida albicans* biofilms to antifungal agents in vitro. *Antimicrob. Agents Chemother.* **39**:2128–2131.

27. **Hawser, S. P., G. S. Baillie, and L. J. Douglas.** 1998. Production of extracellular matrix by *Candida albicans* biofilms. *J. Med. Microbiol.* **47**:253–256.

28. **Holmes, A. R., R. D. Cannon, and H. F. Jenkinson.** 1995. Interactions of *Candida albicans* with bacteria and salivary molecules in oral biofilms. *J. Ind. Microbiol.* **15**:208–213.

29. **Holmes, A. R., P. K. Gopal, and H. F. Jenkinson.** 1995. Adherence of *Candida albicans* to a

cell surface polysaccharide receptor on *Streptococcus gordonii. Infect. Immun.* **63**:1827–1834.

30. **Holmes, A. R., R. McNab, and H. F. Jenkinson.** 1996. *Candida albicans* binding to the oral bacterium *Streptococcus gordonii* involves multiple adhesin-receptor interactions. *Infect. Immun.* **64**:4680–4685.

31. **Hostetter, M. K.** 1999. Integrin-like proteins in Candida spp. and other microorganisms. *Fungal Genet. Biol.* **28**:135–145.

32. **Hube, B., and J. Naglik.** 2001. *Candida albicans* proteinases: resolving the mystery of a gene family. *Microbiology* **147**:1997–2005.

33. **Jabra-Rizk, M. A., W. A. Falkner, Jr., W. G. Merz, J. I. Kelley, A. A. M. A. Baqui, and T. F. Meiller.** 1999. Coaggregation of *Candida dubliniensis* with *Fusobacterium nucleatum. J. Clin. Microbiol.* **37**:1464–1468.

34. **Jenkinson, H. F., and D. R. Demuth.** 1997. Structure, function and immunogenicity of streptococcal antigen I/II polypeptides. *Mol. Microbiol.* **23**:183–190.

35. **Jenkinson, H. F., and R. J. Lamont.** 1997. Streptococcal adhesion and colonization. *Crit. Rev. Oral Biol. Med.* **8**:175–200.

36. **Jenkinson, H. F., H. C. Lala, and M. G. Shepherd.** 1990. Coaggregation of *Streptococcus sanguis* and other streptococci with *Candida albicans. Infect. Immun.* **58**:1429–1436.

37. **Jimenez-Lucho, V., V. Ginsburg, and H. C. Krivan.** 1990. *Cryptococcus neoformans, Candida albicans,* and other fungi bind specifically to the glycosphingolipid lactosylceramide (Galβ1-4Glcβ1-1Cer), a possible adhesion receptor for yeasts. *Infect. Immun.* **58**:2085–2090.

38. **Johansson, I., P. Bratt, D. I. Hay, S. Schluckebier, and N. Stromberg.** 2000. Adhesion of *Candida albicans,* but not *Candida krusei,* to salivary statherin and mimicking host molecules. *Oral Microbiol. Immunol.* **15**:112–118.

39. **Kamma, J. J., M. Nakou, and P. C. Baehni.** 1999. Clinical and microbiological characteristics of smokers with early onset periodontitis. *J. Periodontal Res.* **34**:25–33.

40. **Lamont, R. J., and H. F. Jenkinson.** 1998. Life below the gum line: pathogenic mechanisms of *Porphyromonas gingivalis. Microbiol. Mol. Biol. Rev.* **62**:1244–1263.

41. **Lamont, R. J., and H. F. Jenkinson.** 2000. Adhesion as an ecological determinant in the oral cavity, p. 131–168. *In* H. K. Kuramitsu and R. P. Ellen (ed.), *Oral Bacterial Ecology: The Molecular Basis.* Horizon Scientific Press, Wymondham, United Kingdom.

42. **Lana, M. A., A. P. Ribeiro-Sobrinho, R. Stehling, G. D. Garcia, B. K. Silva, J. S. Hamdan, J. R. Nicoli, M. A. Carvalho, and**

L. D. Farias. 2001. Microorganisms isolated from root canals presenting necrotic pulp and their drug susceptibility in vitro. *Oral Microbiol. Immunol.* **16:**100–105.

43. **Lendenmann, U., and F. G. Oppenheim.** 1998. Protein structure and function: histatins, p. 198–210. *In* B. Guggenheim, and S. Shapiro (ed.), *Oral Biology at the Turn of the Century.* Karger, Basel, Switzerland.

44. **Leonhardt, A., S. Renvert, and G. Dahlen.** 1999. Microbial findings at failing implants. *Clin. Oral Implants Res.* **10:**339–345.

45. **Liu, B., S. A. Rayment, C. Gyurko, F. G. Oppenheim, G. D. Offner, and R. F. Troxler.** 2000. The recombinant N-terminal region of human salivary mucin MG2 (MUC7) contains a binding domain for oral streptococci and exhibits anti-candidacidal activity. *Biochem. J.* **345:**557–564.

46. **Maki, D. G., and P. A. Tambyah.** 2001. Engineering out the risk of infection with urinary catheters. *Emerg. Infect. Dis.* **7:**1–6.

47. **Marco, F., S. R. Lockhart, M. A. Pfaller, C. Punjol, M. S. Rangel-Frausto, T. Wiblin, H. M. Blumberg, J. E. Edwards, W. Jarvis, L. Saiman, J. E. Patterson, M. G. Rinaldi, R. P. Wenzel, and D. R. Soll.** 1999. Elucidating the origins of nosocomial infections with *Candida albicans* by DNA fingerprinting with the complex probe Ca3. *J. Clin. Microbiol.* **37:**2817–2818.

48. **Marrie, T. J., J. Y. Sung, and J. W. Costerton.** 1990. Bacterial biofilm formation on nasogastric tubes. *J. Gastroenterol. Hepatol* **5:**503–506.

49. **Matthews, R., and J. Burnie.** 1996. Antibodies against *Candida:* potential therapeutics? *Trends Microbiol.* **4:**354–358.

50. **Millan, R. S., N. Elguezabal, P. Regulez, M. D. Moragues, G. Quindos, and J. Ponton.** 2000. Effect of secretory IgA on the adhesion of *Candida albicans* to polystyrene. *Microbiology* **146:**2105–2112.

51. **Millsap, K. W., R. Bos, H. C. van der Mei, and H. J. Busscher.** 1999. Adhesion and surface aggregation of *Candida albicans* from saliva on acrylic surfaces with adhering bacteria as studied in a parallel plate flow chamber. *Ant. Van Leeuwenhoek* **75:**351–359.

52. **Nair, R. G., and L. P. Samaranayake.** 1996. The effect of oral commensal bacteria on *Candida* adhesion to human buccal epithelial cells in vitro. *J. Med. Microbiol.* **45:**179–185.

53. **Nikawa, H., H. Nishimura, T. Yamamoto, T. Hamada, and L. P. Samaranayake.** 1996. The role of saliva and serum in *Candida albicans* biofilm formation on denture acrylic surfaces. *Microb. Ecol. Health Dis.* **9:**35–48.

54. **O'Sullivan, J. M., R. D. Cannon, P. A. Sullivan, and H. F. Jenkinson.** 1997. Identification of salivary basic proline-rich proteins as receptors for *Candida albicans* adhesion. *Microbiology* **143:**341–348.

55. **O'Sullivan, J. M., H. F. Jenkinson, and R. D. Cannon.** 2000. Adhesion of *Candida albicans* to oral streptococci is promoted by selective adsorption of salivary proteins to the streptococcal cell surface. *Microbiology* **146:**41–48.

56. **Prakobphol, A., F. Xu, V. M. Hoang, T. Larsson, J. Bergstrom, I. Johansson, L. Frangsmyr, U. Holmskov, H. Leffler, C. Nilsson, T. Boren, J. R. Wright, N. Stromberg, and S. J. Fisher.** 2000. Salivary agglutinin, which binds *Streptococcus mutans* and *Helicobacter pylori,* is the lung scavenger receptor cysteine-rich protein gp-340. *J. Biol. Chem.* **275:**39860–39866.

57. **Prigent-Combaret, C., O. Vidal, C. Dorel, and P. Lejeune.** 1999. Abiotic surface sensing and biofilm-dependent regulation of gene expression in *Escherichia coli. J. Bacteriol.* **181:**5993–6002.

58. **Sen, B. H., K. E. Safavi, and L. S. W. Spangberg.** 1997. Colonization of *Candida albicans* on cleaned human dental hard tissues. *Arch. Oral Biol.* **42:**513–520.

59. **Sheng, W. H., W. J. Ko, J. T. Wang, S. C. Chang, P. R. Hseuh, and K. T. Luh.** 2000. Evaluation of antiseptic-impregnated central venous catheters for prevention of catheter-related infection in intensive care unit patients. *Diagn. Microbiol. Infect. Dis.* **38:**1–5.

60. **Singleton, D. R., J. Masuoka, and K. C. Hazen.** 2001. Cloning and analysis of a *Candida albicans* gene that affects cell surface hydrophobicity. *J. Bacteriol.* **183:**3582–3588.

61. **Socransky, S. S., A. D. Haffajee, M. A. Cugini, C. Smith, and R. J. Kent, Jr.** 1998. Microbial complexes in subgingival plaque. *J. Clin. Periodontol.* **25:**134–144.

62. **Staab, J. F., S. D. Bradway, P. L. Fidal, and P. Sundstrom.** 1999. Adhesive and mammalian transglutaminase substrate properties of *Candida albicans* Hwp1. *Science* **283:**1535–1538.

63. **Sziegoleit, F., A. Sziegoleit, and W.-E. Wetzel.** 1999. Effect of dental treatment and/or local application of amphotericin B to carious teeth on oral colonization by *Candida. Med. Mycol.* **37:**345–350.

64. **Tosh, F. D., and L. J. Douglas.** 1992. Characterization of a fucoside-binding adhesin of *Candida albicans. Infect. Immun.* **60:**4734–4739.

65. **Van der Mei, H. C., R. H. Free, G. J. Elving, R. van Weissenbruch, F. W. J. Albers, and H. J. Busscher.** 2000. Effect of probiotic bacteria on prevalence of yeasts in oropharyngeal

biofilms on silicone rubber voice prostheses in vitro. *J. Med. Microbiol.* **49:**713–718.

66. **Waltimo, T. M., E. K. Siren, H. L. Torkko, I. Olsen, and M. P. Haapasalo.** 1997. Fungi in therapy-resistant periodontitis. *Int. Endod. J.* **30:**96–101.

67. **Xu, Y., I. Ambudkar, H. Yamagishi, W. Swaim, T. J. Walsh, and B. C. O'Connell.** 1999. Histatin-3 mediated killing of *Candida albicans:* effect of extracellular salt concentration on binding and internalization. *Antimicrob. Agents Chemother.* **43:**2256–2262.

POLYMICROBIAL DISEASES AS A RESULT OF MICROBE-INDUCED IMMUNOSUPPRESSION

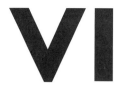

VIRUS-INDUCED IMMUNOSUPPRESSION

Jane E. Libbey and Robert S. Fujinami

19

INTRODUCTION

The History of Measles Virus

Measles virus (MV) naturally infects only humans and occasionally other primates (33). Because of the absence of a reservoir other than humans and the ability to induce lifelong immunity, MV can only maintain itself in human populations of greater than 200,000 individuals capable of sustaining a continuous person-to-person transmission (10). Thus, measles is a relatively new disease of humans, most likely evolving from an animal morbillivirus such as rinderpest virus of cattle (64).

Measles, as a disease of civilization, most likely first appeared in the early population centers of northern Africa, Mesopotamia, and India (33; A. Zahoor, 1997, http://www.erols.com/zenithco/razi.html). An Arab physician first recognized measles as distinct from smallpox in the 9th century. European and Far Eastern records show epidemics of illnesses characterized by a rash between A.D. 1 and 1200. European records of the 11th and 12th centuries show repeated epidemics identified as measles. Measles was first described as a disease of childhood in 1224 (33). Francis Home, a Scottish physician, formally showed measles to be caused by an infectious agent, by transmitting the disease via blood from measles patients to naïve individuals, in 1757 (71). James Lucas, an English surgeon, first described complications of measles in 1790 (54). Peter Panum, a young Danish physician, described the highly contagious nature, the 14-day incubation period, and the induction of lifelong immunity and postulated a respiratory route of infection for measles in 1846 (68).

In Vienna, von Pirquet first described measles virus-induced immunosuppression, as represented by the disappearance of delayed-type hypersensitivity (DTH) skin test responses to tuberculin in 1908 (84). This tuberculin skin response was only transiently impaired during the course of acute measles infection (84). von Pirquet's work with measles virus provided the first evidence that viruses have the ability to suppress the immune system.

Part of the difficulty encountered in examining measles virus is its limited host range. It was not until Goldenberger and Anderson (30) successfully passaged measles virus in macaque monkeys that any sort of laboratory system for the examination of measles existed. Research on measles virus has greatly advanced since Enders and Peebles (21) successfully grew measles

Jane E. Libbey and Robert S. Fujinami, Department of Neurology, University of Utah School of Medicine, Salt Lake City, UT 84132.

Polymicrobial Diseases, Edited by Kim A. Brogden and Janet M. Guthmiller, © 2002 ASM Press, Washington, D.C.

virus in tissue culture. Enders et al. (20) went on to develop a live virus vaccine for measles, which was further attenuated to produce the Schwarz vaccine used today (77). When used in a vigorous immunization regimen, this vaccine dramatically reduced the incidence of measles in the United States and other countries.

A Description of Measles Virus

MV belongs to the family *Paramyxoviridae,* subfamily *Paramyxovirinae,* genus *Morbillivirus* (72). Other members of the *Morbillivirus* genus, specifically canine distemper virus and rinderpest virus, have also been shown to cause immunosuppression (50, 60).

MV is an enveloped, negative-sense, single-stranded, nonsegmented RNA virus with a genome of approximately 15,890 nucleotides (Fig. 1). The viral genome comprises six genes separated by conserved noncoding sequences containing termination, polyadenylation, and initiation signals. MV replicates in the cytoplasm of infected cells (90). The viral genome is transcribed into seven monocistronic mRNAs, resulting in a gradient of mRNA abundance. Control regions comprising 50 nucleotides at the 3′ end and 50 nucleotides at the 5′ end, termed the leader and trailer, respectively, function in transcription to control viral gene expression and in replication to initiate encapsidation (52). The seven mRNAs are translated into eight proteins, most of which are structural and found in the virion (90).

The hemagglutinin (H) protein is a type II integral membrane glycoprotein that is incorporated as a spike in the virus envelope. This protein mediates attachment to cells through a cellular receptor (52). The H protein can cause the agglutination of primate erythrocytes and can elicit neutralizing antibodies (52, 90). The MV hemagglutinin protein is different from other paramyxovirus hemagglutinins in that the MV H protein does not contain neuraminidase activity (90).

The fusion (F) protein is a type I integral membrane glycoprotein that is also incorporated as a spike in the virus envelope (52). This protein mediates the fusion of the viral envelope to the cell plasma membrane. It also has the ability to fuse cells into syncytia and thus spread the virus intercellularly. The F protein, like the H protein, also elicits antibodies (90). The F protein is translated as an F_0 precursor that is cleaved by a cellular protease, furin in the *trans*-Golgi, into F_1 and F_2, which are linked by a disulfide bond (12, 89). Some nonpermissive host cells are unable to cleave F_0 and thus produce noninfectious virions (26, 90). The N-terminal 20 amino acids of the F protein are a highly conserved, hydrophobic region named the fusion peptide. This fusion peptide inserts into target membranes allowing membrane fusion to proceed (52).

The nucleoprotein (N) is associated with the RNA along with two other proteins, L and P, to form the nucleocapsid. The nucleocapsid does not disassemble upon infection of cells,

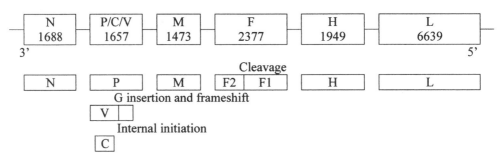

FIGURE 1 MV genome. The structure of the MV RNA and resultant viral proteins is shown.

but acts as a template for RNA synthesis. The transcribed RNA, which is mRNA, is translated into viral proteins. When the concentration of the N protein reaches a critical level, there is a switch from transcription of viral mRNAs to replication of full-length, positive-sense viral RNA, which in turn acts as a template for the production of full-length, negative-sense viral genomic RNA (90).

The large (L) protein is the least abundant viral protein, with only 50 copies per virion. The L protein, together with the P protein, forms the viral polymerase/transcriptase. The L protein also encodes the guanylyl- and methyltransferase activities required for mRNA capping (52).

The phosphoprotein (P), together with the L protein, forms the viral polymerase. The gene that encodes the P protein also encodes two other proteins, C via an internal initiation site for translation and V via the insertion of a nontemplated G nucleotide during transcription that results in a frameshift (90). The C and V proteins are thought to act to either speed up or slow down viral replication by either decreasing mRNA synthesis, C, or decreasing genome replication, V (52).

The matrix (M) protein is the most abundant protein in the virion. The M protein is peripherally associated with the nucleocapsid and the cell plasma membrane, where H and F proteins are located. The M protein inhibits transcription of the nucleocapsid during viral assembly, and the resultant virion is released by budding from the plasmid membrane (52).

MEASLES VIRUS-INDUCED IMMUNOSUPPRESSION

Immunologic Paradox

MV infection produces an immune system paradox. MV infection, while inducing lifelong immunity, also suppresses the immune system leading to an increase in susceptibility to other, secondary infections (24, 67, 91). In vitro research has shown that MV infection of cell cultures makes the cells more susceptible to a secondary bacterial invasion (13). The immune suppression appears coincident with the marked activation of the immune system, in the form of MV-specific responses, which in turn is coincident with the onset of clinical disease, i.e., rash. Immune suppression can continue for many weeks after the apparent recovery from measles (47). Therefore, MV infection results in both immune activation and immune suppression at the same time. Immune suppression is apparent in vivo in such forms as the loss of the DTH skin test response, the impairment of the production of antibody and cellular immune responses to new antigens, reactivity of tuberculosis, and remission of immune mediated diseases such as juvenile rheumatoid arthritis (15, 16, 84, 95). Immune suppression is apparent in vitro in such forms as suppressed lymphoproliferative responses to mitogens, abnormal lymphokine production, and inhibition of antigen-specific proliferation of T lymphocytes (9, 40, 87).

Secondary bacterial, protozoal, or viral infections occur because of immunosuppression by MV infection. These infections can result in pneumonia, chronic pulmonary disease, otitis media, laryngotracheobronchitis, adult respiratory distress syndrome, hepatitis and diarrhea (7, 29). Secondary infections are more common in underdeveloped countries. These secondary infections account for most of the morbidity and mortality associated with acute measles (7). Much research has been done to determine whether a correlation exists between malnutrition and/or overcrowding, which in turn results in a more intensive exposure to measles, and measles mortality (1, 2, 4, 5, 28). A natural epidemic of measles virus in a rhesus monkey colony showed that enteric organisms normally carried in healthy individuals became serious pathogens during the viral infection (58). Some of the bacteria that can be involved in superinfections in measles patients are *Streptococcus pneumoniae, Haemophilus influenzae, Staphylococcus aureus, Morganella morganii, Pseudomonas aeruginosa, Chlamydia trachomatis,* and *Streptococcus pyogenes* (7, 56, 94). Some of the viruses that can be involved in superinfections include adenovirus and herpes simplex virus (7, 88, 92). Although acute measles infection causes a relatively high mortality, there was no increase in mortality of those who survived a measles infection found in the postmeasles period as compared with uninfected community controls (6).

Recovery from MV infection depends on both the cell-mediated immune system and the humoral immune system (3). The role of the cell-mediated immune system in MV infection has been known since the work of Burnet (14). He described the course of MV infection in individuals with immunological abnormalities. In individuals with congenital agammaglobulinemia, lack of humoral immunity, measles follows its normal course, whereas in individuals with cortisone-treated acute leukemia, lack of cell-mediated immunity, measles results in fatal giant cell pneumonia without a rash (14). Kiepiela and colleagues demonstrated that MV causes a defect in the T-cell population, specifically the T-helper cell population, the severity of which could be correlated with the severity of the measles disease (46). Patients with a severe depletion of the T-helper cell population had an elevated level of the complement component C3, which in turn is an index of a poor prognosis (46).

The role of humoral immunity in MV infection was explored by determining the beneficial therapeutic effects of antibodies and the correlation between outcome and antibody response (3). It has been found that passive immunization with pooled normal human immunoglobulin will abort the disease if given promptly and will modify the disease if given a few days later, as well as modify or interfere with measles immunization (51, 79, 90). Also, maternal antibodies are sufficient to protect infants from MV infection (8, 11). Antibodies in a natural infection are first detectable when the rash appears (70, 74), and the failure to mount an adequate antibody response results in a poor prognosis (17). The antibody titers after vaccination can be as much as 10 times lower than the titer induced by natural infection, yet long-term immunity is still induced (90).

Models of Immunosuppression

Although MV-induced immunosuppression has been known since the days of von Pirquet (84), the mechanisms involved remain elusive. Many groups around the globe are studying MV-induced immunosuppression. The next section and Table 1 summarize the many approaches being used by various groups to determine the mechanism of MV-induced immunosuppression.

Fujinami and colleagues have approached the problem of MV-induced immunosuppression by examining the affect of MV infection on T and B cells. They have studied the production of cytokines by T lymphocytes and the role of a soluble factor in suppression (9, 27, 81). The study examining cytokine production determined that there is no generalized inhibition of cytokine production leading to generalized immunosuppression (9). MV infection of antigen-specific activated T cells caused no significant alteration in the production of interferon gamma (IFN-γ), interleukin-2 (IL-2), IL-6, or IL-10, although there was a 50% reduction in the production of IL-4. However, the expression of the IL-2 receptor alpha (IL-2Rα) subunit was decreased in infected, antigen-specific activated T cells. The block in expression of the IL-2Rα subunit by activated T cells may be one mechanism for

TABLE 1 Potential mechanisms of MV-induced immunosuppression

Model of immunosuppression	Reference(s)
Cytokine production	9
Soluble immunosuppressive factor	27, 81
Type 1 to type 2 shift	32, 35, 85
IL-12	43, 44, 61
Lymphoproliferative effect: cell cycle block	57, 59, 62
Host-pathogen interaction: transgenic mice	69
MV proteins	55
SLAM receptor	41, 82
Fas-mediated apoptosis, DCs	78
MV infection of DCs	48

the suppression of proliferation following MV infection (9).

Through the study of in vitro infected peripheral blood mononuclear cells (PBMC), it was shown that the virus-infected cells secreted an immunosuppressive factor, which was not IFN-γ, IFN-α, or prostaglandin E (75). Studies by Fujinami's group have further examined the role of a soluble factor in immunosuppression, and these studies show that both MV-infected T and B cells produce a soluble factor, present in the supernatants, which in turn can suppress the proliferation of uninfected T and B cells (27, 81). The suppression of proliferation by the supernatants is not due to infectious virus, IL-10, or transforming growth factor beta (TGF-β). The soluble factor is larger than 100 kDa; however, trypsin digestion reveals an antiproliferative activity associated with a factor of less than 10 kDa, and heat treatment at 56°C results in loss of activity. These data support the idea that the soluble factor may be a new cytokine (81). This soluble factor also has the ability to mirror the effects of MV infection of B cells, which results in the inhibition of antigen presentation (27).

Griffin and colleagues have approached the problem of MV-induced immunosuppression by examining the immune responses during MV infection. Various studies of humans have shown that the T-cell-driven immune response is activated during measles infection. There is an elevation in the plasma levels of the soluble forms of the T-cell surface molecules CD4, CD8, IL-2R, and β_2-microglobulin and of the T-cell products IL-2, IL-4, and INF-γ (34, 36–39). The plasma also contains elevated levels of proliferating CD8 T cells (86). Therefore, immunosuppression is occurring even though substantial immune activation is present. The MV-specific immune response that is induced is effective in clearing the virus and in inducing long-term immunity. Analysis of the in vitro abnormalities suggests defects in the responses of both monocytes and lymphocytes which may be due to infection of these cells leading to cell lysis, via apoptosis, or functional alterations (22, 32). Increases in IL-1 and decreases in tumor necrosis factor alpha (TNF-α) may result from direct infection of monocytes (87). Although T cells have not been shown to be infected in vivo, the numbers of T cells decrease during measles even though a normal proportion of CD4 and CD8 lymphocytes is maintained; therefore, abnormalities in T-cell responses may be secondary to other changes (86). One of the mechanisms suggested for immunosuppression is the presence of elevated levels of IL-4 which functions to suppress macrophage activation and DTH responses (34, 87). The analysis of the cytokine pattern present during MV infection suggests an initial type 1 immune response during viral clearance followed by a prolonged type 2 response; DTH responses depend on the production of type 1 cytokines (43).

Karp and colleagues have approached the problem of MV-induced immunosuppression by examining the role of IL-12 and the complement system during MV infection. IL-12 activity is critical for both protective and pathological cellular immune responses, and as such, is tightly regulated (61). The prime producers of IL-12 in vivo are monocytes/macrophages and dendritic cells (DCs), which are also the main immune cells productively, infected with MV in vivo (44). MV infection of primary human monocytes suppresses the stimulated production of IL-12 (45). This suppression of IL-12 did not appear to be dependent on either an endogenous soluble inhibitor or a productive infection with MV. A direct interaction between MV and CD46, the cellular receptor for MV, was suggested to cause the suppression of IL-12 production even if no productive MV infection results (45). This hypothesis is supported by the suppression of IL-12 production seen as a result of antibody-mediated cross-linking of CD46 on the surface of primary human monocytes. Likewise, complement activation products that interact with CD46 also suppress the stimulated production of IL-12 (45). MV also suppresses the production of IL-12 by DCs (25). The ability of MV infection to suppress the production of IL-12 may be one mechanism by which MV induces immunosuppression, because IL-12 is required for most DTH responses (44). This requirement for IL-12 in DTH responses may in turn be due to the requirement for IL-12 in the development of type 1 immune responses (43). However, suppression of IL-12 does not explain the in vitro lymphoproliferative defects caused by MV infection, nor has the suppression of IL-12 yet been shown to occur in vivo (44, 61).

Oldstone and colleagues have approached the problem of MV-induced immunosuppression by examining both the in vitro lymphoproliferative defect and the host-pathogen interactions. The suppressed lymphoproliferative responses to mitogens in vitro has been shown to be caused by a block in the cell cycle at late G_1 or G_0 (57, 59, 62).

The host-pathogen interactions are being examined via transgenic mice. Mice transgenic for CD46, the human MV receptor, have been used to study the pathogenesis of MV infection (69). Immunosuppression in the transgenic mice has been shown to occur as seen by: (i) a reduction of the CD8[+] cytotoxic T lymphocyte (CTL) response against viral challenge with viruses such as lymphocytic choriomeningitis virus (LCMV) and vaccinia virus (VV), (ii) the inability to generate antibodies against antigens, and (iii) the susceptibility of the transgenic mice to secondary bacterial infections (69).

Horvat and colleagues have approached the problem of MV-induced immunosuppression by examining the role of MV proteins in the generation of immunosuppression in vivo (55). They have studied the DTH response mediated by CD4[+] T cells and the contact hypersensitivity (CHS) response mediated by CD8[+] T cells, two types of T-cell-dependent inflammatory reactions. They demonstrated that inactivated MV (thus absence of viral replication) efficiently suppresses these inflammatory responses in mice after the MV envelope proteins, F and H, and N protein have interacted with their cellular receptors, CD46 and FcγR, respectively. CD46 appears to be expressed on DCs as well as an additional cell type, while FcγR is expressed on DCs (55).

Two groups, Yanagi and colleagues and Richardson and colleagues, have approached the problem of MV-induced immunosuppression by examining the receptor used by MV to bind to cells. CD46 has been identified as the MV receptor yet MV strains isolated in B95a cells or human B cell lines did not grow in CD46[+] cell lines (18, 49, 63). Through the use of two different versions of functional expression cloning, the human signaling lymphocytic activation molecule (SLAM) gene was identified as the cellular receptor for MV strains that cannot use CD46 (41, 82). Unlike CD46, which is ubiquitously expressed, SLAM is constitutively expressed on immature thymocytes, CD45RO[high] memory T cells, and some B cells and is induced on activated T and B cells (53, 93). The pattern for SLAM expression is consistent with the lymphoid tropism of MV infection. Binding of MV to SLAM on the cell surface may cause either the destruction of SLAM[+] cells or may impair the lymphocyte activation by affecting the signals induced through SLAM, resulting in immunosuppression (93). Type 1 immune cells express more SLAM than type 2 immune cells; therefore, the destruction of SLAM[+] cells could favor the type 1 to type 2 immune response shift suggested previously (41).

Servet-Delprat and colleagues approached the problem of MV-induced immunosuppression by examining Fas-mediated apoptosis of MV-infected DCs and activation of bystander uninfected DCs in vitro (78). They determined that the Fas-mediated apoptosis, induced by MV replication, of infected DCs helps mediate the release of infectious MV particles. They also found that apoptotic MV-infected DCs induce the maturation of uninfected DCs via a bystander mechanism of contact with or engulfment of infected apoptotic DCs. These two occurrences may explain how both a specific immune response to measles (DC activation) and immunosuppression (DC apoptosis) can occur simultaneously after MV infection (78).

Klagge and colleagues approached the problem of MV-induced immunosuppression by also examining DCs and the affect of MV infection on them in vitro (48). They determined that the release, induced by MV infection, of INF-α/β by DCs contributes to DC maturation. However, MV-infected DCs expressing the MV F and H glycoproteins on their surface inhibit mitogen-induced proliferation of T cells. Therefore, the immunosuppressive activity of the glycoproteins on the cell surface appears to overcome the promotion of DC maturation by soluble mediators (48). This same group showed that the expression of the MV F and H glycoproteins on peripheral blood lymphocytes (PBLs), used as presenter cells, reduced the proliferation of naïve PBLs to various stimuli by means of surface contacts (76).

POTENTIAL THERAPIES

Measles itself can be treated by the administration of immunoglobulin, as discussed above, and interferon, vitamin A, and ribavirin (42, 56). Interferon is thought to reduce virus replication by inhibiting infection of uninfected cells by virions (31). For reasons that are as yet unexplained, the administration of vitamin A decreases the mortality due to MV infection. Ribavirin, a synthetic nucleoside analog structurally related to guanosine and inosine, has in vitro activity against MV replication (56). Measles pneumonia may be life threatening in immunocompromised adults, and ribavirin has been used in vivo to treat measles pneumonia in oncology and HIV-infected patients, and in immunocompetent individuals (23, 42, 73, 80).

The secondary infections, which occur as a result of MV-induced immunosuppression, can themselves be treated. Secondary infections due to bacteria can be treated with antibiotics. Secondary infections due to viruses can be treated with antiviral drugs.

The most efficient way to treat measles, and the resultant immunosuppression and secondary infections, is by prevention. Prior to the introduction of the measles vaccine, the United States alone had almost 4 million cases of measles annually. Following the introduction of the measles vaccine in the United States, the incidence of measles decreased dramatically, to a low of 1,497 cases in 1983 (56). Measles has not been eradicated, however. Outbreaks continue to occur in the United States in preschool-age children who have not received vaccination and in adolescents of high school and college age who have received only a single dose of the vaccine (56). On the basis of the presence of these outbreaks, a two-dose vaccination schedule was implemented in the United States in 1989, and a two-dose vaccination schedule is supported worldwide by the World Health Organization (56, 83). Through the use of the two-dose vaccination strategy, it is feasible to raise the level of vaccination coverage such that the virus transmission is interrupted and measles could be essentially eradicated (65, 66). Eradication of measles is feasible because measles is only transmitted from human to human, so 100% vaccination is not necessary. It is only necessary to increase the overall immunity level to a level where the number of susceptible individuals in the population is too low to sustain measles virus transmission (19).

SUMMARY

Many laboratories are studying the immunosuppression induced by MV infection. One theory about the mechanism is that the viral infections shift the immune response to a type 2 immune response (32, 35, 85). This mechanism was explored further to demonstrate that the interaction of MV with its cellular receptor, CD46, results in the suppression of IL-12 which is required for type 1 immune responses (43, 45). Another theory about the mechanism is that an as-yet-unidentified soluble factor is able to inhibit lymphoproliferation (27, 81). Other groups are addressing the role that the MV proteins play in immunosuppression (48, 55, 76), while others are examining the role of the alternate MV receptor, SLAM, in immunosuppression (41, 82). Yet another group is examining the Fas-mediated apoptosis of

MV-infected DCs as a means of explaining the presence of both a specific immune response and immunosuppression (78). Regardless of the extensive work that has been done on MV-induced immunosuppression, the exact molecular mechanism remains unresolved and may be multifactorial.

ACKNOWLEDGMENTS

We thank Kathleen Borick for preparation of the manuscript.

This research is supported by NMSS grant RG29258.

REFERENCES

1. **Aaby, P.** 1988. Malnutrition and overcrowding/intensive exposure in severe measles infection: review of community studies. *Rev. Infect. Dis.* **10**:478–491.
2. **Aaby, P., J. Bukh, G. Hoff, J. Leerhoy, I. M. Lisse, C. H. Mordhorst, and I. R. Pedersen.** 1986. High measles mortality in infancy related to intensity of exposure. *J. Pediatr.* **109**:40–44.
3. **Aaby, P., J. Bukh, G. Hoff, I. M. Lisse, and A. J. Smits.** 1987. Humoral immunity in measles infection: a critical factor? *Med. Hypotheses* **23**:287–301.
4. **Aaby, P., J. Bukh, I. M. Lisse, and A. J. Smits.** 1984. Overcrowding and intensive exposure as determinants of measles mortality. *Am. J. Epidemiol.* **120**:49–63.
5. **Aaby, P., and J. Leeuwenburg.** 1990. Patterns of transmission and severity of measles infection: a reanalysis of data from the Machakos area, Kenya. *J. Infect. Dis.* **161**:171–174.
6. **Aaby, P., I. M. Lisse, K. Molbak, K. Knudsen, and H. Whittle.** 1996. No persistent T lymphocyte immunosuppression or increased mortality after measles infection: a community study from Guinea-Bissau. *Pediatr. Infect. Dis. J.* **15**:39–44.
7. **Abramson, O., R. Dagan, A. Tal, and S. Sofer.** 1995. Severe complications of measles requiring intensive care in infants and young children. *Arch. Pediatr. Adolesc. Med.* **149**:1237–1240.
8. **Albrecht, P., F. A. Ennis, E. J. Saltzman, and S. Krugman.** 1977. Persistence of maternal antibody in infants beyond 12 months: mechanism of measles vaccine failure. *J. Pediatr.* **91**:715–718.
9. **Bell, A. F., J. B. Burns, and R. S. Fujinami.** 1997. Measles virus infection of human T cells modulates cytokine generation and IL-2 receptor alpha chain expression. *Virology* **232**:241–247.
10. **Black, F. L.** 1966. Measles endemicity in insular populations: critical community size and its evolutionary implication. *J. Theor. Biol.* **11**:207–211.
11. **Black, F. L.** 1989. Measles active and passive immunity in a worldwide perspective. *Prog. Med. Virol.* **36**:1–33.
12. **Bolt, G., and I. R. Pedersen.** 1998. The role of subtilisin-like proprotein convertases for cleavage of the measles virus fusion glycoprotein in different cell types. *Virology* **252**:387–398.
13. **Bukholm, G., K. Modalsli, and M. Degre.** 1986. Effect of measles-virus infection and interferon treatment on invasiveness of *Shigella flexneri* in HEp2-cell cultures. *J. Med. Microbiol.* **22**:335–341.
14. **Burnet, F. M.** 1968. Measles as an index of immunological function. *Lancet* **ii**:610–613.
15. **Christensen, P. E., H. Schmidt, H. O. Bang, V. Andersen, B. Jordal, and O. Jensen.** 1953. An epidemic of measles in southern Greenland, 1951. Measles in virgin soil. II. The epidemic proper. *Acta Med. Scand.* **144**:430–449.
16. **Coovadia, H. M., M. A. Parent, W. E. Loening, A. Wesley, B. Burgess, F. Hallett, P. Brain, J. Grace, J. Naidoo, P. M. Smythe, and G. H. Vos.** 1974. An evaluation of factors associated with the depression of immunity in malnutrition and in measles. *Am. J. Clin. Nutr.* **27**:665–669.
17. **Coovadia, H. M., A. Wesley, and P. Brain.** 1978. Immunological events in acute measles influencing outcome. *Arch. Dis. Child.* **53**:861–867.
18. **Dorig, R. E., A. Marcil, A. Chopra, and C. D. Richardson.** 1993. The human CD46 molecule is a receptor for measles virus (Edmonston strain). *Cell* **75**:295–305.
19. **Dowdle, W. R., and W. A. Orenstein.** 1994. Quest for life-long protection by vaccination. *Proc. Natl. Acad. Sci. USA* **91**:2464–2468.
20. **Enders, J. F., S. L. Katz, M. V. Milovanovic, and A. Holloway.** 1960. Studies of an attenuated measles-virus vaccine: I. Development and preparation of the vaccine: technics for assay of effects of vaccination. *N. Engl. J. Med.* **263**:153–159.
21. **Enders, J. F., and T. C. Peebles.** 1954. Propagation in tissue culture of cytopathic agents from patients with measles. *Proc. Soc. Exp. Biol. Med.* **86**:277–286.
22. **Esolen, L. M., S. W. Park, J. M. Hardwick, and D. E. Griffin.** 1995. Apoptosis as a cause of death in measles virus-infected cells. *J. Virol.* **69**:3955–3958.
23. **Fernandez, H., G. Banks, and R. Smith.** 1986. Ribavirin: a clinical overview. *Eur. J. Epidemiol.* **2**:1–14.

24. **Fireman, P., G. Friday, and J. Kumate.** 1969. Effect of measles vaccine on immunologic responsiveness. *Pediatrics* **43:**264–272.

25. **Fugier-Vivier, I., C. Servet-Delprat, P. Rivailler, M. C. Rissoan, Y. J. Liu, and C. Rabourdin-Combe.** 1997. Measles virus suppresses cell-mediated immunity by interfering with the survival and functions of dendritic and T cells. *J. Exp. Med.* **186:**813–823.

26. **Fujinami, R. S., and M. B. A. Oldstone.** 1981. Failure to cleave measles virus fusion protein in lymphoid cells. *J. Exp. Med.* **154:**1489–1499.

27. **Fujinami, R. S., X. Sun, J. M. Howell, J. C. Jenkin, and J. B. Burns.** 1998. Modulation of immune system function by measles virus infection: role of soluble factor and direct infection. *J. Virol.* **72:**9421–9427.

28. **Garenne, M., and P. Aaby.** 1990. Pattern of exposure and measles mortality in Senegal. *J. Infect. Dis.* **161:**1088–1094.

29. **Gavish, D., Y. Kleinman, A. Morag, and T. Chajek-Shaul.** 1983. Hepatitis and jaundice associated with measles in young adults. An analysis of 65 cases. *Arch. Intern. Med.* **143:**674–677.

30. **Goldenberger, J., and J. F. Anderson.** 1911. An experimental demonstration of the presence of the virus of measles in the mixed buccal and nasal secretions. *JAMA* **57:**496–578.

31. **Greenberg, S. B.** 1991. Viral pneumonia. *Infect. Dis. Clin. N. Am.* **5:**603–621.

32. **Griffin, D. E.** 1995. Immune responses during measles virus infection. *Curr. Top. Microbiol. Immunol.* **191:**117–134.

33. **Griffin, D. E., and W. J. Bellini.** 1996. Measles virus, p. 1267–1312. *In* B. N. Fields, D. M. Knipe, and P. M. Howley (ed.), *Fields Virology,* 3rd ed. Lippincott-Raven Publishers, Philadelphia, Pa.

34. **Griffin, D. E., and B. J. Ward.** 1993. Differential CD4 T cell activation in measles. *J. Infect. Dis.* **168:**275–281.

35. **Griffin, D. E., B. J. Ward, and L. M. Esolen.** 1994. Pathogenesis of measles virus infection: an hypothesis for altered immune responses. *J. Infect. Dis.* **170**(Suppl. 1)**:**S24–S31.

36. **Griffin, D. E., B. J. Ward, E. Jauregui, R. T. Johnson, and A. Vaisberg.** 1989. Immune activation in measles. *N. Engl. J. Med.* **320:**1667–1672.

37. **Griffin, D. E., B. J. Ward, E. Jauregui, R. T. Johnson, and A. Vaisberg.** 1990. Immune activation during measles: interferon-γ and neopterin in plasma and cerebrospinal fluid in complicated and uncomplicated disease. *J. Infect. Dis.* **161:**449–453.

38. **Griffin, D. E., B. J. Ward, E. Jauregui, R. T. Johnson, and A. Vaisberg.** 1990. Natural killer cell activity during measles. *Clin. Exp. Immunol.* **81:**218–224.

39. **Griffin, D. E., B. J. Ward, E. Juaregui, R. T. Johnson, and A. Vaisberg.** 1992. Immune activation during measles: β₂-microglobulin in plasma and cerebrospinal fluid in complicated and uncomplicated disease. *J. Infect. Dis.* **166:**1170–1173.

40. **Hirsch, R. L., D. E. Griffin, R. T. Johnson, S. J. Cooper, I. Lindo de Soriano, S. Roedenbeck, and A. Vaisberg.** 1984. Cellular immune responses during complicated and uncomplicated measles virus infections of man. *Clin. Immunol. Immunopathol.* **31:**1–12.

41. **Hsu, E. C., C. Iorio, F. Sarangi, A. A. Khine, and C. D. Richardson.** 2001. CDw 150(SLAM) is a receptor for a lymphotropic strain of measles virus and may account for the immunosuppressive properties of this virus. *Virology* **279:**9–21.

42. **Kaplan, L. J., R. S. Daum, M. Smaron, and C. A. McCarthy.** 1992. Severe measles in immunocompromised patients. *JAMA* **267:**1237–1241.

43. **Karp, C. L.** 1999. Measles: immunosuppression, interleukin-12, and complement receptors. *Immunol. Rev.* **168:**91–101.

44. **Karp, C. L., and M. Wills-Karp.** 2001. Complement and IL-12: yin and yang. *Microb. Infect.* **3:**109–119.

45. **Karp, C. L., M. Wysocka, L. M. Wahl, J. M. Ahearn, P. J. Cuomo, B. Sherry, G. Trinchieri, and D. E. Griffin.** 1996. Mechanism of suppression of cell-mediated immunity by measles virus. *Science* **273:**228–231.

46. **Kiepiela, P., H. M. Coovadia, and P. Coward.** 1987. T helper cell defect related to severity in measles. *Scand. J. Infect. Dis.* **19:**185–192.

47. **Kipps, A., L. Stern, and E. G. Vaughan.** 1966. The duration and the possible significance of the depression of tuberculin sensitivity following measles. *S. Afr. Med. J.* **40:**104–108.

48. **Klagge, I. M., V. ter Meulen, and S. Schneider-Schaulies.** 2000. Measles virus-induced promotion of dendritic cell maturation by soluble mediators does not overcome the immunosuppressive activity of viral glycoproteins on the cell surface. *Eur. J. Immunol.* **30:**2741–2750.

49. **Kobune, F., H. Sakata, and A. Sugiura.** 1990. Marmoset lymphoblastoid cells as a sensitive host for isolation of measles virus. *J. Virol.* **64:**700–705.

50. **Krakowka, S., R. J. Higgins, and A. Koestner.** 1980. Canine distemper virus: review of structural and functional modulations in lymphoid tissues. *Am. J. Vet. Res.* **41:**284–292.

51. **Krugman, S.** 1963. Medical progress: the clinical use of gamma globulin. *N. Engl. J. Med.* **269:** 195–201.

52. **Lamb, R. A., and D. Kolakofsky.** 1996. *Paramyxoviridae:* the viruses and their replication, p. 1177–1204. *In* B. N. Fields, D. M. Knipe, and P. M. Howley (ed.), *Fields Virology,* 3rd ed. Lippincott-Raven Publishers, Philadelphia, Pa.

53. **Liszewski, M. K., T. W. Post, and J. P. Atkinson.** 1991. Membrane cofactor protein (MCP or CD46): newest member of the regulators of complement activation gene cluster. *Annu. Rev. Immunol.* **9:**431–455.

54. **Lucas, J.** 1790. An account of uncommon symptoms succeeding the measles; with additional remarks on the infection of measles and smallpox. *Lond. Med. J.* **11:**325–331.

55. **Marie, J. C., J. Kehren, M. C. Trescol-Biemont, A. Evlashev, H. Valentin, T. Walzer, R. Tedone, B. Loveland, J. F. Nicolas, C. Rabourdin-Combe, and B. Horvat.** 2001. Mechanism of measles virus-induced suppression of inflammatory immune responses. *Immunity* **14:**69–79.

56. **Mason, W. H.** 1995. Measles. *Adolesc. Med.* **6:**1–14.

57. **McChesney, M. B., A. Altman, and M. B. A. Oldstone.** 1988. Suppression of T lymphocyte function by measles virus is due to cell cycle arrest in G1. *J. Immunol.* **140:**1269–1273.

58. **McChesney, M. B., R. S. Fujinami, N. W. Lerche, P. A. Marx, and M. B. A. Oldstone.** 1989. Virus-induced immunosuppression: infection of peripheral blood mononuclear cells and suppression of immunoglobulin synthesis during natural measles virus infection of rhesus monkeys. *J. Infect. Dis.* **159:**757–760.

59. **McChesney, M. B., J. H. Kehrl, A. Valsamakis, A. S. Fauci, and M. B. A. Oldstone.** 1987. Measles virus infection of B lymphocytes permits cellular activation but blocks progression through the cell cycle. *J. Virol.* **61:** 3441–3447.

60. **McChesney, M. B., and M. B. A. Oldstone.** 1989. Virus-induced immunosuppression: infections with measles virus and human immunodeficiency virus. *Adv. Immunol.* **45:**335–380.

61. **Mosser, D. M., and C. L. Karp.** 1999. Receptor mediated subversion of macrophage cytokine production by intracellular pathogens. *Curr. Opin. Immunol.* **11:**406–411.

62. **Naniche, D., S. I. Reed, and M. B. A. Oldstone.** 1999. Cell cycle arrest during measles virus infection: a G0-like block leads to suppression of retinoblastoma protein expression. *J. Virol.* **73:**1894–1901.

63. **Naniche, D., G. Varior-Krishnan, F. Cervoni, T. F. Wild, B. Rossi, C. Rabourdin-Combe, and D. Gerlier.** 1993. Human membrane cofactor protein (CD46) acts as a cellular receptor for measles virus. *J. Virol.* **67:**6025–6032.

64. **Norrby, E., H. Sheshberadaran, K. C. McCullough, W. C. Carpenter, and C. Orvell.** 1985. Is rinderpest virus the archevirus of the Morbillivirus genus? *Intervirology* **23:**228–232.

65. **Omer, M. I.** 1999. Measles: a disease that has to be eradicated. *Ann. Trop. Paediatr.* **19:**125–134.

66. **Orenstein, W. A., P. M. Strebel, M. Papania, R. W. Sutter, W. J. Bellini, and S. L. Cochi.** 2000. Measles eradication: is it in our future? *Am. J. Public Health* **90:**1521–1525.

67. **Osler, W.** 1904. *The Principles and Practices of Medicine,* 5th ed., p. 88. D. Appleton and Company, New York, N.Y.

68. **Panum, P.** 1938. Observations made during the epidemic of measles on the Faroe Islands in the year 1846. *Med. Classics* **3:**829–886.

69. **Patterson, J. B., M. Manchester, and M. B. A. Oldstone.** 2001. Disease model: dissecting the pathogenesis of the measles virus. *Trends Mol. Med.* **7:**85–88.

70. **Perry, K. R., D. W. Brown, J. V. Parry, S. Panday, C. Pipkin, and A. Richards.** 1993. Detection of measles, mumps, and rubella antibodies in saliva using antibody capture radioimmunoassay. *J. Med. Virol.* **40:**235–240.

71. **Plotkin, S. A.** 1967. Vaccination against measles in the 18th century. *Clin. Pediatr.* **6:**312–315.

72. **Rima, B., D. J. Alexander, M. A. Billeter, P. L. Collins, D. W. Kingsbury, M. A. Lipkind, Y. Nagai, C. Orvell, C. R. Pringle, and V. ter Meulen.** 1995. Paramyxovirus taxonomy, p. 268–274. *In* F. A. Murphy, C. M. Fauquet, D. H. L. Bishop, S. A. Ghabiral, A. W. Jarvis, G. P. Martelli, M. A. Mayo, and M. D. Summers (ed.), *Virus Taxonomy. Sixth Report of the International Committee on Taxonomy of Viruses.* Springer-Verlag Publishers, New York, N.Y.

73. **Ross, L. A., K. S. Kim, W. H. Mason, Jr., and E. Gomperts.** 1990. Successful treatment of disseminated measles in a patient with acquired immunodeficiency syndrome: consideration of antiviral and passive immunotherapy. *Am. J. Med.* **88:**313–314.

74. **Rossier, E., H. Miller, B. McCulloch, L. Sullivan, and K. Ward.** 1991. Comparison of immunofluorescence and enzyme immunoassay for detection of measles-specific immunoglobulin M antibody. *J. Clin. Microbiol.* **29:**1069–1071.

75. **Sanchez-Lanier, M., P. Guerin, L. C. McLaren, and A. D. Bankhurst.** 1988.

Measles virus-induced suppression of lymphocyte proliferation. *Cell. Immunol.* **116:**367–381.

76. **Schlender, J., J. J. Schnorr, P. Spielhoffer, T. Cathomen, R. Cattaneo, M. A. Billeter, V. ter Meulen, and S. Schneider-Schaulies.** 1996. Interaction of measles virus glycoproteins with the surface of uninfected peripheral blood lymphocytes induces immunosuppression in vitro. *Proc. Natl. Acad. Sci. USA* **93:**13194–13199.

77. **Schwarz, A. J. F.** 1962. Preliminary tests of a highly attenuated measles vaccine. *Am. J. Dis. Child.* **103:**216–219.

78. **Servet-Delprat, C., P. O. Vidalain, O. Azocar, F. Le Deist, A. Fischer, and C. Rabourdin-Combe.** 2000. Consequences of Fas-mediated human dendritic cell apoptosis induced by measles virus. *J. Virol.* **74:**4387–4393.

79. **Siber, G. R., B. G. Werner, N. A. Halsey, R. Reid, J. Almeido-Hill, S. C. Garrett, C. Thompson, and M. Santosham.** 1993. Interference of immune globulin with measles and rubella immunization. *J. Pediatr.* **122:**204–211.

80. **Stogner, S. W., J. W. King, C. Black-Payne, and J. Bocchini.** 1993. Ribavirin and intravenous immune globulin therapy for measles pneumonia in HIV infection. *South Med. J.* **86:**1415–1418.

81. **Sun, X., J. B. Burns, J. M. Howell, and R. S. Fujinami.** 1998. Suppression of antigen-specific T cell proliferation by measles virus infection: role of a soluble factor in suppression. *Virology* **246:**24–33.

82. **Tatsuo, H., N. Ono, K. Tanaka, and Y. Yanagi.** 2000. SLAM (CDw150) is a cellular receptor for measles virus. *Nature* **406:**893–897.

83. **Tulchinsky, T. H., G. M. Ginsberg, Y. Abed, M. T. Angeles, C. Akukwe, and J. Bonn.** 1993. Measles control in developing and developed countries: the case for a two-dose policy. *Bull. W. H. O.* **71:**93–103.

84. **von Pirquet, C.** 1908. Verhalten der kutanen tuberkulin-reaktion wahrend der Masern. *Dtsch. Med. Wochenschr.* **34:**1297–1300.

85. **Ward, B. J., and D. E. Griffin.** 1993. Changes in cytokine production after measles virus vacci-

nation: predominant production of IL-4 suggests induction of a Th2 response. *Clin. Immunol. Immunopathol.* **67:**171–177.

86. **Ward, B. J., R. T. Johnson, A. Vaisberg, E. Jauregui, and D. E. Griffin.** 1990. Spontaneous proliferation of peripheral mononuclear cells in natural measles virus infection: identification of dividing cells and correlation with mitogen responsiveness. *Clin. Immunol. Immunopathol.* **55:**315–326.

87. **Ward, B. J., R. T. Johnson, A. Vaisberg, E. Jauregui, and D. E. Griffin.** 1991. Cytokine production *in vitro* and the lymphoproliferative defect of natural measles virus infection. *Clin. Immunol. Immunopathol.* **61:**236–248.

88. **Warner, J. O., and W. C. Marshall.** 1976. Crippling lung disease after measles and adenovirus infection. *Br. J. Dis. Chest* **70:**89–94.

89. **Watanabe, M., A. Hirano, S. Stenglein, J. Nelson, G. Thomas, and T. C. Wong.** 1995. Engineered serine protease inhibitor prevents furin-catalyzed activation of the fusion glycoprotein and production of infectious measles virus. *J. Virol.* **69:**3206–3210.

90. **White, D. O., and F. J. Fenner.** 1994. *Paramyxoviridae,* p. 456–474. *Medical Virology,* 4th ed. Academic Press, San Diego, Calif.

91. **Whittle, H. C., A. Bradley-Moore, A. Fleming, and B. M. Greenwood.** 1973. Effects of measles on the immune response of Nigerian children. *Arch. Dis. Child.* **48:**753–756.

92. **Whittle, H. C., J. S. Smith, O. I. Kogbe, J. Dossetor, and M. Duggan.** 1979. Severe ulcerative herpes of mouth and eye following measles. *Trans. R. Soc. Trop. Med. Hyg.* **73:**66–69.

93. **Yanagi, Y.** 2001. The cellular receptor for measles virus—elusive no more. *Rev. Med. Virol.* **11:**149–156.

94. **Yetgin, S., and C. Altay.** 1980. Defective bactericidal function of polymorphonuclear neutrophils in children with measles. *Acta Paediatr. Scand.* **69:**411–413.

95. **Yoshioka, K., H. Miyata, and S. Maki.** 1981. Transient remission of juvenile rheumatoid arthritis after measles. *Acta Paediatr. Scand.* **70:**419–420.

HUMAN IMMUNODEFICIENCY VIRUS, *PNEUMOCYSTIS CARINII, TOXOPLASMA GONDII,* AND *LEISHMANIA* SPECIES

Raul E. Isturiz and Eduardo Gotuzzo

20

Human immunodeficiency virus (HIV) type 1 and 2 (HIV-1 and HIV-2) infections have had a profound impact on morbidity and mortality worldwide (84, 86). Two decades after the description of the first cases, the disease has spread to an estimated 60 million people worldwide (85). AIDS has evolved from an illness of men who have sex with men and of injection drug users into a large and expanding pandemic of heterosexually transmitted disease affecting men, women, and children across the globe (Table 1). Since the beginning of the epidemic, the modes of transmission of HIV have been known and have remained unchanged, but the relative importance of each mode varies considerably between regions and even between countries. Sexual contact (male to male and heterosexual) predominates, followed by injection drug use, but transmission through blood, blood products, body fluids, and organs as well as perinatal transmission continues to occur, albeit at a lesser scale in western societies. HIV-1 exhibits genetic diversity (38) and is currently divided into 10 subtypes, with M being the major subtype and O and N important, although infrequent, because they may not be detected by standard serological tests (77). More than 90% of infected individuals, particularly young adults, live in underprivileged areas of the world (85), where few have access to modern high-efficiency combination therapy. These patients experience the natural course of HIV infection and AIDS. They suffer from the strongest subversion of their immune systems, which makes them highly susceptible to opportunistic pathogens. Immunosuppression, the hallmark of HIV infection, is associated with the primary acquisition and growth of pathogens as well as the reactivation of latent infections. Opportunistic diseases resulting from immunosuppression occur more frequently in HIV-infected patients than in other immunosuppressed patient groups and may exhibit unique clinical characteristics. In the United States, the incidence of AIDS-related opportunistic infections appears to be leveling off after a dramatic increase and later decline (A. D. McNaghten, L. Hanson, A. K. Nakashima, and D. L. Swerdlow, *Annu. Meet. Infect. Dis. Soc. Am.,* p. 751, 2001).

This chapter concentrates on the interaction between HIV-1, immune suppression and reconstitution, and opportunistic microbes

Raul E. Isturiz, Centro Medico de Caracas and Centro Medico Docente La Trinidad, Caracas, Venezuela. *Eduardo Gotuzzo,* Alexander von Humboldt Institute of Tropical Medicine, Universidad Peruana Cayetano Heredia, Lima, Peru.

Polymicrobial Diseases, Edited by Kim A. Brogden and Janet M. Guthmiller,
© 2002 ASM Press, Washington, D.C.

TABLE 1 HIV infection data[a]

Parameter	No. of persons (millions)
People living with HIV/AIDS	
Total	40.0
Adults	37.2
Women	17.6
Children <15 yr old	2.7
Sub-Saharan Africa	28.1
North Africa and the Middle East	0.4
Latin America	1.4
Caribbean	0.4
North America	0.9
Western Europe	0.6
Eastern Europe and Central Asia	1.0
East Asia and the Pacific	1.0
Southeast Asia	6.1
New HIV infections in 2001.	5.0
Deaths due to HIV/AIDS in 2001.	3.0
Cumulative no. of deaths due to HIV/AIDS.	20.0
People infected through December 2001	60.0

[a] Modified from reference 85.

such as *Pneumocystis carinii, Toxoplasma gondii,* and *Leishmania* species.

HIV INFECTION AND AIDS

HIV-1 and HIV-2 are enveloped retroviruses containing two copies of positive-sense, single-stranded genomic RNA that is reverse transcribed to DNA for integration into the human genome (31). CD4[+] T lymphocytes are the preferred targets of infection, but macrophages and other cells may be infected as well. Cell entry is accomplished by a complex interaction between M-tropic HIV envelope molecules, the cellular structure, and a relevant coreceptor molecule, usually CCR5. Transmission into a new host is almost always followed by replication of M-tropic strains in that individual. Abnormalities in all aspects of immune defense are present in AIDS patients, including impaired T- and B-lymphocyte function and antigen-presenting cell ability as well as dysfunction of NK cells, monocytes/macrophages, dendritic cells, and neutrophils. However, progressive CD4[+] T-lymphocyte defects, both in number and in function, constitute the hallmark of AIDS. In fact, the loss of

immune competence can be estimated by the measurement of decreasing numbers of peripheral CD4[+] T cells and of their progressive loss of in vitro proliferative responses to recall antigens, alloantigens, and mitogens (16). The mechanisms of helper T-cell death and dysfunction appear to be multiple (17). Cellular activation, production of T-tropic HIV strain CC chemokines, and dysregulation of proinflammatory cytokine production contribute to HIV pathogenesis by enhancing viral replication, further suppressing the human antiviral response, and inducing cytopathic effects (17).

Despite a variety of measurable cellular and humoral immune responses that may partially control virus replication, progression of immunosuppression and disease ensues, with no correlation with the vigor of the response mounted by the host. This fact constitutes a major obstacle to the development of immunotherapy and vaccines against HIV. Insight has been gained by studying noninfected exposed individuals as well as infected nonprogressors (6, 57, 66).

The natural history of HIV in humans has been used for the development of a clinical classification and surveillance system. The first stage is a primary infection that can show no symptoms or is manifested by the acute retroviral syndrome, a nonspecific and clinically variable mononucleosis-like illness accompanied by high levels of viral load and mild, transient immune suppression. This is followed by a stage of asymptomatic infection during which active viral replication, widespread dissemination of virus, and seeding of organs occur despite the absence of symptoms. As the immune system is progressively ablated poorly differentiated stages of early symptomatic disease (i.e., persistent generalized lymphadenopathy, constitutional disease, wasting, and manifestations of diseases of the mouth, musculoskeletal system, skin, lung, kidney, eye, and heart) occur, followed by advanced immunodeficiency characterized by opportunistic, infectious, or malignant complications. Seropositivity, defined as a repeatedly reactive enzyme-linked immunosorbent assay (ELISA) confirmed by detection of two or more antibodies to HIV (p24, gp41, gp120, and gp160) by a more specific test such as the Western blot (10), is the rule except in the first 2 to 8 weeks after infection and in the very late stages. False-positive Western blot tests are rare (0.0004%) in blood donors (41). Highly sensitive and specific rapid tests that detect HIV-1 and HIV-2 antibodies are available (40). False-negatives are seen in patients with agammaglobulinemia, in other patients in the period between HIV acquisition and antibody response, and in patients with HIV-1 genetic variants and occur in 1 of 500,000 units of donated blood. Subtypes O (genetically very close to HIV-2) and N pose diagnostic problems.

The period from initial infection to disease or death in the absence of specific therapy has been estimated to be from 7 to 12 years (1). Throughout this time, including any time of benefit from antiretroviral drugs, the $CD4^+$-lymphocyte count (estimating the extent of immune compromise as well as the risk of opportunistic infections and neoplasms) and the HIV RNA level or viral load in plasma (indicating the replicative rate and threat to the immune system) are the best and most widely used laboratory prognostic markers for assessment of disease progression.

Management of HIV infection is very complex and has evolved rapidly. The understanding of viral replication dynamics, antiviral drug efficacy, pharmacokinetics, interactions, and toxicities has permitted the design of highly active but complex antiretroviral regimens. Highly active antiretroviral therapy (HAART) has been responsible for a drop in mortality rates from 29.4/100 person-years in 1995 to 8.8/100 person-years in 1997 (65) and an extension of the time required to develop AIDS, but there have been failures. Therapy should be started when the patient has quantifiable virus in plasma, and, since lack of compliance guarantees failure and facilitates HIV resistance, when the patient is ready to cope with difficult drug regimens (76). Most authorities consider initiation of antiretroviral combinations in asymptomatic naive patients at plasma viral loads of ≥30,000 (branched DNA) or ≥55,000 (reverse transcriptase PCR) copies/ml, irrespective of $CD4^+$ T-cell counts (82), as well as for patients with $CD4^+$-T-cell counts of ≤350 irrespective of viral loads in plasma (7). This is usually accomplished by use of a combination of two nucleoside reverse transcriptase inhibitors (NRTIs) plus a protease inhibitor or, alternatively, two NRTIs plus one nonnucleoside reverse transcriptase inhibitor (NNRTI) or three NRTIs (7). Certain combinations, combinations of two drugs, and monotherapy are not recommended. Failure of initial therapy is possible, and treatment options that call for major changes in the combination regimens have been designed (7, 8). Treatment options are also available for patients with the acute retroviral syndrome or with recent exposure to HIV and for prevention of perinatal transmission to the fetus. Resistant HIV can be detected by phenotypic and genotypic laboratory methods. Patients are closely monitored by their physicians, in areas including measurements of viral loads and $CD4^+$ T-cell counts, use of appropriate vaccines, prophylactic therapy, and many other medical and psychosocial aspects related to AIDS. Quality of life issues are always relevant. Prophylaxis of some opportunistic infections will be addressed in detail later in this chapter.

P. carinii

Infection by *P. carinii,* a ubiquitous fungus of global distribution but unknown habitat (68, 81), is a major cause of disease and lethality in AIDS patients, especially those not receiving HAART. This opportunistic pathogen poses a threat not only directly, but also by enhancing HIV replication (15). Healthy and presumably not-healthy humans are exposed to the organism early in life, as demonstrated by the large proportion of the normal population that exhibits serum anti-*Pneumocystis* antibodies (68). Reactivation of a latent infection and de novo exposure to the organisms have been implicated as pathogenic mechanisms (24). After being inhaled, the tropic yeast cell forms adhere tightly to alveolar type I pneumocytes, where the organisms tend to form clumps. Fungal growth is achieved by binary fission of yeast cells and probably sexual reproduction (55). For respiratory colonization and disease production, adherence between fungal polypeptide adhesins and the host's extracellular matrix proteins, such as fibronectin, vitronectin, and laminin (62, 87), surfactant proteins A and D, and the mannose receptor (26, 50) must occur. Different immune mechanisms participate in resistance against colonization and infection. $CD4^+$ T cells and macrophages, cell lines that are depleted or poorly functional in AIDS patients, are essential for fungal elimination (33–35). $CD4^+$ T cells act either by cytokine production (11, 12) and consequent induction of effector functions in other cells or by direct interactions through accessory receptors and coreceptors. In animals, the pivotal role of $CD4^+$ T-cells has been demonstrated by cell depletion and reconstitution experiments. Evidence of the importance of $CD4^+$ T-cells in humans has been based on the analysis of immune defects and their relationship to the development of pneumocystosis. Since the 1980s, HIV infection has superseded all other conditions as the most common predisposing illness for development of pulmonary and extrapulmonary pneumocystosis. $CD4^+$ T-cell counts of $\leq200/mm^3$ have strong positive predictive values that still define the need for prophylaxis in HIV patients. The decline in $CD4^+$-T-cell numbers and function in HIV patients has been extensively documented. Macrophages act by intra- or extracellular killing of the fungus, but this interaction is more complex and probably involves blastogenic responses (32) as well as formation of macrophages around yeast cells in a way analogous to granuloma formation (4). Disruption of this process in AIDS is likely to interfere with the immune response and lead to impaired clearance of the fungus. Recent evidence suggests that alveolar macrophages from persons with advanced HIV infection demonstrate a specific impairment of the gp-A- and mannose receptor-mediated oxidative burst response to *P. carinii* in vitro (43), which may contribute to the pathogenesis of pneumonia and perhaps extrapulmonary disease in these patients. The defect may also be found in neutrophils from AIDS patients with previous *P. carinii* pneumonia. In experiments, the defect was correctable in vitro by priming of the white blood cells with recombinant granulocyte and granulocyte-macrophage colony-stimulating factors (G-CSF/GM-CSF) (47). In vivo, quantitative differences in phagocytosis and degradation of *P. carinii* by alveolar macrophages may explain the large numbers of extracellular organisms found in bronchoalveolar lavage (BAL) specimens from AIDS patients (88). Impaired local or systemic humoral immunity also plays a role (24, 25, 71). Lower levels of immunoglobulin G (IgG) antibodies against *P. carinii* in HIV-infected patients (46) may contribute to the increased prevalence and severity of the disease.

In AIDS patients, proliferating *P. carinii* clumps gradually fill alveolar spaces, and then a characteristic foamy, eosinophilic exudate develops. As an indicator of fungal burden, cluster ratios appear to be more sensitive than organism counts for BAL specimens (80). Hyaline membrane formation, edema, and interstitial fibrosis follow. An interstitial pneumonia ensues.

Pneumocystis carinii pneumonia in AIDS patients often has an insidious onset and presents with progressive dry cough, retrosternal inspiratory discomfort, and shortness of breath, as well as constitutional symptoms such as fever, sweats, fatigue, and weight loss. Pleuritic chest pain is uncommon. The chest examination may be normal or rales are heard during inspiration, which may be incomplete. The chest radiograph, although also normal at times, is often helpful, demonstrating fine, heterogeneous, diffuse interstitial infiltrates extending from the hilar to the peripheral regions of both lungs. Atypical infiltrates, pneumothoraces, nodules, cavities, and effusions are seen sporadically, especially in patients receiving prophylactic inhaled pentamidine. Some degree of hypoxemia and elevation of lactic dehydrogenase levels in serum are common. In fact, the degree of hypoxemia on presentation is a prognostic indicator. High-resolution computerized tomography (CT), technetium-99 lung scans, and pulmonary function studies may prove helpful in diagnosis of pulmonary disease. Extrapulmonary pneumocystosis, commonly encountered in the lymph nodes, spleen, liver, bone marrow, gastrointestinal tract, eyes, thyroid, adrenal glands, and kidneys, may occur with or without lung involvement, most often in advanced patients receiving no systemic prophylaxis. Biopsy reveals eosinophilic foamy material and numerous fungal forms.

P. carinii cannot be cultured. Identification of the fungus from clinical specimens relies on a variety of procedures. Methenamine silver and Wright-Giemsa stains and their variants are widely used among pathology laboratories; immunofluorescence, also popular, appears to be more sensitive, and PCR appears to be even more so. In general, the more invasive the method of collection of the respiratory specimen, the better the diagnostic accuracy. Induced sputum, fiberoptic bronchoscopy, and BAL (instead of brushing) are preferred. Open-lung biopsy, performed infrequently, constitutes the current diagnostic "gold standard." Less invasive methods such as detection of antigenemia (42, 72) and serum antibodies (24, 42, 46, 72) are imperfect and seldom utilized. *S*-Adenosylmethionine levels are considered a promising diagnostic tool, but more-extensive studies are needed.

In HIV patients, untreated pneumocystosis progresses to death, but the prognosis is greatly improved by optimal management. Trimethoprim-sulfamethoxazole has been the drug of choice, but gene mutations that result in sulfonamide resistance have appeared (36, 56), which has made some experts utilize other regimens, such as dapsone plus trimethoprim and other drugs. Steroids are used to treat hypoxemic patients and to prevent the clinical relapse associated with the rapid death of *P. carinii* forms that occurs during treatment. The management of pulmonary pneumocystosis may be complicated by the simultaneous presence of other respiratory infections, the severity of the underlying immune suppression, and previous lung diseases. Recovery from pneumocystosis is common. Relapses and reinfections occur, and pneumothorax is a well-described complication after recovery. In patients receiving HAART, prophylaxis for *P. carinii* need not be lifelong, and the suggested threshold of 200 CD4$^+$ cells/μl can continue to be used in most cases for decisions regarding starting, discontinuation, and restarting of appropriate regimens.

An emerging clinical entity, immunorestitution disease (29), defined as an acute symptomatic or paradoxical deterioration of a pre-existing infection that follows the recovery of the immune system secondary to HAART, may be caused by *P. carinii* (13, 29).

T. gondii

Toxoplasmosis, a worldwide coccidian zoonosis with many animal reservoirs, is also a major cause of concern for HIV-infected patients. It commonly presents as a life-threatening disease of the central nervous system and other organs, more often in patients not receiving HAART or correct prophylaxis and having low CD4$^+$-T-cell counts. Humans can be infected with *T.*

gondii, an intracellular parasite, by ingestion of cysts and oocysts in raw or undercooked meats such as lamb, beef, pork, and venison or soil-contaminated foods or by transplacental vertical transmission (58), but in persons with AIDS, *T. gondii* causes disease mainly by reactivation of an infection acquired earlier in life (73). After ingestion, the parasite infects replication-permissive circulating monocytes in the intestinal lamina propria, which may transport the organism progressing to gastrointestinal lymphatics and later to various organs and tissues. Necrosis due to death of parasitized cells and lymphocytic infiltration follows. In immunocompetent hosts, replication of tachyzoites is controlled, and tissues are restored to anatomical integrity; cysts containing bradyzoites remain, rarely causing inflammation, mass effect, or clinical manifestations (67). Disruption of cyst forms followed by proliferation of the parasite and tissue destruction follows dissemination in individuals with deficient cell-mediated immunity (30, 63); thus, the incidence of toxoplasmosis in AIDS patients correlates with the prevalence of IgG antitoxoplasma antibodies and immune deficiency. Serologic surveys demonstrate variable rates of prevalence in healthy humans, ranging from negligible to >90% in different areas of the world (23, 75, 78). In AIDS patients, the incidence of toxoplasma encephalitis (TE) varies among different geographical regions and ethnic groups, probably reflecting differences in the prevalence of previous exposure and seropositivity (51, 73). The risk of clinical disease, essentially TE, among seropositive HIV-infected persons correlates well with their level of CD4$^+$ T cells (48), typically below 100/μl. Further, with severe depletion of T cells, blastogenic responses to *T. gondii* trophozoites are lost (9). Decreased in vitro lymphocyte proliferative responses and gamma interferon (IFN-γ) in the presence of *Toxoplasma* antigen have been recently found in seropositive HIV-1-infected patients, in inverse relation to CD4$^+$-T-cell counts (28). Prostaglandin E2 may reduce toxoplasmastatic activity of monocytes and monocyte-derived macrophages (19). Immune reconstitution under HAART restored the immune defects (28). GM-CSF-mediated toxoplasmastatic activity of monocytes from AIDS patients is reduced (20). Elaboration of protective cytokines, including interleukin 2 and IFN-γ, appears to be critical for disease control, and in AIDS patients, impaired production of both is documented (60, 61). AIDS patients with toxoplasmic lymphadenopathy have lower levels of IFN-γ than immunocompetent individuals (5). The pathogenesis of defective cytokine production remains unclear but appears to be related to an impaired CD40 ligand trimer signal (83).

Clinically, cerebral disease is most common, a multifocal necrotizing encephalitis characterized by enlarging necrosis and microglial nodules (64, 75). Less commonly, retinochoroiditis, pneumonitis, myocarditis, disseminated disease, and a sepsis-like syndrome have been reported (54). Altered mental status, focal neurological signs and symptoms, headache, and seizures, with or without fever and of subacute onset, are the main clinical features of TE. Some patients present with confusion, stupor, and coma. Meningeal signs are uncommon. The CD4$^+$-T-cell count is <100/μl for about 80% of patients. The main differential diagnosis is cerebral lymphoma, and less commonly other enhancing lesions such as metastatic carcinoma, tuberculoma, and brain abscess are diagnosed. Multiple, spherical, ring enhancing lesions with cortical, corticomedullary, and basal ganglia localizations are frequently seen by imaging procedures (14, 49). Magnetic resonance imaging (MRI) exhibits superior sensitivity and shows more extensive disease than is suspected clinically or evidenced by CT; therefore, MRI can be used as the initial procedure, especially when CT is negative or shows a single suggestive lesion (14, 49). MRI detection of single lesions does not separate TE from lymphoma, and a differentiating procedure is required. Brain biopsy is the gold standard, but positron emission tomography (70), radionuclide scanning magnetic resonance spectroscopy, and thallium-201 single-photon emission CT (79) have been used and continue to be studied.

Examination of cerebrospinal fluid is seldom rewarding and shows mononuclear pleocytosis and proteinorrhachia. Finding intrathecally produced antitoxoplasmal IgG supports the diagnosis but is not necessarily more useful than a positive dye test. *T. gondii* DNA can be detected in serum by PCR (27), which may be useful for monitoring the response to treatment.

The antitoxoplasma plasma IgG antibody titer is useful for confirming previous toxoplasma infection, and the titer has some prognostic value; however, no single test is perfect, and there is not one that reliably distinguishes active from latent or subclinical infection. Testing positive for IgG and negative for IgM is common in immunosuppressed patients. A negative test weights heavily against active reactivation toxoplasmosis. A panel of tests to measure different antibodies that have different time-related patterns is available. A complete description of each serological test is beyond the scope of this chapter and can be found in reference 59.

Untreated cerebral toxoplasmosis in AIDS patients is lethal, but treatment is highly successful. In vitro growth of *Toxoplasma* organisms is markedly and continuously inhibited 1 day after initiation of therapy with pyrimethamine-sulfadiazine; the inhibition does not correlate well with the levels of pyrimethamine in blood and seems potentiated by sulfadiazine more than by macrolides (21). The note of response to empirical treatment is over 85% by day 7; hence, a diagnostic biopsy can be avoided if a response is documented (Editorial, *Lancet* **340**:1135, 1992). Dementia appears to be a more common late sequela than previously thought. Pyrimethamine combined with sulfadiazine and folinic acid or trimethoprim-sufamethoxazole is the primary suggested regimen. Pyrimethamine and folinic acid plus clindamycin, clarithromycin, azithromycin, or dapsone are an alternative regimen.

Seropositive individuals who have $CD4^+$-T-cell counts of $<100/\mu l$ should receive prophylaxis against TE. Trimethoprim-sul-famethoxazole and dapsone-pyrimethamine as for *P. carinii* are recommended. Prophylaxis can be discontinued in patients who have responded to HAART with an increase in $CD4^+$-T-cell counts to above $200/\mu l$ for 3 months and reintroduced if the $CD4^+$-T-cell count decreases to <100 to $200/\mu l$. After initial therapy for TE, suppressive treatment is necessary for life unless immune reconstitution is achieved. During pregnancy, pyrimethamine treatment is best avoided. Infants born to women seropositive for HIV and toxoplasmosis should be evaluated for congenital toxoplasmosis.

Leishmania donovani and *Leishmania infantum*

Visceral leishmaniasis, a vector-borne intramacrophage protozoosis, has emerged as an opportunistic HIV coinfection in the Mediterranean Basin (2), especially in southern France, Spain, and Italy (37), where a novel artificial (syringes instead of sand flies), epidemic (unusually large numbers of cases and the proportion of adults with visceral leishmaniasis that are coinfected with HIV), and anthroponotic (the reservoir for parasites is human drug addicts) cycle has been proposed (3), in contrast to the zoonotic transmission cycle. Furthermore, *L. donovani* has been considered a cofactor in the pathogenesis of HIV infection because its lipophosphoglycan up-regulates HIV-1 transcription in $CD4^+$ T cells. The immunopathogenic mechanisms of *Leishmania*-HIV interaction have been recently reviewed in detail (89). *L. infantum* (of the *L. donovani* species complex) is endemic in rural areas of France, extending to the Mediterranean littoral and to the Middle East into western China, and with canine reservoirs constitutes the predominant coinfection species. The coinfection has been reported in 33 countries (22), mostly in southern Europe, where 25 to 70% of leishmaniasis patients are coinfected with HIV and 1.5 to 9% of patients with AIDS have leishmaniasis (90). Although children are sometimes coinfected, the age range is usually 29 to 33 years. There are more cases of coinfection caused by intravenous drug use (50 to 92%) than by any sexual transmission (5 to 40%); transfusion accounts for 4 to 13% of cases, and unknown causes account for 3%.

L. infantum strains isolated from individuals coinfected with HIV show great enzymatic variability in Spain and Italy and less in France, especially in the southern areas; this heterogeneity includes many known and even newly described zymodemes (39). Interestingly, sequential isolates from the same individual belong to the same zymodeme, suggesting relapse rather than reinfection (74). Common strains or cutaneous strains (for example, *Vinnia braziliensis*) of low virulence may cause widespread disease.

For HIV patients, questions concerning the incubation period and primary infection versus reactivation of a previous infection remain, and asymptomatic leishmania infections have been described (18).

Each infection (HIV and *Leishmania* spp.) induces immunological responses and eventually immune suppression. HIV-induced T-cell-mediated immunosuppression favors visceral dissemination of leishmaniasis. The CD4$^+$-T-cell count is below 200/μl for up to 90% of patients (2); therefore, over two-thirds of cases present clinically with typical disseminated visceral disease in which amastigotes can be identified in virtually any body organ. However, rare manifestations, such as aplastic anemia, cutaneous leishmaniasis (including diffuse cutaneous and atypical disease), mucocutaneous leishmaniasis, and combinations are seen, less frequently. Splenomegaly may be absent. Gastrointestinal complaints may be important symptoms (44). The level of coexistence of other opportunistic infections is unusually high, around 50%.

Although parasites abound in tissues in HIV-infected patients coinfected with *Leishmania* spp., making parasitological diagnosis relatively simple, serological tests that detect antibody may be negative, especially for patients infected first with HIV and in later stages of AIDS. Levels of antibodies, when present, are lower than those of immunocompetent in-

dividuals (53). Up to 20% of coinfected patients showed negative results with all methods utilized, including indirect immunofluorescence, ELISA, and Western blotting, when a diagnostic serology panel was used (69). Western blotting is the most sensitive. A defect in antigen presentation by macrophages or in T- and B-lymphocyte cooperation may be responsible for lower or nonexistent antibody levels (45, 52). Direct microscopic examination, culture in NNN medium, and PCR are clinically in use. They are commonly performed with bone marrow samples, the diagnostic gold standard, but the observation of parasitized macrophages in peripheral blood is encouraging as a simpler method.

Treatment of leishmaniasis in HIV-infected patients with pentavalent antimonial salts alone or combined with allopurinol, aminosidine, or IFN-γ, as well as therapy with lipid (effective and less toxic) and nonlipid amphotericin B, can proceed in a standard fashion (2), but toxicity is greater than in immunocompetent individuals. Pentamidine is toxic, and ketoconazole and itraconazole are likely to fail. Treatment, when successful, may need to be prolonged to avoid relapses. Prophylaxis could be helpful.

REFERENCES

1. **Alcabes, P., A. Munoz, D. Vlahov, and G. H. Friedland.** 1993. Incubation period of human immunodeficiency virus. *Epidemiol. Rev.* **15:**303–318.
2. **Alvar, J., C. Canavate, B. Gutierrez-Solar, M. Jimenez, F. Laguna, R. Lopez-Velez, R. Molina, and J. Moreno.** 1997. Leishmania and human immunodeficiency virus coinfection: the first 10 years. *Clin. Microbiol. Rev.* **10:**298–319.
3. **Alvar, J., B. Gutierrez-Solar, I. Pachon, E. Calbacho, M. Ramirez, R. Valles, J. L. Guillen, C. Canavate, and C. Amela.** 1996. AIDS and *Leishmania infantum.* New approaches for a new epidemiological problem. *Clin. Dermatol.* **14:**541–546.
4. **Blumenfeld, W., O. McCook, and J. M. Griffiss.** 1991. In vitro aggregation of macrophages around human-derived *Pneumocystis carinii. J. Protozool.* **38:**32S–33S.
5. **Canessa, A., V. Del Bono, F. Miletich, and V. Pistoia.** 1992. Serum cytokines in toxoplas-

mosis: increased levels of interferon-gamma in immunocompetent patients with lymphadenopathy but not in AIDS patients with encephalitis. *J. Infect. Dis.* **165:**1168–1170.

6. **Cao, Y., L. Qin, L. Zhang, J. Safrit, and D. D. Ho.** 1995. Virologic and immunologic characterization of long-term survivors of human immunodeficiency virus type 1 infection. *N. Engl. J. Med.* **332:**201–208.

7. **Carpenter, C. C., D. A. Cooper, M. A. Fischl, J. M. Gatell, B. G. Gazzard, S. M. Hammer, M. S. Hirsch, D. M. Jacobsen, D. A. Katzenstein, J. S. Montaner, D. D. Richman, M. S. Saag, M. Schechter, R. T. Schooley, M. A. Thompson, S. Vella, P. G. Yeni, and P. A. Volberding.** 2000. Antiretroviral therapy in adults: updated recommendations of the International AIDS Society–USA Panel. *JAMA* **283:**381–390.

8. **Carpenter, C. C., M. A. Fischl, S. M. Hammer, M. S. Hirsch, D. M. Jacobsen, D. A. Katzenstein, J. S. Montaner, D. D. Richman, M. S. Saag, R. T. Schooley, M. A. Thompson, S. Vella, P. G. Yeni, and P. A. Volberding.** 1998. Antiretroviral therapy for HIV infection in 1998: updated recommendations of the International AIDS Society–USA Panel. *JAMA* **280:**78–86.

9. **Carrega, G., A. Canessa, P. Argenta, M. Cruciani, and D. Bassetti.** 1995. T cell blastogenic responses to *Toxoplasma gondii* trophozoites among HIV-infected patients. *AIDS Res. Hum. Retrovir.* **11:**741–746.

10. **Centers for Disease Control and Prevention.** 1989. Interpretation and use of the Western blot assay for serodiagnosis of human immunodeficiency virus type 1 infections. *Morb. Mortal. Wkly. Rep.* **38:**1–7.

11. **Chen, W., E. A. Havell, and A. G. Harmsen.** 1992. Importance of endogenous tumor necrosis factor alpha and gamma interferon in host resistance against *Pneumocystis carinii* infection. *Infect. Immun.* **60:**1279–1284.

12. **Chen, W., E. A. Havell, L. L. Moldawer, K. W. McIntyre, R. A. Chizzonite, and A. G. Harmsen.** 1992. Interleukin 1: an important mediator of host resistance against *Pneumocystis carinii*. *J. Exp. Med.* **176:**713–718.

13. **Cheng, V. C., K. Y. Yuen, W. M. Chan, S. S. Wong, E. S. Ma, and R. M. Chan.** 2000. Immunorestitution disease involving the innate and adaptive response. *Clin. Infect. Dis.* **30:**882–892.

14. **Ciricillo, S. F., and M. L. Rosenblum.** 1990. Use of CT and MR imaging to distinguish intracranial lesions and to define the need for biopsy in AIDS patients. *J. Neurosurg.* **73:**720–724.

15. **Clarke, J. R., and D. Israel-Biet.** 1996. Interactions between opportunistic microorganisms and HIV in the lung. *Thorax* **51:**875–877.

16. **Clerici, M., N. I. Stocks, R. A. Zajac, R. N. Boswell, D. R. Lucey, C. S. Via, and G. M. Shearer.** 1989. Detection of three distinct patterns of T helper cell dysfunction in asymptomatic, human immunodeficiency virus-seropositive patients. Independence of CD4$^+$ cell numbers and clinical staging. *J. Clin. Invest.* **84:**1892–1899.

17. **Cohen, O., C. Cicala, M. Vaccarezza, and A. S. Fauci.** 2000. The immunology of human immunodeficiency virus infection, p. 1374–1397. *In* G. L. Mandell, J. E. Bennett, and R. F. Dolin (ed.), *Principles and Practice of Infectious Diseases,* 5th ed. Churchill Livingstone, Philadelphia, Pa.

18. **Condom, M. J., B. Clotet, G. Sirera, F. Milla, and M. Foz.** 1989. Asymptomatic leishmaniasis in the acquired immunodeficiency syndrome (AIDS). *Ann. Intern. Med.* **111:**767–768.

19. **Delemarre, F. G., A. Stevenhagen, F. P. Kroon, M. Y. van Eer, P. L. Meenhorst, and R. van Furth.** 1995. Reduced toxoplasmastatic activity of monocytes and monocyte-derived macrophages from AIDS patients is mediated via prostaglandin E2. *AIDS* **9:**441–445.

20. **Delemarre, F. G., A. Stevenhagen, F. P. Kroon, and R. van Furth.** 1998. Reduced toxoplasmastatic activity of monocytes from AIDS patients: a role for granulocyte-macrophage colony-stimulating factor. *Scand. J. Immunol.* **47:**163–166.

21. **Derouin, F., L. Gerard, R. Farinotti, C. Maslo, and C. Leport.** 1998. Determination of the inhibitory effect on Toxoplasma growth in the serum of AIDS patients during acute therapy for toxoplasmic encephalitis. *J. Acquir. Immune Defic. Syndr. Hum. Retrovirol.* **19:**50–54.

22. **Desjeux, P., B. Piot, K. O'Neill, and J. P. Meert.** 2001. Co-infections of leishmania/HIV in south Europe. *Med. Trop.* **61:**187–193.

23. **Desmonts, G., and J. Couvreur.** 1974. Toxoplasmosis in pregnancy and its transmission to the fetus. *Bull. N. Y. Acad. Med.* **50:**146–159.

24. **Elvin, K., A. Bjorkman, N. Heurlin, B. M. Eriksson, L. Barkholt, and E. Linder.** 1994. Seroreactivity to *Pneumocystis carinii* in patients with AIDS versus other immunosuppressed patients. *Scand. J. Infect. Dis.* **26:**33–40.

25. **Elvin, K., C. Lidman, E. Tynell, E. Linder, and A. Bjorkman.** 1994. Natural history of asymptomatic and symptomatic *Pneumocystis carinii* infection in HIV infected patients. *Scand. J. Infect. Dis.* **26:**643–651.

26. **Ezekowitz, R. A., D. J. Williams, H. Koziel, M. Y. Armstrong, A. Warner, F. F. Richards, and R. M. Rose.** 1991. Uptake of

Pneumocystis carinii mediated by the macrophage mannose receptor. *Nature* **351**:155–158.

27. **Foudrinier, F., D. Aubert, D. Puygauthier-Toubas, C. Rouger, I. Beguinot, P. Halbout, P. Lemaire, C. Marx-Chemla, and J. M. Pinon.** 1996. Detection of *Toxoplasma gondii* in immunodeficient subjects by gene amplification: influence of therapeutics. *Scand. J. Infect. Dis.* **28**:383–386.

28. **Fournier, S., C. Rabian, C. Alberti, M. V. Carmagnat, J. F. Garin, D. Charron, F. Derouin, and J. M. Molina.** 2001. Immune recovery under highly active antiretroviral therapy is associated with restoration of lymphocyte proliferation and interferon-gamma production in the presence of *Toxoplasma gondii* antigens. *J. Infect. Dis.* **183**:1586–1591.

29. **French, M. A., and P. Price.** 2001. Immune restoration disease in HIV-infected patients after antiretroviral therapy. *Clin. Infect. Dis.* **32**:325–326.

30. **Frenkel, J. K., B. M. Nelson, and J. Arias-Stella.** 1975. Immunosuppression and toxoplasmic encephalitis: clinical and experimental aspects. *Hum. Pathol.* **6**:97–111.

31. **Greene, W. C.** 1991. The molecular biology of human immunodeficiency virus type 1 infection. *N. Engl. J. Med.* **324**:308–317.

32. **Hagler, D. N., G. S. Deepe, C. L. Pogue, and P. D. Walzer.** 1988. Blastogenic responses to *Pneumocystis carinii* among patients with human immunodeficiency (HIV) infection. *Clin. Exp. Immunol.* **74**:7–13.

33. **Hanano, R., and S. H. Kaufmann.** 1998. Immune responses to naturally acquired *Pneumocystis carinii* in gene disruption mutant mice. *Res. Immunol.* **149**:429–435, 514.

34. **Hanano, R., and S. H. Kaufmann.** 1998. *Pneumocystis carinii* and the immune response in disease. *Trends Microbiol.* **6**:71–75.

35. **Hanano, R., K. Reifenberg, and S. H. Kaufmann.** 1998. Activated pulmonary macrophages are insufficient for resistance against *Pneumocystis carinii*. *Infect. Immun.* **66**:305–314.

36. **Helweg-Larsen, J., T. L. Benfield, J. Eugen-Olsen, J. D. Lundgren, and B. Lundgren.** 1999. Effects of mutations in *Pneumocystis carinii* dihydropteroate synthase gene on outcome of AIDS-associated *P. carinii* pneumonia. *Lancet* **354**:1347–1351.

37. **Herwaldt, B. L.** 1999. Leishmaniasis. *Lancet* **354**:1191–1199.

38. **Hu, D. J., T. J. Dondero, M. A. Rayfield, J. R. George, G. Schochetman, H. W. Jaffe, C. C. Luo, M. L. Kalish, B. G. Weniger, C. P. Pau, C. A. Schable, and J. W. Curran.** 1996. The emerging genetic diversity of HIV.

The importance of global surveillance for diagnostics, research, and prevention. *JAMA* **275**:10–216.

39. **Jimenez, M. I., F. Laguna, F. de la Torre, F. Solis, F. Pratlong, and J. Alvar.** 1995. New *Leishmania (Leishmania) infantum* zymodemes responsible for visceral leishmaniasis in patients coinfected with HIV in Spain. *Trans. R. Soc. Trop. Med. Hyg.* **89**:33.

40. **Kassler, W. J., C. Haley, W. K. Jones, A. R. Gerber, E. J. Kennedy, and J. R. George.** 1995. Performance of a rapid, on-site human immunodeficiency virus antibody assay in a public health setting. *J. Clin. Microbiol.* **33**:2899–2902.

41. **Kleinman, S., M. P. Busch, L. Hall, R. Thomson, S. Glynn, D. Gallahan, H. E. Ownby, and A. E. Williams for the Retrovirus Epidemiology Donor Study.** 1998. False-positive HIV-1 test results in a low-risk screening setting of voluntary blood donation. *JAMA* **280**:1080–1085.

42. **Kovacs, J. A., J. L. Halpern, J. C. Swan, J. Moss, J. E. Parrillo, and H. Masur.** 1988. Identification of antigens and antibodies specific for *Pneumocystis carinii*. *J. Immunol.* **140**:2023–2031.

43. **Koziel, H., X. Li, M. Y. Armstrong, F. F. Richards, and R. M. Rose.** 2000. Alveolar macrophages from human immunodeficiency virus-infected persons demonstrate impaired oxidative burst response to *Pneumocystis carinii* in vitro. *Am. J. Respir. Cell Mol. Biol.* **23**:452–459.

44. **Laguna, F., J. Garcia-Samaniego, V. Soriano, E. Valencia, C. Redondo, M. J. Alonso, and J. M. Gonzalez-Lahoz.** 1994. Gastrointestinal leishmaniasis in human immunodeficiency virus-infected patients: report of five cases and review. *Clin. Infect. Dis.* **19**:48–53.

45. **Lane, H. C., H. Masur, L. C. Edgar, G. Whalen, A. H. Rook, and A. S. Fauci.** 1983. Abnormalities of B-cell activation and immunoregulation in patients with the acquired immunodeficiency syndrome. *N. Engl. J. Med.* **309**:453–458.

46. **Laursen, A. L., and P. L. Andersen.** 1998. Low levels of IgG antibodies against *Pneumocystis carinii* among HIV-infected patients. *Scand. J. Infect. Dis.* **30**:495–499.

47. **Laursen, A. L., J. Rungby, and P. L. Andersen.** 1995. Decreased activation of the respiratory burst in neutrophils from AIDS patients with previous *Pneumocystis carinii* pneumonia. *J. Infect. Dis.* **172**:497–505.

48. **Leport, C., G. Chene, P. Morlat, B. J. Luft, F. Rousseau, S. Pueyo, R. Hafner, J. Miro, J. Aubertin, R. Salamon, J. L. Vilde, ANRS 005-ACTG 154 Group Members, Agence Nationale de Recherche sur le SIDA,**

and **AIDS Clinical Trial Group.** 1996. Pyrimethamine for primary prophylaxis of toxoplasmic encephalitis in patients with human immunodeficiency virus infection: a double-blind, randomized trial. *J. Infect. Dis.* **173:**91–97.

49. **Levy, R. M., C. M. Mills, J. P. Posin, S. G. Moore, M. L. Rosenblum, and D. E. Bredesen.** 1990. The efficacy and clinical impact of brain imaging in neurologically symptomatic AIDS patients: a prospective CT/MRI study. *J. Acquir. Immune Defic. Syndr.* **3:**461–471.

50. **Limper, A. H.** 1995. Adhesive glycoproteins in the pathogenesis of *Pneumocystis carinii* pneumonia: host defense or microbial offense? *J. Lab. Clin. Med.* **125:**12–13.

51. **Luft, B. J., and J. S. Remington.** 1992. Toxoplasmic encephalitis in AIDS. *Clin. Infect. Dis.* **15:**211–222.

52. **Macatonia, S. E., R. Lau, S. Patterson, A. J. Pinching, and S. C. Knight.** 1990. Dendritic cell infection, depletion and dysfunction in HIV-infected individuals. *Immunology* **71:**38–45.

53. **Mary, C., D. Lamouroux, S. Dunan, and M. Quilici.** 1992. Western blot analysis of antibodies to *Leishmania infantum* antigens: potential of the 14-kD and 16-kD antigens for diagnosis and epidemiologic purposes. *Am. J. Trop. Med. Hyg.* **47:**764–771.

54. **Masur, H.** 2000. Management of opportunistic infections associated with human immunodeficiency virus infection, p. 1500–1519. *In* G. L. Mandell, J. E. Bennett, and R. F. Dolin (ed.), *Principles and Practice of Infectious Diseases,* 5th ed. Churchill Livingstone, Philadelphia, Pa.

55. **Matsumoto, Y., and Y. Yoshida.** 1984. Sporogony in *Pneumocystis carinii:* synaptonemal complexes and meiotic nuclear divisions observed in precysts. *J. Protozool.* **31:**420–428.

56. **Meshnick, S. R.** 1999. Drug-resistant *Pneumocystis carinii. Lancet* **354:**1318–1319.

57. **Meyer, L., M. Magierowska, J. B. Hubert, C. Rouzioux, C. Deveau, F. Sanson, P. Debre, J. F. Delfraissy, I. Theodorou, and the SEROCO Study Group.** 1997. Early protective effect of CCR-5 delta 32 heterozygosity on HIV-1 disease progression: relationship with viral load. *AIDS* **11:**F73–F78.

58. **Minkoff, H., J. S. Remington, S. Holman, R. Ramirez, S. Goodwin, and S. Landesman.** 1997. Vertical transmission of toxoplasma by human immunodeficiency virus-infected women. *Am. J. Obstet. Gynecol.* **176:**555–559.

59. **Montoya, J. G., and J. S. Remington.** 2000. *Toxoplasma gondii,* p. 2858–2888. *In* G. L. Mandell, J. E. Bennett, and R. F. Dolin (ed.), *Principles and Practice of Infectious Diseases,* 5th ed. Churchill Livingstone, Philadelphia, Pa.

60. **Murray, H. W., B. Y. Rubin, H. Masur, and R. B. Roberts.** 1984. Impaired production of lymphokines and immune (gamma) interferon in the acquired immunodeficiency syndrome. *N. Engl. J. Med.* **310:**883–889.

61. **Murray, H. W., K. Welte, J. L. Jacobs, B. Y. Rubin, R. Mertelsmann, and R. B. Roberts.** 1985. Production of and in vitro response to interleukin 2 in the acquired immunodeficiency syndrome. *J. Clin. Investig.* **76:**1959–1964.

62. **Narasimhan, S., M. Y. Armstrong, K. Rhee, J. C. Edman, F. F. Richards, and E. Spicer.** 1994. Gene for an extracellular matrix receptor protein from *Pneumocystis carinii. Proc. Natl. Acad. Sci. USA* **91:**7440–7444.

63. **Navia, B. A., C. K. Petito, J. W. Gold, E. S. Cho, B. D. Jordan, and R. W. Price.** 1986. Cerebral toxoplasmosis complicating the acquired immune deficiency syndrome: clinical and neuropathological findings in 27 patients. *Ann. Neurol.* **19:**224–238.

64. **Nebuloni, M., A. Pellegrinelli, A. Ferri, A. Tosoni, S. Bonetto, P. Zerbi, R. Boldorini, L. Vago, and G. Costanzi.** 2000. Etiology of microglial nodules in brains of patients with acquired immunodeficiency syndrome. *J. Neurovirol.* **6:**46–50.

65. **Palella, F. J., Jr., K. M. Delaney, A. C. Moorman, M. O. Loveless, J. Fuhrer, G. A. Satten, D. J. Aschman, S. D. Holmberg, and the HIV Outpatient Study Investigators.** 1998. Declining morbidity and mortality among patients with advanced human immunodeficiency virus infection. *N. Engl. J. Med.* **338:**853–860.

66. **Pantaleo, G., S. Menzo, M. Vaccarezza, C. Graziosi, O. J. Cohen, J. F. Demarest, D. Montefiori, J. M. Orenstein, C. Fox, L. K. Schrager, et al.** 1995. Studies in subjects with long-term nonprogressive human immunodeficiency virus infection. *N. Engl. J. Med.* **332:** 209–216.

67. **Pavesio, C. E., M. L. Chiappino, P. Y. Setzer, and B. A. Nichols.** 1992. *Toxoplasma gondii:* differentiation and death of bradyzoites. *Parasitol. Res.* **78:**1–9.

68. **Peglow, S. L., A. G. Smulian, M. J. Linke, C. L. Pogue, S. Nurre, J. Crisler, J. Phair, J. W. Gold, D. Armstrong, and P. D. Walzer.** 1990. Serologic responses to *Pneumocystis carinii* antigens in health and disease. *J. Infect. Dis.* **161:**296–306.

69. **Piarroux, R., F. Gambarelli, H. Dumon, M. Fontes, S. Dunan, C. Mary, B. Toga, and M. Quilici.** 1994. Comparison of PCR with direct examination of bone marrow aspiration, myeloculture, and serology for diagnosis of visceral leishmaniasis in immunocompromised patients. *J. Clin. Microbiol.* **32:**746–749.

70. **Pierce, M. A., M. D. Johnson, R. J. Maciunas, M. J. Murray, G. S. Allen, M. A. Harbison, J. L. Creasy, and R. M. Kessler.** 1995. Evaluating contrast-enhancing brain lesions in patients with AIDS by using positron emission tomography. *Ann. Intern. Med.* **123:**594–598.

71. **Pifer, L. L., H. B. Niell, S. B. Langdon, S. Baltz, S. T. Clark, C. C. Edwards, and D. R. Woods.** 1987. Evidence for depressed humoral immunity to *Pneumocystis carinii* in homosexual males, commercial plasma donors, and patients with acquired immunodeficiency syndrome. *J. Clin. Microbiol.* **25:**991–995.

72. **Pifer, L. W., B. L. Wolf, J. J. Weems, Jr., D. R. Woods, C. C. Edwards, and R. E. Joyner.** 1988. *Pneumocystis carinii* antigenemia in acquired immunodeficiency syndrome. *J. Clin. Microbiol.* **26:**1357–1361.

73. **Porter, S. B., and M. A. Sande.** 1992. Toxoplasmosis of the central nervous system in the acquired immunodeficiency syndrome. *N. Engl. J. Med.* **327:**1643–1648.

74. **Pratlong, F., J. P. Dedet, P. Marty, M. Portus, M. Deniau, J. Dereure, P. Abranches, J. Reynes, A. Martini, M. Lefebvre, et al.** 1995. Leishmania-human immunodeficiency virus coinfection in the Mediterranean basin: isoenzymatic characterization of 100 isolates of the Leishmania infantum complex. *J. Infect. Dis.* **172:**323–326.

75. **Remington, J. S., R. McLeod, and G. Desmonts.** 1995. Toxoplasmosis, p. 140–266. *In* J. S. Remington and J. O. Klein (ed.), *Infectious Diseases of the Fetus and Newborn Infants.* W. B. Saunders, Philadelphia, Pa.

76. **Sherer, R.** 1998. Adherence and antiretroviral therapy in injection drug users. *JAMA* **280:**567–568.

77. **Simon, F., P. Mauclere, P. Roques, I. Loussert-Ajaka, M. C. Muller-Trutwin, S. Saragosti, M. C. Georges-Courbot, F. Barre-Sinoussi, and F. Brun-Vezinet.** 1998. Identification of a new human immunodeficiency virus type 1 distinct from group M and group O. *Nat. Med.* **4:**1032–1037.

78. **Sinibaldi, J., and I. De Ramirez.** 1992. Incidence of congenital toxoplasmosis in live Guatemalan newborns. *Eur. J. Epidemiol.* **8:**516–520.

79. **Skiest, D. J., W. Erdman, W. E. Chang, O. K. Oz, A. Ware, and J. Fleckenstein.** 2000. SPECT thallium-201 combined with Toxoplasma serology for the presumptive diagnosis of focal central nervous system mass lesions in patients with AIDS. *J. Infect.* **40:**274–281.

80. **Smulian, A. G., M. J. Linke, M. T. Cushion, R. P. Baughman, P. T. Frame, M. N. Dohn, M. L. White, and P. D. Walzer.** 1994. Analysis of *Pneumocystis carinii* organism burden, viability and antigens in bronchoalveolar lavage fluid in AIDS patients with pneumocystosis: correlation with disease severity. *AIDS* **8:**1555–1562.

81. **Smulian, A. G., D. W. Sullivan, M. J. Linke, N. A. Halsey, T. C. Quinn, A. P. MacPhail, M. A. Hernandez-Avila, S. T. Hong, and P. D. Walzer.** 1993. Geographic variation in the humoral response to *Pneumocystis carinii. J. Infect. Dis.* **167:**1243–1247.

82. **Stephenson, J.** 2001. New HIV therapy guidelines. *JAMA* **285:**1281.

83. **Subauste, C. S., M. Wessendarp, A. G. Smulian, and P. T. Frame.** 2001. Role of CD40 ligand signaling in defective type 1 cytokine response in human immunodeficiency virus infection. *J. Infect. Dis.* **183:**1722–1731.

84. **UNAIDS and World Health Organization.** 1998. *AIDS Epidemic Update.* UNAIDS, Geneva, Switzerland.

85. **UNAIDS and World Health Organization.** 2001. *AIDS Epidemic Update.* UNAIDS, Geneva, Switzerland.

86. **UNAIDS and World Health Organization.** 1998. *Report on the Global HIV/AIDS Epidemic.* UNAIDS, Geneva, Switzerland.

87. **Walzer, P. D.** 1986. Attachment of microbes to host cells: relevance of *Pneumocystis carinii. Lab. Invest.* **54:**589–592.

88. **Wehle, K., M. Schirmer, J. Dunnebacke-Hinz, T. Kupper, and P. Pfitzer.** 1993. Quantitative differences in phagocytosis and degradation of *Pneumocystis carinii* by alveolar macrophages in AIDS and non-HIV patients in vivo. *Cytopathology* **4:**231–236.

89. **Wolday, D., N. Berhe, H. Akuffo, and S. Britton.** 1999. Leishmania-HIV interaction: immunopathogenic mechanisms. *Parasitol. Today* **15:**182–187.

90. **World Health Organization.** 1995. *Report on the Consultative Meeting on leishmaniasis/HIV Coinfection,* p. 35. World Health Organization, Rome, Italy.

CONCLUDING
PERSPECTIVE

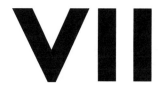

POLYMICROBIAL DISEASES: CURRENT AND FUTURE RESEARCH

Kim A. Brogden and Janet M. Guthmiller

21

According to the developing concept of polymicrobial diseases, some diseases in both animals and humans result from infections by multiple pathogens. In chapter 17, Soll defines polymicrobial diseases as those diseases that can occur with organisms from different kingdoms, from different genera in a kingdom, from different species in a genus, from different strains in a species, and finally from different substrains in a strain. In chapter 1, Brogden reviews the literature and provides lists of the many diseases induced by multiple pathogens. Although the concept of polymicrobial diseases is not new, this book provides a unique collection of polymicrobial diseases and categorizes the diseases in animals and humans on the basis of etiology, i.e., diseases that originate from polyviral infections, polybacterial infections, viral and bacterial infections, and polymicrobial mycotic infections, and those that result from microbe-induced immunosuppression. Chapter 1 concludes with a section on the common underlying mechanisms of pathogenesis.

In assembling the text, it became obvious that research of polymicrobial diseases still requires extensive study. In some areas, current research focuses on identifying the spectrum of etiologic agents involved. These include many polymicrobial diseases in animals (e.g., chapters 3, 10, 12, and 13) and humans (e.g., chapters 5 to 7 and 15 to 18). In other areas, research has progressed beyond the identification of etiologic agents to focus on mechanisms of microbial interaction, host response to infection, and mechanisms of disease pathogenesis. These include hepatotropic viral diseases (chapter 4), periodontal diseases (chapter 8), abscesses (chapter 9), otitis media (chapter 14), respiratory diseases (chapters 11 to 13), and disease resulting from microbe-induced immunosuppression (chapters 19 and 20). As research continues, we anticipate advances in several key areas including those discussed below.

NEW POLYMICROBIAL DISEASES

The number of polymicrobial diseases will undoubtedly increase. In animals, new polymicrobial diseases are likely to include poult enteritis mortality syndrome (PEMS) in turkeys (17, 41, 52), papillomatous digital dermatitis in dairy cattle (5, 14, 50), postweaning multisystemic wasting syndrome in pigs (1, 2, 23), and

Kim A. Brogden, Respiratory Diseases of Livestock Research Unit, National Animal Disease Center, USDA Agricultural Research Service, Ames, IA 50010. *Janet M. Guthmiller,* Department of Periodontics and Dows Institute for Dental Research, College of Dentistry, University of Iowa, Iowa City, IA 52252.

acute interstitial pneumonia in cattle (20). In humans, new polymicrobial diseases may include multiple sclerosis (6, 18, 32), Alzheimer's disease (53), atherosclerosis (34), and other chronic diseases (22, 53). Chronic diseases, such as atherosclerosis, have complex causal mechanisms, which include an infectious hypothesis (34). As one example, *Chlamydia pneumoniae,* cytomegalovirus, herpes simplex virus type 1, *Porphyromonas gingivalis,* and *Streptococcus sanguis* were detected in carotid plaques (8), and from one to four organisms were found in the same specimen. These microorganisms were localized in plaque shoulders and lymphohistiocytic infiltrates associated with ulcer and thrombus formation and found adjacent to areas of strong labeling for apoptotic bodies. The data provided evidence that multiple infectious agents may be found in atherosclerotic plaques, and sometimes in the same specimen (8). The data do not confirm pathogenic potential of individual organisms but do suggest possible synergy between organisms and a cumulative infection in atherogenesis (34).

Finally, there is optimism that an infectious etiology, possibly polymicrobial in nature, will be found for Kawasaki disease, sarcoidosis, multiple sclerosis, neurodegenerative disorders, arthritis, inflammatory bowel disease, and autoimmune disease (22, 34, 53).

ETIOLOGIC AGENTS

Identification of new etiologic agents involved in polymicrobial diseases will require improved analytic tools. Current reagents and methods are not sufficient to prove or refute a potential polymicrobial etiology of many chronic diseases, including atherosclerosis (34). Culturing fastidious agents is difficult; serology relies on tedious, reagent- and reader-dependent immunofluorescent assays; and immunocytochemistry can be subjective. The practical diagnostic usefulness of molecular assays has consistently fallen short, in part, because these methods are time consuming and expensive, and they require the assistance and interpretation of experienced technologists, who tend to be in short supply (7). Despite this, molecular

assays can detect pathogens in situations where current tests are unsatisfactory or simply not available and have shown promise in large research-oriented clinical laboratories.

Studies utilizing molecular techniques have shown that bacterial diversity in host tissues is severely underestimated in reports based entirely on microbial culture (3, 35, 38, 39). In chapter 14, Bakaletz points out that the "advent of more sophisticated, specific, and sensitive assays for the detection of viral and bacterial DNA and/or RNA lent further support for" multiple predisposing agents in these diseases. Conventional techniques can differentiate among organisms in different kingdoms, genuses, or species. However, more sophisticated tests are required to further differentiate strains within a species or substrains within a strain. These latter assays include restriction endonuclease analysis (33), Southern blot hybridization (30), ribotyping (33), species-specific probes, PCR (22), random amplified polymorphic DNA techniques (42), multilocus enzyme electrophoresis (42), and multilocus sequence typing (45). In the future, microarrays and gene expression microarrays have enormous potential to come into routine clinical use (7).

Improved Detection of Conventional Agents

The methodologies above will reveal a more accurate prevalence of conventional agents in many polymicrobial diseases. As one example, adenovirus (27, 28), bovine viral diarrhea virus (16, 29), parainfluenza virus 3 (16), bovine respiratory syncytial virus (16, 29), bovine coronavirus (46), and other cytocidal viruses (46) will likely be found to have increasingly important roles in respiratory disease and gastroenteritis in cattle. In humans, routine molecular testing is already identifying viruses not readily cultured from patients (7). Amplification assays are being used to detect and quantitate human immunodeficiency virus (HIV) and hepatitis C virus in patients with infections. Both of these agents are involved in polymicrobial diseases (chapters 4, 5, and 20). Finally, molecular assays for cytomegalovirus, herpes simplex virus, and hepatitis B virus will probably be adopted in clinical laboratories in the near future (7).

Detection of New Agents

Additional etiologic agents will emerge as new approaches are used to detect difficult-to-culture or nonculturable microorganisms. Again, periodontal disease serves as an example. A recent study used molecular methods to obtain full 16S rRNA sequences for cultivable and not-yet-cultivated bacterial species in subgingival plaque from individuals with various forms of periodontitis and acute necrotizing ulcerative gingivitis. The predominant subgingival microbial community consisted of 347 species from 9 bacterial phyla and 68 unseen species, for an estimated total of 415 species in the subgingival plaque (38). The roles of these newly recognized organisms (38) or other recently isolated organisms like *Dialister pneumosintes* (10), *Capnocytophaga granulosa* (9), *Capnocytophaga haemolytica* (9), *Desulfomicrobium orale* sp. nov. (26), and viruses (chapter 16) in the pathogenesis of periodontal disease are yet to be determined.

Additional viruses, like the "small round virus" and astrovirus were recently found to be associated with PEMS in turkeys (2, 41). Again, the extent to which these newly recognized viruses affect the pathogenesis of PEMS is yet to be determined.

MECHANISMS OF POLYMICROBIAL DISEASE PATHOGENESIS

In chapter 1, Brogden proposes several mechanisms of polymicrobial disease pathogenesis that were drawn from the numerous reports describing polymicrobial diseases in animals and humans. These include (i) factors that can predispose the host to polymicrobial disease, (ii) microbial alterations in mucosa during infection that favors the colonization of other microorganisms, (iii) synergistic triggering of proinflammatory cytokines by microorganisms that can increase the severity of disease, reactivate latent infections, or favor the colonization of other microorganisms, (iv) the sharing of determinants among organisms which allows

nonpathogenic or weakly pathogenic microorganisms to cause disease, and (v) weakening of the immune system by one organism that allows the colonization of other microorganisms. Smith proposed mechanism iv in 1982 (44). His theory described how nonpathogenic or weakly pathogenic microorganisms could interact synergistically to cause harmful, even fatal, infections (44) and is applicable here. In the future, all the proposed mechanisms will likely be revised or refined as additional results become available on the etiology and pathogenesis of polymicrobial diseases.

Predisposing Factors

Stress, physiological abnormalities, metabolic diseases, alterations in life styles, and heritability are all known to increase the susceptibility of animals and humans to polymicrobial infection; however, in many cases, the underlying reasons for this are not understood. In chapter 8, Guthmiller and Novak discuss smoking and diabetes as two clearly defined risk factors for periodontal disease and the fact that periodontal disease may be attributed to as much as a 50% heritability component. A recent study showed that the molecular by-products of smoking interfered with mechanisms normally containing the growth of such pathogenic subgingival bacteria as *P. gingivalis, Prevotella intermedia,* and *Actinobacillus actinomycetemcomitans* (13). In chapter 7, Hay describes a situation in which carcinogens, such as benzo[*a*]pyrene diol epoxide, present in cigarette smoke can induce lysogeny in human vaginal lactobacilli, resulting in conditions favoring the colonization of other organisms leading to bacterial vaginosis. Psychological, physiological, and physical predisposing factors are difficult to assess (47), but as research progresses, indicators that will help to delineate the mechanisms predisposing animals and humans to polymicrobial disease will be identified (24).

Interactions among Etiologic Agents

True synergistic and mutualistic interactions among microorganisms are just now being described, and this will be an intense area of future research, as exemplified below. Receptors, which account for specific microbial interactions, and parameters for metabolic interdependence are being identified, explaining the occurrence of various microbial combinations.

In chapter 13, Brockmeier et al. describe research showing sequential colonization of organisms in models of the porcine respiratory disease complex. In these studies, *Pasteurella multocida* could not be isolated from pigs challenged with *P. multocida* alone but could be isolated from pigs challenged sequentially with porcine reproductive and respiratory syndrome virus, *Bordetella bronchiseptica*, and *P. multocida*. This may be due to two recently discovered filamentous hemagglutinins in *P. multocida* (31), similar to that of *Bordetella* spp., that facilitate binding of heterologous species of bacteria like *Haemophilus influenzae, Streptococcus pneumoniae,* or *Staphylococcus aureus* (49). Whether *P. multocida* and *B. bronchiseptica* cocolonize via similar mechanisms remains to be seen.

Some polymicrobial diseases are being considered as biofilm diseases. In chapter 14, Bakaletz introduces the hypothesis that otitis media is likely a true "biofilm disease," explaining the inherently high resistance of etiologic agents to antibodies and antimicrobials. In chapter 8, Guthmiller and Novak describe periodontal disease as a true mixed biofilm disease, whereby specific mechanisms are just being described to explain microbial attachment and interdependence (25, 36). Biofilm development on oral surfaces first involves interaction of gram-positive commensal organisms, e.g., streptococci and *Actinomyces* spp., with the salivary pellicle coating the tissue surface (12). These primary colonizing organisms then provide an attachment substrate for the ordered accumulation of other gram-positive and gram-negative bacterial spp. in the mixed milieu of subgingival plaque.

Attachment is not enough and interspecies and intergeneric cooperation among microorganisms is critical to their survival. In a rapidly developing area, a current hypothesis suggests that biofilm architecture may be influenced to a high degree by metabolic interdependence

among organisms. This was recently demonstrated in mixed species biofilms by laser confocal microscopy (37). Coadherence of *Streptococcus gordonii, Streptococcus oralis,* and *Actinomyces naeslundii* was dependent on the order in which they were added to a flow cell (37). Without *S. gordonii, A. naeslundii* could not multiply, but with *S. gordonii,* a mutually beneficial metabolic collaboration developed and *A. naeslundii* was found to coadhere. Synergy was also exhibited by the *A. naeslundii-S. oralis* interaction, and both strains grew luxuriantly.

With the availability of bacterial genome sequences and microarray technology, we anticipate that the genetic basis for these specific interactions will be found. This information is just beginning to be described for single-species biofilms (51) and will soon be expanded to mixed culture biofilms. Such information will show if many of these interactions are mutualistic or independent (37).

Host Response to Infection

Little is known whether or not the host response to polymicrobial infections differs from the host response to individual etiologic agent infections. In vivo models of polymicrobial infection will allow us to better assess these responses. Various technologies, such as DNA microarrays, are also now available (11) and can be used to identify host genes that are essential for the life cycle of microorganisms, those that are important in antimicrobial defense, or genes that may be activated nonspecifically in polymicrobial infections. For example, microarray analysis of host-commensal microbial relationships in the intestine recently revealed an unanticipated breadth of an organism's impact on expression of genes involved in modulating fundamental intestinal functions (21). In germfree mice colonized with *Bacteroides thetaiotaomicron,* expression of ~71 genes involved in several important intestinal functions were altered, including nutrient absorption, mucosal barrier fortification, xenobiotic metabolism, angiogenesis, and postnatal intestinal maturation. Similar studies with other organisms induced different responses, suggesting that variations between in-dividuals may be partly due to differences in their resident gut flora (21).

Viral infections have also been shown to have a profound effect on host gene expression. In a recent study by Prosniak et al. (40), approximately 39 genes were activated by rabies virus infection. These included genes involved in regulation of cell metabolism, protein synthesis, synaptic activity, and cell growth and differentiation. Such regulation of host genes and their resultant products may be involved in the replication and spread of rabies virus in the brain.

Another example is the interaction of *Bordetella pertussis* with a human bronchial epithelial cell line (4). The early transcriptional response in cells to this pathogen was characterized by altered expression of cytokines, DNA-binding proteins, and NF-κB-regulated genes.

Future research evaluating host genomic transcriptional profiling, in combination with functional assays to evaluate subsequent biological events, will provide insight into the complex interaction of host and pathogen. Future research will also need to assess specific mechanisms resulting in the breakdown in host defense as well as identification of host-derived biologic markers with diagnostic potential. These studies will reveal contributions by the host genes in the pathogenesis of polymicrobial diseases and may ultimately assist in better strategies for prophylaxis and/or treatment.

PROPHYLAXIS AND/OR TREATMENT OF POLYMICROBIAL DISEASES

Many mixed microbial infections fail to respond to antimicrobial treatment (15, 19, 43, 48), and the reasons are not well known. One possible explanation is that the organisms occur in biofilms. In chapter 14, Bakaletz points out that biofilms are inherently highly resistant to the action of antibodies and antimicrobial agents, a view shared by others (51). Differences in susceptibility among bacteria in a free-floating planktonic state and as a biofilm were recently shown by using DNA microarrays (51).

Only about 1% of genes showed differences in expression between these two growth modes, ~0.5% of genes were activated, and ~0.5% of the genes were repressed in biofilms. None of the conventional genes involved in antimicrobial resistance were activated. However, other genes (e.g., *tolA* and *rpoS*) were activated in *Pseudomonas aeruginosa* biofilms, possibly contributing to their resistance to aminoglycosides. Similar analysis of other organisms may provide insights into their resistance to antimicrobials and host immune defenses.

CONCLUSIONS

Rapid technological advancements will help us to define more clearly the etiology of currently described polymicrobial diseases and assist us in identifying additional polymicrobial diseases. It is likely that the roles of some etiologic agents will be clarified and new agents will be identified. Simultaneously, work will begin to characterize specific mechanisms of microbial interaction and the factors that lead to microbial synergy and mutualism. DNA microarrays of organisms in these diseases may provide insights into their resistance to antimicrobials and host immune defenses, potential avenues of therapeutic treatment. Arrays containing expressed sequence tags will begin to identify host response to infection, hopefully to reveal markers of infection, mechanisms of disease pathogenesis, and therapeutic avenues to reduce inflammation.

The field of polymicrobial diseases will continue to grow, and significant advances will be made. This will require a multidisciplinary approach using experts from many specialized disciplines to recognize polymicrobial diseases, understand their complex etiology, establish methods for their study, identify mechanisms of disease pathogenesis, and assess appropriate methods of treatment.

REFERENCES

1. **Allan, G. M., F. McNeilly, J. Ellis, S. Krakowka, B. Meehan, I. McNair, I. Walker, and S. Kennedy.** 2000. Experimental infection of colostrum deprived piglets with porcine circovirus 2 (PCV2) and porcine repro-

ductive and respiratory syndrome virus (PRRSV) potentiates PCV2 replication. *Arch. Virol.* **145:** 2421–2429.

2. **Allan, G. M., F. McNeilly, B. M. Meehan, J. A. Ellis, T. J. Connor, I. McNair, S. Krakowka, and S. Kennedy.** 2000. A sequential study of experimental infection of pigs with porcine circovirus and porcine parvovirus: immunostaining of cryostat sections and virus isolation. *J. Vet. Med. Ser. B* **47:**81–94.

3. **Aul, J. J., K. W. Anderson, R. M. Wadowsky, W. J. Doyle, L. A. Kingsley, J. C. Post, and G. D. Ehrlich.** 1998. Comparative evaluation of culture and PCR for the detection and determination of persistence of bacterial strains and DNAs in the Chinchilla laniger model of otitis media. *Ann. Otol. Rhinol. Laryngol.* **107:** 508–513.

4. **Belcher, C. E., J. Drenkow, B. Kehoe, T. R. Gingeras, N. McNamara, H. Lemjabbar, C. Basbaum, and D. A. Relman.** 2000. The transcriptional responses of respiratory epithelial cells to Bordetella pertussis reveal host defensive and pathogen counter-defensive strategies. *Proc. Natl. Acad. Sci. USA* **97:**13847–13852.

5. **Brown, C. C., P. D. Kilgo, and K. L. Jacobsen.** 2000. Prevalence of papillomatous digital dermatitis among culled adult cattle in the southeastern United States. *Am. J. Vet. Res.* **61:**928–930.

6. **Cermelli, C., and S. Jacobson.** 2000. Viruses and multiple sclerosis. *Viral Immunol.* **13:**2551–2567.

7. **Check, W.** 2001. Nucleic acid-based tests move slowly into clinical labs. *ASM News* **67:**560–565.

8. **Chiu, B.** 1999. Multiple infections in carotid atherosclerotic plaques. *Am. Heart. J.* **138:**S534–S536.

9. **Ciantar, M., D. A. Spratt, H. N. Newman, and M. Wilson.** 2001. Capnocytophaga granulosa and Capnocytophaga haemolytica: novel species in subgingival plaque. *J. Clin. Periodontol.* **28:**701–705.

10. **Contreras, A., N. Doan, C. Chen, T. Rusitanonta, M. J. Flynn, and J. Slots.** 2000. Importance of Dialister pneumosintes in human periodontitis. *Oral. Microbiol. Immunol.* **15:**269–272.

11. **Cummings, C. A., and D. A. Relman.** 2000. Using DNA microarrays to study host-microbe interactions. *Emerg. Infect. Dis.* **6:**513–522.

12. **Demuth, D. R., D. C. Irvine, J. W. Costerton, G. S. Cook, and R. J. Lamont.** 2001. Discrete protein determinant directs the species-specific adherence of *Porphyromonas gingivalis* to oral streptococci. *Infect. Immun.* **69:**5736–5741.

13. **Eggert, F. M., M. H. McLeod, and G. Flowerdew.** 2001. Effects of smoking and treatment status on periodontal bacteria: evidence that smoking influences control of periodontal bacteria at the mucosal surface of the gingival crevice. *J. Periodontol.* **72:**1210–1220.

14. **el-Ghoul, W., and B. I. Shaheed.** 2001. Ulcerative and papillomatous digital dermatitis of the pastern region in dairy cattle: clinical and histopathological studies. *Dtsch. Tierarztl. Wochenschr.* **108:**216–222.

15. **Ernould, J. C., K. Ba, and B. Sellin.** 1999. Increase of intestinal schistosomiasis after praziquantel treatment in a Schistosoma haematobium and Schistosoma mansoni mixed focus. *Acta Trop.* **73:** 143–152.

16. **Fulton, R. W., C. W. Purdy, A. W. Confer, J. T. Saliki, R. W. Loan, R. E. Briggs, and L. J. Burge.** 2000. Bovine viral diarrhea viral infections in feeder calves with respiratory disease: interactions with Pasteurella spp., parainfluenza-3 virus, and bovine respiratory syncytial virus. *Can. J. Vet. Res.* **64:**151–159.

17. **Guy, J. S., L. G. Smith, J. J. Breslin, J. P. Vaillancourt, and H. J. Barnes.** 2000. High mortality and growth depression experimentally produced in young turkeys by dual infection with enteropathogenic Escherichia coli and turkey coronavirus. *Avian Dis.* **44:**105–113.

18. **Haahr, S., and M. Munch.** 2000. The association between multiple sclerosis and infection with Epstein-Barr virus and retrovirus. *J. Neurovirol.* **6**(suppl. 2):S76–S79.

19. **Hament, J. M., J. L. Kimpen, A. Fleer, and T. F. Wolfs.** 1999. Respiratory viral infection predisposing for bacterial disease: a concise review. *FEMS Immunol. Med. Microbiol.* **26:**189–195.

20. **Hjerpe, C. A.** 1983. Clinical management of respiratory disease in feedlot cattle. *Vet. Clin. N. Am. Large Anim. Pract.* **5:**119–142.

21. **Hooper, L. V., M. H. Wong, A. Thelin, L. Hansson, P. G. Falk, and J. I. Gordon.** 2001. Molecular analysis of commensal host-microbial relationships in the intestine. *Science* **291:**881–884.

22. **Kellam, P.** 1998. Molecular identification of novel viruses. *Trends Microbiol.* **6:**160–165.

23. **Kennedy, S., D. Moffett, F. McNeilly, B. Meehan, J. Ellis, S. Krakowka, and G. M. Allan.** 2000. Reproduction of lesions of postweaning multisystemic wasting syndrome by infection of conventional pigs with porcine circovirus type 2 alone or in combination with porcine parvovirus. *J. Comp. Pathol.* **122:**9–24.

24. **Knowles, T. G., S. N. Brown, P. D. Warriss, A. J. Phillips, S. K. Dolan, P. Hunt, J. E. Ford, J. E. Edwards, and P. E. Watkins.** 1995. Effects on sheep of transport by road for up to 24 hours. *Vet. Rec.* **136:**431–438.

25. **Kolenbrander, P. E.** 2000. Oral microbial communities: biofilms, interactions, and genetic systems. *Annu. Rev. Microbiol.* **54:**413–437.

26. **Langendijk, P. S., E. M. Kulik, H. Sandmeier, J. Meyer, and J. S. van der Hoeven.** 2001. Isolation of Desulfomicrobium orale sp. nov. and Desulfovibrio strain NY682, oral sulfate-reducing bacteria involved in human periodontal disease. *Int. J. Syst. Evol. Microbiol.* **51:** 1035–1044.

27. **Lehmkuhl, H. D., R. E. Briggs, and R. C. Cutlip.** 1998. Survey for antibodies to bovine adenoviruses in six- to nine-month-old feedyard cattle. *Am. J. Vet. Res.* **59:**1579–1580.

28. **Lehmkuhl, H. D., R. C. Cutlip, J. T. Meehan, and B. M. DeBey.** 1997. Pathogenesis of infection induced by an adenovirus isolated from a goat. *Am. J. Vet. Res.* **58:**608–611.

29. **Liu, L., H. D. Lehmkuhl, and M. L. Kaeberle.** 1999. Synergistic effects of bovine respiratory syncytial virus and non-cytopathic bovine viral diarrhea virus infection on selected bovine alveolar macrophage functions. *Can. J. Vet. Res.* **63:**41–48.

30. **Lockhart, S. R., C. Pujol, S. Joly, and D. R. Soll.** 2001. Development and use of complex probes for DNA fingerprinting the infectious fungi. *Med. Mycol.* **39:**1–8.

31. **May, B. J., Q. Zhang, L. L. Li, M. L. Paustian, T. S. Whittam, and V. Kapur.** 2001. Complete genomic sequence of Pasteurella multocida, Pm70. *Proc. Natl. Acad. Sci. USA* **98:** 3460–3465.

32. **Moses, H., Jr., and S. Sriram.** 2001. An infectious basis for multiple sclerosis: perspectives on the role of Chlamydia pneumoniae and other agents. *BioDrugs* **15:**199–206.

33. **Murphy, G. L., L. C. Robinson, and G. E. Burrows.** 1993. Restriction endonuclease analysis and ribotyping differentiate *Pasteurella haemolytica* serotype A1 isolates from cattle within a feedlot. *J. Clin. Microbiol.* **31:**2303–2308.

34. **O'Conner, S., C. Taylor, L. A. Campbell, S. Epstein, and P. Libby.** 2001. Potential infectious etiologies of atherosclerosis: a multifactorial perspective. *Emerg. Infect. Dis.* **7:**780–788.

35. **Okamoto, Y., K. Kudo, K. Shirotori, M. Nakazawa, E. Ito, K. Togawa, J. A. Patel, and P. L. Ogra.** 1992. Detection of genomic sequences of respiratory syncytial virus in otitis media with effusion in children. *Ann. Otol. Rhinol. Laryngol. Suppl.* **157:**7–10.

36. **O'Toole, G., H. B. Kaplan, and R. Kolter.** 2000. Biofilm formation as microbial development. *Annu. Rev. Microbiol.* **54:**49–79.

37. **Palmer, R. J., Jr., K. Kazmerzak, M. C. Hansen, and P. E. Kolenbrander.** 2001. Mu-tualism versus independence: strategies of mixed-species oral biofilms in vitro using saliva as the sole nutrient source. *Infect. Immun.* **69:**5794–5804.

38. **Paster, B. J., S. K. Boches, J. L. Galvin, R. E. Ericson, C. N. Lau, V. A. Levanos, A. Sahasrabudhe, and F. E. Dewhirst.** 2001. Bacterial diversity in human subgingival plaque. *J. Bacteriol.* **183:**3770–3783.

39. **Post, J. C., J. J. Aul, G. J. White, R. M. Wadowsky, T. Zavoral, R. Tabari, B. Kerber, W. J. Doyle, and G. D. Ehrlich.** 1996. PCR-based detection of bacterial DNA after antimicrobial treatment is indicative of persistent, viable bacteria in the chinchilla model of otitis media. *Am. J. Otolaryngol.* **17:**106–111.

40. **Prosniak, M., D. C. Hooper, B. Dietzschold, and H. Koprowski.** 2001. Effect of rabies virus infection on gene expression in mouse brain. *Proc. Natl. Acad. Sci. USA* **98:**2758–2763.

41. **Qureshi, M. A., M. Yu, and Y. M. Saif.** 2000. A novel "small round virus" inducing poult enteritis and mortality syndrome and associated immune alterations. *Avian Dis.* **44:**275–283.

42. **Schloter, M., M. Lebuhn, T. Heulin, and A. Hartmann.** 2000. Ecology and evolution of bacterial microdiversity. *FEMS Microbiol. Rev.* **24:** 647–660.

43. **Schutten, M., M. E. van der Ende, and A. D. Osterhaus.** 2000. Antiretroviral therapy in patients with dual infection with human immunodeficiency virus types 1 and 2. *N. Engl. J. Med.* **342:**1758–1760.

44. **Smith, H.** 1982. The role of microbial interactions in infectious disease. *Philos. Trans. R. Soc. Lond. B* **297:**551–561.

45. **Smith, J. M., E. J. Feil, and N. H. Smith.** 2000. Population structure and evolutionary dynamics of pathogenic bacteria. *Bioessays* **22:**1115–1122.

46. **Storz, J., C. W. Purdy, X. Lin, M. Burrell, R. E. Truax, R. E. Briggs, G. H. Frank, and R. W. Loan.** 2000. Isolation of respiratory bovine coronavirus, other cytocidal viruses, and Pasteurella spp from cattle involved in two natural outbreaks of shipping fever. *J. Am. Vet. Med. Assoc.* **216:**1599–1604.

47. **Swanson, J. C.** 1995. Farm animal well-being and intensive productive systems. *J. Anim. Sci.* **73:**2744–2751.

48. **Thibault, V., Y. Benhamou, C. Seguret, M. Bochet, C. Katlama, F. Bricaire, P. Opolon, T. Poynard, and H. Agut.** 1999. Hepatitis B virus (HBV) mutations associated with resistance to lamivudine in patients coinfected with HBV and human immunodeficiency virus. *J. Clin. Microbiol.* **37:**3013–3016.

49. **Tuomanen, E.** 1986. Piracy of adhesins: attachment of superinfecting pathogens to respiratory cilia by secreted adhesins of *Bordetella pertussis. Infect. Immun.* **54:**905–908.

50. **Walker, R. L., D. H. Read, K. J. Loretz, and R. W. Nordhausen.** 1995. Spirochetes isolated from dairy cattle with papillomatous digital dermatitis and interdigital dermatitis. *Vet. Microbiol.* **47:**343–355.

51. **Whiteley, M., M. G. Bangera, R. E. Bumgarner, M. R. Parsek, G. M. Teitzel, S.** **Lory, and E. P. Greenberg.** 2001. Gene expression in Pseudomonas aeruginosa biofilms. *Nature* **413:**860–864.

52. **Yu, M., M. M. Ismail, M. A. Qureshi, R. N. Dearth, H. J. Barnes, and Y. M. Saif.** 2000. Viral agents associated with poult enteritis and mortality syndrome: the role of a small round virus and a turkey coronavirus. *Avian Dis.* **44:**297–304.

53. **Zimmer, C.** 2001. Do chronic diseases have an infectious root? *Science* **293:**1974–1977.

INDEX

Note: Page numbers followed by "f" indicate figures; page numbers followed by "t" indicate tables.